THE
ALTERNATIVE
ADVISOR

THE
ALTERNATIVE
ADVISOR

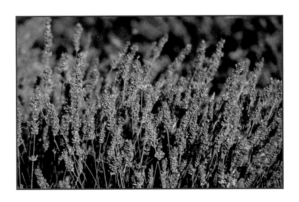

BY THE EDITORS OF TIME-LIFE BOOKS
ALEXANDRIA, VIRGINIA

Consultants

 ZOË BRENNER
LAc, Dipl Ac and Dipl Ch (NCCA), FNAAOM
has practiced acupuncture since 1977 and Chinese herbal medicine since 1984. She teaches Oriental medicine and the history and philosophy of Chinese medicine at the Traditional Acupuncture Institute in Columbia, Maryland, and lectures in other schools around the United States.

 DWIGHT C. BYERS
began teaching with his aunt, Eunice Ingham, who pioneered and developed the original Ingham method of reflexology. Byers now serves as president of the International Institute of Reflexology in St. Petersburg, Florida, which offers seminars worldwide.

 DEBORAH CAPLAN, MA, PT
is a licensed physical therapist and a certified teacher of the Alexander technique. She studied with F. M. Alexander and is a founding member of the American Center for the Alexander Technique, Inc. The author of Back Trouble, she specializes in teaching the Alexander technique to people with back problems.

 JOHN G. COLLINS, ND, DHANP
teaches dermatology and homeopathy at the National College of Naturopathic Medicine in Portland, Oregon. He also has a private practice in Gresham, Oregon.

 KYLE H. CRONIN, ND
specializes in women's healthcare in her medical practice in Phoenix. Dr. Cronin is also cofounder of Southwest College of Naturopathic Medicine and Health Sciences, where she is dean of Curricular Development.

 BARBARA CROWE, RMT-BC
teaches music therapy at Arizona State University, Tempe. She frequently gives presentations on music therapy and sound healing and is writing a book on the theory of music therapy. She is past president of the National Association for Music Therapy.

 PALI C. DELEVITT, PhD
consults on alternative therapies at the cancer center of the University of Virginia, where she also teaches in the School of Medicine. Dr. Delevitt has consulted on curriculum development for the medical schools of Columbia University, Emory University, and Indiana University.

 ADRIANE FUGH-BERMAN, MD
is chair of the National Women's Health Network, a science-based advocacy group. An expert on herbs and nutritional medicine, she has lectured internationally on diverse alternative medicine issues and formerly directed field investigations for the National Institutes of Health Office of Alternative Medicine.

 ELLIOT GREENE, MA
is past president of the American Massage Therapy Association and currently maintains a private practice in Silver Spring, Maryland. Certified in therapeutic massage by the National Certification Board for Therapeutic Massage and Bodywork, he has spent more than 24 years in the field. He was formerly on the board of directors of the National Wellness Coalition.

 GARY KAPLAN, DO
is a family physician and a specialist in chronic pain medicine. He is president of the Medical Acupuncture Research Foundation and serves on the clinical faculty of Georgetown University Medical School. Dr. Kaplan is director of the Kaplan Clinic in Arlington, Virginia, where he is in private practice.

 CHRISTOPHER M. KIM, MD
is past president of the American Apitherapy Society, an organization that informs the public on the therapeutic uses of bee venom and other bee products. A pain-medicine specialist, Dr. Kim is medical director of the Monmouth Pain Institute in Red Bank, New Jersey, and president of the International Pain Institute.

Consultants

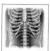

DANA J. LAWRENCE, DC, FICC
has been a faculty member at the National College of Chiropractic in Lombard, Illinois, for more than 17 years. He is the director of the college's Department of Publication and Editorial Review, and editor of its Journal of Manipulative and Physiological Therapeutics.

JEFFREY MIGDOW, MD
has been practicing holistic medicine for 17 years. In his medical practice, Dr. Migdow counsels patients on lifestyle and recommends a wide variety of homeopathic, nutritional, and other therapies. He is also a director of yoga-teacher training at the Kripalu Center for Yoga and Health in Lenox, Massachusetts. He began his yoga training more than 20 years ago and has been teaching yoga for 10 years.

DONALD G. MURPHY, PhD
is a basic scientist who retired from the National Institutes of Health after a career in biomedical research and research administration. He is a martial arts master instructor with experience in aikido, jujitsu, judo, tae kwon do, qigong, and t'ai chi. Dr. Murphy provides experiential training in life force (bioenergy, chi, ki) and is an adjunct faculty member at the Uniformed Services University of the Health Sciences in Bethesda, Maryland.

CHRISTINA PUCHALSKI, MD, OCDS
utilizes her patients' spiritual background in her work as an internist and primary care physician at the George Washington University Hospital in Washington, D.C. Dr. Puchalski was instrumental in creating and integrating a course on spirituality and medicine into the curriculum at George Washington University Medical School.

BEVERLY RUBIK, PhD
is founding director of the Institute for Frontier Science in Philadelphia. Her interests in alternative medicine include light therapy, bio-electromagnetic therapy, spiritual healing, acupuncture, and homeopathy.

KURT SCHNAUBELT, PhD
founded and directs the Pacific Institute of Aromatherapy in San Rafael, California. Drawing on his background in chemistry, Dr. Schnaubelt has written numerous articles and books on scientifically based aromatherapy.

J. JAMISON STARBUCK, JD, ND
practices family medicine in Missoula, Montana. A former practicing attorney, she is past president of the American Association of Naturopathic Physicians and a member of the Homeopathic Academy of Naturopathic Physicians.

MICHAEL A. TANSEY, PhD
is a pioneer researcher and authority on biofeedback, EEG neurofeedback, and the Instrumental Cartography of Consciousness. He is past president of the Society for the Study of Neuronal Regulation.

DICK W. THOM, DDS, ND
teaches clinical and physical diagnosis at the National College of Naturopathic Medicine in Portland, Oregon. He is also a clinic supervisor at the Portland Naturopathic Clinic and maintains a general family practice at Natural Choices Health Clinic in Beaverton, Oregon.

ROBERT C. WARD, DO, FAAO
teaches osteopathic manipulative medicine and family medicine at Michigan State University's College of Osteopathic Medicine. He was in private family practice for 14 years prior to teaching.

KENNETH G. ZYSK, PhD
researches Ayurvedic medicine as the project director of the Indic Traditions of Healthcare at Columbia University. Dr. Zysk also teaches in the Department of Near Eastern Languages and Literature at New York University, and in the Department of Religion at Columbia University. He is senior editor of a series of books on Indian and Tibetan medicine for the University of California Press.

TIME® LIFE BOOKS

TIME-LIFE BOOKS IS A DIVISION
OF TIME LIFE INC.

TIME LIFE INC.
PRESIDENT and CEO: George Artandi

TIME-LIFE BOOKS
Publisher/Managing Editor: Neil Kagan

TIME-LIFE CUSTOM PUBLISHING
Vice President and Publisher: Terry Newell
Vice President of Sales and Marketing: Neil Levin
Director of Special Sales: Liz Ziehl
Editor for Special Markets: Anna Burgard
Production Manager: Carolyn Mills Bounds
Quality Assurance Manager: James King

Pre-press services by the Time-Life
Imaging Center

Books produced by Time-Life Custom Publishing are available at special bulk discount for
promotional and premium use. Custom adapta-
tions can also be created to meet your specific
marketing goals. Call 1-800-323-5255.

EDITORIAL STAFF

EDITOR
Robert Somerville

Deputy Editor
Tina S. McDowell

Design Director
Tina Taylor

Text Editor
Jim Watson

Associate Editors/Research and Writing
Nancy Blodgett
Stephanie Summers Henke

Technical Art Assistant
Dana R. Magsumbol

Senior Copyeditors
Anne Farr
Mary Beth Oelkers-Keegan

Picture Coordinator
Lisa Groseclose

Editorial Assistant
Patricia D. Whiteford

SPECIAL CONTRIBUTORS
John Drummond, Rebecca Mowrey,
Monika Thayer (design)

Gretchen Case, Patti Cass, Juli Duncan,
Kevan Miller (research)

Lisa Ann Clark, Patricia Daniels, Silvia Hines,
Susan Perry (text)

Elizabeth Moore, Jacqueline Shaffer (art models)

Barbara L. Klein (index)

CORRESPONDENTS
Maria Vincenza Aloisi (Paris)
Christine Hinze (London)
Christina Lieberman (New York)

Cover photograph courtesy of PhotoDisc
Cover design by Anna Burgard

ISBN 0-7370-0045-7

The Library of Congress has cataloged the trade
version of this titles as follows:

Library of Congress Cataloging-in-Publication Data
The alternative advisor:
the complete guide to natural therapies
and alternative treatments/
by the editors of Time-Life Books.
p. cm.
Includes bibliographical references and index.
ISBN 0-7835-4907-5
1. Alternative medicine.
2. Self-care, Health.
I. Time-Life Books.
R733.A454 1997
615.5—dc21   96-49614 CIP

Contents

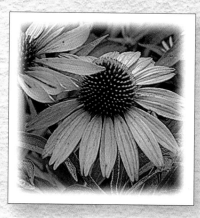

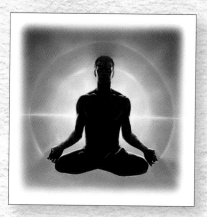

Contents

Introduction 12

A-Z Guide to Alternative Therapies 14

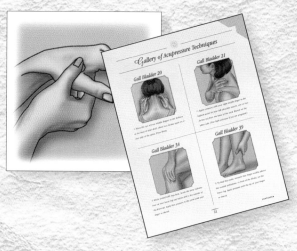

Acupressure **16**

Gallery of Acupressure Techniques . . . **18**

Acupuncture **32**

   Meridians and Acupoints **34**

Apitherapy **36**

Aromatherapy **38**

   The 15 Most Effective Essential Oils . **40**

Ayurvedic Medicine **42**

Bodywork **47**

   Alexander Technique **47**

   Aston-Patterning **49**

   Feldenkrais Method **50**

   Hellerwork **51**

   Myotherapy **52**

   Reiki **53**

   Rolfing **54**

   Therapeutic Touch **55**

   Trager Psychophysical Integration . . . **56**

Chinese Medicine **57**

Chiropractic **61**

Energy Medicine **64**

Flower Remedies **66**

   39 Essential Flower Remedies **68**

Herbal Therapies **70**

The 75 Most Effective Herbs **74**

Homeopathy **104**

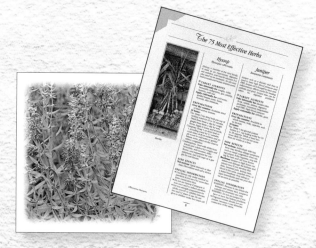

Contents

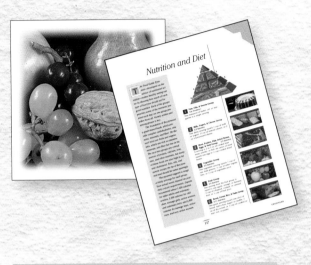

The 30 Most Effective
Homeopathic Remedies **107**

Hydrotherapy **117**

Light Therapy **119**

Massage **121**

Gallery of Massage Techniques . . . **124**

Mind/Body Medicine **130**

    ■ Biofeedback **132**

    ■ Guided Imagery **133**

    ■ Hypnotherapy **135**

    ■ Meditation **136**

    ■ Relaxation Techniques **138**

    ■ Spiritual Healing and Prayer **140**

Naturopathic Medicine . . . **141**

Nutrition and Diet **144**

    ■ The Food Guide Pyramid **147**

    ■ Diet Plans **148**

The 32 Most Common
Vitamins and Minerals **152**

Osteopathy **163**

Qigong **165**

Reflexology **167**

    ■ Reflexology Areas **169**

Sound Therapy **170**

T'ai Chi **172**

Gallery of T'ai Chi Positions **174**

Yoga **182**

Gallery of Yoga Positions **184**

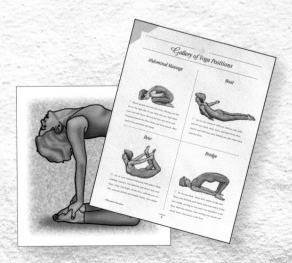

Contents
CONTINUED

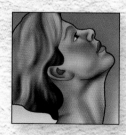

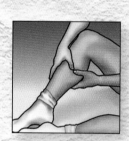

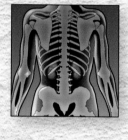

Common Ailments 194

Allergies 196

Anemia. 198

Angina 200

Arthritis. 202

Asthma. 206

Atherosclerosis. 208

Athletic Injuries. 210

Back Problems 214

Bladder Infections. 216

Breast Problems 218

Bronchitis 220

Bursitis 222

Cancer 224

Carpal Tunnel Syndrome . . . 228

Cholesterol Problems 230

Chronic Fatigue Syndrome . . . 232

Circulatory Problems 234

Common Cold 236

Conjunctivitis 238

Constipation 240

Cough. 242

Depression. 244

Diabetes. 246

Diarrhea. 248

Earache 250

Endometriosis 252

Fever and Chills 254

Flu 256

Food Poisoning 258

Gas and Gas Pains. 260

Glaucoma. 262

Gout 264

Gum Problems. 266

Hay Fever. 268

Headache. 270

Hearing Problems 274

Heartburn 276

Heart Problems. 278

Hemorrhoids 282

High Blood Pressure. 284

Immune Problems. 286

Incontinence 288

Indigestion 290

Insomnia 292

Contents

Irritable Bowel Syndrome. . . . 294

Kidney Disease 296

Laryngitis. 298

Ménière's Disease 300

Menopause 302

Menstrual Problems 304

Mononucleosis 308

Motion Sickness 310

Multiple Sclerosis 312

Muscle Cramps 314

Nausea. 316

Neuralgia 318

Osteoporosis. 320

Pain, Chronic. 322

Pneumonia. 324

Poison Ivy 326

Premenstrual Syndrome. 328

Prostate Problems 330

Rashes and Skin Problems . . . 332

Seasonal Affective Disorder . . 336

Sexually Transmitted Diseases. 338

Shingles 340

Sinusitis 342

Sore Throat 344

Stomach Ulcers 346

Stress 348

Sty 350

Sunburn. 352

Tendinitis. 354

Thyroid Problems 356

TMJ Syndrome 358

Tonsillitis. 360

Toothache 362

Vaginal Problems. 364

Varicose Veins 366

Warts 368

Yeast Infections. 370

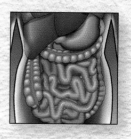

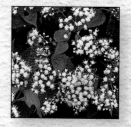

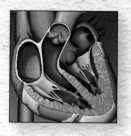

■ **ESSENTIAL FIRST AID** 372
   ■ Conventional Medicine Chest 379
   ■ Alternative Medicine Chest 380

Glossary 381
Bibliography 387
Index 391
Acknowledgments/Picture Credits/Abbreviations 400

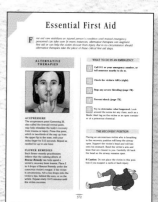

Essential First Aid

Introduction

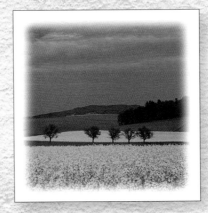

In my work as a physician—and as a practitioner of alternative medicine—I am constantly reminded of the importance of keeping an open mind when it comes to finding what's best for my patients. Years of experience have shown me that no single approach to healthcare has all the answers; the search for healing solutions often requires a willingness to look beyond one remedy or system of treatment. At the same time, I also feel a deep responsibility to be selective—to recognize important distinctions among the vast array of treatment options available. Because the same therapy can affect different patients in different ways, an approach that works for one person may do nothing for another. My job, then, is not just to seek out which remedies are available or safe, but to prescribe the course of treatment that best suits the patient's condition and lifestyle. I've discovered, though, that I can't do this job alone. Whatever the therapy, patients respond dramatically better to treatment when they take an active, confident role in their own healthcare.

More than ever before, taking such an active role in your own health requires a good working knowledge of alternative medicine—practical knowledge that this book is expressly intended to give you. While conventional physicians generally view health as the absence of disease, alternative practitioners think of it as a balancing of body, mind, and spirit. Central to alternative medicine is the principle of holism, or the idea that all aspects of a person are interrelated; disharmony in one aspect upsets the balance and stresses the body, eventually leading to illness.

Alternative practitioners use a number of methods to bolster the body's own defenses and restore balance to help overcome disease. Among these therapies are ancient healing systems that were ignored by Western society but are now being rediscovered for their powerful therapeutic ability.

The Alternative Advisor offers an in-depth look at the wide variety of healing approaches—some dating to the dawn of civilization—that are used to treat ailments ranging in severity from the common cold to skin cancer. Part one of the book addresses the pros and cons of particular therapies, explaining their origins, who can benefit from them, and specifically how they are used both to treat ailments and to help maintain wellness. Part two, "Common Ailments," is an alphabetical listing of more than 80 health disorders. Each entry explains the ailment in detail, its causes and its mechanisms, and gives a selection of alternative therapies that can be used to treat it.

Besides the variety and scope of its treatment options, what I find particularly impressive about The Alternative Advisor is its pervading sense of responsibility—its honest recognition that alternative methods are not always sufficient on their own, and that in some cases the best medicine is so-called conventional treatment. In other words, when conventional medications or treatments such as surgery are necessary, this book does not hesitate to say so. The authors and editors take great pride in presenting an objective, reasoned look at alternative medicine. I share that pride and sense of responsibility, and I know that my fellow consultants do as well. After all, the health of our patients depends on it.

Alternative medicine has flowered in the past few decades as more and more people seek to avoid the drugs and surgery of conventional healthcare—or at the very least supplement them with other approaches. Already, thousands of medical doctors (including myself) have incorporated alternative therapies into their practices. Health insurance companies now cover certain alternative methods, including acupuncture, which has been used in China for millennia but was practically unknown in this country until 20 years ago. Indeed, the face of healthcare is changing, moving toward a more open-minded view of nonconventional remedies—some new, some long forgotten. Ironic as it sounds, it looks as though the future of medicine may well lie in these healing traditions of the past. Knowing more about them—and having practical advice about how to use them at your fingertips—may be one of the best things you can do for your health.

—*Jeffrey Migdow, MD*
Former Medical Director, Kripalu Center for Yoga and Health

A-Z Guide to *Alternative Therapies*

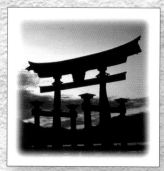

In this section, 24 alternative therapies are arranged by name in alphabetical order. Most are listed individually, but in some cases a few similar or related techniques are grouped together under a single umbrella heading. Bodywork, for instance, is a general category for various therapies that involve bodily manipulation or techniques for improving posture and movement. Examples include Hellerwork and Reiki. (Note: Massage and chiropractic, though generally considered to be bodywork techniques, are listed separately.) Therapies that rely on the healing power of the mind—biofeedback, guided imagery, and hypnotherapy, to name a few—are discussed under the group heading Mind/Body Medicine. If you're not sure where to look for a particular therapy, you can find it easily in the index.

Each entry offers a comprehensive, "big picture" look at a given therapy as well as a close examination of its various elements. An introduction sets the stage, defining the technique and explaining its working principles. Next comes a brief review of the technique's historical origins, identifying the key players and explaining how their methods evolved over the decades or millennia into the therapy as practiced today.

Under "What It's Good For," you'll find general information about how this therapy acts on the body to improve health. Specific disorders commonly treated with this method are listed as "Target Ailments," each of which is the subject of a full entry elsewhere in the book (see Common Ailments, beginning on page 194). "Preparations/Techniques" delves into the nuts and bolts of the therapy; here you'll learn such things as how healing substances are prepared and administered, and what techniques or equipment is used. Under "Visiting a Professional," you'll find out what you can expect when visiting a practitioner's office. Because wellness is a big part of alternative medicine, most entries describe how a given therapy helps promote and maintain lasting good health. "What the Critics Say" attempts to characterize—and occasionally rebut—criticisms that have been leveled against this form of therapy. A special "Licensed & Insured?" box explains the licensing requirements for practitioners and whether their services are covered by health insurance, and another box labeled "For More Info" lists addresses and phone numbers of organizations you can contact to learn more about the topic.

Besides the alphabetized list of therapies, this first section of *The Alternative Advisor* also features 10 illustrated galleries that give practical, in-depth information about selected remedies and therapeutic techniques. The acupressure, t'ai chi, and yoga galleries, for example, show exactly how and where to apply healing pressure to the body or how to perform certain positions for relaxation and good health. Another gallery provides step-by-step instruction in therapeutic massage, while others explore such health-related topics as vitamins and minerals, herbs, essential oils, and homeopathic remedies.

How to Choose a Practitioner

When searching for an alternative practitioner, you may want to begin with a recommendation from a conventional doctor. Illness-related self-help groups and books on alternative healing can also be good sources for names. You may find that family and friends can provide valuable opinions based on their experience with particular practitioners. In your search, don't hesitate to act on personal considerations such as a preference for a male or female practitioner, or an older or younger one. If you have beliefs or philosophies that play a major role in your healthcare, be sure that you choose a provider who will respect your views.

You should fully investigate any alternative practitioner's background and experience and be aware of any licensing requirements in your state or district. Be extremely suspicious of anyone who expresses hostility or derision toward mainstream medicine or makes grandiose claims for a cure. A conscientious practitioner understands that every therapy has its limitations. Get explicit information about the treatment you will receive, and remember that you are in charge of the entire treatment process. Above all, trust your own instincts and judgment. ■

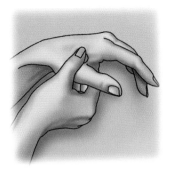

Target Ailments

- Allergies
- Arthritis
- Asthma
- Athletic Injuries
- Back Problems
- Chronic Fatigue Syndrome
- Common Cold
- Constipation
- Diarrhea
- Earache
- Headache
- Immune Problems
- Indigestion
- Insomnia
- Motion Sickness
- Nausea
- Pain, Chronic
- TMJ Syndrome
- Toothache

See Common Ailments, beginning on page 194.

Acupressure

An integral part of the traditional practice of Chinese medicine (pages 57-60), acupressure has become increasingly popular and accepted in the West. Its simple, noninvasive techniques have shown beneficial effects for a wide array of health problems—even if the theory behind it remains questionable to many conventional medical practitioners.

Like acupuncture (pages 32-33), acupressure is based on the concept of chi (sometimes spelled "qi"), defined in Chinese medicine as an essential life force that flows through the body, circulating through invisible passageways called meridians (see the illustrations on pages 34-35). The movement, or flow, of chi is said to vary with the mental, physical, and spiritual changes of daily living. According to this theory, when chi flows freely and evenly, harmony and good health are possible; however, if chi circulation is stagnant, overstimulated, or unbalanced, illness is likely.

The invisible meridians carrying chi are said to reside within the body's interior. However, there are specific places on the skin, called acupoints, where chi may be accessed and guided using deep, focused finger pressure. By improving chi circulation, practitioners encourage the harmonious equilibrium of mind and body believed to be essential for physical and spiritual health. And once this internal harmony is achieved, they claim, the body is able to invoke its self-healing capabilities.

Origins

The various therapeutic techniques of Chinese medicine, including acupressure, are among the most ancient healing approaches in the world, dating back some 5,000 years. Acupressure itself probably originated as a combination of acupuncture and massage.

What It's Good For

Acupressure techniques address hundreds of ailments. In addition to those listed at left, studies have shown that acupressure can hasten recuperation from stroke and surgery. And at some hospitals, elastic acupressure wristbands (designed to relieve motion sickness) are used to reduce the

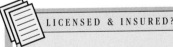

LICENSED & INSURED?

No. Although acupuncturists are licensed, acupressurists are not. Acupressure is often viewed by insurance companies as massage; as such, it may or may not be covered. Contact your insurance provider for more-specific information.

Acupressure

anesthesia-induced nausea that often follows surgery. Acupressure can also be valuable during pregnancy, as it may relieve morning sickness, indigestion, and backache; alleviate the pain of childbirth; and enhance recuperation. But be sure to read the caution at right.

Preparations/Techniques

Acupressure can be performed by a trained specialist or by patients in their own homes. A specialist can provide comprehensive treatment, which involves the redirecting of chi around the meridians; the American Association of Oriental Medicine can help you locate a good practitioner. To try acupressure yourself for local, symptomatic relief, first identify which acupoints you will use. This may be a single point, or several points in a specific order *(see the Gallery of Acupressure Techniques, pages 18-31)*. Locate the first acupoint with your fingertips, then press lightly with one finger. Gradually increase the pressure until you are comfortably pressing as firmly as you can. Hold this pressure steadily until you begin to feel a very faint, even pulse at the acupoint. (This usually takes three to 10 minutes, or longer for severe problems.) When you're ready to release, reduce the pressure from the acupoint very slowly. You may occasionally feel some discomfort, but if the pressure is actually painful, ease up. There is no "correct" amount of pressure that you should strive for; everyone's needs are different, and the amount required at one acupoint will vary from that needed at another.

For best results, apply pressure to the same acupoints on both sides of the body; when working with a series of acupoints, complete the set on one side of the body before continuing to the other side. In some forms of acupressure, such as shiatsu, pressure is applied sequentially, from one end of the meridian to the other. To work on hard-to-reach spots (such as your back), either ask a partner for help, or place a tennis or golf ball on the floor and then lie on top of it.

Wellness

Beyond its many potential healing effects, acupressure may also be beneficial in maintaining overall good health. Acupressure releases tension in muscle fibers, promoting the movement of blood and nutrients to the tissues. Many people report acupressure induces peaceful rejuvenation and clarity of thought, as well as improved athletic performance.

What the Critics Say

Because no one is certain just how acupressure works, its critics typically claim that it is simply not effective, offering the placebo effect to explain its success. Studies testing the placebo effect do not support this criticism, however. ∎

CAUTION

If you have a serious illness, ask your doctor before using acupressure. Never press on an open wound, swollen or inflamed skin, bruises, varicose veins, or a lump. Avoid sites of recent surgery and sites of a suspected bone injury. If you have atherosclerosis, avoid direct pressure on the carotid arteries. If you are pregnant, avoid pressure to the lower abdomen, and don't use points Spleen 6 or Large Intestine 4 (some believe these points can induce miscarriage).

FOR MORE INFO

Following is a list of organizations you can contact to learn more about acupressure:

American Association of Oriental Medicine
433 Front Street
Catasauqua, PA 18032
(610) 433-2448
fax: (610) 264-2768
e-mail: AAOM1@aol.com

National Certification Commission for Acupuncture and Oriental Medicine
PO Box 97075
Washington, DC 20090-7075
(202) 232-1404
fax: (202) 462-6157

Gallery of Acupressure Techniques

Bladder 10

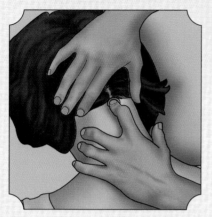

■ *Locate the ropy muscles one-half inch below the base of the skull. Press inward using the thumb or a finger.*

Bladder 13

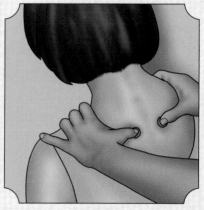

■ *Use your thumbs or fingers to press into the muscles one-half inch outward from either side of the spine and one finger width below the upper tip of the shoulder blade.*

Bladder 23

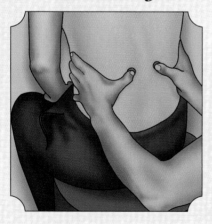

■ *This point site is level with the space between the second and third lumbar vertebrae. Find BL 23 by aligning your thumbs or fingers about an inch outward from either side of the spine, just behind the navel, then press inward.*

Bladder 25

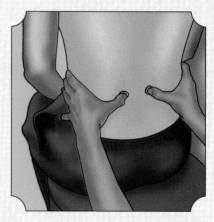

■ *With your thumbs or fingers, press into the muscles about an inch outward from either side of the spine, about midway between BL 23 (left) and the bottom of the spine. The point is level with the fourth and fifth lumbar vertebrae.*

Gallery of Acupressure Techniques

Bladder 32

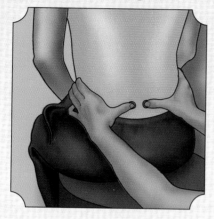

■ At the base of the spine, directly above the tailbone, use your thumbs or fingers to press into the muscles one-half inch outward from either side of the spine.

Bladder 40

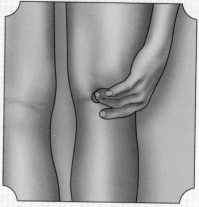

■ With your leg slightly bent, find the fold on the back of your knee where the knee bends. Use your middle finger to press inward on the fold, between the two tendons.

Conception Vessel 4

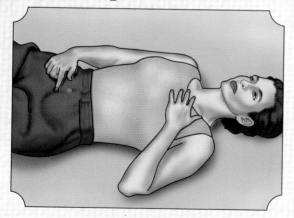

■ Locate this point, which lies just below CV 6 (right), by measuring four finger widths down from the navel on the midline of the abdomen. With your index finger, gradually press as deep as possible on the point site.

Conception Vessel 6

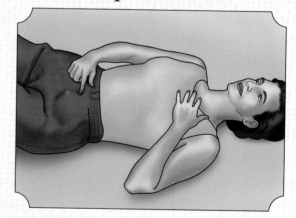

■ Measure three finger widths below the navel—or about one finger width up from CV 4 (left)—then press inward on this point as far as you can, using your index finger. Inhale slowly and deeply, relaxing as you exhale.

CONTINUED

Gallery of Acupressure Techniques

Conception Vessel 12

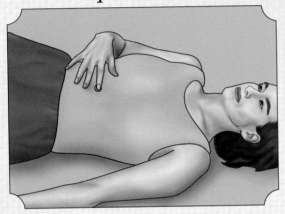

■ This point lies four thumb widths above the navel along the midline of the belly, about halfway between the navel and the bottom of the breastbone. Press softly inward, using your index finger.

Conception Vessel 17

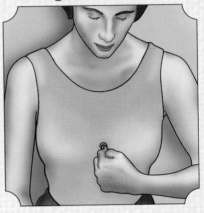

■ Place your index finger in the center of your chest, midway between the nipples, and press lightly.

Conception Vessel 22

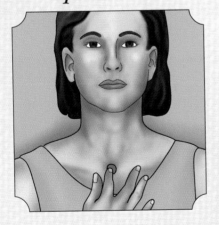

■ This point lies directly below the Adam's apple, midway between the collarbones in the large hollow at the base of the throat. Place the tip of your index or middle finger on the point site and press downward lightly.

Gall Bladder 2

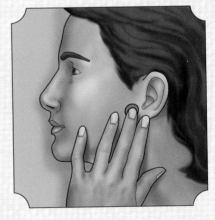

■ Open your mouth and, feeling along the jawbone, locate the depression directly in front of your ears. Place the tips of your middle fingers about one-half inch below the base of the depression. Close your mouth and press steadily on the point.

Gallery of Acupressure Techniques

Gall Bladder 20

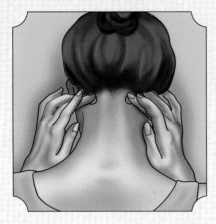

■ *Place the tips of your middle fingers in the hollows at the base of your skull, about two inches apart on either side of the spine. Press firmly.*

Gall Bladder 21

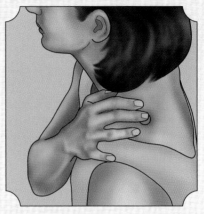

■ *Apply pressure with your right middle finger to the highest point on your left shoulder muscle, one or two inches out from the base of the neck. Repeat on the other side. (Use light pressure if you are pregnant.)*

Gall Bladder 34

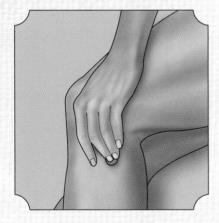

■ *While seated with legs bent, locate the bony indentation on your lower leg just below and to the outside of the kneecap. Apply firm pressure to the point with your finger or thumb.*

Gall Bladder 39

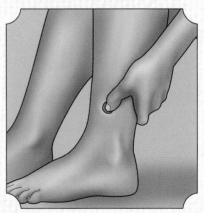

■ *To find this point, measure four finger widths above the outside anklebone, in front of the fibula, on the lower leg. Apply pressure with the tip of your finger or thumb.*

CONTINUED

Gallery of Acupressure Techniques

Governing Vessel 4

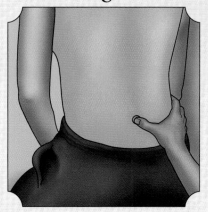

■ Press hard with your thumb on the midline of the spine, directly behind the navel. The point is located between the second and third lumbar vertebrae.

Governing Vessel 14

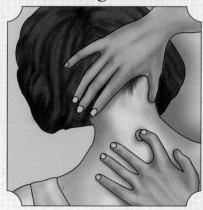

■ Tilt your head and locate the seventh cervical vertebra, the most prominent bone on the back of your neck. Have a helper press the thumb or index finger hard between this bone and the first thoracic vertebra below it.

Governing Vessel 20

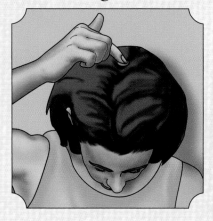

■ This point is located on the flat spot at the top of the head, midway along an imaginary line connecting the upper part of the ears. Apply pressure with your thumb or index finger. (Do not press this point if you have high blood pressure.)

Governing Vessel 24.5

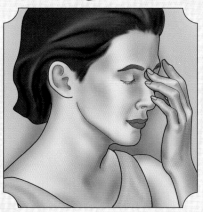

■ Place the tip of your middle finger at the top of the bridge of the nose, between your eyebrows. Press lightly.

Gallery of Acupressure Techniques

Governing Vessel 25

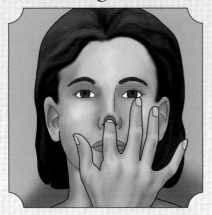

■ Lightly press the tip of your nose with the end of your finger.

Heart 3

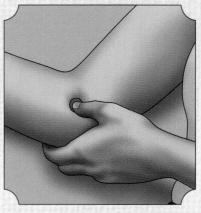

■ On the inside of the upper arm, use your thumb to apply pressure next to the tendon in the indentation near the inside elbow crease, in line with the little finger.

Heart 7

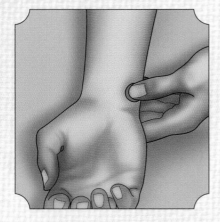

■ This point is located on the crease along the inside of the wrist, directly in line with the little finger. Squeeze firmly, using the thumb and index finger of your other hand.

Kidney 1

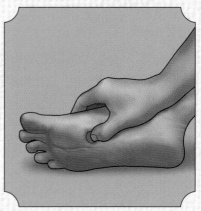

■ Use one or both thumbs to press just behind the ball of the foot, in the slight indentation of the back of the large pad that corresponds to the big toe. (Do not use this point if you have low blood pressure.)

CONTINUED

Gallery of Acupressure Techniques

Kidney 3

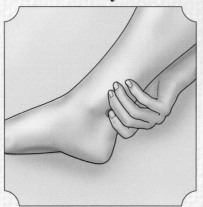

■ *This point lies midway between the inside anklebone and the Achilles tendon at the back of the ankle. Apply pressure with your thumb or index finger. (Avoid using this point after the third month of pregnancy.)*

Large Intestine 4

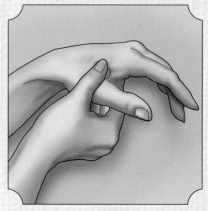

■ *Use the thumb and index finger of your right hand to squeeze the webbing between the thumb and index finger of your left hand. Switch hands and repeat. (Do not apply pressure to this point if you are pregnant.)*

Large Intestine 10

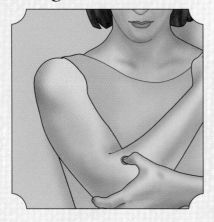

■ *With your arm bent and your palm down, measure two thumb widths below the edge of the elbow crease. The point site lies in the groove between the muscles on the outside of the arm. Press hard with your thumb, then repeat on the other arm.*

Large Intestine 11

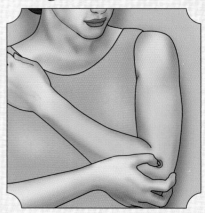

■ *With your arm bent, use your thumb to press deeply on the outer edge of the elbow crease. Repeat on the other arm.*

Gallery of Acupressure Techniques

Large Intestine 20

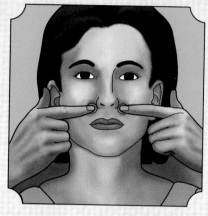

■ Using your index or middle fingers, press hard on the outer edge of the nostrils at the base of the nose.

Liver 2

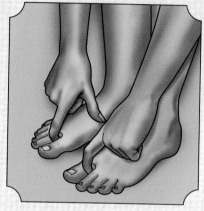

■ On the top of each foot, use your index finger to press into the webbing between the big toe and the second toe.

Liver 3

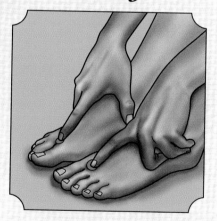

■ Place your index fingers next to the large knuckle of each big toe, then press into the groove on top of the foot between the big toe and the second toe.

Liver 8

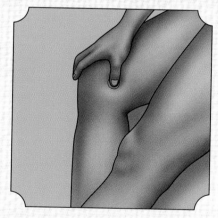

■ Bend the right knee and place your right thumb just above the knee crease on the inside of the leg. The point lies just below the knee joint (swing your leg a few times to help locate it). Press, then repeat on the other leg.

CONTINUED

Gallery of Acupressure Techniques

Lung 1

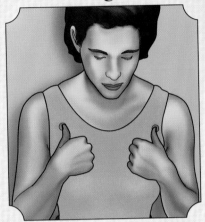

■ Place the thumb or index finger of each hand about one-half inch below the large hollow under the collarbone, on the outer part of the chest near the shoulder. Apply pressure gently.

Lung 5

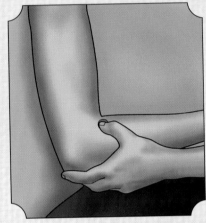

■ Bend your right elbow and make a fist. Place your left thumb on the outside crease (thumb side) of the elbow alongside the taut tendon and press firmly. Repeat on the other arm.

Lung 7

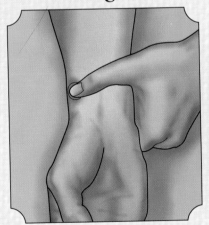

■ On the thumb side of the inner forearm, measure two finger widths above the crease in the wrist. Apply steady, firm pressure to the point site with your thumb, then repeat on the other arm.

Lung 10

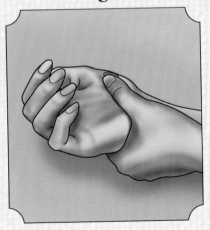

■ On the palm side of the hand, locate this point at the center of the pad at the base of the thumb. Apply pressure with your other thumb while taking several deep breaths.

Gallery of Acupressure Techniques

Pericardium 3

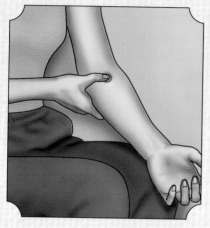

■ Locate the point along the biceps tendon at the elbow crease, in a direct line with your ring finger. Use your thumb to apply firm pressure, then repeat on the other arm.

Pericardium 6

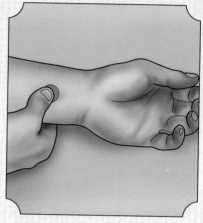

■ To find this point, measure two finger widths above the center of the wrist crease on the inside of your arm. With your thumb, press between the two bones of the forearm. Repeat on the other arm.

Small Intestine 3

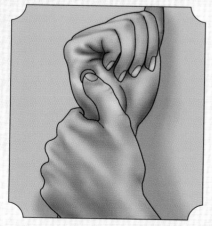

■ Make a loose fist, then twist your wrist to view the side of your little finger. Using your thumb, apply pressure to the side of your palm just below the knuckle of the little finger, between the bone and muscle.

Small Intestine 17

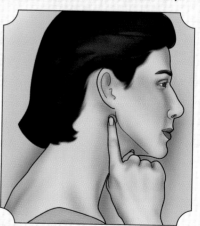

■ Place your index fingers just below your earlobes, in the indentations at the back of the jawbone. Apply light pressure while breathing deeply.

CONTINUED

Gallery of Acupressure Techniques

Spleen 3

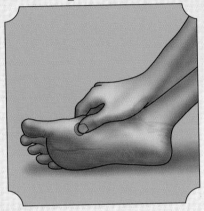

■ Locate the indentation on the inside of the foot, just behind the bulge made by the large joint of the big toe. Maintain steady pressure on the point site with your thumb. Repeat on the other foot.

Spleen 4

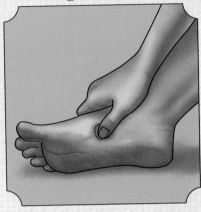

■ On the inside arch of your foot, measure one thumb width back from the ball of the foot. Apply pressure to this point with your thumb, and then repeat on the other foot.

Spleen 6

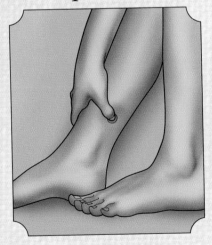

■ Measure four finger widths up from the top of the right inside anklebone. With your thumb, press near the edge of the shinbone. Repeat on the other leg. (Do not apply pressure to this point if you are pregnant.)

Spleen 8

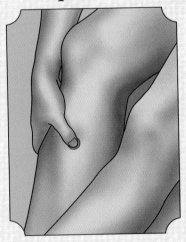

■ On the inside of the lower leg, locate the depression four finger widths below the knee. Press firmly between your calf muscle and your leg bone.

Gallery of Acupressure Techniques

Spleen 9

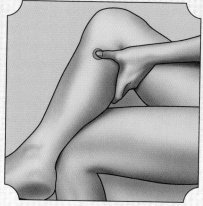

■ Place your thumb in the depression between the tibia and calf muscle on the inside of your leg, just below the knee joint. Press under the large bulge of the bone.

Spleen 10

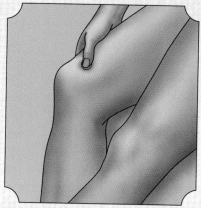

■ Bend your knee slightly to find this point, located two thumb widths up from the top of your knee, in line with the inner edge of the kneecap. Press on the bulge of the muscle with your thumb.

Spleen 12

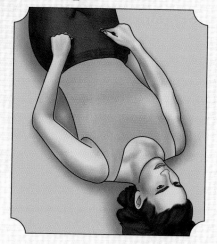

■ In the pelvic area, use your fingertips to press the middle of the crease where the leg joins the trunk of the body.

Stomach 2

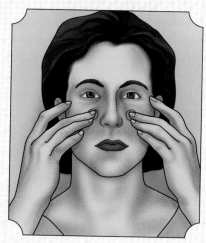

■ Measure one finger width below the lower ridge of the eye sockets, in line with the pupils. Press into the indentation of the cheeks.

CONTINUED

Gallery of Acupressure Techniques

Stomach 3

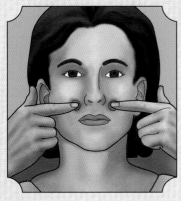

■ Place your index fingers at the bottom of your cheekbones, directly under the pupils of your eyes, then press firmly.

Stomach 7

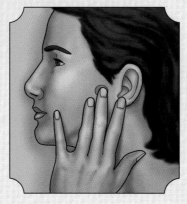

■ With your middle finger, feel on either side of your jaw one thumb width in front of your ears. Press the point site in the slight indentation along the upper jaw line.

Stomach 25

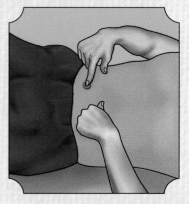

■ Place the index fingers of both hands two finger widths from your navel on either side. Press down firmly and breathe deeply.

Stomach 36

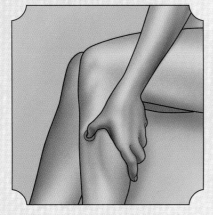

■ Measure four finger widths below the kneecap just outside the shinbone (flex your foot; you should feel a muscle bulge at the point site). Press the point steadily with a finger or thumb, then repeat on the other leg.

Stomach 44

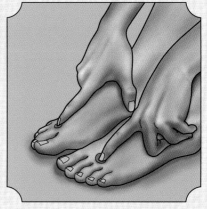

■ Using your index fingers, press lightly on the webbing between the second and third toes of each foot.

Gallery of Acupressure Techniques

Triple Warmer 3

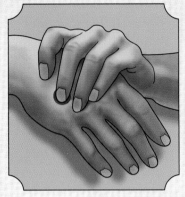

■ On the back of the hand, press firmly into the furrow just below the fourth and fifth knuckles (between the ring and little fingers). Repeat on the other hand.

Triple Warmer 5

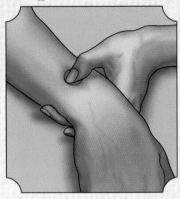

■ Center your thumb on the top of your forearm, two thumb widths from the wrist joint, and press firmly. Repeat on the other arm.

Triple Warmer 6

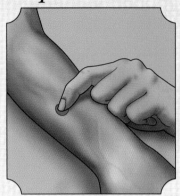

■ Measure about three finger widths from the wrist on the top of the forearm, then press this point with your thumb or index finger. Repeat on the other arm.

Triple Warmer 17

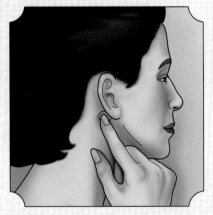

■ Using the tips of your index or middle fingers, find the hollows behind the earlobes where the ears meet the jawbone. Press lightly and breathe deeply.

Hiccup 1

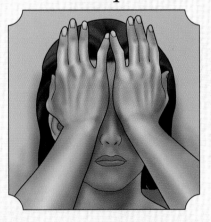

■ To stop hiccups, place your palms over both eyes, with heels resting on your cheekbones. Massage gently by pressing the pads below your thumbs toward your palms, then follow instructions for Governing Vessel 25.

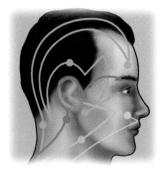

Target Ailments

- Arthritis
- Asthma
- Athletic Injuries
- Back Problems
- Bursitis
- Chronic Fatigue Syndrome
- Common Cold
- Depression
- Earache
- Gout
- Headache
- Hemorrhoids
- Indigestion
- Insomnia
- Nausea
- Pain, Chronic
- Sinusitis
- Sore Throat
- Stress
- Tendinitis
- Toothache

See Common Ailments, beginning on page 194.

Acupuncture

T *he healing technique of acupuncture, like other therapeutic approaches in the traditional practice of Chinese medicine (pages 57-60), is founded on the principle that internal harmony is essential for good health. Fundamental to this harmony is the concept of chi (sometimes spelled "qi"), a vital energy or life force that ebbs and flows with changes in a person's mental, physical, and spiritual well-being. Chi is said to circulate through the body within 14 invisible channels called meridians (see the illustrations on pages 34-35), forming a network called the web of life. A balanced, freely flowing chi is said to generate good health, while a sluggish, blocked, or overstimulated chi is believed to cause illness. Acupuncturists strive to encourage proper chi circulation by manipulating it at "chi gateways" just below the skin; the manipulation is achieved by inserting hair-thin needles at these gateways, which are more commonly known as acupoints. The stimulation that results is said to enable a person to achieve internal harmony, a state that allows the body's self-healing mechanisms to engage.*

Origins

Acupuncture has been practiced in China for about 4,500 years. Its spread to the West has been relatively slow but steady. The first real surge in popularity in the United States came in 1971, following a story by a *New York Times* journalist who had been successfully treated for pain with acupuncture during a visit to China.

What It's Good For

Traditionally, acupuncturists have treated scores of different illnesses, as indicated by the list at left, which represents only a sampling of them. Although acupuncture's primary use in the United States has been to alleviate pain, its therapeutic applications have been gradually expanding. Today,

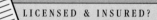

LICENSED & INSURED?

YES! *Currently 33 states and the District of Columbia have set standards for acupuncturists. Choose a practitioner who is a physician or who is board-certified in acupuncture by the National Certification Commission for Acupuncture and Oriental Medicine. For help finding a certified acupuncturist in your area, contact the American Association of Oriental Medicine.*

In 1996 the FDA classified acupuncture needles as a type of medical device. This indirectly boosts acupuncture's credibility and increases the likelihood that your insurance provider will pay for your acupuncture treatments. Coverage varies tremendously. Your provider's claims office is your best information source.

Acupuncture

acupuncture is employed in treating addictions, controlling weight, and enhancing recuperation following surgery or stroke.

Visiting a Professional

In order to properly evaluate your needs, during a first visit an acupuncturist will observe you closely, check your pulse, look at your tongue, and ask many questions about your health and your lifestyle. These are customary diagnostic routines employed by practitioners of all forms of Chinese medicine.

After this evaluation, the therapy itself can begin. Typically, the acupuncturist inserts acupuncture needles into the skin at the appropriate acupoints, then twirls them and, possibly, applies a gentle electric current (which is believed to enhance effectiveness). The needles may penetrate as little as a fraction of an inch (on the fingertips, for example) or as much as three or four inches (where a thick layer of fat or muscle exists). The procedure usually causes little pain, although patients often feel numbness where the needles are inserted, and perhaps a bit of tingling.

In addition to—or sometimes instead of—inserting needles, acupuncturists may opt for a treatment called moxibustion. This consists of applying heat directly above acupuncture points by means of small bundles of smoldering herbs, usually mugwort leaf. The practitioner may also employ acupressure *(pages 16-17)*.

Wellness

Because acupuncture's ultimate goal is to maximize the body's own healing abilities, it is little surprise that acupuncture treatments are considered helpful in maintaining as well as restoring health. Indeed, acupuncturists are trained to recognize so-called disharmonies early, often before they develop into full-blown disease.

What the Critics Say

Although the American Medical Association does not officially sanction acupuncture, more than 2,000 of the United States' 12,000 acupuncturists are MDs. But many physicians find it hard to accept acupuncture's invisible energy-path theory of effectiveness. The "placebo effect" is most often cited as the reason acupuncture works—an argument that has not, however, held up to scientific testing. Some say that the pain of inserting acupuncture needles distracts the patient from his or her original pain, but this would not account for acupuncture's reputed success in treating other, painless ailments; also, properly inserted needles are not usually painful.

Research indicates that acupuncture stimulates the body to release its own natural painkillers (endorphins and enkephalins), as well as an anti-inflammatory agent (cortisol). Whether enough of these natural chemicals are released to account for acupuncture's apparent success has yet to be determined. ∎

CAUTION

While acupuncture can help one manage the pain of labor and delivery, it is generally not recommended for other purposes during pregnancy because it may stimulate uterine contractions and could induce labor.

FOR MORE INFO

Following is a list of organizations you can contact to learn more about acupuncture:

National Acupuncture and Oriental Medicine Alliance
14637 Starr Road, SE
Olalla, WA 98359
(206) 851-6896
fax: (206) 851-6883

American Association of Oriental Medicine
433 Front Street
Catasauqua, PA 18032
(610) 433-2448
fax: (610) 264-2768
e-mail AAOM1@aol.com

American Academy of Medical Acupuncture
5820 Wilshire Blvd, Suite 500
Los Angeles, CA 90036
(800) 521-2262
fax: (213) 937-0959
e-mail: KCKD71F@prodigy.com

National Certification Commission for Acupuncture and Oriental Medicine
PO Box 97075
Washington, DC 20090-7075
(202) 232-1404
fax: (202) 462-6157

CONTINUED

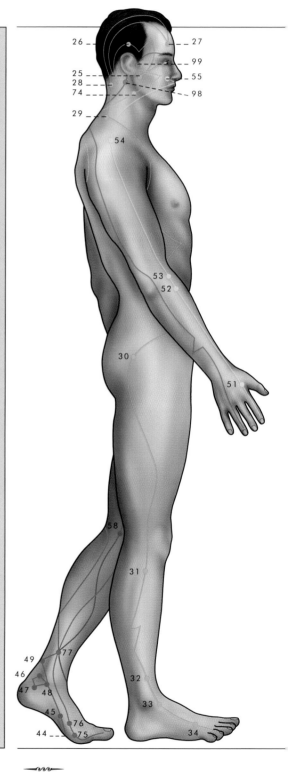

Meridians and Acupoints

Chinese medicine teaches that energy flowing through invisible channels in the body called meridians may be manipulated by pressure (acupressure), the insertion of fine needles (acupuncture), or warmth (moxibustion) to treat disease and improve health. Meridians and related acupoints are listed below. For more information, see the Gallery of Acupressure Techniques, pages 18-31.

Bladder
1 BL 1
2 BL 2
3 BL 7
4 BL 10
5 BL 13
6 BL 23
7 BL 25
8 BL 27
9 BL 28
10 BL 29
11 BL 30
12 BL 31
13 BL 32
14 BL 33
15 BL 34
16 BL 40
17 BL 57
18 BL 58
19 BL 60

Conception Vessel
20 CV 4
21 CV 6
22 CV 12
23 CV 17
24 CV 22

Gall Bladder
25 GB 2
26 GB 8
27 GB 14
28 GB 20
29 GB 21
30 GB 30
31 GB 34
32 GB 39
33 GB 40
34 GB 41

Governing Vessel
35 GV 4
36 GV 14

37 GV 16
38 GV 20
39 GV 24.5
40 GV 25
41 GV 26

Heart
42 HE 3
43 HE 7

Kidney
44 KI 1
45 KI 2
46 KI 3
47 KI 5
48 KI 6
49 KI 7
50 KI 27

Large Intestine
51 LI 4
52 LI 10
53 LI 11
54 LI 15
55 LI 20

Liver
56 LV 2
57 LV 3
58 LV 8

Lung
59 LU 1
60 LU 5
61 LU 6
62 LU 7
63 LU 9
64 LU 10

Pericardium
65 PE 3
66 PE 6
67 PE 7

Small Intestine
68 SI 3
69 SI 4
70 SI 5
71 SI 8
72 SI 10
73 SI 11
74 SI 17

Spleen
75 SP 3
76 SP 4
77 SP 6
78 SP 8
79 SP 9
80 SP 10
81 SP 12
82 SP 16

Stomach
83 ST 2
84 ST 3
85 ST 6
86 ST 7
87 ST 16
88 ST 18
89 ST 25
90 ST 35
91 ST 36
92 ST 40
93 ST 44

Triple Warmer
94 TW 3
95 TW 4
96 TW 5
97 TW 15
98 TW 17
99 TW 21

Acupuncture

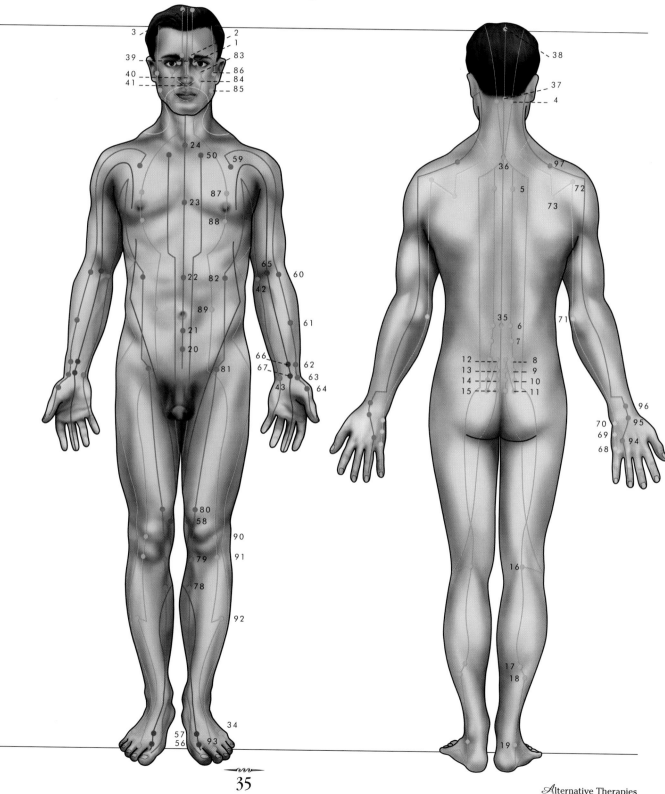

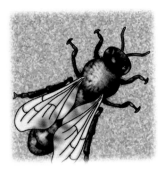

Target Ailments

For Bee Venom Therapy:

- Arthritis
- Bursitis
- Headache
- Menopause
- Multiple Sclerosis
- Premenstrual Syndrome
- Tendinitis

See Common Ailments, beginning on page 194.

$\mathcal{A}$pitherapy

A pitherapy is the therapeutic use of any of the products of the honeybee. Honey itself, for example, has been shown to have antiseptic and antibacterial properties, as does a substance known as propolis, which is made by bees from tree resin and is used to cement the hive together. Bee pollen has high concentrations of vitamins and minerals and so is sometimes incorporated into nutritional therapy, while royal jelly—a potent food made specially for the queen bee—is reputed to have energizing effects and to stimulate hormone production.

Perhaps most surprising and controversial are reports of success in the use of honeybee venom—administered either by injection or directly by stinging—to reduce symptoms such as pain and inflammation in chronic illnesses.

Bee Venom Therapy

Although by definition a poison, bee venom contains among its active ingredients the peptide melittin, a potent anti-inflammatory agent. Inside the body, melittin stimulates the adrenal glands to produce cortisol, a natural steroid with powerful healing properties and none of the complications of synthetic steroids. When venom is introduced into tissues that are already inflamed by disease, the area becomes further inflamed in reaction to the venom, but at the same time the body's anti-inflammatory agents are called into action; as they work to shrink the swelling caused by the venom, these agents are also thought to help reduce the inflammation resulting from the original condition.

Origins

Apitherapy dates back to the ancient civilizations of Greece and China. Bee stings were used by the Greek physicians Hippocrates and Galen, and apitherapy is mentioned in both the Bible and the Koran. Phillip Terc, an Austrian physician, initiated the modern study of intentional bee stings with his 1888 work entitled "Report about a Peculiar Connection between the Beestings and Rheumatism." Medical and lay practitioners today number in the thousands.

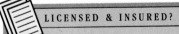

LICENSED & INSURED?

Bee venom therapy does not require a licensed practitioner. But when a physician administers the treatment (using either live bees or a hypodermic needle), the procedure may be covered by medical insurance as part of an office visit. Although bee venom presently is approved by the U.S. Food and Drug Administration only as a desensitizing agent, some physicians have won approval to use it as an "investigational new drug."

Apitherapy

What It's Good For

Raw (unheated, unfiltered) honey can be used topically as a wound or burn dressing. Bee pollen is a potent dietary supplement and may also be helpful in treating seasonal allergies. The germ-fighting properties of propolis make it effective for treating sore throat, colds, and flu. Royal jelly, long a staple of folk medicines and also sometimes used in cosmetics, has been used to treat vascular diseases and illnesses that cause weakness or tiredness.

Venom therapy may help reduce pain and swelling in osteoarthritis, rheumatoid arthritis, and other inflammatory and degenerative diseases. It is also used to treat various autoimmune diseases. Because of anecdotal reports of significant symptom reduction in multiple sclerosis, venom therapy is being used extensively by patients with that disease, and research is under way to document the therapy's effects. Additionally, venom therapy may help alleviate migraine headaches.

Preparations/Techniques

Most honeybee products are available in commercial preparations and are either applied topically or taken internally by mouth. Bee venom is delivered at specific sites related to the illness or at acupuncture points, and is administered either through a hypodermic needle or directly by the bee in the form of stings. Some physicians perform the treatment—a must in the case of injection—but the therapy is also sometimes administered by beekeepers, patients themselves, or a partner.

When the stinging method is used, a supply of bees is kept in a jar containing honey; each bee is removed with tweezers and held over the specified area of the body until it stings. The stinger is removed after three to five minutes. The number and frequency of stings depend on the patient and the specific problem.

Injections cost more than stinging, and it is not known whether the processing of the venom reduces its healing effect. On the other hand, bee stings are extremely painful, and the amount of venom cannot be standardized. A less painful method, used infrequently in the United States, involves removing the stinger from the bee and applying it to the skin.

What the Critics Say

Because most of the evidence for the efficacy of bee venom therapy consists of anecdotes rather than double-blind studies, many Western physicians remain skeptical. Some say multiple sclerosis naturally waxes and wanes and that the benefits reported may be due to either natural remission or the placebo effect. Critics have pointed to occurrences of localized infection and scarring, which result from leaving the stinger in for too long. ∎

CAUTION

Bee venom can cause a serious and potentially fatal allergic reaction, including severe respiratory distress and shock. Before beginning treatment, you should be allergy-tested; also, be sure an emergency bee sting allergy kit containing epinephrine is on hand during treatment. You should not be concerned about minor swelling and itching caused by the venom; this is a desirable inflammatory response necessary to the healing process.

FOR MORE INFO
Following is a list of organizations you can contact to learn more about apitherapy:

The American Apitherapy Society
PO Box 54
Hartland Four Corners, VT 05049
(802) 436-2708
fax: (802) 436-2827

The Multiple Sclerosis Association of America
706 Haddonfield Road
Cherry Hill, NJ 08002
(800) 833-4672
(609) 488-4500

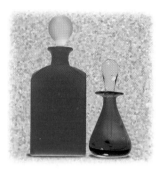

Target Ailments

- Bladder Infections
- Bronchitis
- Common Cold
- Conjunctivitis
- Depression
- Flu
- Gas and Gas Pains
- Immune Problems
- Indigestion
- Insomnia
- Laryngitis
- Menopause
- Motion Sickness
- Muscle Cramps
- Nausea
- Sexually Transmitted Diseases
- Stress
- Tendinitis
- Tonsillitis
- Yeast Infections

See Common Ailments, beginning on page 194.

$\mathcal{A}$romatherapy

Aromatherapy is the therapeutic use of essential oils—concentrated, fragrant extracts of plants—to promote relaxation and help relieve various symptoms. Suppliers of aromatherapy oils extract them from specific parts of plants—the roots, bark, stalks, flowers, leaves, or fruit—by two methods: Distillation uses successive evaporation and condensation to pull the oils from the plants; cold-pressing squeezes rinds or peels through a machine to press out the oils. Users then administer the oils in several ways, generally by applying them to the skin or inhaling their scents.

Some practitioners believe the oils have both physical and ethereal (spiritual) qualities and effects. They assert that the oils work on the emotions because the nerves involved in the sense of smell are directly linked to the brain's limbic system, which governs emotion, and that the active components of the oils give them specific therapeutic value, with antiseptic, antibacterial, and antiviral effects common to many of them.

Origins

Ancient people used aromatic substances for medicinal, cosmetic, and religious purposes. In the 10th century, the Arab doctor Avicenna described methods of distilling plants, although there is evidence that what came to be known as aromatherapy may have been known even in ancient times.

French chemist René-Maurice Gattefossé, who worked in a perfume factory, inaugurated the modern scientific use of essential oils in the 1920s and coined the term *aromatherapy*. After burning his hand in a chemical explosion, he quickly healed it without infection or scarring by applying lavender oil, which happened to be nearby. Gattefossé went on to classify the oils and their properties.

Aromatherapy gained widespread popularity in the United Kingdom and France in the 1980s, but it is less well known and researched in North America.

What It's Good For

Aromatherapists believe that all the oils affect the emotions in some way and that many also work on physical ailments. They think that as well as relieving stress, some oils may improve sluggish circulation, relieve pain, reduce swelling, or cleanse the body of impurities. Others are used to

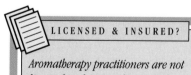

LICENSED & INSURED?

Aromatherapy practitioners are not licensed in the United States today, although licensed healthcare providers may include aromatherapy as one of their techniques.

Aromatherapy

treat bacterial or viral infections, burns, hypertension, arrhythmias, respiratory conditions, insomnia, depression, and many other ailments.

Although patients with asthma may benefit from aromatherapy, they should use the oils only under a practitioner's supervision.

Preparations/Techniques

Essential oils may be applied externally and used in massage, or incorporated into compresses and ointments. They may also be inhaled or taken internally (orally, rectally, or vaginally). Remember to follow all dilution, dosage, and treatment guidelines as well as the cautions on the chart on the following pages.

A common aromatherapy technique is to dilute the oils in a vegetable carrier oil, such as safflower or sweet almond oil, for an aromatherapy massage. You can use basic massage strokes on yourself or a partner *(see the Gallery of Massage Techniques, pages 124-129)* to encourage relaxation or relieve specific problems. If you are prone to allergic reactions, test the oils first by putting a drop of oil on the inside of your elbow and waiting 24 hours for any reaction. During the massage, the skin absorbs the oil at the same time that the user inhales it.

Another way to use the oils is in an aromatic warm bath, which adds the therapeutic qualities of water to those of the oils. You may also apply hot or cold compresses, creams, or lotions made from the oils directly to the skin. For respiratory conditions, insomnia, depression, or stress, try breathing in the aromas using a steam inhaler or a fan-assisted apparatus. Remember to close your eyes when inhaling.

Buy oils from a reputable company and don't shop by price alone, because adulteration with chemicals and cheaper herbs is common. Consult a qualified health practitioner before taking oils internally. Some oils, such as thuja, wormwood, mugwort leaf, tansy, hyssop, sage, and eucalyptus, should never be taken internally.

Wellness

Essential oils are often incorporated into wellness programs because they are easy and pleasant to use. Aromatherapists believe that regular use can reestablish balance and harmony within the body as well as soothe the mind and emotions.

What the Critics Say

Critics from conventional medicine point to the general lack of research in the field and to unscientific pronouncements of its proponents, such as references to ethereal effects and to the so-called subtle parts of the plants. Critics with a holistic viewpoint have faulted aromatherapy because the whole plant is not used. They note that chemical changes occur after a flower is cut that may adversely affect the therapeutic value of a given type of plant. ∎

CAUTION

Because the oils used in aromatherapy are available over the counter, some people may assume that they are all safe. However, they can have potentially serious side effects, including neurotoxicity and inducement of abortion, as well as skin reactions, allergies, and liver damage. Overexposure to oils by inhalation can produce headache and fatigue. It's best to have a healthcare professional supervise you when you use oils.

FOR MORE INFO

Following is a list of organizations you can contact to learn more about aromatherapy:

National Association for Holistic Aromatherapy
PO Box 17622
Boulder, CO 80308-7622
(800) 566-6735

Pacific Institute of Aromatherapy
PO Box 6723
San Rafael, CA 94903
(415) 479-9121
fax: (415) 479-0119

CONTINUED

The 15 Most Effective Essential Oils

Name	Parts Used	Properties	Target Ailments
Bay laurel *Native to the Mediterranean, this hardy evergreen shrub or tree has dark green leaves and black berries. Its oil is greenish yellow and has a powerful spicy scent.*	BERRIES DRIED LEAVES YOUNG TWIGS	An overall strengthener; can be an antiseptic, diuretic, or sedative, and may help to expel gas and clear the lungs.	**Bay laurel** helps in digestive problems and appetite loss, relieves chronic bronchitis, colds, flu, and tonsillitis, and treats scabies and lice. It also aids in rheumatic aches and pains and reduces swollen lymph nodes. CAUTION: Use in moderation. Avoid if pregnant.
Clary sage *This southern European plant has small blue or white flowers and large, hairy leaves. The oil is colorless or pale yellow-green and is used extensively in foods and drinks.*	FLOWERING TOPS LEAVES	A powerful, quick-acting relaxant; has warming effects; eases inflammation; anticonvulsive and antiseptic.	**Clary sage** soothes anxiety and stress, relieves menstrual and menopausal symptoms, and treats burns and eczema. CAUTION: Avoid during pregnancy or if you have high blood pressure. Do not drink alcohol while using.
Eucalyptus globulus *This native Australian evergreen is cultivated in several areas, including the state of California. The oil ranges from clear to yellow and has a penetrating smell.*	LEAVES TWIGS	Strongly antiseptic; antibacterial; expectorant; has stimulating, astringent, and analgesic actions.	**Eucalyptus globulus** reduces fever; fights colds, flu, sinusitis, and cough; helps relieve the symptoms of bronchitis; and is helpful in skin conditions such as boils and pimples. CAUTION: Do not take internally.
Everlasting *This strongly scented herb, with multi-branched stem and bright flowers, is native to the Mediterranean region and grows wild in the Pacific Northwest.*	FLOWERS FLOWERING TOPS	Anti-inflammatory and painkilling properties; prevents internal hemorrhage and swelling after injury.	**Everlasting** is effective in skin conditions such as scarring, sunburn, and wounds. It relieves congestion of the liver or spleen, helps in bronchitis and flu, and is used to treat tendinitis, arthritic pain, and muscle aches, sprains, and strains.
German chamomile *Native to Europe and Asia, this widely cultivated aromatic herb has feathery leaves and white flowers, and produces an inky blue strong-scented oil.*	FLOWERS	Anti-inflammatory, sedative, and painkilling properties; also antiallergic and antiseptic.	**German chamomile** alleviates digestive upsets, menstrual and menopausal problems, inflamed skin, burns, acne, boils, sunburn, and cuts. It aids in arthritis and muscular pain, and helps to relieve symptoms of hay fever and bronchitis.
Lavender *Native to the Mediterranean, this evergreen shrub is now grown worldwide. You may release its familiar aroma by rubbing a flower or leaf between the fingers. The oil is clear or yellow-green.*	FLOWERING TOPS	Known for its calming, soothing, and balancing effects; also has analgesic and antiseptic properties.	**Lavender** relieves headache, depression, insomnia, stress, muscular aches and sprains, menstrual pain, and nausea. It also soothes skin conditions such as cuts, wounds, insect bites, burns, and athlete's foot.
Lemon-scented eucalyptus *This tall evergreen, sometimes called a gum tree, is native to Australia. Its colorless or pale yellow oil has long been used for sachets in linen closets.*	LEAVES TWIGS	Sedative, anti-inflammatory, antiseptic, and deodorant action; can kill bacteria, viruses, and fungi.	**Lemon-scented eucalyptus** soothes mosquito bites and skin irritations. It also helps athlete's foot and herpes sores and relieves muscle tension and stress. CAUTION: Do not take internally.

Aromatherapy

Name	Parts Used	Properties	Target Ailments
Niaouli *Principally from Australia, this evergreen has a spongy bark and white flowers. The yellow or greenish oil has a camphorous odor and is found in health aids such as toothpaste.*	LEAVES YOUNG TWIGS	Antiseptic, analgesic, and anti-allergic properties, as well as tissue-stimulating action helpful for healing.	■ **Niaouli** combats allergies, bronchitis, colds, and flu; cleans minor wounds and burns; aids in acne, boils, and insect bites; and helps relieve muscle aches and pains as well as toothache. It may also be used to treat bladder infection.
Palmarosa *Native to India and Pakistan, this wild tropical grass has a long stem and aromatic leaves. The oil is pale yellow or olive in color, with a sweet floral scent.*	FLOWERS LEAVES	Antiviral, antibacterial, and antiseptic properties, as well as an overall strengthening effect.	■ **Palmarosa** is diluted with almond oil to treat skin conditions such as cuts and wounds, acne, dermatitis, cold sores, and scars. It also relieves symptoms of flu, fights intestinal and other infections, and is helpful in stress-related conditions.
Peppermint *This perennial herb native to Europe and western Asia is cultivated around the world. Its oil is colorless, pale yellow, or green and is a popular flavoring agent.*	FLOWERING TOPS LEAVES	Produces a warming effect (after an initial cooling action) and can relieve pain; also stimulates the liver.	■ **Peppermint** relieves indigestion, nausea, and headache. It is helpful for neuralgia and muscle pain, and can aid in bronchitis, sinusitis, and motion sickness. CAUTION: Use in moderation. Do not give to children under 30 months of age.
Rosemary *This Mediterranean evergreen shrub has silvery green leaves and pale blue flowers. The oil is colorless to pale yellow-green; its scent is minty in oils of good quality.*	FLOWERING TOPS LEAVES	A stimulant that invigorates the whole body and helps eliminate toxins; antiseptic and diuretic properties.	■ **Rosemary** is effective for indigestion, gas, and liver problems. It fights bronchitis and flu, reduces fluid retention, and helps treat depression. CAUTION: Avoid during pregnancy or if you have epilepsy or high blood pressure.
Tarragon *This bushy perennial plant native to Asia and Europe has narrow green leaves and small flowers. The colorless oil has an aroma similar to anise and is a popular food seasoning.*	LEAVES	Antispasmodic, diuretic, and mild laxative properties; stimulant.	■ **Tarragon** helps with menstrual and menopausal symptoms and with digestive ailments such as gas, indigestion, hiccups, and loss of appetite. It can aid in stress-related problems and in overcoming shock. CAUTION: Avoid during pregnancy.
Tea tree *Native to New South Wales, Australia, the tea tree or shrub has small, narrow leaves and yellow or purple flowers. Its tart oil ranges from colorless to pale yellow-green.*	LEAVES TWIGS	Antiseptic action against bacteria, fungi, and viruses; soothing to the skin and mucous membranes.	■ **Tea tree** fights colds, flu, tonsillitis, bronchitis, and sinusitis, and can treat skin ailments such as abscesses, acne, and burns. It also helps clear vaginal thrush, vaginitis, and bladder infections, and helps control *Candida* infection.
Thyme *This evergreen shrub native to the Mediterranean area has gray-green leaves and clusters of purple or white flowers. The oil's natural color varies from red- or orange-brown to yellow.*	FLOWERING TOPS LEAVES	Strongly stimulating, antiseptic, and antibacterial properties; also has antispasmodic and digestive actions.	■ **Thyme** helps in laryngitis and coughs and fights skin, bladder, and other infections. It relieves joint pain, treats diarrhea and gas, and can help to expel intestinal worms. CAUTION: Avoid during pregnancy or if you have high blood pressure.
Ylang-ylang *Native to the Philippines, ylang-ylang is a tall tropical tree with large, fragrant flowers. The clear or yellow oil, used in perfumes and soaps, has a sweet, spicy aroma.*	FRESH FLOWERS	Both stimulant and sedative properties; also can regulate heart action.	■ **Ylang-ylang** helps with acne and oily skin and aids in depression, insomnia, impotence, and other stress-related disorders. It can be a backup therapy for high blood pressure. CAUTION: Overuse can cause headache or nausea.

Target Ailments

- Allergies
- Angina
- Arthritis
- Cancer
- Cholesterol Problems
- Chronic Fatigue Syndrome
- Common Cold
- Constipation
- Depression
- Diabetes
- Diarrhea
- Flu
- Gas and Gas Pains
- Headache
- Heartburn
- High Blood Pressure
- Immune Problems
- Insomnia
- Irritable Bowel Syndrome
- Premenstrual Syndrome

See Common Ailments, beginning on page 194.

Ayurvedic Medicine

Ayurvedic medicine is a system of diagnosis and treatment *that has been practiced in India for more than 2,500 years. The term "ayurveda" comes from the Sanskrit roots āyuh, which means longevity, and veda, meaning knowledge. Ayurvedic theory holds that the human body represents the entire universe in microcosmic form, and that we come to know how we function as organisms only by observing and understanding the world around us. The key to health is maintaining a balance between the microcosmic body and the macrocosmic world, a relationship that is expressed in the concept of three physiological principles called doshas. The role of the Ayurvedic physician is to restore and maintain, through different types of therapies, diet, lifestyle, and natural medicines, the balance of the three doshas that is appropriate for a given individual.*

The Three Doshas

According to Ayurvedic theory, every person contains some amount of the universe's five basic elements: earth, air, fire, water, and ether (or space). To describe and understand the combination of these elements that makes up each unique individual—and thereby to gain insights into aspects of personality as well as of physiology—Ayurvedic healers rely on the concept of *doshas.*

Doshas are general categories; each dosha consists of one or more of the universe's five basic elements. Ayurvedic practitioners recognize three main types of dosha: *vata, pitta,* and *kapha.* Together these are called the *tridosha.*

Vata, "wind," is a combination of ether (space) and air. As such, vata is associated with lightness and dispersion, and this concept encompasses both the movement of fluids and cells through the body and the flow of thoughts through the mind. According to Ayurvedic principles, people who are strongly influenced by vata are said to be active and often restless. Creative people often have a strong vata component in their makeup.

Pitta, "bile," is composed of fire (some descriptions also mention wa-

LICENSED & INSURED?

No. There is currently no licensing board for Ayurvedic practitioners and no recognized form of certification, though the need for some form of regulation is growing as Ayurveda increases in popularity. Insurance providers are generally reluctant to pay for Ayurvedic therapies, although your expenses may be covered if your treatment is performed by a licensed physician. Ask your insurance provider's claims representative for information about your coverage.

Ayurvedic Medicine

ter). The key to this dosha is the concept of transformation—apparent in such physical processes as the digestion of food to produce energy. Pitta is said to be the controlling force behind all of the body's metabolic activities. Persons primarily influenced by pitta are thought to be doers, in the sense of being quick to change things as needs arise. They also may be extremely competitive or aggressive.

Kapha, "phlegm," is made up of earth and water elements. Structure is integral to kapha, as this dosha is said to provide the body's physical strength, stability, and wound-healing abilities. A predominantly kapha person might be relatively heavy and muscular, and would be likely to be characterized as having a stable, tranquil personality.

Doshic Balance

A given individual's natural constitution—known in Ayurvedic medicine as that person's *prakriti*—is a unique balance of the three doshas. Each person's prakriti is said to be present at the moment of conception. While every prakriti contains a certain amount of vata, pitta, and kapha, one dosha usually predominates. According to Ayurveda, your prakriti not only describes your constitution but also regulates your physical, emotional, and mental processes. By living a lifestyle that conforms to your specific prakriti, you can achieve optimum health. If, however, in the course of your daily life you subject yourself to overeating, stress, inadequate or excessive sleep, or other similar conditions, you can excite one or more of the doshas, causing a disruption of your doshic balance (and therefore your prakriti), which is virtually guaranteed to lead to illness.

Ayurvedic practitioners advocate diets and lifestyles that reinforce the doshic balance, and encourage close vigilance (through body and mind-awareness techniques such as meditation) to identify imbalances. When an imbalance is detected and confirmed by an Ayurvedic practitioner, immediate corrective measures are prescribed using Ayurvedic therapies and remedies.

Origins

Historical evidence suggests that the medical system we now call Ayurveda began in India around the sixth century BC, coinciding roughly with the lifetime of the Buddha (although some scholars contend that it began much earlier). According to tradition, holy men, or *rishis,* gathered together in a hermitage high in the Himalayas to compile the healing wisdom they had attained via divine inspiration. Their medical knowledge was then transmitted to the people as part of the sacred Hindu scriptures known as the Vedas. The rishis intended that Ayurveda would maximize wellness of the body and the mind, and that this would create an unencumbered path to a person's spiritual fulfillment.

> ## CAUTION
>
> Some Ayurvedic preparations contain harmful substances such as lead, mercury, and arsenic. Although these substances may be described as "inactivated" and therefore safe, their safety has not been proved: Avoid all preparations containing even minute amounts of heavy metals or dangerous chemicals. Ayurvedic medicine is a comprehensive system of healthcare; however, it is not always appropriate for treating serious injuries or problems that require surgery.

CONTINUED

Ayurvedic Medicine CONTINUED

Through the centuries, Ayurvedic philosophy has spread worldwide. In the last few hundred years, foreign influence in India has overshadowed much traditional knowledge, including Ayurveda. The last 35 years or so, however, have witnessed a powerful resurgence in interest, among both practitioners and patients. In India today, Ayurveda is a popular—though not exclusive—choice for 80 percent of the population; conventional Western-style allopathic medicine, homeopathy, Arabic Unani medicine, and Siddha medicine, in the south, are also commonly practiced.

Ayurveda is steadily growing in popularity in the United States, where two types of Ayurvedic medicine coexist: traditional Ayurveda and Maharishi Ayur-Veda. Traditional Ayurveda is based on the ancient textbooks of the master physicians Caraka, Sushruta, and Vagbhata. Many traditional practitioners have been trained in India's Ayurveda colleges. They practice largely on their own in the United States, as there is currently no unifying professional organization.

Maharishi Ayur-Veda is a modern effort by Maharishi Mahesh Yogi (the Indian teacher who introduced transcendental meditation to the United States in the 1960s) to blend traditional Ayurvedic medicine with transcendental meditation. Maharishi Ayur-Veda practitioners are trained in North America, and this is the more popular type of Ayurvedic medicine in the United States. (Maharishi Ayur-Veda is also the name of a company that sells Ayurvedic products and services.)

What It's Good For

While its primary focus is preventive, Ayurveda also encompasses healing remedies for hundreds of ailments. Practitioners especially recommend Ayurvedic therapies for the relief of chronic, metabolic, and stress-related problems. Numerous studies are under way to determine if Ayurvedic remedies may inhibit breast cancer; increase mobility and reduce the pain of arthritis; allay chemotherapy's side effects; hasten recuperation following conventional surgery; decrease serum cholesterol; alleviate symptoms of Parkinson's disease; reduce insulin dependence for diabetics; and assist in recovery from heroin addiction.

Two Forms of Treatment

Ayurvedic practitioners use many preparations and techniques, including hatha-yoga *(see Yoga, pages 182-183),* sounds, scents, foods, spices, colors, minerals, medicines, and gems. These can be separated into two basic types of Ayurvedic treatment: constitutional and therapeutic.

Constitutional treatments encompass adjustments in lifestyle and the taking of preparations that are believed to enhance and preserve good health. These preventive measures might include engaging in *pranayama,* or breathing exercises; readjusting your sleeping and eating schedules to correspond with your prakriti;

Ayurvedic Medicine

performing Ayurvedic massage (called *abhyanga*) to reestablish your energy flow, or *prana;* or taking regular herbal supplements called *rasayanas* to cleanse your body and harmonize your prakriti. The principal form of constitutional treatment is known as *panchakarma,* and it can last anywhere from three days to three weeks. It is an intensive and individualized five-step cleansing process that incorporates a special diet and various massages, herbal treatments, and evacuation procedures, all with the goal of purifying the body and the mind.

Therapeutic treatments are specific healing regimens. According to Ayurvedic theory, all disease originates in the gastrointestinal tract, and is ultimately caused by decreased enzyme activity and poor digestion. Improperly digested foods are said to form a sludgelike substance called *ama* that blocks the body's digestive and energy channels. Practitioners use therapeutic treatments (called *anamaya*) to fight disease by ridding the body of ama and reestablishing a balanced prakriti.

These treatments might include medicinal remedies (selected from some 8,000 herbal, mineral, fruit, and vegetable preparations used in Ayurvedic practice); cleansing procedures such as therapeutic vomiting (inducing vomiting to expel toxins) or herbal enemas; and bloodletting, which is believed to detoxify the blood.

Dietary change is by far the most common form of constitutional and therapeutic treatment. Certain foods are credited with the ability to strengthen or weaken the doshas, and practitioners often suggest specific diets to help reestablish a patient's prakriti.

Visiting a Professional

Ayurveda dictates that every person is responsible for his or her own health. This is not to negate the value of the practitioner-patient relationship, however. Although Ayurvedic preparations are available to everyone, it is difficult (if not impossible) to identify

---

OF SPECIAL INTEREST

Healing Elements

Using medicinal herbs and prescribing nutritional changes are not the only healing techniques espoused by Ayurvedic practitioners. Colors, aromas, gems, and stones are also believed to activate the body's healing potential. When worn or held close to the body, certain stones and gems are said to release their healing energy and engage the body's own energy centers. Aromas are said to help soothe the mind—a belief shared by practitioners of aromatherapy (pages 38-39)—and to pacify disturbed doshas. The seven colors of the rainbow are believed to be related to the tridosha, and therefore to be helpful in balancing the prakriti. To take advantage of color therapy, practitioners may advise patients to drink water from a glass wrapped in colored paper. The color's power is said to infuse the water and be transported to the person who drinks it.

CONTINUED

Ayurvedic Medicine CONTINUED

what you need without a practitioner's help. And when illness strikes, a practitioner's advice is essential.

Expect your first visit with your *vaidya,* or Ayurvedic doctor, to last 45 to 90 minutes. In determining your unique tridosha and prakriti, he or she will ask many questions about your emotional, spiritual, and physical health, your diet, and your lifestyle. You may also be asked to complete a written questionnaire that delves further into your physical and spiritual health.

Your vaidya will check your pulse to help establish your prakriti and determine your overall condition; rates, intensities, and rhythms of an individual's pulse are believed to indicate specific physical, mental, and metabolic conditions. The practitioner will observe you closely, paying particular attention to the condition of your tongue, skin, lips, eyes, and nails. Some practitioners also rely on laboratory analysis of blood, urine, and stools to help in diagnosing your prakriti.

After determining your constitution, your vaidya will use an integrative approach to consider your specific physical, emotional, mental, and spiritual needs, and recommend treatments to harmonize your lifestyle with your prakriti.

Wellness

Preventive medicine is the central tenet of Ayurvedic healing. According to Ayurveda, health is achieved and maintained by first identifying a person's prakriti and then assigning the proper constitutional or therapeutic remedies to maintain his or her doshic balance. Practitioners encourage their patients to stay in close contact, so that therapies and regimens may be adjusted as needed.

What the Critics Say

Ayurveda's use of nonstandard techniques of diagnosis and treatment and its reliance on organic medicines tend to make conventional Western physicians and scientists uneasy. But not all conventional physicians oppose Ayurveda. Some doctors have received introductory Ayurvedic training and use Ayurveda to complement their conventional-style practices. As Ayurveda's popularity continues to increase within the general population of the United States, this trend is likely to continue.

Some criticism of Ayurveda is directed specifically toward the Maharishi Ayur-Veda system. Detractors allege that the promoters of Maharishi Ayur-Veda may be more interested in selling medicine than in healing. Some insist that descriptions of Maharishi Ayur-Veda's power and potential have been wildly exaggerated. Others question whether Maharishi Ayur-Veda represents authentic Ayurvedic science. Still, Maharishi Ayur-Veda is the most popular form of Ayurvedic medicine in the United States. Both traditional Ayurveda and Maharishi Ayur-Veda therapies are currently being investigated in scientific laboratories around the world. ■

FOR MORE INFO

Following is a list of organizations you can contact to learn more about Ayurvedic medicine:

Ayurvedic Institute
11311 Menaul NE, Suite A
Albuquerque, NM 87112
(505) 291-9698

Indic Traditions of Healthcare
Dharam Hinduja Indic Research
Center Columbia University
Mail Code 3367
1102 International Affairs Building
New York, NY 10027
(212) 854-5300
fax: (212) 854-2802
e-mail: dhirc@columbia.edu

$\mathcal{B}$odywork

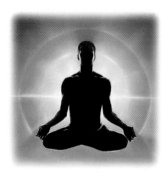

B odywork is an umbrella term for the many techniques that promote relaxation and treat ailments (especially those of the musculoskeletal system) through lessons in proper movement and posture, exercise, massage, and various other forms of bodily manipulation. These techniques can be divided into three broad categories—massage, movement awareness and structural realignment, and energy balancing—although the majority include more than one of these elements. Most take a holistic view of health and emphasize treatment of the mind as well as of the body. Skeptics point out, however, that therapeutic claims made for these techniques are usually based on anecdotal observation rather than on controlled scientific studies.

Some of the many bodywork techniques are explored in detail below and on the following pages. Massage, which is generally considered a form of bodywork, is described separately on pages 121-123.

$\mathcal{A}$lexander Technique

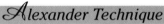

This form of bodywork was developed in the late 1800s by an Australian Shakespearean actor named Frederick Matthias Alexander, whose voice often became hoarse during performances, jeopardizing his career. When the rest and medication prescribed by his physician failed to provide a reliable cure, Alexander decided to find out for himself the cause of his vocal problem. Using a mirror, he studied the way he spoke and concluded that he was unconsciously tensing his body in a way that was interfering with the correct relationship between his head, neck, and back—and that this tension was affecting his voice. In the course of finding a way to correct this damaging habit, Alexander developed the muscle-releasing and postural technique that bears his name. Although he cured his propensity to hoarseness and returned to the stage, Alexander eventually left acting—and Australia—to teach his technique to others in England and America.

What It's Good For • The Alexander technique teaches people how to release painful muscle tension, improve posture, and move with greater ease. Old, damaging habits of sitting, moving, and speaking are replaced with new, more efficient ones. People who practice the technique find it reduces stress and fatigue.

Target Ailments

■ Arthritis

■ Athletic Injuries

■ Back Problems

■ Bursitis

■ Pain, Chronic

■ Tendinitis

See Common Ailments, beginning on page 194.

CONTINUED

Bodywork CONTINUED

Because it improves postural habits, the technique can also help relieve back, knee, and other pain caused by the improper use of muscles; it is especially helpful for disk problems and sciatica. The technique has also been effective in relieving the discomfort associated with arthritis, bursitis, and other conditions involving muscles and joints.

Preparations/Techniques • The Alexander technique is traditionally taught in one-on-one lessons, although some instructors also offer group classes. Basic to the technique is learning how to release your neck muscles so that your head can balance freely on top of your neck. This, in turn, allows your back to lengthen, eliminating compression in the spine.

During a lesson, the teacher will analyze the way you sit, stand, walk, and bend. He or she will then use verbal instructions and gentle touch to guide you into releasing muscle tension, improving posture, and moving with more freedom. You will learn to apply this improved use of your body to everyday tasks, from sitting in a chair to carrying packages to talking on the phone. The Alexander technique does not involve exercises. However, you will learn to apply it to any sport or exercise program you do on a regular basis. Advocates believe this will help you avoid injury and also increase the benefit you receive from your regular exercise program.

Lessons in the Alexander technique generally last 30 to 45 minutes. Wear loose, nonrestrictive clothing. Your instructor will work with you while you are lying on a table and also while you are moving about.

Wellness • Practitioners of this technique believe it promotes wellness by helping people learn how to move within their physical environment in a relaxed and efficient manner that promotes healthy mental and physical functioning.

What the Critics Say
Although correcting poor posture has been known to help prevent back and neck pain, the specific therapeutic benefits of the Alexander technique have not been demonstrated in controlled scientific studies. One study has shown that the technique can be beneficial to healthy adults by enabling them to breathe more efficiently, but it involved only a small number of participants.

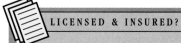

LICENSED & INSURED?

Practitioners must complete a three-year, 1,600-hour instructional program at an approved school to obtain a certification to practice the Alexander technique. Some insurance companies will cover a portion of the cost of Alexander technique therapy if you first get a referral from your physician.

CAUTION

You should avoid bodywork that involves massage if you have an open wound, a bone fracture or dislocation, an infectious disease, a contagious skin condition, severe varicose veins, or any heart problem. Some health professionals are concerned that the deep massage associated with some of these techniques may cause existing cancer cells to metastasize, or spread, in the body. If you have cancer, you may want to ask your bodywork practitioner to consult with your oncologist before undergoing one of these techniques.

FOR MORE INFO
Contact the following organization to learn more about the Alexander technique:

North American Society of Teachers of the Alexander Technique
(800) 473-0620
e-mail: nastat@ix.netcom.com

Bodywork

Aston-Patterning

This type of bodywork was developed in the 1970s by a California dancer named Judith Aston. A decade earlier, two separate car accidents had left her with a disabling back injury. At a doctor's suggestion, Aston went to see Ida Rolf, whose unique form of deep massage and postural retraining known as Rolfing (page 54) helped Aston regain full body movement. Aston began working with Rolf to develop a movement maintenance program that would help people sustain structural changes brought about by Rolfing. She eventually broke away from Rolfing to develop and teach her own form of bodywork.

What It's Good For • Practitioners claim it can help relieve acute or chronic pain such as that caused by poor posture or muscle tension. They also believe it can improve balance, increase strength and endurance, and relieve fatigue. The goal is to help people find more comfortable and efficient ways to work, play, and rest.

Preparations/Techniques • Aston-Patterning is generally taught in one-on-one sessions with a trained practitioner. Each session can last from one to two hours and may include any or all of the following components: movement education, or neurokinetics, which involves learning how to decrease body tension and move more efficiently; three types of bodywork that release tensions held in different body structures; ergonomic training, which teaches how to modify home and work environments in ways that encourage good posture and efficient movement; and fitness training, which helps to stretch, loosen, and tone muscles throughout the body.

Wellness • Like most alternative therapies, Aston-Patterning focuses on promoting health and well-being—goals it seeks to achieve by improving how the body moves and functions.

What the Critics Say
Critics note that Aston-Patterning's therapeutic effectiveness has not been demonstrated in controlled studies.

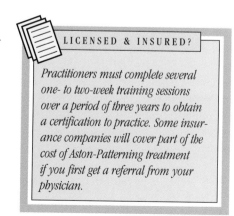

LICENSED & INSURED?

Practitioners must complete several one- to two-week training sessions over a period of three years to obtain a certification to practice. Some insurance companies will cover part of the cost of Aston-Patterning treatment if you first get a referral from your physician.

Target Ailments

■ Athletic Injuries

■ Back Problems

■ Stress

See Common Ailments, beginning on page 194.

FOR MORE INFO
Contact the following organization to learn more about Aston-Patterning:

The Aston Training Center
PO Box 3568
Incline Village, NV 89450
(702) 831-8228

CONTINUED

Bodywork CONTINUED

Target Ailments

■ Back Problems

■ Insomnia

■ Multiple Sclerosis

■ Pain, Chronic

■ Stress

See Common Ailments, beginning on page 194.

See Common Ailments, beginning on page 194.

Feldenkrais Method

This bodywork technique was developed by Moshe Feldenkrais, a Russian-born Israeli physicist who became interested in the physics of body movement during the 1940s, after experiencing a disabling knee injury. He drew on the earlier work of Frederick Matthias Alexander (pages 47-48)—as well as on his own intense study of anatomy, biochemistry, neurophysiology, and other sciences related to human movement—to create this system for improving posture, movement, and breathing.

What It's Good For • Feldenkrais practitioners claim the method can help people with chronic musculoskeletal problems, such as back or knee pain. They also report success helping people overcome some of the physical limitations brought on by an injury or by a chronic medical condition, such as cerebral palsy or multiple sclerosis. Other benefits cited include improved digestion, more restful sleep, greater mental alertness, increased energy, and reduced stress.

Preparations/Techniques • The Feldenkrais method teaches how to recognize and then break improper habits of movement. You can learn the technique through a group class or one-on-one lessons. In group classes a practitioner verbally guides students through a sequence of movements designed to teach how to relax and abandon habitual patterns of movement that reveal unconscious tension. Private lessons provide similar guidance, although here the practitioner also uses slow, gentle touch to help you feel exactly where and how your body is tensing and moving incorrectly. Both types of sessions last about 45 minutes to an hour. You'll also learn exercises to practice at home.

Wellness • Feldenkrais practitioners believe that by helping people release unnecessary muscle tension and move in a freer and more graceful way, injuries and stress-related illness can be prevented.

What the Critics Say
The small amount of objective research that has been done on the therapeutic benefits of the Feldenkrais method has been inconclusive.

FOR MORE INFO
Contact the following organization to learn more about the Feldenkrais method:

The Feldenkrais Guild
524 SW Ellsworth Street
PO Box 489
Albany, OR 97321
(800) 775-2118

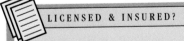

LICENSED & INSURED?

Practitioners must complete 800 hours of instruction over a period of three to four years to obtain a certification to practice. Insurance companies usually do not cover the cost of Feldenkrais treatments.

Bodywork

𝓗ellerwork

Hellerwork was developed by Joseph Heller, a former aerospace engineer who began studying with Ida Rolf in the early 1970s. At the time, Rolfing (page 54) did not include movement education, which Heller thought essential for helping people break old, destructive movement patterns. Nor did it include an exploration of the psychological dynamics behind such habits, which Heller believed was also necessary to root out tension. So in 1978 Heller founded his own method, which includes deep massage, movement education, and therapeutic discussion.

What It's Good For • Hellerwork is based on the premise that a misaligned body limits movement and flexibility, leading to fatigue, physical deterioration, and premature aging. By realigning the body, Hellerwork is thought to release chronic tension and increase flexibility, which in turn reduces stress, increases energy, and creates an overall feeling of youthfulness.

Preparations/Techniques • The Hellerwork program consists of eleven 90-minute private sessions, each with a theme, such as "reaching out," and concentrating on a different part of the body. Each session begins with a deep connective-tissue massage to reduce body tension and realign the musculoskeletal system. Movement lessons follow on how to sit, stand, bend, and walk with more fluidity and balance. The practitioner will also ask about emotional patterns that may have led to physical tension. You may be asked, for example, about how easy or difficult it is for you to be assertive or to reach out to others. The therapy, however, does not require you to answer any questions that you find too painful or uncomfortable.

Wellness • Practitioners believe Hellerwork promotes wellness by breaking the muscular rigidity caused by unconscious habits, so people can better align themselves with gravity and move with more ease and energy.

What the Critics Say
The therapeutic benefits of this technique have not been demonstrated in controlled studies.

LICENSED & INSURED?

Practitioners must complete 1,250 hours of study and training with certified Hellerwork trainers to obtain a certification to practice. Some insurance companies will cover part of the cost of Hellerwork treatments, especially if performed by a physical therapist, as long as you first get a referral from your physician.

Target Ailments

■ Athletic Injuries

■ Back Problems

■ Carpal Tunnel Syndrome

■ Stress

See Common Ailments, beginning on page 194.

FOR MORE INFO
Contact the following organization to learn more about Hellerwork:

Hellerwork International
406 Berry Street
Mount Shasta, CA 96067
(800) 392-3900; (916) 926-2500
e-mail: hwork@snowcrest.net

CONTINUED

Bodywork CONTINUED

Target Ailments

- Arthritis
- Athletic Injuries
- Back Problems
- Carpal Tunnel Syndrome
- Headache
- Menstrual Problems
- Multiple Sclerosis
- TMJ Syndrome

See Common Ailments, beginning on page 194.

Myotherapy

The term "myotherapy" is used here to refer specifically to the technique known formally as Bonnie Prudden Myotherapy. It is an offshoot of trigger point injection therapy, a medical treatment developed in the 1940s that involved injecting saline and the drug procaine directly into painful muscles, or "trigger points," to get them to relax. In 1976 physical fitness pioneer Bonnie Prudden discovered that the injections were unnecessary, as simple manual pressure on the trigger points could produce similar results. This finding led to the development of her form of myotherapy—a deep-pressure massage used to reduce tension and pain originating in specific points in the muscle layers of the body.

What It's Good For • Practitioners claim this therapy is beneficial for a variety of muscle-related conditions, including back, shoulder, and neck pain; headaches; repetitive motion injuries; menstrual cramps; sports injuries; and TMJ syndrome. They say it can also help relieve pain associated with such diseases as arthritis, multiple sclerosis, and lupus. Practitioners emphasize, however, that myotherapy does not cure disease, but rather helps relieve pain and ease recovery.

Preparations/Techniques • Sessions last about an hour. The therapist will ask questions about your sports activities, occupation, injuries, and illnesses, and will test your muscles' strength and flexibility. Then, using fingers, knuckles, and elbows, the therapist will apply pressure to trigger points—those areas in your muscles that the therapist believes are responsible for your pain. Treatment is followed by passive stretching of affected muscles. You will be given corrective exercises to do at home to help keep your muscles free of spasms and pain.

Wellness • Myotherapists believe that by reducing pain and helping to restore the body's full range of motion, they can improve an individual's overall health and sense of well-being.

What the Critics Say
Critics point out that massaging trigger points is not unique to this therapy alone.

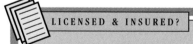

LICENSED & INSURED?

Practitioners must complete a 1,300-hour training program at the Bonnie Prudden School for Physical Fitness and Myotherapy to obtain a certification to practice. Some insurance companies will cover part of the cost of treatments if you first get a referral from your physician.

FOR MORE INFO
Contact the following organization to learn more about myotherapy:

Bonnie Prudden Pain Erasure
7800 East Speedway Boulevard
Tucson, AZ 85710
(520) 529-3979
(800) 221-4634

Bodywork

Reiki

Reiki (pronounced ray-key) practitioners claim this ancient form of healing originated in Tibet thousands of years ago and was rediscovered in the mid-1800s by Mikao Usui, an educator at a Christian seminary in Kyoto, Japan. According to Reiki tradition, Usui spent 21 days fasting on a sacred mountain outside Kyoto, where he experienced a vision that revealed how the universal life energy described in ancient Sanskrit writings could be activated through a hands-on approach to healing. Usui named this healing method Reiki, after the healing aspect of the energy.

What It's Good For • Reiki is used to treat a wide variety of conditions, from minor ailments such as heartburn to chronic diseases such as arthritis.

Preparations/Techniques • Only a trained practitioner may administer Reiki. During a healing session, the practitioner will gently lay his or her hands over the chakras, or energy centers, of your body to enable healing energy to flow more fully into your body. Treatments last from 30 to 60 minutes and are usually carried out in four sessions over four successive days. For some conditions, people receive treatments once a week for one or two months. You will be instructed to drink substantial quantities of water and herb tea during the treatment period to help cleanse your body of toxins. You may be told to avoid stimulants, such as coffee and white sugar, which can interfere with the cleansing process.

Wellness • Reiki practitioners believe the body becomes ill when the universal life energy is out of balance. Thus, by bringing balance and harmony to the body, Reiki enables the body and the mind to heal and remain healthy.

What the Critics Say
Evidence of Reiki's benefits is mainly anecdotal; very few controlled studies of it have been done. Because Reiki is often used to treat illnesses, critics worry that seriously ill patients will not receive the conventional medical care they need. Competent Reiki practitioners, however, do not discourage their patients from receiving such care.

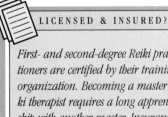

LICENSED & INSURED?

First- and second-degree Reiki practitioners are certified by their training organization. Becoming a master Reiki therapist requires a long apprenticeship with another master. Insurance companies usually do not cover the cost of Reiki treatments.

Target Ailments

■ Arthritis

■ Athletic Injuries

■ Chronic Fatigue Syndrome

■ Heartburn

■ Indigestion

■ Insomnia

■ Irritable Bowel Syndrome

■ Pain, Chronic

■ Stress

See Common Ailments, beginning on page 194.

FOR MORE INFO
Following is a list of organizations you can contact to learn more about Reiki:

The Reiki Alliance
PO Box 41
Cataldo, ID 83810-1041
(208) 682-3535

Reiki Outreach International
PO Box 609
Fair Oaks, CA 95628
(916) 863-1500
fax: (916) 863-6464

The Reiki Center of Los Angeles
16161 Ventura Blvd., Suite 802
Encino, CA 91436
(818) 981-9100
e-mail: joyce@Reiki-Center.Org

CONTINUED

Bodywork CONTINUED

See Common Ailments, beginning on page 194.

Target Ailments

- Athletic Injuries
- Back Problems
- Carpal Tunnel Syndrome
- Stress

Rolfing

This form of bodywork was developed in the 1940s and 1950s by Ida Rolf, a biochemist who wanted to improve the health of her friends and family and cure her own spinal curvature problem. After much study she decided that many physical and mental problems are caused by the body being out of alignment with gravity. She felt that by deeply massaging the fascia—the connective tissue enclosing muscles—most bodies could be brought back into alignment. This deep massage was called structural integration, but it became better known by its trademarked name, Rolfing.

What It's Good For • Rolfing is said to ease chronic pain and stiffness, especially that caused by poor posture. Many athletes, dancers, musicians, and others seeking to improve physical performance in their professions and daily activities say they have been helped by Rolfing. Rolfers also claim the technique can help ease anxiety caused by chronic stress.

Preparations/Techniques • Rolfing is usually applied in 10 one-hour sessions. In each session, a specific area is massaged, or "manipulated." Rolfers use their fingers, knuckles, and elbows during the sometimes painful manipulations. The intent is to loosen adhesions in the fascia and bring the head, shoulders, thorax, pelvis, and legs into improved alignment with gravity. In a separate program, patients are instructed on how to move their body in more efficient ways.

Wellness • Rolfers believe that stretching and lengthening the fascia, and thus bringing the body into proper alignment with gravity, helps keep the body in a state that is free of stress.

What the Critics Say
Critics point out that no large, controlled studies of Rolfing have been carried out. One study of 10 cerebral palsy patients had mixed results. Critics are also concerned that some Rolfers use the technique to treat depression and other psychological disorders but are not qualified to do so.

FOR MORE INFO

Contact the following organization to learn more about Rolfing:

The Rolf Institute
205 Canyon Boulevard
Boulder, CO 80306
(800) 530-8875
e-mail: Rolf Inst@aol.com

LICENSED & INSURED?

Rolfing practitioners must complete a two- to three-year training program at the Rolf Institute and 400 additional hours of classwork to obtain a certification to practice. Some insurance companies will cover part of the cost of Rolfing treatments if you first get a referral from your physician.

Bodywork

Therapeutic Touch

During the 1970s Dolores Krieger, a nursing professor at New York University, brought together a variety of ancient "hands-on" healing practices into a modern technique she called therapeutic touch. Like many of its older predecessors, therapeutic touch is based on the premise that disease reflects a blockage in the flow of energy that surrounds and permeates the body. Krieger devised a four-step process by which a therapeutic touch practitioner could detect and free these blockages, thus healing the body.

What It's Good For • Therapeutic touch practitioners claim it can be used to ease a variety of ailments, including arthritis, chronic back pain, headaches, constipation, and colic in babies. Practitioners also report it can help wounds and broken bones to heal faster and can reduce fevers. Therapeutic touch is frequently used to reduce stress and anxiety. It has been used in some hospitals, for example, to relax people before and after surgery and to alleviate pain.

Preparations/Techniques • Despite its name, therapeutic touch does not involve actual physical contact. Each session begins with the practitioner assuming a relaxed, meditative state. The practitioner then moves his or her hands in slow, rhythmic motions two to six inches above the patient in an effort to detect blockages in the body's energy field that may be causing or contributing to illness. When perceiving a blockage, the practitioner "unruffles" the field with a downward sweep of the hands. After this, the practitioner transfers energy to the patient via what is called noncontact touch. Sessions last about 20 minutes. Once you become proficient in the technique, you can practice it on yourself and on others.

Wellness • Therapeutic touch is most commonly used to relieve pain and other symptoms of illness, but some practitioners also use the technique to help prevent the body from becoming ill in the first place.

What the Critics Say
Although conceding that the technique may comfort some patients, critics of therapeutic touch say that its healing value has not been demonstrated in well-designed, controlled scientific studies.

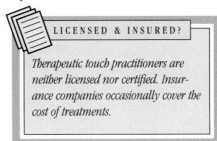

LICENSED & INSURED?

Therapeutic touch practitioners are neither licensed nor certified. Insurance companies occasionally cover the cost of treatments.

Target Ailments

- Arthritis
- Back Problems
- Bronchitis
- Bursitis
- Cancer
- Circulatory Problems
- Constipation
- Endometriosis
- Headache
- Heart Problems
- High Blood Pressure
- Immune Problems
- Menopause
- Menstrual Problems
- Pain, Chronic
- Stress

See Common Ailments, beginning on page 194.

FOR MORE INFO
Contact the following organization to learn more about therapeutic touch:

Nurse Healers Professional Associates
1211 Locust Street
Philadelphia, PA 19107
(215) 545-8079

CONTINUED

Bodywork CONTINUED

Target Ailments

■ Back Problems

■ Headache

■ Multiple Sclerosis

■ Pain, Chronic

■ TMJ Syndrome

See Common Ailments, beginning on page 194.

Trager Psychophysical Integration (Trager Approach)

This type of bodywork was first developed in the 1920s by a young Miami boxer named Milton Trager, who was told by relatives and friends that he had an uncanny knack for massaging away their aches and pains. He eventually gave up boxing to become a physical therapist and later a physician, and over the next seven decades treated thousands of patients with his unique and gentle form of massage. In the 1970s Trager began teaching his technique to others, who now offer it in the United States and other countries to people seeking relief from chronic pain and other ailments.

What It's Good For • The Trager approach is used in the treatment of all kinds of chronic pain, including back pain, headaches, muscle spasms, and TMJ syndrome. A few small studies have shown it to be beneficial for some people with severe neuromuscular problems produced by injury or with such diseases as multiple sclerosis or muscular dystrophy.

Preparations/Techniques • Sessions last 60 to 90 minutes. The patient lies or sits on a table while the practitioner applies gentle touch and rhythmic rocking and shaking movements to the body to relax and loosen joints and muscles. Practitioners work in a meditative state called hook-up, which enables them to better sense minute responses of the patient's body. Patients are also taught a series of exercises to practice at home. Called mentastics, they are intended to help identify and correct chronic tension patterns that affect posture and movement.

Wellness • Trager practitioners believe that this form of movement reeducation brings people into a relaxed and physically graceful state that enhances wellness and helps make the body more resistant to injury and illness.

What the Critics Say
Because large, controlled studies involving the Trager approach to bodywork have never been conducted, its ability to help people suffering from chronic pain or other ailments cannot be stated with any degree of certainty.

FOR MORE INFO

Contact the following organization to learn more about the Trager approach:

The Trager Institute
21 Locust Avenue
Mill Valley, CA 94941-2806
(415) 388-2688
e-mail: Trager D@aol.com

LICENSED & INSURED?

Trager practitioners must complete more than 200 hours of training at the Trager Institute to obtain a certification to practice. Some insurance companies will cover part of the cost of Trager treatments if you first get a referral from your physician.

Chinese Medicine

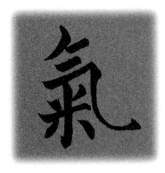

Chinese medicine is an ancient system of healthcare that uses a variety of techniques—including acupuncture (pages 32-33), acupressure (pages 16-17), herbal therapy (pages 70-73), qigong (pages 165-166), and massage (pages 121-123)—to treat disorders by restoring the balance of vital energies in the body.

Unlike Western medicine, which tends to focus on specific parts of the body immediately affected by disease or injury, Chinese medicine takes a more global, holistic approach to healthcare, fashioning remedies to treat the entire body rather than just its component parts. Practitioners of Chinese medicine think of the human body not as a bundle of cells, bones, and tissues but rather as a complex system of interrelated processes—an ecosystem unto itself, constantly influenced by the push and pull of opposing forces within it. These physicians regard the human being as both a part of nature and a separate entity, complete and self-contained. It is, they believe, a microcosm of the grand cosmic order, moved by the same rhythms and cycles that shape the natural world. At the core of Chinese medicine is the belief that disease is the result of disturbances in the flow of a bodily energy called chi or qi (pronounced "chee") or a lack of balance in the complementary states of yin (characterized by darkness and quiet) and yang (characterized by light and activity).

Chi and the Dynamics of Yin and Yang

Defined in early Chinese writings as "basic stuff," chi is thought to be the force that animates life and enlivens all activity. Powerful yet invisible, chi cannot be isolated, measured, or quantified; it is known not through direct observation but through its observable effects. Just as blood courses through the vessels of the circulatory system, chi flows through the body primarily by way of invisible channels called meridians. Practitioners of Chinese medicine believe that maintaining the proper movement of chi through these meridians is essential to good health.

Wellness also requires preserving a delicate balance, or equilibrium, between the contrasting states of yin and yang. Translated literally, the Chinese character for *yin* depicts the shady side of the mountain, *yang* the sunny side; together they symbolize the dual nature of all things. According to Chinese theory, yin and yang coexist harmoniously in the body. Polar opposites, they represent alternate phases in the natural cycle, contradicting and at the same time complementing one another. In a healthy body, the darkness and inactivity of yin are perfectly counterbalanced by the

Target Ailments

- Allergies
- Arthritis
- Asthma
- Bursitis
- Common Cold
- Constipation
- Depression
- Diarrhea
- Earache
- Flu
- Headache
- Hemorrhoids
- High Blood Pressure
- Insomnia
- Menstrual Problems
- Nausea
- Pain, Chronic
- Sore Throat
- Stomach Ulcers
- Stress
- Vaginal Problems

See Common Ailments, beginning on page 194.

CONTINUED

Chinese Medicine

lightness and activity of yang. Just as day melts into night and night into day, the body fluctuates cyclically between yin and yang. Any deviation from this orderly course causes a yin-yang disharmony, resulting in disease.

Origins

Rooted in the philosophies of Taoism, Buddhism, and Confucianism, Chinese medicine has been practiced in China for more than 2,500 years, although the underlying principles of herbal therapy and acupuncture are even older. According to legend, the philosophical and practical groundwork of Chinese herbal medicine was laid by Emperor Shen Nung, the "Divine Farmer" who became fascinated with the apparent healing properties of certain plants. He spent years testing the efficacy of these herbs, and his observations led him to develop a theory involving nature's "opposing principles." In the centuries that followed, Chinese thinkers refined and elaborated on these principles, which came to be called yin and yang. The philosophy grew and flourished in China and from there spread throughout much of eastern Asia. It arrived with Chinese immigrants in the United States in the mid-1800s but remained relatively unknown among Americans until just a few decades ago.

What It's Good For

Chinese medicine is used to treat a full spectrum of conditions. In recent years these methods have been subjected to increasingly rigorous study in China and elsewhere. Evidence indicates that, although some may not perform as claimed, a number of these remedies do seem to work. For example, acupuncture has been shown to be effective in the treatment of nausea, asthma, and migraines. In other studies, researchers have found that the management of chronic pain and drug addiction is more successful when acupuncture is included in a comprehensive treatment plan.

Preparations/Techniques

Chinese medicine recognizes more than 6,000 healing substances, although only a few hundred are in practical use today. Following a sophisticated classification system, herbs are grouped according to four basic properties, or "essences"— hot, cold, warm, and cool. In general, practitioners choose plants for their ability to restore balance in individuals whose conditions are said to show signs of excessive heat or cold. For example, a hot herb such as cinnamon bark might be recommended for a condition described as cold; the cool herb chrysanthemum flower might be prescribed for a condition characterized as warm.

Herbs are further categorized according to their "flavor"—pungent, sour, sweet, bitter, or salty. An herb's taste indicates its action in the body, particularly on the movement and direction of chi. Each flavor is said to have a strong influence on

Chinese Medicine

a certain major organ system: Pungent herbs are associated with the lungs, sour with the liver, sweet with the spleen or pancreas, bitter with the heart, salty with the kidneys. It is important to note that the Chinese notion of body organs is much broader than the Western. The Chinese term for *heart,* for instance, encompasses not only the physical organ itself but also the general order and clarity of the mind.

Because many Chinese herbs work best when taken with others, practitioners almost always prescribe herbs in combination, occasionally blending as many as 15 in a single preparation. Some plants are used to disperse chi that has become stagnant or misdirected. Others help summon scattered reserves of chi, while still others provide nourishment or rid the body of noxious substances.

Herbs are prepared in a variety of ways. Many are cooked and made into soup or tea. In some cases the raw plants are ground into a powder, then combined with honey or some other binding agent and pressed into a pill. A number of herbs are cooked and processed into a powder and are then either mixed with warm water and swallowed or taken as capsules. Some herbs are made into pastes that are applied to the skin, while others are extracted in alcohol and used as tinctures. Mixing herbs is an extremely tricky business. Certain Chinese herbs can be poisonous in large amounts, so you should always check with a qualified practitioner for the proper dosages.

Before prescribing any type of treatment, a practitioner performs an evaluation of the patient's overall physical and mental makeup, or "individual conformation." According to Chinese theory, a single symptom by itself is meaningless; it acquires significance only in terms of how it relates to a host of other signs. The evaluation consists of four basic techniques, or stages: looking, listening and smelling (in Chinese, these are expressed by the same word), asking, and touching.

An experienced practitioner can gather a great deal of information by observing the patient's general appearance, posture, facial color, and behavior. For more detailed information, the physician looks for more specific signs, such as the alertness of the eyes and the color of the skin and nails. Crucial to the diagnosis is a careful evaluation

LICENSED & INSURED?

In the United States, practitioners of Chinese medicine usually operate under the title of "licensed" or "certified" acupuncturist. Many conventional doctors have incorporated acupuncture into their practices, and some states allow chiropractic and naturopathic physicians to use the technique.

Few insurance providers reimburse patients for the cost of herbal treatments. But a number of companies do cover acupuncture, in some cases only if performed by a conventional medical doctor. In early 1996, the FDA removed a label classifying acupuncture needles as experimental devices, possibly clearing the way for broader insurance coverage.

CONTINUED

Chinese Medicine CONTINUED

of the patient's tongue, which is considered to be an excellent barometer of disharmonies in the body. To trained eyes, the shape, movement, color, texture, and moistness of the tongue—even its coating—speak volumes about the patient's condition. A red, dry tongue, for example, suggests the presence of heat; a purple tongue may indicate stagnant chi. During their examinations, practitioners take pulse readings at three points on each wrist; each point is believed to reveal conditions in different parts of the body. They also look for clues in bodily secretions, the sound of the voice, and any unusual odors emanating from the patient's body.

Chinese Medicine and Wellness

Preventing disease and preserving the conditions of good health are among the fundamental aims of Chinese medicine. More than a system of after-the-fact healing techniques, it is a philosophy of life grounded on the assumption that illness is much easier to prevent than to cure. Besides providing treatment to overcome disease, practitioners strive to arm the body against conditions that bring about ill health. Historically, Chinese medical professionals have rejected the notion of quick cures, insisting that disease is caused by deep-rooted imbalances that must be treated continuously over time. (In ancient China, doctors were paid only if their patients stayed healthy.) Herbal therapy, in particular, is often prescribed to be used on a regular basis to correct small energy imbalances before they can erupt into major problems. Many Chinese herbs can be taken or eaten daily as a preventive measure in much the same way as vitamins or nutritional supplements.

What the Critics Say

Many of those raised in the tradition of Western medicine dismiss Chinese medicine as so much superstition and hocus-pocus—a vague, primitive, and quasi-religious set of beliefs founded not on the principles of hard science and logical reasoning but on irrational faith and mysticism. They refute claims that Chinese medicine is appropriate for all ailments, and they attribute any positive results to other causes or to simple good luck. Nonetheless, recent studies have shown that Chinese medical techniques can be effective. Acupuncture, in particular, has proved to be especially beneficial in chronic pain management, stroke rehabilitation, drug addiction, and nausea relief. Inserting needles in the skin evidently releases endorphins and other chemicals that serve as the body's natural painkillers, although how acupuncture provides long-term pain management is unclear.

Barriers are gradually falling, and now certain medical practices of the East are starting to gain formal acceptance in cultures of the West. In one sign of this newfound recognition, the World Health Organization of the United Nations lists about 50 diseases for which it considers acupuncture an appropriate treatment. ■

FOR MORE INFO

Following is a list of organizations you can contact to learn more about Chinese medicine:

**American Academy
of Medical Acupuncture**
5820 Wilshire Blvd., Suite 500
Los Angeles, CA 90036
(800) 521-2262
fax: (213) 937-0959
e-mail: KCKD71@prodigy.com

**Council of Colleges of Acupuncture
and Oriental Medicine**
1010 Wayne Avenue, Suite 1270
Silver Spring, MD 20910
(301) 608-9175
fax: (301) 608-9576

**National Acupuncture
Detoxification Association**
(addictive and mental disorders)
PO Box 1927
Vancouver, WA 98668-1927
phone and fax: (360) 260-8620
e-mail: NADAclear@aol.com

**National Acupuncture
and Oriental Medicine Alliance**
14637 Starr Road, SE
Olalla, WA 98359
(206) 851-6896
fax: (206) 851-6883

**National Certification Commission
for Acupuncture
and Oriental Medicine**
PO Box 97075
Washington, DC 20090-7075
(202) 232-1404
fax: (202) 462-6157

Chiropractic

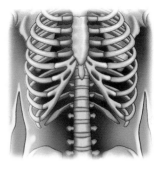

Chiropractic is based on the concept that the human body has an innate self-healing ability and seeks homeostasis, or balance. According to general chiropractic theory, the nervous system plays an important role in maintaining homeostasis—and hence health. But "subluxations" (misalignments of bones within joints) or "fixations" (abnormalities of motion) are said to interfere with the flow of nervous impulses and diminish the body's ability to stay healthy. Through manipulation of the bones and their associated muscles and joints, particularly the spine, chiropractors work to correct these misalignments, thereby improving the function of the neuromusculoskeletal system and restoring homeostasis. The term chiropractic is derived from the Greek words "cheir" (hand) and "practikos" (done by).

Today, chiropractors are divided into two major camps. On one side are the straights—traditional chiropractors who adhere to the philosophy that subluxations are at the root of disease and that manipulation is the best treatment. On the other side are the mixers, so named because their approach represents a mix of traditional and progressive techniques.

Although chiropractic is often considered alternative medicine, it is gaining wider acceptance, in part because of recent clinical studies showing these methods to be effective in treating problems such as acute lower back pain and headache.

Origins

Chiropractic originated in 1895, when Daniel David Palmer, a magnetic healer who practiced laying on of hands in Davenport, Iowa, cured a janitor's deafness by pushing on a malpositioned vertebra in the man's back. To Palmer, this was proof that misalignments in the spine could impair health and that realigning the spine enhanced health by restoring the flow of nerve impulses throughout the body.

Two years later Palmer founded the first chiropractic school, and it was here, under the management of his son, that the schism currently dividing

LICENSED & INSURED?

YES! *The services of chiropractors are covered by Medicare and, in many states, by Medicaid and most major private insurance plans. Chiropractic is taught in special five-year colleges and licensed in all 50 states according to standards established by the Council of Chiropractic Education and the Federation of Chiropractic Licensing Boards.*

Target Ailments

- Arthritis
- Asthma
- Back Problems
- Bursitis
- Carpal Tunnel Syndrome
- Chronic Fatigue Syndrome
- Earache
- Headache
- High Blood Pressure
- Menstrual Problems
- Muscle Cramps
- Neuralgia
- Pain, Chronic
- Premenstrual Syndrome
- Sprains and Strains
- Tendinitis
- TMJ Syndrome

See Common Ailments, beginning on page 194.

CONTINUED

Chiropractic CONTINUED

the profession began to form. Dissatisfied with the Palmers' teachings—particularly their claims about the role of subluxations in disease—a faculty member named John Howard broke away to start his own chiropractic college (now the National College of Chiropractic) and, using Palmer's theories, to develop a program that was more firmly grounded in rational thought and solid scientific evidence. Within a decade, a number of other chiropractic schools had emerged. Practitioners who allied themselves with the Palmers became known as the straights; those who departed from the original concept were dubbed the mixers.

The straight-mixer split began a debate within the chiropractic community over the scope of its techniques and the profession's relationship with conventional medicine. While the straights concentrate almost exclusively on manipulation, the mixers employ manipulation along with a broad range of other therapeutic methods, including massage, physical therapy, and nutritional therapy.

What It's Good For

Straight chiropractors believe that chiropractic manipulation can provide relief from every type of ailment, from asthma to impotence. The mixers, on the other hand, maintain that chiropractic is appropriate only for certain conditions and is particularly effective in the treatment of acute lower back pain, musculoskeletal problems, headache, and neck pain.

- **Back pain:** Studies show that spinal manipulation can relieve acute lower back pain, the most common reason that people make their first visit to a chiropractor.
- **Neck pain:** Chiropractic adjustment can often help correct painful misalignments in the neck, including those caused by whiplash injury.
- **Headache:** Spinal manipulation has been shown to decrease the frequency and intensity of migraine and tension headaches.
- **Other conditions:** Scientific studies and anecdotal evidence suggest that chiropractic can be beneficial in the treatment of otitis media, digestive problems, dysmenorrhea, hypertension, disk problems, scoliosis, sprains and some sports injuries, frozen shoulder, tennis elbow, carpal tunnel syndrome, abnormal jaw function, respiratory problems, enuresis, and arthritis in the wrist, hand, or hip.

Visiting a Professional

Your first visit to a chiropractor usually begins with a general evaluation and case history: While noting your posture and gait, the practitioner will ask you about the problem and how it began, and about your medical history and lifestyle.

For the actual examination, you will be asked to wear a hospital gown. The

Chiropractic

chiropractor will palpate, or feel, your vertebrae to detect misplacement of bones or muscle weakness, and may perform a reflex test to check nerve function. You will then be instructed to bend forward, backward, and sideways while the chiropractor palpates your vertebrae and joints to determine their range of motion. The doctor may also take x-rays in order to discover any joint problems that could be worsened by manipulation.

Next, the doctor will make a diagnosis and determine a treatment plan, which may begin right away or on your second visit. In chiropractic treatment the practitioner adjusts your joints using a small controlled thrust that moves the joint slightly beyond its restricted range of motion; before making the adjustment, however, the doctor may massage the area around the joint in order to loosen tight muscles and ligaments.

If the chiropractor is adjusting your spine, you will need to lie on a padded table on your stomach or side. For an adjustment of your neck, you will be asked to sit upright. (While adjustments are being made, you may hear the joints crack just as your knuckles do when they crack.) The treatments are painless, and many patients feel improvement within nine to 12 sessions.

Wellness

Unless you have a musculoskeletal problem, chiropractic may not fit into your long-term wellness plan: Some chiropractors insist that manipulation should be used to treat only specific problems, and that manipulating a healthy spine or joint accomplishes nothing. Others, however, argue that periodic chiropractic adjustments should be part of a preventive health maintenance program.

What the Critics Say

- Some medical doctors maintain that misaligned vertebrae—the chiropractor's clue to health problems—are common, often harmless, and do not require treatment.
- Critics charge that frequent visits to a chiropractor are useless, whether as a preventive measure or to treat a specific condition such as back pain—which, they say, usually clears up on its own.
- Those critical of chiropractic often point out that quadriplegics can have healthy internal organs despite their extensive nerve damage. This fact, they maintain, disproves the assertion that a sound nervous system is the key to overall health.
- A number of critics argue that chiropractors should restrict their practice to treating back pain, since there is insufficient evidence to show that manipulation provides relief from any other condition. ■

FOR MORE INFO
Following is a list of organizations you can contact to learn more about chiropractic medicine:

American Chiropractic Association
1701 Clarendon Boulevard
Arlington, VA 22209
(703) 276-8800
fax: (703) 243-2593
e-mail: amerchiro@aol.com
(advocates mixer principles)

International Chiropractors Association
1110 North Glebe Road, Suite 1000
Arlington, VA 22201
(703) 528-5000
(advocates straight principles)

World Federation of Chiropractic
78 Glencairn Avenue
Toronto, Ontario M4R1M8
(416) 484-9978
fax: (416) 484-9665

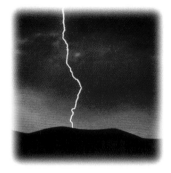

Target Ailments

■ Headache

■ Irritable Bowel Syndrome

■ Pain, Chronic

■ Premenstrual Syndrome

■ Stress

See Common Ailments, beginning on page 194.

Energy Medicine

E nergy medicine, also known as energy therapy or biofield therapeutics, is based on the premise that the human body is composed of various energy fields and that people fall ill when the energy in those fields becomes blocked, out of balance, or otherwise disturbed. Energy therapists attempt to restore health by first detecting and then removing the blockages.

Some energy therapists use special devices to diagnose and treat disturbed energy fields; others rely on various methods of healing touch, such as therapeutic touch (page 55), Reiki (page 53), and polarity therapy (described below).

The Vital Flow of Energy

Many ancient healing methods view health and sickness in terms of energy flow. Traditional Chinese medicine *(pages 57-60),* for example, posits illness as being the result of disturbances in a type of energy called *chi.* The Japanese healing technique of shiatsu *(page 17)* attempts to correct imbalances in an energy force called *ki.* And Ayurvedic medicine *(pages 42-46),* a form of healing practiced for thousands of years in India, uses body postures, breathing exercises, and meditative techniques to stimulate the flow of a variety of body energies.

Modern energy therapy has borrowed elements from these traditional approaches. The points and meridians (or energy "pathways") described in acupuncture *(pages 32-35),* for example, are often used as treatment sites by energy therapists. But some modern energy therapies have identified unique patterns of energy flow. Polarity therapy, for example, cites five currents of energy within the body, with specific points along the currents said to hold either positive or negative charges; to balance the body's energy flow, polarity therapists place their hands on points with opposite charges, creating a current.

Origins

The earliest reference to energy healing can be found in Chinese medical texts written 2,500 to 5,000 years ago. Hippocrates also described the healing powers of "the force that flows from many people's hands." In the late 1700s, an Austrian physician named Franz Mesmer popularized the technique of laying on of hands in Europe and America with his "magnetic

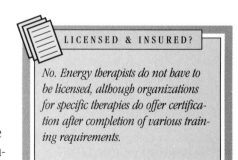

LICENSED & INSURED?

No. Energy therapists do not have to be licensed, although organizations for specific therapies do offer certification after completion of various training requirements.

Energy Medicine

healing" treatments. The technique gained renewed popularity during the 1970s when Dolores Krieger, a nursing professor at New York University, began teaching a hands-on healing method she called therapeutic touch.

What It's Good For

Energy therapy is used for a variety of conditions. As a group, the techniques are reported to be most effective for healing wounds, reducing pain, and relieving anxiety. Some practitioners of energy therapy have also reported consistent success treating PMS, migraine, irritable bowel syndrome, eating disorders, and posttraumatic stress disorder. Energy therapy is also used to help people overcome addictions, and to ease the pain and anxiety of pregnancy, childbirth, and surgical treatment.

Preparations/Techniques

Energy therapists use a variety of techniques to balance and release the body's flow of energy. Most involve the practitioner's placing his or her hands either directly on or very near the patient's body. The hands do not always touch the body because energy fields are said to extend outward from the body for several inches.

Practitioners first attempt to detect subtle clues, such as changes in body temperature or sensations of "electricity" or "magnetism," that indicate where your body's energy needs to be unblocked or rebalanced. Some practitioners diagnose with measuring instruments known as electroacupuncture biofeedback machines, which are said to measure electrical energy disturbances at acupuncture points.

In general, there are two views about how energy therapy heals. One is that the practitioner directs or modifies the patient's energy field in a way that facilitates healing. The other is that the source of the healing comes not from the practitioner directly, but from a universal energy field or higher spiritual power. Some practitioners meditate or pray before starting a treatment; others go into a deep meditative state during it. Some also practice mental healing—a technique in which the practitioner actively focuses his or her intention on becoming a vehicle for healing the patient.

Wellness

Practitioners believe that these techniques free the body's flow of energy, thus relieving stress, increasing vitality, and contributing to overall wellness.

What the Critics Say

Critics point out that energy therapy has not undergone rigorous scientific study; indeed, the very existence of bodily energy fields is widely considered unproved. In addition, most reports of energy medicine's success in healing have been anecdotal, and some critics hold that positive results are due to the placebo effect. ■

FOR MORE INFO
Following is a list of organizations you can contact to learn more about energy medicine:

American Polarity Therapy Association
2888 Bluff Street, Suite 149
Boulder, CO 80301
(303) 545-2080
fax: (303) 545-2161

International Society for the Study of Subtle Energies and Energy Medicine
356 Goldco Circle
Golden, CO 80403-1347
(303) 278-2228
e-mail: 74040.1273@compuserve.com

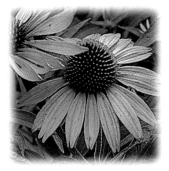

Target Ailments

- Athletic Injuries

- Back Problems

- Chronic Fatigue Syndrome

- Depression

- Headache

- Immune Problems

- Insomnia

- Pain, Chronic

- Premenstrual Syndrome

- Stress

See Common Ailments, beginning on page 194.

Flower Remedies

F lower remedies, also called flower essences, are specially prepared liquid concentrates made by soaking flowers in pure spring water. The concentrates are diluted and sipped to treat various emotional and physical disorders. The fundamental theory behind flower-essence therapy is that physical ailments and disease, as well as psychological problems, arise from emotional disturbances; diagnosis and treatment thus involve an evaluation of personality, state of mind, and emotional makeup.

Like homeopathic remedies (pages 104-106), flower essences are diluted to such a degree that they do not work on a biochemical level. Practitioners say they contain specific aspects of the plants' energy, which affect the energy field of the person taking them. In this way, the flower remedies are believed to help people work with and integrate their emotions; a typical treatment might, for example, aim to develop in a fearful person the courage to face his or her fear.

Origins

Although healing with flowers goes back to ancient times, the specific use of flower concentrates to treat emotions and attitudes was developed in the 1930s by the English bacteriologist and homeopathic physician Edward Bach. After careful observation of his patients, Bach concluded not only that links existed between certain personality traits and certain illnesses but also that people with similar personalities reacted to their illnesses similarly. He searched for natural agents that would deal with the emotional precursors to disease and eventually discovered the flower essences, whose specific qualities he determined through intuition and experimentation on himself.

Today, many companies produce versions of flower essences. Among the major, well-established lines are the original 38 English essences of Dr. Bach, available from several different sources; North American flower essences, a group of over 100 remedies sometimes called California remedies; and a series of Rose essences, some of which are designated as addressing specific functions of the body.

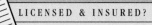

LICENSED & INSURED?

There is no licensing of practitioners, but licensed healthcare providers might use flower essences as part of a treatment that may be covered by insurance. Depending on the manufacturer, some flower essences are sold as dietary supplements. Others are enrolled in the official homeopathic pharmacopoeia and classified as homeopathic medicines.

Flower Remedies

What It's Good For

Proponents say flower remedies are helpful for numerous physical ailments and emotional states. Each of Bach's original 38 remedies corresponds to a negative mood or state of mind. The 38 are divided into seven groups of emotions: fear, uncertainty, insufficient interest in present circumstances, loneliness, oversensitivity to influences and ideas, despondency and despair, and overconcern for the welfare of others. Within each of the seven groups are subcategories of the emotion, each with a specific remedy. For example, subcategories under fear include terror, fear of an unknown cause, and fear for other people.

The group of English remedies includes a combination formula of five of the 38 essences that is said to be beneficial for a variety of problems, such as physical injury, shock, pain, or severe emotional upset. Among the brand names for this combination are Rescue Remedy, Five Flower Formula, and Calming Essence.

Preparations/Techniques

The remedies, usually obtained in liquid concentrate form (called the stock) and preserved in alcohol or vinegar, may be bought at health food stores and some pharmacies, by mail order, or through a practitioner. Preparation of the essences is a complex process that takes into account a variety of factors, including the plants' environment and the climatic conditions at the time of collection and concentration.

You can match your own emotions and state of mind with those listed in the chart on pages 68-69 to choose one or more remedies (up to six at a time) for yourself or your children. To administer, place 2 to 4 drops of the stock under your tongue four times daily or place several drops in a large glass of water and sip a few times a day. Flower essences may also be used topically or added to baths.

Visiting a Professional

If you are unfamiliar with these remedies, it may be helpful to seek out a practitioner at first. The practitioner is likely to choose your remedies by observing you and asking you questions, and possibly by evaluating the results of certain physical tests.

What the Critics Say

Critics point out that claims of effectiveness are based on intuition rather than science and therefore are unsubstantiated. Some say any reported positive effects are due to the placebo effect; however, proponents point to benefits experienced by animals and children, who presumably would not be susceptible to the placebo effect. Proponents also claim there is no evidence of side effects, ill effects following a wrong diagnosis, or harmful interactions with any other medicines. ∎

CAUTION

Some practitioners say that the essences may bring unresolved emotional issues to the surface for consideration, which may be psychologically unsettling, yet beneficial in the long run.

People who are sensitive to the alcohol in some remedies can dilute the remedy or use a few drops on the wrist or lips rather than ingesting.

FOR MORE INFO

Contact the following organizations to learn more about flower essences:

Flower Essence Society
PO Box 459
Nevada City, CA 95959
(800) 736-9222; (916) 265-9163
(North American and English essences)

Perelandra Ltd.
PO Box 3603
Warrenton, VA 20188
(540) 937-2153
fax: (540) 937-3360
(Rose essences)

Nelson Bach USA Ltd.
Wilmington Technology Park
100 Research Drive
Wilmington, MA 01887
(800) 334-0843
(the official Bach flower Essences)

Ellon USA, Inc.
644 Merrick Road
Lynbrook, NY 11563
(800) 423-2256
(English essences)

CONTINUED

Flower Remedies CONTINUED

39 Essential Flower Remedies

This chart lists the 38 Bach essences plus the combination formula Rescue Remedy. Each entry describes—in language typically used by practitioners—the mental and emotional states for which that remedy is said to be beneficial. Up to six Bach remedies may be taken at a time. The illustrations show four common herbs from which additional essences—beyond Bach's originals—have been developed.

Agrimony
Proclivity to conceal worry and deny pain, restlessness, distressed by arguments and confrontation.

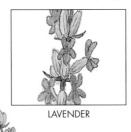

LAVENDER

Aspen
Unexplained anxiety, apprehension, fears of unknown origin, tending to have nightmares.

Beech
Intolerant, critical, dissatisfied, negative, unwilling to make allowances.

Centaury
Weak-willed, submissive, easily influenced or imposed upon, difficulty saying no.

Cerato
Distrust of self and own ability, overdependent on the advice of others.

Cherry Plum
Desperation, fear of emotional breakdown, uncontrolled and irrational thoughts.

Chestnut Bud
Failure to learn from experience, lack of observation, repeating mistakes.

Chicory
Possessiveness, self-love, self-pity, controlling, demanding, attention-seeking.

Clematis
Indifference, daydreaming, inattention, absorbed in own thoughts, impractical.

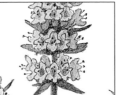

PEPPERMINT

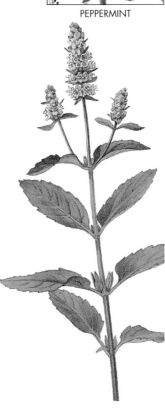

Crab Apple
Self-disgust, shame, feeling of uncleanness.

Elm
Occasional feelings of inadequacy, being overwhelmed by responsibility.

Gentian
Doubt, depression, discouragement after setback, skepticism, negativity.

Gorse
Hopelessness, despair, resignation, loss of will, pessimism, defeatism.

Heather
Self-centered, talking incessantly about oneself, obsessed with own problems.

Holly
Hatred, envy, jealousy, suspicion, strong negativity, feeling cut off from love.

Honeysuckle
Nostalgia, homesickness, living in the past, regretful, loss of interest in the present.

Hornbeam
Fatigue, feeling of

Flower Remedies

being burdened, temporary mental and physical exhaustion, procrastination.

Impatiens
Impatience, irritability, intolerance, impulsivity, nervous tension, overexertion.

Larch
Lack of confidence, despondency, self-censorship, feelings of inferiority.

Mimulus
Fear or anxiety of known things, timidity, shyness, nervousness.

Mustard
Deep depression of unknown cause, sadness that comes and goes unexpectedly.

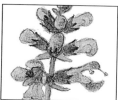

SAGE

Oak
Plodding, uncomplaining, inflexible, overachieving, obstinate.

Olive
Complete exhaustion, depletion after illness or long-term stress.

Pine
Self-reproach, guilt, self-blame, inability to accept self, apologetic.

Red Chestnut
Excessive fear or anxiety for loved ones, anticipation of trouble.

Rock Rose
Sudden alarm, terror, panic, hysteria, nightmares, feelings of horror.

Rock Water
Self-repression, self-denial, self-martyrdom, perfectionism, obsessiveness.

Scleranthus
Uncertainty, indecision, hesitancy, confusion, wavering, lack of mental clarity.

Star-of-Bethlehem
Grief, distress, past or

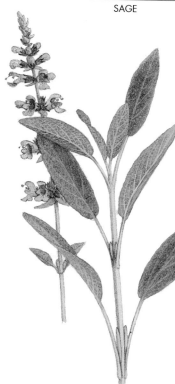

RESCUE REMEDY
Star-of-Bethlehem, Rock Rose, Impatiens, Cherry Plum, Clematis
Trauma, terror, panic, stress, desperation, disorientation.

---

present trauma such as that sustained from bad news, accident, or fright.

Sweet Chestnut
Extreme mental anguish, utter dejection, hopelessness, despair.

Vervain
Overenthusiastic, tendency to impose will, argumentative, fanatical, overbearing.

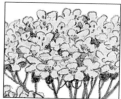

YARROW

Vine
Dominating others, tyrannical, ambitious, arrogant, inflexible, ruthless.

Walnut
Difficulty in adjusting to transition or change, including relocation, a new job, divorce, menopause, or puberty.

Water Violet
Pride, aloofness, self-reliance, noninterfering, enjoys being alone.

White Chestnut
Persistent unwanted thoughts, internal arguments, worry, preoccupation.

Wild Oat
Dissatisfaction due to uncertainty regarding career, lack of direction or commitment.

Wild Rose
Resignation, apathy, surrender, failure to make effort, lack of hope.

Willow
Resentment, bitterness, grumbling, self-pity, blaming others, dissatisfaction, victim role.

Alternative Therapies

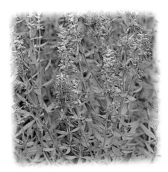

Target Ailments

Herbs are used for ailments affecting all body systems.

- ■ Cardiovascular System
- ■ Digestive System
- ■ Immune System
- ■ Musculoskeletal System
- ■ Nervous System
- ■ Reproductive System
- ■ Respiratory System
- ■ Skin
- ■ Urinary System

See Common Ailments, beginning on page 194.

Herbal Therapies

H *erbal medicines are prepared from a wide variety of plant materials—frequently the leaves, stems, roots, and bark, but also the flowers, fruits, twigs, seeds, and exudates (material that oozes out, such as sap). They generally contain several biologically active ingredients and are used primarily for treating chronic or mild conditions, although on occasion they are employed as complementary or supportive therapy for acute and severe diseases.*

Across the spectrum of alternative medicine, the use of herbs is varied: Western herbology, Chinese medicine, and Ayurvedic medicine differ in the way practitioners diagnose diseases and prescribe herbal remedies. Naturopathic physicians may use herbs from any of these systems.

Western Herbs

Medicinal plants in the group known as Western herbs bear English as well as Latin names and are categorized in several ways. Normalizers, or tonics, have a gentle, healing effect on the body. Another type, called effectors, have powerful actions and are used to treat illnesses. Herbs are also frequently grouped into more than 20 categories according to how they affect the body. Some of these categories are familiar—anti-inflammatories, diuretics, laxatives. Other, less well known classes include diaphoretics (herbs that promote perspiration and therefore the elimination of waste products through the skin) and nervines (herbs that act to strengthen the nervous system).

In many cases, herbs are also grouped according to the body systems they affect. The cardiovascular system, for example, responds well to herbs that strengthen blood vessels; these herbs include ginkgo, buckwheat, and linden. The digestive system, on the other hand, benefits from the relaxing effects of chamomile. Individual herbs can act on a body system in different ways. For instance, the sedative valerian, the cardiotonic herb hawthorn, and the herb St.-John's-wort, which has an antidepressant effect, invoke distinct responses from the nervous system.

LICENSED & INSURED?

Naturopaths and acupuncturists are licensed on a state-by-state basis, and in some states their services are covered by medical insurance. However, Ayurvedic physicians and clinical or medical herbalists are not licensed, and insurance companies usually do not provide coverage for their services.

Traditional Chinese Herbs

Another group of herbs, used by practitioners of Chinese medicine, are

Herbal Therapies

part of a larger system of healing that attempts to help the body correct energy imbalances *(see Chinese Medicine, pages 57-60)*. Chinese herbs are classified according to certain active characteristics (such as heating, cooling, moisturizing, or drying) and are prescribed according to how they influence the various organ systems. Practitioners of Chinese medicine also recognize five herb "tastes"—sweet, sour, salty, pungent, and bitter—each of which is associated with a particular physiological action. Chinese herbal prescriptions usually contain several herbs, perhaps as many as a dozen. These combinations are chosen not only for their effect on specific diseases but also for their ability to balance potential side effects and direct the therapy to a certain area of the body.

Origins

People have used plants for medicine since before recorded history, and all known cultures have long histories of folk medicine that include the use of herbs. Physical evidence of the existence of herbal remedies was found in the burial site of a Neanderthal man who lived more than 60,000 years ago.

Early observations of the characteristics of herbs and the way certain plants affected animals and humans were amassed in collections called pharmacopoeias or materia medicas. Many traditional herbalists believed that a healing energy inherent in the plants, and not the chemical constituents alone, accounted for the beneficial effects—a theory that is being explored by some contemporary practitioners.

Ancient cultures such as those of Greece and Rome developed well-defined herbal pharmacopoeias, and some herbal knowledge came to Europe from the Middle East during the Crusades. In the United States, herbs were used for many years to prevent various ailments and treat minor emergencies. In fact, American physicians relied on herbal preparations as primary medicines through the 1930s.

During the latter part of the 20th century, the use of plant remedies declined with advancements in medical technology and developments in the production of new pharmaceuticals. A 1992 report on alternative medicine prepared for the National Institutes of Health expressed concern that our knowledge of herbs—as medicinal plants and as unique species—may soon be lost. Recently, however, interest in herbal therapy has increased dramatically, partly in response to the growing perception that medicinal drugs are expensive, may cause side effects or allergic reactions, and are not capable of curing every disease.

What It's Good For

Herbal therapy offers remedies for virtually every ailment affecting all body systems. For a list of specific herbs and some of their medicinal uses, see The 75 Most Effective Herbs, on pages 74-103.

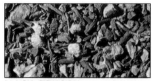

BLACK COHOSH

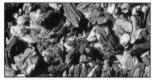

DANDELION

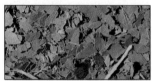

EUCALYPTUS

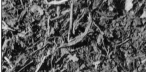

NETTLE

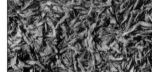

RED CLOVER

TURMERIC

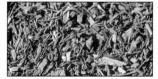

VALERIAN

Dried Herbs • *The leaves and other parts of medicinal plants, including those shown above, are sold in many forms.*

CONTINUED

Herbal Therapies CONTINUED

Preparations/Techniques

Herbs are available in various forms at health food stores and pharmacies, and many can be ordered by mail. Although Chinese herbs can usually be bought at Asian food stores, these products are more likely to be dispensed by practitioners, who are familiar with the combination formulas. Many practitioners of Chinese medicine also dispense Western herbs.

Herbal remedies can be prepared at home in a variety of ways, using either fresh or dried ingredients. Herbal teas, or infusions, can be steeped to varying strengths. Roots, bark, or other plant parts can be simmered into strong solutions called decoctions. Honey or sugar can be added to infusions and decoctions to make syrups. You can also buy many herbal remedies over the counter in the form of pills, capsules, or powders, or in more concentrated liquid forms called extracts and tinctures. Certain herbs can be applied topically as creams or ointments, soaked into cloths and used as compresses, or applied directly to the skin as poultices.

Visiting a Professional

Because some herbs can be toxic or carcinogenic, all medicinal plants should be used only under the guidance of a healthcare practitioner who is familiar with herbal medicine. The major professional herbalists in the U.S. include naturopathic physicians specializing in botanical medicine, acupuncturists trained in Chinese herbal medicine, Ayurvedic doctors, and trained medical or clinical herbalists.

Practitioners select a plant or formula that is appropriate for the patient rather than for just the complaint alone. Typically, the herbalist will take your personal and family history and may either perform a physical examination or request the results of a recent exam. He or she may evaluate any personal, social, or lifestyle factors that affect your health, then make recommendations regarding diet, exercise, or other lifestyle modifications. The practitioner will then suggest one or more remedies deemed appropriate for your condition. The exact form and dosage will depend on the strength of the herb, the effects desired, your age, and your constitution. In the case of Chinese medicine, the choice of herbs is based on a diagnostic system that evaluates specific individual characteristics, including the pulse rate and the appearance of the tongue *(see Chinese Medicine, pages 57-60)*.

Wellness

Herbs can be of great value when used in a program of self-care and preventive medicine. But because they vary in strength from gentle remedies that can be eaten like food to potential lethal poisons, medicinal plants should always be used under the supervision of a professional. A practitioner can advise which of the milder "ton-

Herbal Therapies

ic" herbs, such as dandelion and nettle, are safe and appropriate for your condition. A number of culinary herbs—including thyme and rosemary, which act as digestive stimulants and antiseptics—may also be used in a preventive health program.

What the Critics Say

Those suspicious of herbal therapy often point to the widespread availability of what they consider inaccurate or deceptive information about herbs. Although herbs cannot legally be labeled as to their efficacy in fighting diseases, advocacy literature—some of it carrying extreme claims of therapeutic effectiveness—may be sold alongside herbs on store shelves. Sometimes dangerous herbs are recommended, and in other cases herbs are said to be imbued with magical or mystical properties. Such claims draw fire from critics either because they are unscientific or because they leave the erroneous impression that potentially dangerous plants are harmless.

Herbal therapy also is criticized because medicinal plants have not been tested for efficacy according to rigid pharmaceutical standards. However, these tests are very expensive. Because herbs are natural products and cannot be patented, any company paying for such testing would likely never recover its losses. Furthermore, there's continuing debate over whether such testing should be performed on the entire herb or only on its active ingredients. Some remedies depend on the actions of several components (or several herbs) working together. Another problem is that sometimes an herb's active ingredients are not known.

Proponents of herbal therapy point out that the pharmaceutical industry grew out of herbal treatment and that plant extracts are still used to make drugs. For example, digitalis, used to treat heart disease, comes from the foxglove, and morphine comes from the opium poppy. About 25 percent of today's prescription drugs are at least partially derived from plants. ∎

OF SPECIAL INTEREST

Using Herbs Safely

Purchasing herbs is generally safer than harvesting your own plants. Many herbalists also advise against collecting your own herbs from the wild. Plants have natural variations that can be misleading, and the consequences of a mistake can be severe: A number of people have died from ingesting toxic wild plants believed to be benign substances. Because all forms of herbs lose potency over time, you should look for a source that provides the freshest possible product.

If you consistently develop nausea, diarrhea, or headache within two hours of taking an herb, discontinue its use immediately. Call your practitioner if the symptoms are prolonged. Women who are pregnant or breastfeeding are advised not to take medicinal amounts of herbs without first consulting a healthcare professional.

FOR MORE INFO
Following is a list of organizations you can contact to learn more about herbal therapy:

The American Herbalist Guild
PO Box 746555
Arvada, CO 80006
(303) 423-8800

Herb Research Foundation
1007 Pearl Street, Suite 200
Boulder, CO 80302
(303) 449-2265

National Acupuncture and Oriental Medicine Alliance
14637 Starr Road, SE
Olalla, WA 98359
(206) 851-6896

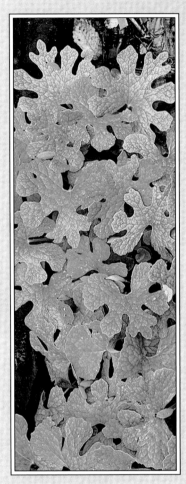

Bloodroot

Aloe
Aloe barbadensis

The translucent gel obtained from the inner leaves of this tropical herb works externally to relieve minor burns, skin irritations, and infections; taken internally, it provides relief from stomach disorders. Among its ingredients are several that reduce inflammation. Aloe gel is also used as a beauty aid and moisturizer because it contains polysaccharides, which act as emollients.

■ TARGET AILMENTS
Take internally for digestive disorders, gastritis, stomach ulcers.
Apply externally for minor burns, infected wounds, insect bites, irritated skin or eyes, bruises, chickenpox, sunburn, poison ivy, acne.

PREPARATIONS
Over the counter: Aloe is available as powder, fluidextract, powdered capsules, or bottled gel.
At home:
Eyewash: Dissolve ½ tsp powdered aloe gel in 1 cup water. Add 1 tsp boric acid to accelerate the healing process. Pour through a coffee filter before applying to the eyes.
Bath: Add 1 to 2 cups gel to a warm bath to relieve sunburn or skin lesions.
Combinations: Use aloe gel externally with wheat-germ oil and safflower flower to reduce bruising.

SIDE EFFECTS
Not serious: The use of aloe may result in allergic dermatitis, intestinal cramps, or diarrhea. Try a lower dosage or stop using the product.

SPECIAL INFORMATION
☙ If you are pregnant or have a gastrointestinal illness, consult an herbalist or a licensed healthcare professional before taking aloe internally.

Astragalus
Astragalus membranaceus

The perennial plant astragalus, or milk-vetch root, has sprawling stems and pale yellow blooms. Western herbalists believe that substances known as polysaccharides in this herb stimulate the immune system and generally strengthen the body, promoting tissue regeneration, speeding metabolism, and increasing energy. The herb is also used in traditional Chinese medicine.

■ TARGET AILMENTS
Take internally for general weakness and fatigue, loss of appetite, spontaneous perspiration, diarrhea, blood abnormalities, chronic colds and flu, AIDS, cancer. (Take with conventional medical treatment.)

PREPARATIONS
Over the counter: Astragalus is available as prepared tea, fluidextract, capsules, and dried root.
At home:
Chinese: Combine 1 part honey, 4 parts dried root, and a small amount of water in a wok or skillet. Allow mixture to simmer until the water evaporates and the herbs are slightly brown.
Combinations: For spontaneous perspiration, astragalus is mixed with Asian ginseng. As an immune system stimulant, the herb is combined with siler (Ledebouriella divaricata). Blood abnormalities are treated with a mix of astragalus and dong quai. Herbalists combine astragalus and atractylodes (white) for diarrhea.
Western: Boil 1 oz astragalus root in 1 cup water for 15 to 20 minutes to make a tea.

SIDE EFFECTS
None expected.

SPECIAL INFORMATION
☙ Pregnant women should check with their practitioners before using astragalus.

The 75 Most Effective Herbs

Black Cohosh
Cimicifuga racemosa

The knotty black rhizome and root of black cohosh contain substances that act like the female hormone estrogen. It is prescribed for several menstrual and menopausal conditions. The herb also acts as a sedative and is believed to promote urination, dry up discharges of fluid, aid in expelling mucus from the lungs, and relieve coughing spasms.

■ TARGET AILMENTS
Take internally for menstrual discomfort, menopause, PMS, headache, bleeding gums, coughs.
Apply externally for sciatica, neuralgia, muscle spasms, rheumatism.

PREPARATIONS
Over the counter: Black cohosh is available as tincture, syrup, capsules, fluidextract, and also as dried root and rhizome.
At home:
Decoction: Boil ½ tsp powdered rootstock per cup of water for 30 minutes and let cool. Add lemon and honey. Take as much as a cup per day, 2 tbsp at a time.

SIDE EFFECTS
Not serious: Prolonged use may irritate the uterus.
Serious: Overdoses or prolonged use can cause dizziness, diarrhea, nausea, vomiting, abdominal pain, headaches, joint pains, and lowered heart rate. It can contribute to abnormal blood clotting, liver problems, and breast tumors. If any symptoms develop, stop using black cohosh and call your doctor immediately.

SPECIAL INFORMATION
WARNING: Because it can cause serious side effects, use black cohosh only under medical supervision. Do not use if you have heart problems.
❧ Do not use if you are pregnant or if you have been told not to take contraceptive pills.

Black Walnut
Juglans nigra

Native Americans used the bark of the black walnut, a tree that grows in the eastern U.S., to treat skin problems such as ringworm. They drank a tea made from the bark as a laxative, and they chewed on the bark to relieve headache pain. Today black walnut's bark, leaves, fruit rind, and liquid extracts are prescribed by herbalists for constipation, fungal and parasitic infections, and mouth sores. Black walnut is rich in tannins and contains a large amount of iodine, which makes it a good antiseptic. Also, the herb is believed to relieve toxic blood conditions. And some evidence indicates that, if used internally over a long period, the herb will help eliminate warts caused by viruses.

■ TARGET AILMENTS
Take internally for constipation, intestinal worms and parasites, warts, mouth sores.
Apply externally for ringworm, scabies, eczema, herpes, psoriasis, sores, pimples, athlete's foot, jock itch, cold sores.

PREPARATIONS
Over the counter: Black walnut is available as tincture, extract, dried bark, leaves, and fruit rind.
At home:
Decoction: Simmer the bark in boiling water for 10 to 15 minutes. Take 1 tbsp three or four times a day.
Gargle: Use the decoction as a mouthwash or gargle to treat mouth sores.
Extract: Rub on the affected area twice a day.
Poultice: Make a poultice from the green rind of black walnut and apply to the sites of ringworm.

SIDE EFFECTS
None expected.

Bloodroot
Sanguinaria canadensis

Named for the crimson extract made from its root, bloodroot not only looks forbidding but is potentially toxic and can cause severe side effects if ingested in excess. For this reason, herbalists prescribe the root of this perennial plant primarily as an external remedy to relieve eczema, venereal blisters, rashes, and other skin disorders. Bloodroot is a major ingredient in many mouthwashes and toothpastes because of its ability to kill the bacteria that can lead to gingivitis (gum disease) and the buildup of plaque.

■ TARGET AILMENTS
Take internally for gingivitis. (Use as toothpaste and mouthwash.)
Apply externally for fungus, athlete's foot, venereal blisters, rashes, eczema, ringworm, warts.

PREPARATIONS
Over the counter: Bloodroot is available as tincture and dried root.
At home:
Tea: Boil 1 oz bloodroot in 1 cup water for 15 to 20 minutes. Drink three times daily.
Combinations: With horehound and elecampane to relieve congestion; with red sage and a pinch of cayenne to treat pharyngitis.

SIDE EFFECTS
Serious: At high doses, internal use can cause burning in the stomach, vomiting, nausea, slowing of the heart rate, impaired vision, intense thirst, and dizziness. Stop using immediately if these symptoms develop, and consult your practitioner.

SPECIAL INFORMATION
WARNING: Bloodroot is potentially toxic. Take it internally only under the supervision of an herbalist or licensed healthcare professional.
❧ Avoid using bloodroot internally during pregnancy.

CONTINUED

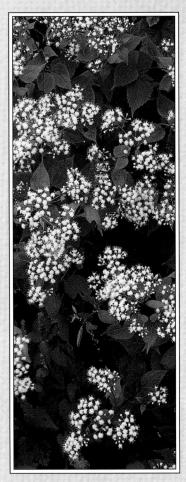

Boneset

Boneset
Eupatorium perfoliatum

Boneset, also called sweat plant and feverwort, was first used by Native Americans and then by the colonists to treat fever-producing illnesses. Today herbalists still recommend the herb for the aches and pains that accompany fever, especially during bouts of influenza, and to help clear mucus from the respiratory tract. It is also often used for arthritis and rheumatism.

■ TARGET AILMENTS
Take internally for fever, colds, flu, coughs, upper respiratory tract congestion, arthritis, and rheumatism.

PREPARATIONS
Over the counter: Available in health food stores as dried leaves and flowers, and as tincture.
At home:
Infusion: Pour 1 cup boiling water onto 2 to 3 tsp dried herb; let steep 10 to 15 minutes. Drink as hot as possible. For fever or flu, drink a cup every half hour, up to 4 cups in 6 hours. Do not exceed 6 cups in a 24-hour period. To mask boneset's very bitter taste, mix it with an herbal tea or add honey and lemon.

SIDE EFFECTS
Not serious: Large doses can cause nausea or diarrhea. Do not exceed the recommended dosage; call your doctor if you experience adverse reactions.

SPECIAL INFORMATION
WARNING: Do not use fresh boneset. It contains a toxic chemical called tremerol that can cause vomiting, rapid breathing, and at high doses, possibly coma and death. Drying boneset removes the tremerol.
• Do not take boneset for more than two weeks at a time. If you have a history of alcoholism or liver problems, consult your herbalist before taking boneset; it is toxic to the liver.

Bupleurum
Bupleurum chinense

Bupleurum, sometimes called hare's ear or thorowax root, is often used in Chinese medicine to reduce certain types of fever and to treat irritability.

■ TARGET AILMENTS
Take internally for low-grade fevers; malaria; alternating chills and fever, typically accompanied by a bitter taste in the mouth, pain in the side, irritability, vomiting, or difficulty in breathing; prolapse of the uterus; vertigo combined with chest pain, and tenderness in the side or breast, often accompanied by irritability; menstrual problems; pressure in the chest, bloated abdomen, nausea, and indigestion.

PREPARATIONS
The root is available in bulk in Chinese pharmacies, Asian markets, and some Western health food stores. Chinese pharmacies also offer mixtures containing the root.

Combinations: White peony root mixed with bupleurum is prescribed for vertigo, chest pain, and painful menstruation. Irregular menstruation, PMS, and certain kinds of depression may be treated with a blend of bupleurum and field mint. Bupleurum is often combined with bitter orange fruit to relieve pressure in the chest, abdominal pain, and irregular bowel movements, and to improve poor appetite. For information on specific dosages and additional herbal combinations, consult your Chinese medicine practitioner.

SIDE EFFECTS
Not serious: Too large a dose can cause nausea.

SPECIAL INFORMATION
• Clinical tests have indicated that the herb might be useful in treating tuberculosis, influenza, and polio.

The 75 Most Effective Herbs

Burdock
Arctium lappa

Herbalists have long prescribed burdock root for a wide range of illnesses. Today, some use it to treat urinary tract infections, arthritis, external wounds, and skin ulcers. This herb works best in conjunction with conventional medical treatment. Burdock got its name from its tenacious burrs and from "dock," the Old English word for plant.

■ TARGET AILMENTS

Take internally for fungal and bacterial infections; skin disorders, such as eczema and psoriasis, which cause dry, scaly skin; urinary tract infections; rheumatism; arthritis.

Apply externally for wounds and skin conditions.

PREPARATIONS

Over the counter: Burdock is available as dried powder, slices of root, and tincture.

At home:

Decoction: Add 1 tsp burdock root to 3 cups water; boil for 30 minutes. Drink up to 3 cups a day to treat genital and urinary tract irritations.

Compress: Soak a clean cloth in burdock tea and place it on the skin to speed healing of wounds and skin ulcers.

Combinations: Burdock, mixed with yellow dock, red clover, or cleavers, can be taken orally for skin disorders. Consult an herbalist for more information.

SPECIAL INFORMATION

WARNING: Because it stimulates the uterus, do not use if pregnant.

ᴥ Do not give burdock to children younger than two years of age. Older children and people over 65 should start with lower-strength doses, increasing them if needed.

ᴥ Doses higher than recommended may cause stomach discomfort.

Calendula
Calendula officinalis

The therapeutic use of calendula, whose medically active parts are its flowers, originated in ancient Egypt. One variety is the common marigold. A natural antiseptic and anti-inflammatory agent, calendula is one of the best herbs for treating wounds, skin abrasions, and infections. Taken internally, it also alleviates indigestion as well as other gastrointestinal disorders. Calendula's healing power appears to come from components known as terpenes. One of these is recognized as a sedative and for its healing effect on ulcers.

■ TARGET AILMENTS

Take internally for indigestion, gastric and duodenal ulcers, gallbladder problems, irregular or painful menstruation.

Apply externally for cuts, wounds, sores, and burns; skin rashes from measles, chickenpox, and other eruptive skin diseases; diaper rash; athlete's foot and other fungal infections.

PREPARATIONS

Over the counter: Available as lotion, ointment, oil, tincture, and fresh or dried leaves and florets.

At home:

Rub lotions, ointments, and oils on injuries, rashes, and infections.

Poultice: Mash up the leaves, then apply directly to minor burns or scalds.

Tea: Steep 1 oz dried herb in 1 pt boiling water. For acute internal symptoms, drink two to four times a day until symptoms lessen.

Combinations: A mixture of goldenseal, calendula, and myrrh makes an antiseptic lotion.

SPECIAL INFORMATION

ᴥ Calendula flowers can be made into an oil for external use and to ease earaches and other infections.

Catnip
Nepeta cataria

Herbalists have used the flowers and leaves of catnip, an aromatic member of the mint family, for more than 2,000 years. Today it is prescribed for easing digestion, calming nerves, and relieving muscle spasms, including menstrual cramps. Cats are strongly attracted to catnip and may become intoxicated by eating it, but the herb has no such effect on humans.

■ TARGET AILMENTS

Take internally for indigestion, gas, tension, difficulty in sleeping, colds, flu, bronchial congestion, fever, colic in infants, menstrual cramps.

Apply externally for cuts and scrapes.

PREPARATIONS

Over the counter: Catnip is available in dried bulk flowers and leaves, tincture, and tea bags.

At home: To treat minor cuts and scrapes, press crushed catnip leaves into them before washing and bandaging them.

Tea: Pour 1 cup boiling water onto 2 tsp dried leaves and steep for 10 to 15 minutes. Drink three times a day.

Combinations: Mix with boneset, elder, yarrow, or cayenne for colds.

SIDE EFFECTS

Not serious: Catnip can produce an upset stomach. If this occurs, discontinue use and call your doctor.

SPECIAL INFORMATION

ᴥ Avoid catnip during pregnancy.

ᴥ Infants with colic can be given weak, cool infusions. For older children and people over 65, start treatment with weak preparations and increase the strength as necessary.

CONTINUED

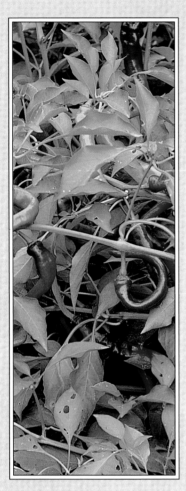

Cayenne

Cayenne

Capsicum annuum var. annuum

Regarded by herbalists as a powerful tonic, cayenne stimulates the heart and promotes blood circulation, improves digestion, and boosts energy. Like other species of hot pepper, such as tabasco, cayenne contains the natural stimulant known as capsaicin. Widely grown in Central and South America in pre-Columbian times, cayenne was carried to Spain and Europe after the early voyages of discovery.

■ TARGET AILMENTS
Take internally for poor circulation, indigestion, gas, physical or mental exhaustion, and lowered vitality, particularly in the elderly.
Apply externally for pain, including that of arthritis and diabetes, strains, sore muscles and joints, the need to stimulate blood flow or to stop external bleeding.

PREPARATIONS
Over the counter: Available as powder, capsules, tincture, or oil.
At home:
Rub the oil on sprains, swelling, sore muscles, and joints to ease pain.
Infusion: Pour 1 cup boiling water onto ½ to 1 tsp cayenne powder and steep for 10 minutes. Mix 1 tbsp of the infusion with hot water and drink as needed.
Gargle: Combine cayenne with myrrh to treat laryngitis and to use as an antiseptic wash.

SIDE EFFECTS
Not serious: In large doses, cayenne can produce vomiting, stomach pain, and a type of intoxication. Do not exceed prescribed dosages.

SPECIAL INFORMATION
☛ Hot and spicy as a tea or tincture, cayenne can cause mild nausea at first. It's best to start with a small amount and work up gradually to the recommended dosage.

Chamomile

Matricaria recutita

Of the three types of chamomile plant, the most popular and thoroughly studied is German chamomile, used medicinally around the world for thousands of years. Modern herbalists have identified elements in the oil of the chamomile flower that appear to calm the central nervous system, relax the digestive tract, and speed healing.

■ TARGET AILMENTS
Take internally for stomach cramps, gas and nervous stomach, indigestion, ulcers, menstrual cramps, insomnia, colic, bladder problems. Use as a gargle for gingivitis and sore throat.
Apply externally for swelling and joint pain, sunburn, cuts and scrapes, teething pain, varicose veins, hemorrhoids.

PREPARATIONS
Over the counter: Available as prepared tea, tincture, essential oil, and dried or fresh flowers.
At home:
Tea: Pour 8 oz boiling water over 2 tsp chamomile flowers and steep for 10 minutes. Drink 1 cup three or four times daily.
Fomentation: Apply three or four times daily to sore muscles; sore, swollen joints; varicose veins; and burns and skin wounds.
Herbal bath: Add no more than 2 drops essential oil of chamomile to bathwater.

SIDE EFFECTS
None expected.

SPECIAL INFORMATION
☛ Allergies to chamomile are rare. However, anyone allergic to other plants in the daisy family should be alert to possible allergic reactions to chamomile.

The 75 Most Effective Herbs

Chaste Tree
Vitex agnus-castus

Since ancient times, herbalists have used the berries of the chaste tree to manipulate the functioning of the female reproductive system. Chaste tree's natural compounds seem to aid in regulating the menstrual cycle by bringing into balance the female sex hormones, estrogen and progesterone. In addition to menstrual irregularities, chaste tree is prescribed for premenstrual syndrome and menopausal symptoms. It also aids in readjusting the body after withdrawal from long-term use of birth-control pills, in preventing miscarriage in the first three months of pregnancy, and in promoting lactation. Used by Roman matrons and medieval monks to dampen sexual ardor, chaste tree has also, paradoxically, had a reputation as an aphrodisiac.

■ TARGET AILMENTS
Take internally for PMS, menstrual irregularities, symptoms of menopause, prevention of miscarriage, promotion of lactation, hormone-related constipation, endometriosis, fibroid cysts in smooth muscle tissue, teenage acne.

PREPARATIONS
Over the counter: Chaste tree is available as berries, powder, dried herb, capsules, and tincture.
At home:
Tea: Pour 1 cup boiling water onto 1 tsp ripe berries; infuse for 10 to 15 minutes. Drink three times a day.

SPECIAL INFORMATION
- Chaste tree seems to regulate hormonal imbalances within 10 days, and relief from PMS may be noticeable by the second menstrual cycle. For optimal benefit, however, the herb should be taken for six months or longer.
- Discontinue the herb after the third month of pregnancy, since it may cause premature milk production.

Chinese Foxglove Root
Rehmannia glutinosa

The thick reddish yellow Chinese foxglove root is cooked in wine and used as a tonic. The cooked form of the root is also often used in Chinese medicine for treating disorders that are associated with aging.

■ TARGET AILMENTS
Take internally for lightheadedness, palpitations, blurred vision, or floaters in vision; insomnia; chronic low-grade fever and night sweats; constipation with dry, hard stools; irregular menstruation or uterine bleeding, especially after childbirth; low back pain and weak knees; weak, stiff joints; hearing loss and tinnitus; premature graying of hair.

PREPARATIONS
The prepared root and the raw version are available from Chinese pharmacies, Asian markets, and some Western health food stores. Ask for the cooked version, which is made by soaking the root in rice wine with spices such as cardamom.

Combinations: A mixture with gelatin is prescribed for coughing and vomiting blood, nosebleeds, and uterine bleeding. The cooked root is also combined with cornus and Chinese yam to treat lightheadedness, insomnia, forgetfulness, and related symptoms. See a Chinese medicine practitioner for dosages and further herbal combinations.

SPECIAL INFORMATION
WARNING: Those with digestive problems should use this herb carefully; the cooked herb can distend the abdomen and cause loose stools.
- Grains-of-paradise fruit is often added to preparations of Chinese foxglove root to prevent side effects such as diarrhea, nausea, and abdominal pain.

Chinese Yam
Dioscorea opposita

Chinese yam, a thick, firm root with a white cross section, is used as a tonic. Classified as neutral and sweet in traditional Chinese medicine, the herb is harvested in the winter in the mountains of Hunan and in many other Chinese provinces.

■ TARGET AILMENTS
Take internally for weak digestion with diarrhea and fatigue, reduced appetite, frequent urination, excessive vaginal discharge, chronic coughing and wheezing, symptoms that accompany diabetes.

PREPARATIONS
Chinese yam is available as a fresh or dried vegetable in Chinese pharmacies, Asian food markets, and some Western health food stores. For symptoms of diabetes, slices of the fresh root are steeped in hot water to make an infusion.

Combinations: A mixture of Chinese yam, poria, and atractylodes (white) may be prescribed for loose, watery stools. Chinese yam and codonopsis root make up a preparation used to treat fatigue, general weakness, and poor appetite. Consult a Chinese medicine practitioner for information on proper dosages and other herbal combinations.

SIDE EFFECTS
None expected.

SPECIAL INFORMATION
- If symptoms include abdominal swelling and pain, do not use Chinese yam.

POSSIBLE INTERACTIONS
Do not take Chinese yam with kan-sui root.

CONTINUED

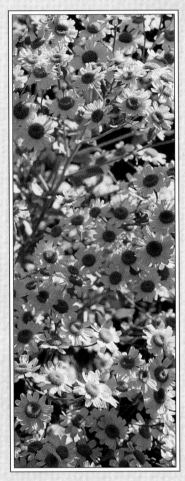

Chamomile

Cinnamon Bark
Cinnamomum cassia

A popular stimulant in Chinese medicine, cinnamon is usually harvested from trees after they are seven years old. Its outer bark is the common spice; the inner bark contains more oil and has stronger medicinal effects. Cinnamon bark is used to treat abdominal disorders, menstrual pain, infertility, and some forms of asthma.

■ TARGET AILMENTS
Take internally for lack of appetite, diarrhea, abdominal discomfort; excessive urination, impotence, and lack of sexual desire; menstrual problems and infertility; wheezing from exposure to cold.

PREPARATIONS
Cinnamon bark is available fresh or dried at Asian food markets and pharmacies and some Western health food stores. It is normally taken in the form of powder, pill, or tincture (crushed bark mixed with alcohol).

Combinations: Used with the roots of Asian ginseng and of Chinese foxglove cooked in wine to treat palpitations of the heart and shortness of breath. Check with a Chinese medicine practitioner on dosages and other combinations.

SIDE EFFECTS
Serious: Large doses can cause changes in breathing, dilation of blood vessels, and convulsions.

SPECIAL INFORMATION
WARNING: Use this herb cautiously if you are pregnant.
WARNING: Do not use the herb when there is fever, inflammation, or hemorrhaging.
ᵛ᷉ In a clinical trial, an alcohol-based preparation of the bark, injected at an acupuncture point associated with the lung, seemed to help bronchial asthma.

Coltsfoot
Tussilago farfara

Coltsfoot has a long history as a cough suppressant and is still used today for that purpose and as a gentle expectorant. It is banned in Canada, but in the United States the FDA classifies it as an herb with "undefined safety." It contains an alkaloid that can seriously damage the liver, and a Japanese study found that the flower buds may be carcinogenic. Many practitioners, however, still routinely use coltsfoot on a short-term basis to treat respiratory ailments.

■ TARGET AILMENTS
Take internally for coughs, asthma, and emphysema.
Apply externally for burns, skin ulcers, inflammations, and insect bites.

PREPARATIONS
Over the counter: Available in tincture, in capsules, and in bulk.
At home:
Tea: Pour 1 cup boiling water onto 1 to 3 tsp dried flowers or leaves and steep for 10 minutes. Drink three times a day, as hot as possible.
Compress: Soak a pad in a coltsfoot infusion for several minutes, wring out, then apply to the affected area.
Combinations: For coughs, take it with white horehound and mullein; for bronchitis, with garlic or echinacea.

SIDE EFFECTS
Serious: Fever, nausea, loss of appetite, diarrhea, jaundice, or abdominal pain may result. Stop taking it and call your doctor now.

SPECIAL INFORMATION
WARNING: Use only as prescribed by a practitioner, for short periods of time. Do not give coltsfoot to children under two, pregnant or nursing women, alcoholics, or anyone with liver disease.

The 75 Most Effective Herbs

Dandelion
Taraxacum officinale

Dandelion has a long history of medicinal use. It acts as a natural diuretic while also supplying potassium, a nutrient that is often lost through diuretic use. The plant is rich in vitamins A and C—antioxidants that are believed to help prevent cancer. The young leaves can be eaten fresh or used in herbal preparations.

■ TARGET AILMENTS
Take internally for poor digestion, gallbladder problems, inflammation of the liver. As a supplemental diuretic, dandelion may help relieve symptoms associated with high blood pressure, congestive heart failure, premenstrual syndrome, menstrual pain, and joint pain.

PREPARATIONS
Over the counter: Available in tincture, prepared tea, capsule, and dried or fresh leaves or roots.
At home:
Tea: Steep 1 tbsp dried or 2 tbsp fresh leaves for each cup of boiling water for 10 minutes. Drink up to 4 cups a day.
Decoction: Simmer 1 tbsp fresh or dried root per cup of water for 15 minutes. Drink up to 4 cups a day.
Nutrition: Add fresh leaves to a salad.

SIDE EFFECTS
Not serious: Allergic dermatitis, stomach upset, diarrhea, flulike symptoms, liver pain. Discontinue use and call your doctor when convenient.

SPECIAL INFORMATION
🍂Consult an herbalist if you plan to use the herb longer than two or three months, or if you are pregnant, have a heart condition, or suffer from stomach discomfort.
🍂Use low doses for adults over 65 and children between two and 12. Do not give to children under two.

Dong Quai
Angelica sinensis

Also known as Chinese angelica root, dong quai is used by Chinese herbalists as a treatment for several gynecological complaints. Look for a long, moist, oily plant as the source of the root, which has brown bark and a white cross section. The herb is characterized in traditional Chinese medicine as sweet, acrid, bitter, and warm.

■ TARGET AILMENTS
Take internally for menstrual problems; poor blood circulation, pale complexion, possible anemia; abscesses, sores; lightheadedness, blurred vision, heart palpitations.

PREPARATIONS
This root is available in bulk and in tablet form at health food stores and Asian markets and pharmacies. You should avoid the herb if it is dry or has a greenish brown cross section.

Combinations: Mixed with astragalus, it provides a tonic for treating fatigue. Blend it with white peony root, Chinese foxglove root cooked in wine, and cnidium root for menstrual irregularities. Dong quai is also combined with honeysuckle flowers and red peony root to form a preparation that reduces swelling and alleviates pain from abscesses and sores. Consult a Chinese practitioner for further information.

SIDE EFFECTS
None expected if used as directed.

SPECIAL INFORMATION
🍂You should not take dong quai during the early stages of pregnancy.
🍂Check with your Chinese medicine practitioner on the use of this herb if you have diarrhea or bloating.
🍂Modern acupuncturists sometimes inject the herb into acupuncture points to treat pain, especially that from neuralgia and arthritis.

Echinacea
Echinacea spp.

Echinacea was frequently used by Native Americans of the southwest plains in poultices, mouthwashes, and teas. Now a popular garden perennial, the plant displays purple blossoms and grows as high as five feet. Herbalists value the dried root of echinacea for its broad-based action against many types of viral and bacterial illnesses, such as colds, bronchitis, ear infections, influenza, and cystitis. Laboratory tests show that echinacea may have antibiotic effects. It seems to bolster the immune system's white blood cells in their battle against foreign microorganisms. It can also be effective as a topical medicine for eczema and other skin problems.

■ TARGET AILMENTS
Take internally for colds, flu, and other respiratory illnesses; mononucleosis; ear infections; blood poisoning; bladder infections.
Apply externally for boils, burns, abscesses, wounds, stings, hives, insect bites, eczema, and herpes.

PREPARATIONS
Over the counter: Available in tea, capsule, tincture, and dried bulk form.
At home:
Tea: Boil 2 tsp dried root in 1 cup water and simmer for 15 minutes. Drink three times daily.
Combinations: Use echinacea with yarrow or uva ursi to treat cystitis.

SIDE EFFECTS
None expected.

SPECIAL INFORMATION
🍂Do not use echinacea continuously for more than a few weeks.
🍂Do not give to children younger than two; start with minimal doses for older children and older adults.
🍂Check with your doctor before using if you are pregnant or nursing.

CONTINUED

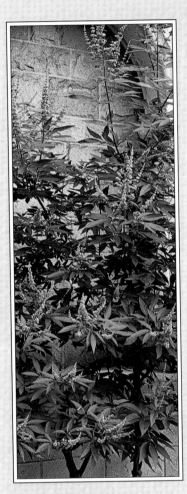

Chaste Tree

Ephedra
Ephedra sinica

Known in China as ma huang, ephedra has long been used there by healers. Its root and other parts have been used in the West as a decongestant and remedy for asthma, hay fever, and colds. Its active ingredients are central nervous system stimulants that open bronchial passages, activating the heart, increasing blood pressure, and speeding up metabolism. For this reason, herbalists warn against excessive use of the herb.

■ TARGET AILMENTS
Take internally for fever, respiratory ailments, hay fever, stomachache.

PREPARATIONS
Over the counter: Available as fluid-extract, tablets, dried bulk herb.
At home:
Chinese: Combine 1 part honey with 4 parts dried herb in a small amount of water. Simmer until water is gone and herbs are slightly brown.
Combinations: For fever and chills, mix with cinnamon twig; for coughing and asthma,with apricot seed; for indigestion, with licorice.
Western: Boil 1 tsp of the herb with 1 cup water for 15 to 20 minutes. Drink up to 2 cups of the tea a day.

SIDE EFFECTS
Serious: Increased blood pressure or heart rate, heart palpitations. If any of these symptoms develop, discontinue use and consult your physician immediately.

SPECIAL INFORMATION
WARNING: Because it can cause side effects—and rarely, death—consult a practitioner before taking, especially if you are on any medication. It may not be safe as a weight-loss aid.
WARNING: Do not use if you are pregnant or have heart disease, diabetes, glaucoma, or hyperthyroidism.
➤ Use mild doses for children or seniors. Do not treat children under two.

Eyebright
Euphrasia officinalis

Eyebright is an herb whose name suggests both its action and its appearance. The red spots on its white or purple flowers seem to resemble bloodshot eyes. Moreover, its dried stems, leaves, and flowers have long been used as a tonic for irritated or infected eyes. Eyebright can be applied to eyes that are itching, red, and tearing from hay fever, other allergies, or colds; it can also alleviate the symptoms of conjunctivitis. Drinking eyebright tea may help to maintain good vision and to diminish nasal congestion and coughs.

■ TARGET AILMENTS
Apply externally for eye irritations from allergies, colds, conjunctivitis.
Take internally for nasal congestion and coughs from colds, sinusitis, or allergies.

PREPARATIONS
Over the counter: Available in bulk, capsules, and tincture.
At home:
Tea: Pour 1 cup boiling water onto 2 tsp dried eyebright and steep for 10 minutes; drink three times daily.
Compress: Boil 1 to 2 tbsp dried eyebright in 1 pt water for 10 minutes. After the water has cooled, strain it, dip a sterile cloth in it and wring it out, then put it on your eyes for 15 minutes a few times a day.
Combinations to be taken orally: For congestion, combine it with goldenrod, elder flowers, or goldenseal. For hay fever, mix it with ephedra. Consult an herbalist for dosages.

SIDE EFFECTS
Not serious: Eyebright may cause a skin rash or nausea. If this occurs, lessen your dose or stop taking completely.

SPECIAL INFORMATION
➤ Consult a practitioner before using eyebright to treat children.

The 75 Most Effective Herbs

Feverfew

Tanacetum parthenium
(or Chrysanthemum parthenium)

Feverfew is a perennial with small-blossoms that resemble daisies. In the late 1970s British researchers found feverfew leaves helpful in treating migraine headaches where other treatments had failed. They believe this relief is due to the chemical parthenolide, which blocks the release of inflammatory substances from the blood. The researchers consider these inflammatory elements to be key components in the onset of a migraine.

■ TARGET AILMENTS
Take internally for migraines.

PREPARATIONS
Over the counter: Available in dry bulk, pills, capsules, and tinctures.
At home: Chew two fresh or frozen leaves a day for migraines. If you find the leaves too bitter, substitute capsules or pills containing 85 mg of the leaf material, but fresh leaves are best for immediate results.

Tea: Steep 2 tsp dried herb in 1 cup boiling water for 5 to 10 minutes; drink 2 to 3 cups per day.

SIDE EFFECTS
Serious: Chewing fresh or dried feverfew may cause internal mouth sores or abdominal pain. If these symptoms develop, discontinue use and notify your doctor.

SPECIAL INFORMATION
- Do not take if you are pregnant.
- Feverfew may interfere with the blood's clotting ability; talk to your doctor before using if you have a clotting disorder or take anticoagulant medicine.
- You may need to take feverfew daily for two to three months before it has any effect.

Ganoderma

Ganoderma lucidum

A variety of mushroom also known as ling zhi in China and as reishi in the West, ganoderma grows in mountainous regions in China. It is a rare fungus that Chinese practitioners value highly for its multiple uses. Practitioners have traditionally used it to treat psychological disturbances as well as respiratory complaints and ulcers. Ganoderma has also been prescribed to boost patients' immune systems.

■ TARGET AILMENTS
Take internally for nervousness, insomnia, dizziness; asthma, allergy-related chronic bronchitis; weakened immune system; tumors; ulcers; poor blood circulation; mushroom poisoning.

PREPARATIONS
Ganoderma can be found in bulk at some health food stores (under the name *reishi*) and at Asian pharmacies and markets. It is also possible to obtain it in pill or tablet form, and in alcohol extracts. Consult a Chinese medicine practitioner for information on appropriate dosages. Unlike most other Chinese herbs, ganoderma is not traditionally combined with other substances.

SIDE EFFECTS
Not serious: Patients may experience dizziness, sore bones, itchy skin, increased bowel movements, hard stools, and pimplelike eruptions when they use ganoderma. Discontinue use of the herb if these symptoms develop.

SPECIAL INFORMATION
- The herb may be useful in conjunction with conventional medical treatment of AIDS and cancer.
- In clinical studies, ganoderma seems to have reduced blood pressure in humans and animals.

Garlic

Allium sativum

The garlic bulb has long been recognized as a medicinal remedy in Chinese and Western cultures. Garlic's active ingredient is allicin, which is also responsible for the herb's pungent smell. In China this herb is prescribed for colds and coughs and for intestinal and digestive disorders. Chinese herbalists believe garlic can be used externally as an antibiotic and antifungal treatment for skin infections. Western herbalists prescribe it for many of the same ailments as their Chinese counterparts. It is also used to reduce cholesterol and to lower blood pressure.

■ TARGET AILMENTS
Take internally for colds, coughs, flu, high cholesterol, high blood pressure, atherosclerosis, digestive disorders, bladder infection, liver and gallbladder problems.
Apply externally for athlete's foot, ringworm, minor skin infections.

PREPARATIONS
Over the counter: Garlic is available as cloves and in tablet form.
At home:
Tincture: Combine 1 cup crushed cloves with 1 qt brandy. Shake daily for two weeks. Take up to 3 tbsp a day.

SIDE EFFECTS
Not serious: Allergic rash from touching or eating the herb.

SPECIAL INFORMATION
- Consult your practitioner before using garlic if you are pregnant.
- Garlic has a blood clot-preventing agent. If you have a blood-clotting disorder, consult an herbalist or a licensed healthcare professional.
- Garlic is thought to function as an adjunct treatment for cardiovascular disease. Consult your practitioner before using it in this capacity.

CONTINUED

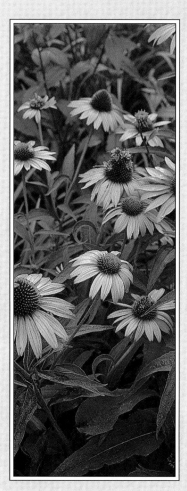

Echinacea

Gentiana
Gentiana scabra

Several varieties of this herb grow throughout China. Gentiana scabra, the most widely used, is a long, thick, yellow root, described as cold by Chinese herbalists. They prescribe the herb primarily for disorders of the liver and organs in the pelvic area. Gentiana tastes so bitter that Chinese herbalists use it as a standard for judging bitterness in plants.

■ TARGET AILMENTS
Take internally for hepatitis, jaundice, and other liver disorders; sexually transmitted diseases, vaginal discharge, inflammation of the pelvis, pain or swelling in the genital area; convulsions.

PREPARATIONS
You can find gentiana in bulk at some health food stores and Asian pharmacies and markets. While the Chinese variety is not available in pills or tablets, the European root can be obtained in that form.

Combinations: Chinese herbalists prescribe a preparation that contains gentiana, sophora root, and plantago seeds for genital itching and vaginal discharge. A combination of gentiana with cattle gallstone and gambir is given for convulsions, especially when the symptoms appear in children. Check with your practitioner for advice on other combinations and dosages.

SIDE EFFECTS
None expected.

SPECIAL INFORMATION
WARNING: Chinese herbalists advise against the use of this root when diarrhea is among the symptoms.
❧ Gentiana is believed to have an antibiotic effect; it is also thought to be toxic to malarial parasites.

Ginger
Zingiber officinale

Ginger not only is a valued culinary seasoning but also is considered a remedy for a range of ailments. Both Chinese and Western herbalists believe it relieves motion sickness and dizziness and improves digestion. Ginger is also said to alleviate menstrual cramps. Its active constituents, gingerols, soothe the abdomen and relieve excess gas. In China, ginger, called gan-jian, is applied to first- and second-degree burns.

■ TARGET AILMENTS
Chinese: vomiting, abdominal pain, menstrual irregularity (take internally); minor burns (apply externally).
Western: motion sickness, digestive disorders, menstrual cramps, colds, flu, arthritis, high cholesterol, high blood pressure (take internally).

PREPARATIONS
Over the counter: Available as fresh or dried root, liquid extract, tablets, capsules, prepared tea.
At home:
Chinese: Wrap fresh roots in five or six layers of rice paper. Bury under warm coals until the paper is blackened. Discard paper before use.
Rub: Treat minor burns by rubbing fresh ginger juice on the wound.
Combinations: For vomiting, ginger is mixed with pinellia root; when there is also severe abdominal pain, the herb is combined with licorice or galanga. A preparation of ginger and chamomile is used to treat menstrual irregularity.
Western: Boil 1 oz dried root in 1 cup water for 15 to 20 minutes for tea.

SIDE EFFECTS
Not serious: Heartburn.

SPECIAL INFORMATION
❧ Ginger may help prevent heart disease and strokes.
❧ If you are pregnant, consult your doctor before using.

Ginkgo
Ginkgo biloba

Chinese herbalists have used the fan-shaped leaves of the ginkgo tree for thousands of years to treat asthma, chilblains, and swelling. Western herbalists value it for its action against vascular diseases. It dilates blood vessels and thereby improves blood flow, especially to areas such as the lower legs and feet, as well as to the brain. Herbalists believe ginkgo can keep blood clots from forming and bronchial tubes from constricting during an asthma attack. It may also help reduce damage from macular degeneration.

■ TARGET AILMENTS
Take internally for vertigo; tinnitus; phlebitis; leg ulcers; cerebral atherosclerosis; diabetic vascular disease; Raynaud's syndrome; headache; depression; lack of concentration or mental and emotional fatigue in the elderly; asthma; clotting disorders, including stroke and heart attack.

PREPARATIONS
Leaves are available in dry bulk, capsules, or tincture. You can find ginkgo biloba extract (GBE) in health food stores. Most herbalists recommend using only over-the-counter ginkgo products.

SIDE EFFECTS
Not serious: Irritability, restlessness, diarrhea, nausea; check with your doctor to see if you should lower your dose or stop taking it completely.

SPECIAL INFORMATION
WARNING: Some people cannot tolerate ginkgo even in small doses.
❧ Do not use if you have a bleeding disorder like hemophilia or are pregnant or nursing.
❧ Do not give ginkgo to children without a doctor's supervision.
❧ Consult a healthcare professional before using it in medicinal amounts.

Ginseng, American
Panax quinquefolius

Native Americans believed American ginseng could alleviate painful childbirths and restore energy in the elderly. American ginseng is identified by a single stalk crowned by delicate chartreuse blooms and crimson berries; its leaflets have sawlike teeth. The active ingredients of American ginseng are panaxosides, which are thought to calm the stomach and the brain and act as a mild stimulant to vital organs. American ginseng is milder than Asian ginseng and is often prescribed for people who consider Asian ginseng too potent. Both American and Asian ginseng are frequently used to treat the elderly.

■ TARGET AILMENTS
Take internally for depression, fatigue, stress, colds, influenza, respiratory problems, inflammation, a damaged immune system.

PREPARATIONS
Over the counter: Ginseng is available as fresh or dried root, root powder, capsules, tablets, prepared tea, freeze-dried root, cured rock candy.
At home:
Decoction: Boil 1 oz fresh root with 1 cup water for 15 to 20 minutes. Drink up to 2 cups a day.

SIDE EFFECTS
Not serious: Headache, insomnia, anxiety, breast soreness, skin rash.
Serious: You may experience asthma attacks, increased blood pressure, heart palpitations, or postmenopausal uterine bleeding. Discontinue use of ginseng and consult your doctor.

SPECIAL INFORMATION
❧ American ginseng is considered an endangered species because of excessive harvesting.

Ginseng, Asian
Panax ginseng

Growing on the mountains of northeast China, Asian ginseng is the most potent and expensive form of ginseng. With its yellow-green flowers and red berries, it looks like American ginseng, but the stalk is longer. Its active constituents are ginsenosides, substances that strengthen the immune system and increase the body's ability to deal with fatigue and stress. Herbalists prescribe Asian ginseng root for fever, colds, coughs, and menstrual irregularities.

■ TARGET AILMENTS
Take internally for depression, fatigue, stress, colds, flu, respiratory problems, inflammation, a damaged immune system.

PREPARATIONS
Over the counter: Ginseng is available as fresh or dried root, root powder, capsules, tablets, prepared tea, freeze-dried root, cured rock candy.
At home:
Decoction: Boil 1 oz fresh root with 1 cup water for 15 to 20 minutes. Drink up to 2 cups a day.

SIDE EFFECTS
Not serious: Headache, insomnia, anxiety, breast soreness, or skin rash.
Serious: Asthma attacks, increased blood pressure, heart palpitations, or postmenopausal uterine bleeding. Stop using ginseng and consult your doctor.

SPECIAL INFORMATION
❧ Use only under the direction of an herbalist or a healthcare professional if you are pregnant or have insomnia, hay fever, fibrocystic breasts, asthma, emphysema, high blood pressure, blood-clotting or heart disorders, or diabetes.

CONTINUED

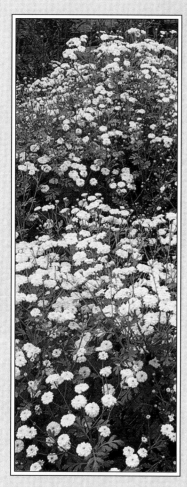

Feverfew

Ginseng, Siberian
Eleutherococcus senticosus

Found in the Siberian regions of Russia and China, Siberian ginseng, also called eleuthero, affects the body in a manner similar to Asian and American ginseng, although its effects are subtler and result in less-pronounced reactions. The active elements of Siberian ginseng are eleutherosides, which stimulate the immune system, increasing the body's resistance to disease, stress, and fatigue. Siberian ginseng has gained popularity as a Western herb because it does not cause the insomnia and anxiety that sometimes occur when Asian or American ginseng is used.

■ TARGET AILMENTS
Take internally for depression, fatigue, stress; colds, influenza, respiratory problems; inflammation, damaged immune system.

PREPARATIONS
Over the counter: Ginseng is available as fresh or dried root, root powder, capsules, tablets, prepared tea, freeze-dried root, cured rock candy.
At home:
Decoction: Boil 1 oz fresh root with 1 cup water for 15 to 20 minutes. Drink up to 2 cups a day.

SIDE EFFECTS
Not serious: Headaches, insomnia, anxiety, breast soreness, skin rashes.
Serious: Asthma attacks, increased blood pressure, heart palpitations, postmenopausal uterine bleeding.

SPECIAL INFORMATION
🍂 Siberian ginseng gained popularity in Russia when an extract was mass-produced and used in a popular colalike drink called Bodust, meaning "vigor."

Goldenseal
Hydrastis canadensis

Herbalists use the dried and powdered rhizomes and roots of the perennial goldenseal to treat several respiratory and skin infections. The herb acts as a stimulant and seems to affect the body's mucous membranes by drying up secretions, reducing inflammation, and fighting infection. Goldenseal also aids digestion and may control postpartum bleeding.

■ TARGET AILMENTS
Take internally for stomach problems; sore throat; infected gums, ears, and sinuses; postpartum bleeding.
Apply externally for eczema, ringworm, contact dermatitis, athlete's foot, impetigo.

PREPARATIONS
Over the counter: Dry root is available in bulk, capsules, and tincture.
At home:
Tea: Pour 1 cup boiling water onto 2 tsp goldenseal; steep for 10 to 15 minutes. Drink three times daily.
Combinations: Use with meadowsweet and chamomile for stomach problems. For a skin wash, mix with distilled witch hazel; for ear infections, make drops using goldenseal and mullein. See your herbalist for exact instructions.

SIDE EFFECTS
Not serious: In high doses, it can irritate the skin, mouth, and throat and cause nausea and diarrhea. If any of these develop, stop taking it.

SPECIAL INFORMATION
🍂 Do not take if you are pregnant.
🍂 Do not use goldenseal without consulting a physician if you have had heart disease, diabetes, glaucoma, a stroke, or high blood pressure.
🍂 Do not give goldenseal to children under two; for older children and older adults, start with small doses.

Gotu Kola
Centella asiatica

The gotu kola plant grows in marshy areas in many parts of the world. Its fan-shaped leaves contain the soothing agent known as asiaticoside. As a result they have been used to treat burns, skin grafts, and episiotomies. Gotu kola may also help heal outbreaks of psoriasis and may help decrease edema and promote blood circulation in the legs. It may therefore be useful in treating phlebitis.

■ TARGET AILMENTS
Take internally for poor circulation in the legs, edema.
Apply externally for burns, cuts, and other skin injuries; psoriasis. (Use a compress.)

PREPARATIONS
Over the counter: Available in dry bulk, capsules, and tincture.
At home:
Tea: Use 1 to 2 tsp dried gotu kola per cup of boiling water; drink twice daily to improve circulation.
Compress: Soak a pad in a tea or in a tincture to help treat wounds or psoriasis. Start with a weak solution and increase the concentration of gotu kola if necessary.

SIDE EFFECTS
Not serious: Gotu kola may cause a skin rash or headaches; in either case, lower your dosage or stop taking it.

SPECIAL INFORMATION
➤ Do not use gotu kola if you are pregnant or nursing, or using tranquilizers or sedatives, since gotu kola may have a narcotic effect.
➤ Do not give gotu kola to children under two. For older children and older adults, start with low-strength doses and increase if necessary.

Hawthorn
Crataegus laevigata
(or C. oxyacantha)

Herbalists use the flowers, fruit, and leaves of the hawthorn, a European shrub with thorny branches. They prescribe the herb as a mild heart tonic. It is thought to dilate the blood vessels, thereby facilitating the flow of blood in the arteries and lowering blood pressure. Hawthorn is also believed to increase the pumping force of the heart muscle and to eliminate arrhythmias. It may have a calming effect on the nervous system and is sometimes recommended as a remedy for insomnia.

■ TARGET AILMENTS
Take internally in conjunction with conventional medical treatment for high blood pressure, clogged arteries, heart palpitations, angina, inflammation of the heart muscle.
Take internally for insomnia and nervous conditions. Use as a gargle for sore throat.

PREPARATIONS
Hawthorn is available as fluidextract, dried berries and leaves, capsules.

SIDE EFFECTS
Serious: Taking large amounts of hawthorn may result in a dramatic drop in blood pressure, which in turn may cause you to feel faint.

SPECIAL INFORMATION
WARNING: Use hawthorn as a heart tonic only if you have been diagnosed with angina, cardiac arrhythmias, or congestive heart failure, and only in consultation with a physician. Do not practice self-diagnosis.
➤ Children and pregnant or nursing women should use hawthorn only under the direction of a medical herbalist or a licensed healthcare professional.

Horsetail
Equisetum arvense

Horsetail has been valued since ancient times for its ability to stem the flow of blood, bind tissues, and increase urine production. It is rich in silica, which helps mend broken bones and form collagen, a constituent of bones and tissue. Herbalists today prescribe horsetail for wounds, urinary problems, benign prostate disorders, and the pain of rheumatism or arthritis.

■ TARGET AILMENTS
Take internally for bladder and kidney problems, prostatitis, ulcers; broken bones or sprains; strengthening bones and nails; joint pain.
Apply externally for sores and inflammation.

PREPARATIONS
Over the counter: Available dried or fresh, in capsules, and in tincture.
At home:
Tea: Steep 2 tsp dried or 1 tbsp fresh herb per cup of boiling water for 15 minutes. Drink cold, up to 4 cups a day, 2 tbsp at a time. Apply to cuts.
Combinations: Use with hydrangea for prostate problems.

SIDE EFFECTS
Not serious: Upset stomach, diarrhea, increased urination. Discontinue and call your doctor.
Serious: Kidney or lower back pain, or pain on urination; cardiac problems. Call your doctor now.

SPECIAL INFORMATION
WARNING: Do not take for more than three days in a row, and follow the given dosage; extended use may cause kidney or cardiac damage.
➤ Use only under a doctor's care. Heart disease or high-blood-pressure patients should use with caution.
➤ Use mild doses for adults over 65 and children ages two to 12. Children under two and pregnant women should not use horsetail.

CONTINUED

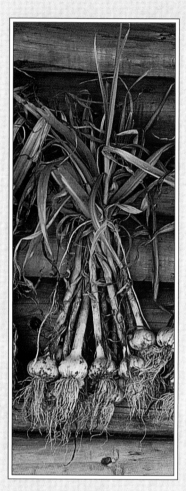

Garlic

Hyssop
Hyssopus officinalis

Hyssop, a member of the mint family, is used as an expectorant, digestive aid, sedative, and muscle relaxant. It is also used as an antiseptic; its oils may heal wounds and herpes simplex sores.

■ TARGET AILMENTS
Take internally for coughs, colds, bronchitis; indigestion, gas; anxiety, hysteria; petit mal seizures.
Apply externally for cold sores, genital herpes sores, burns, wounds, skin irritations.

PREPARATIONS
Over the counter: Available dried or fresh and as tincture.
At home:
Tea: Steep 2 tsp dried herb per cup of boiling water for 10 to 15 minutes. Drink three times a day for cough; gargle three times a day for sore throat. Apply to burns and wounds.
Compress: Steep 1 oz dried herb in 1 pt boiling water for 15 minutes; soak clean cloth in solution and apply warm to cold sores or genital herpes sores; place on the chest to relieve congestion.
Combinations: Used with white horehound and coltsfoot for coughs and bronchitis; with boneset, elder flower, and peppermint for cold symptoms; and with sage as a gargle for sore throats.

SIDE EFFECTS
Not serious: Upset stomach or diarrhea. Discontinue and call a doctor.

SPECIAL INFORMATION
🌙 Use hyssop only under medical supervision if you use it for more than three consecutive days.
🌙 Do not use hyssop if pregnant; it was once used to induce abortion.
🌙 Use low-strength preparations for adults over 65 or children between two and 12 years of age. Do not give to children under two years old.

Juniper
Juniperus communis

Juniper acts as a diuretic and thus is used to treat high blood pressure and PMS. Juniper oil is thought to have anti-inflammatory effects useful for treating arthritis and gout. Juniper teas can be taken for digestive problems.

■ TARGET AILMENTS
Take internally for bladder infections, cystitis, edema; digestive problems; menstrual irregularities and PMS; high blood pressure.
Apply externally for arthritis, gout.

PREPARATIONS
Over the counter: Available in whole berries, bulk, and capsules, and as tincture.
At home:
Tea: Steep 1 tsp ground juniper berries in 1 cup boiling water for 10 to 20 minutes. Drink at least two times daily. Do not use for more than six weeks at a time.

SIDE EFFECTS
Not serious: Individuals with hay fever may develop allergy symptoms such as nasal congestion when taking juniper. If this happens, stop taking the herb and call your doctor.
Serious: Juniper in high doses can irritate and damage the kidneys and urinary tract. If you develop diarrhea, intestinal pain, kidney pain, blood in the urine, purplish urine, or a faster heartbeat, stop taking juniper immediately and see your doctor as soon as possible.

SPECIAL INFORMATION
WARNING: Because it can irritate the kidneys and urinary tract, juniper is suitable for short-term use only.
WARNING: Do not use juniper if you have or have had kidney problems.
🌙 Pregnant women should not use juniper, because it may stimulate contraction of the uterus.

The 75 Most Effective Herbs

Kelp
Fucus spp.

Extracts of iodine-rich kelp, one of the many forms of seaweed, provided an effective goiter remedy for many years. Today some herbalists rely on another component of kelp's stemlike and leaf-like parts, an agent known as sodium alginate. Because of its action, kelp is prescribed to aid in the treatment of heavy-metal environmental pollutants, including barium and cadmium, and to prevent the body from absorbing strontium 90, a radioactive substance created in nuclear power plants.

Some practitioners of alternative medicine also recommend taking kelp supplements for thyroid disorders such as mild hypothyroidism (underactive thyroid).

■ TARGET AILMENTS
Take internally for goiter, hypothyroidism, radiation exposure, heavy-metal environmental pollutants.

PREPARATIONS
Over the counter: Available in dry bulk, capsules, and tincture.
At home:
Infusion: Steep 2 to 3 tsp dried or powdered kelp in 1 cup boiling water for 10 minutes; drink three times daily.

SIDE EFFECTS
None expected.

SPECIAL INFORMATION
WARNING: If you are already taking medication for hyperthyroidism (overactive thyroid), kelp supplements could worsen the condition.
WARNING: Do not gather your own wild kelp for use; coastal colonies may be contaminated by offshore pollutants.
WARNING: Check with your practitioner before using kelp if you have a history of thyroid problems or high blood pressure.

Lavender
Lavandula officinalis

A fragrant herb that scents clothes and helps repel moths, lavender also has medicinal properties. Herbalists prescribe lavender tea and the essential oil of lavender, both made from the plant's flowers, to treat common minor ailments such as insomnia, headache, and nausea. Anecdotal evidence suggests that lavender has a calming effect that relieves anxiety and promotes gastrointestinal relaxation. Its aroma (particularly that of *L. angustifolia*) is thought to stimulate mental processes and help alleviate depression, especially when it is used with other herbs. Like many aromatic essential oils, lavender oil has antiseptic qualities that may kill several types of disease-causing bacteria, and herbalists use it to treat skin ailments such as fungus, burns, wounds, and eczema.

■ TARGET AILMENTS
Take internally for insomnia, depression, or headache, especially when caused by stress; poor digestion, nausea, flatulence, colic.
Apply externally for burns, wounds, eczema, acne, candidiasis, ringworm, rheumatism.

PREPARATIONS
Over the counter: Available in dried bulk, capsules, oil, and tincture.
At home:
Tea: Steep 1 tsp dried flowers in 1 cup boiling water for 10 minutes; drink three times daily.
Oil: To relax, use a few drops of the essential oil in a bath; rub it on your skin to ease rheumatic pains; or use a few drops in a steam inhalation for coughs, colds, and flu.
Combinations: For depression, lavender can be used with rosemary, skullcap, or kola.

SPECIAL INFORMATION
WARNING: Do not use oil of lavender internally.

Licorice
Glycyrrhiza glabra

Licorice is one of the most commonly used medicinal herbs. Its intense sweetness masks the bitterness in any herbal mixture. Chinese and Western herbalists use licorice root as a cough suppressant and also prescribe it for digestive disorders, believing that it acts as a mild laxative and prevents stomach ulcers by forming a protective coating on the stomach wall. Practitioners think that licorice, as an external antibiotic, relieves skin irritations such as eczema and herpes sores.

■ TARGET AILMENTS
Take internally for cough, sore throat, colic, constipation, heartburn, stomach ulcers, arthritis, hepatitis, cirrhosis.
Apply externally for skin infections, eczema, herpes sores.

PREPARATIONS
Over the counter: Available as dried root, liquid extract, and capsules.
At home:
Tea: Prepare by boiling 1 oz licorice root in 1 cup water for 15 to 20 minutes. Drink up to 2 cups daily.
Antibiotic: Sprinkle licorice powder directly on the infection or sore.

SIDE EFFECTS
Not serious: Upset stomach, diarrhea, headache, edema (fluid retention), grogginess, weakness.

SPECIAL INFORMATION
WARNING: Large amounts of licorice taken over a long period can lead to high blood pressure and edema. Consult your practitioner for advice.
➤ Do not use licorice root if you have edema, high blood pressure, kidney disease, or glaucoma.
➤ Avoid the herb if you are pregnant. It increases production of aldosterone, a hormone that regulates the salt and water balance in the body, resulting in a rise in blood pressure.

CONTINUED

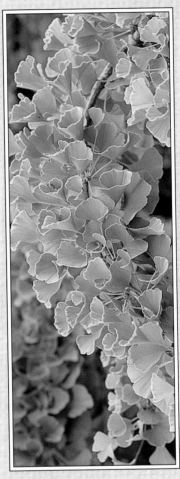

Ginkgo

Lobelia
Lobelia inflata

Lobelia, sometimes called Indian tobacco, is prescribed for both respiratory ailments and external conditions, but it can be extremely toxic. Because it is thought to relax overworked bronchial muscles and promote coughing, lobelia is most widely used to treat respiratory illnesses. Lobelia compresses have been used to treat skin injuries, fungus infections, and muscle strains.

■ TARGET AILMENTS
Take internally for pneumonia, asthma, bronchitis.
Apply externally for bruises, insect bites, poison ivy, fungus infections including ringworm, muscle strains.

PREPARATIONS
Over the counter: Available in dried bulk, capsules, and tincture.
At home:
Tea: Steep ¼ to ½ tsp dried leaves in 1 cup boiling water for 10 to 15 minutes; drink three times daily.
Compress: Soak a piece of cloth in an infusion for several minutes; wring out and apply to affected area.
Combinations: For asthma, use with cayenne, skunk cabbage, and ginger.

SIDE EFFECTS
Serious:
WARNING: Lobelia poisoning can cause nausea, excessive salivation, diarrhea, impaired hearing and vision, weakness, and mental confusion, and if not treated promptly can bring on respiratory failure and even death. If you develop any side effects, call your doctor at once.

SPECIAL INFORMATION
WARNING: Use lobelia only in doses prescribed by your practitioner.
➤ If your practitioner prescribes lobelia for your child, monitor the child frequently for the development of any side effects.

Lycium Fruit
Lycium barbarum
(or *L. chinense*)

Similar in appearance and action, the berries of both Lycium barbarum and Lycium chinense are large, soft, and red. The fruit is sometimes known as wolfberry. In traditional Chinese medical terms, the two herbs are classified as sweet and neutral. Lycium chinense appears largely in Hebei Province, while the more common Lycium barbarum grows in a number of Chinese provinces.

■ TARGET AILMENTS
Take internally for night blindness, tinnitus (ringing in the ears), dizziness, and blurred vision; consumptive coughs; diabetes; sore back, knees, and legs; impotence and nocturnal emission.

PREPARATIONS
Lycium fruit, both fresh and in the form of tablets, can be obtained from Chinese pharmacies, Asian markets, and some Western health food stores. The fruit is usually added to a dish during the last five minutes of cooking.

Combinations: When mixed with cuscuta, eucommia bark, and Chinese foxglove root cooked in wine, lycium fruit is prescribed for impotence, dizziness, and tinnitus. Practitioners also use the fruit to treat consumptive coughs, combining it with ophiopogon tuber, anemarrhena, and fritillaria.

SPECIAL INFORMATION
➤ You should not take this herb if you suffer from an inflammatory ailment, weak digestion, or a tendency to become bloated.
➤ In a laboratory test, lycium was administered intravenously to rabbits; it seemed to reduce the blood pressure of these animals and to calm labored breathing.

The 75 Most Effective Herbs

Magnolia Flower
Magnolia liliflora
(or M. denudata)

More accurately described as magnolia buds, this herb is the unopened magnolia flower. Chinese medicine practitioners prescribe it for blocked nasal and sinus passages. The best-quality buds are green and dry; they should include none of the stems or branches. The herb is characterized in traditional Chinese medicine as acrid and warm. Growing in several Chinese provinces, magnolia is harvested in early spring, before the flowers unfold.

■ TARGET AILMENTS
Take internally for nasal congestion, nasal discharge, sinus headaches, other sinus disorders.

PREPARATIONS
Magnolia buds are available in bulk at Chinese pharmacies, Asian markets, and some Western health food stores.

Combinations: Magnolia flowers are mixed with xanthium, angelica *(Angelica dahurica)*, and field mint to treat nasal congestion and sinus headaches, and with chrysanthemum flowers *(Chrysanthemum morifolium)* and siegesbeckia for frontal sinusitis. Consult an herbal practitioner for details of other mixtures and doses.

SIDE EFFECTS
Not serious: Because of its hairy texture, the herb can irritate the throat. Rub the herb with cotton cloth or place it in cheesecloth before mixing it into a solution. In addition, overdoses can cause dizziness and red eyes.

SPECIAL INFORMATION
☙ In test-tube studies, magnolia flowers seemed to inhibit the growth of several fungi on the skin.

Marsh Mallow
Althaea officinalis

For centuries people in Europe and the Middle East have eaten wild-growing marsh mallow when their crops failed. Today it is still recognized as a wilderness forage food. Herbalists use the roots, and sometimes the leaves, to treat cuts and wounds, mouth sores, stomach distress, and other ailments. And teething, irritable babies and toddlers have traditionally found comfort in sucking on a root of marsh mallow.

The healing substance in marsh mallow is mucilage, a spongy root material that forms a gel when mixed with water and is especially soothing to inflamed mucous membranes. One study suggests that mucilage supports the immune system's white blood cells in their fight against invading microbes. Another trial indicates that marsh mallow may help to lower blood sugar.

■ TARGET AILMENTS
Take internally for sore throat, coughs, colds, flu, bronchitis, sinusitis; upset stomach, peptic ulcers, gastritis, colitis; cystitis, bladder infections, urethritis, kidney stones.
Apply externally for abscesses, boils, skin ulcers, scrapes, cuts, burns, other wounds; varicose veins; dental abscesses and gingivitis.

PREPARATIONS
Over the counter: Available in dried bulk, capsules, tincture.
At home:
Decoction: Simmer 1 to 2 tsp finely chopped or crushed root in 1 cup water for 10 to 15 minutes; drink three times daily. Use the decoction as a gargle for mouth problems.
Gel: Add just enough water to the finely chopped root to give it a gel-like consistency and use for skin problems.

SPECIAL INFORMATION
☙ Marsh mallow can be given in low doses to infants and children.

Milk Thistle
Silybum marianum

Milk thistle is used by herbalists to treat such liver disorders as cirrhosis and hepatitis. The active ingredient, silymarin, found in the seeds, is believed to prompt the growth of new, healthy liver cells without encouraging any malignancy that may be present. It is also thought that silymarin acts as an antioxidant, protecting the liver from damage by free radicals, harmful byproducts of many bodily processes. The use of silymarin by healthy people can greatly increase the liver's content of glutathione, a key agent in detoxifying many potentially harmful substances.

Extracts of silymarin appear to neutralize toxins from the death cup mushroom, which can inflict lethal injury on the liver. Milk thistle also is believed to ease outbreaks of psoriasis, since these may worsen when the liver fails to neutralize certain toxins.

■ TARGET AILMENTS
Take internally for liver problems; inflammation of the gallbladder duct; poisoning from ingestion of the death cup mushroom; psoriasis.

PREPARATIONS
Over the counter: Available in dried bulk, capsules, extract.
At home:
Tea: Steep 1 tsp freshly ground seeds in 1 cup boiling water for 10 to 15 minutes; drink three times daily. Or eat 1 tsp of freshly ground seeds. Milk thistle extract may be more effective than teas, since silymarin is only slightly water soluble. See an herbalist for more information.

SIDE EFFECTS
Not serious: Because taking milk thistle increases bile secretion, you may develop loose stools.

SPECIAL INFORMATION
WARNING: If you think you have a liver disorder, seek medical advice.

CONTINUED

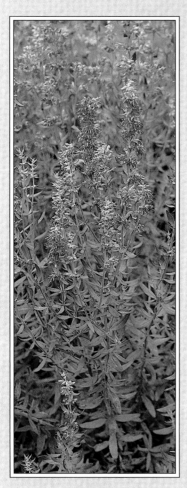

Hyssop

Mugwort Leaf
Artemisia argyi (or A. vulgaris)

Mugwort leaf is prescribed in Chinese medicine for a range of gynecological problems. In China mugwort is harvested at the end of spring or in early summer, when the leaves are growing vigorously but the flowers have not yet bloomed. The best leaves are grayish white with a thick, hairy texture. In Western tradition it is used to aid digestion and combat depression.

■ TARGET AILMENTS
Take internally for excessive menstrual bleeding and cramps, uterine bleeding, vaginal pain and bleeding during pregnancy, threatened miscarriage; a digestive aid; depression.

PREPARATIONS
Leaves are available in bulk at some health food stores and Asian markets and pharmacies. The herb is also sold in pills. The dried, aged, powdered herb can be rolled in tissue paper into a cigarlike cylinder; one end is burned near the site of an injury to increase blood circulation and relieve pain. Acupuncturists sometimes use this technique instead of inserting needles.

Combinations: A mixture with gelatin is prescribed for vaginal bleeding and pain during pregnancy or for spotting between periods. Combining mugwort with dried ginger targets menstrual pain. And a preparation of mugwort leaves and kochia fruit is applied to itching lesions on the skin. For information on dosages and other preparations, check with an herbal practitioner.

SIDE EFFECTS
None expected.

SPECIAL INFORMATION
❧ A clinical trial suggests that crushed fresh leaves may eradicate warts.
❧ The herb seems to indicate an antibiotic effect in test-tube studies.

Mullein
Verbascum thapsus

Mullein is useful in treating diarrhea and hemorrhoids and, as an expectorant, bronchitis and coughs. The dried leaves, flowers, and roots are all used.

■ TARGET AILMENTS
Take internally for respiratory ailments; gastrointestinal problems such as stomach cramps, diarrhea.
Apply externally for external ulcers, tumors, hemorrhoids.

PREPARATIONS
Over the counter: Mullein is available as tincture and as dried leaves, flowers, or roots.
At home:
Tea: Steep 1 to 2 tsp dried leaves, flowers, or roots per cup of boiling water for 10 or 15 minutes. Drink as many as 3 cups a day.
Compress: Soak bandages in a cooled tea made with vinegar; apply to ulcers, tumors, or hemorrhoids.
Inhalant: Boil fresh leaves in water and inhale the steam to relieve coughs and congestion.
Combinations: With elder and red clover to ease painful coughing; with gumweed for asthma; as an extract in olive oil for external ulcers, hemorrhoids, and tumors; with white horehound, coltsfoot, and lobelia for treating bronchitis.

SIDE EFFECTS
Not serious: Mild stomach upset or diarrhea. Reduce dosage or discontinue; consult your doctor when convenient.

SPECIAL INFORMATION
WARNING: If you have a history of cancer, consult your doctor before ingesting this herb; the tannin in mullein may be carcinogenic.
WARNING: Do not ingest the seeds; they are toxic.
WARNING: Do not take mullein if you are pregnant or nursing a baby.

The 75 Most Effective Herbs

Myrrh
Commiphora molmol

Myrrh, an oil found in the bark of certain shrubs, hardens into nuggets, called gum resin, which are powdered to make the healing herb. Myrrh fights infection by stimulating production of white blood cells and by a direct antibacterial action. It is also used as a fragrance in cosmetics and perfumes.

■ TARGET AILMENTS
Take internally for sinusitis, chest congestion, asthma, coughs, colds, boils; use as a mouthwash or gargle for mouth and throat infections.
Apply externally for wounds, abrasions (combine with witch hazel).

PREPARATIONS
Over the counter: Available as tincture and as an ingredient in toothpastes, and as a powder.
At home:
Mouthwash: Steep 1 tsp powdered herb and 1 tsp boric acid in 1 pt boiling water. Let stand 30 minutes and strain; use when cool.
Tea: Steep 1 to 2 tsp powdered herb per cup of boiling water for 10 to 15 minutes. Drink three times a day.

SIDE EFFECTS
Not serious: May cause stomach upset or diarrhea. Use a smaller amount less often or discontinue.
Serious: Large amounts may have a violent laxative action and may cause sweating, vomiting, kidney problems, or accelerated heartbeat. Stop using and call your doctor.

SPECIAL INFORMATION
WARNING: Any resin tends to be hard to eliminate and can cause minor kidney damage if taken internally for extended periods. Consult your physician or herbalist before using if you are pregnant or nursing, or have kidney disease. Do not exceed recommended doses and do not give to children younger than two.

Nettle
Urtica dioica

Notorious for its stinging needles, nettle can be safely ingested when boiled or dried. Herbalists consider nettle a diuretic capable of removing toxins. Nettle has an erect stem and serrated, heart-shaped, dark green leaves.

■ TARGET AILMENTS
Take internally for arthritis, gout, hay fever, premenstrual syndrome, vaginal yeast infections, excessive menstrual flow, hemorrhoids, eczema, diarrhea, chronic cystitis.
Take internally only under a doctor's supervision for high blood pressure, congestive heart failure.

PREPARATIONS
Over the counter: Nettle is available as tincture, capsules, and dried leaves and stems.
At home:
Tea: Steep 1 to 2 tsp dried herb in 1 cup boiling water for 10 minutes. Drink up to 2 cups a day.
Juice: Add 2 tsp juice squeezed from nettle to a vegetable or fruit drink.
Combinations: Nettle combines well with figwort and burdock to treat eczema; take orally as juice or tea.

SIDE EFFECTS
Not serious: Large doses of nettle tea may cause stomach irritation, constipation, burning skin, or urinary suppression. Stop taking the herb and call your doctor.

SPECIAL INFORMATION
WARNING: Do not use uncooked nettle; it may cause kidney damage and other symptoms of poisoning.
WARNING: Nettle is a diuretic, and it may therefore remove potassium from the body. If you use it frequently, eat foods high in potassium.
❧ Do not give nettle to children younger than two years old.
❧ To harvest, wear gloves and long pants and sleeves to avoid the sting.

Notoginseng Root
Panax notoginseng

Notoginseng root is employed in Chinese medicine to stop bleeding, reduce swelling, and alleviate pain from injuries. Unlike Western medications it seems to halt the bleeding without making the blood clot, and to stop the clotting or hematoma without causing bleeding. Practitioners of sports medicine in the West frequently use this herb as a tonic to improve stamina. The best variety, also known as pseudoginseng root (Panax pseudoginseng), is large, solid, and dark brown, with thin skin.

■ TARGET AILMENTS
Take internally for internal bleeding such as nosebleeds and blood in the stool and urine, coughing up blood.
Use both internally and externally for bleeding from injuries; swelling and pain of fractures; falls; contusions and sprains, cuts, and gunshot wounds.

PREPARATIONS
Available in bulk from Chinese pharmacies, Asian markets, and Western health food stores, where it is sold as loose, dried roots or as tablets.

Combinations: Notoginseng can be made into a liniment for swelling and pain and is included in many injury tonics. A preparation containing notoginseng root and bletilla root is prescribed for vomiting, and for coughing up blood, nosebleeds, and blood in the urine. For information on appropriate preparations and doses, check with an herbal practitioner.

SPECIAL INFORMATION
WARNING: Pregnant women should avoid this herb; it may cause a miscarriage under certain conditions.
❧ Notoginseng is sometimes used to treat acute attacks of Crohn's disease.

CONTINUED

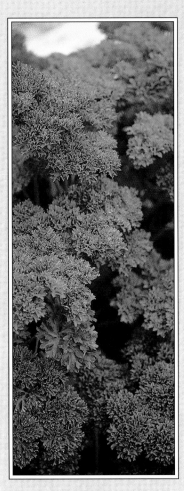

Parsley

Parsley
Petroselinum crispum

Added to salads and cooked foods or used as a garnish, the feathery leaves of parsley are a source of vitamins C and A, as well as a versatile herbal remedy. Because it eases muscle spasms and cramps, parsley is used as a digestive aid, and it is prescribed as a diuretic and mild laxative. Parsley is also considered to be an expectorant.

■ TARGET AILMENTS
Take internally for indigestion, congestion from coughs and colds, asthma, irregular menstruation, premenstrual syndrome, fever.

Take internally under a doctor's supervision for high blood pressure, congestive heart failure.

PREPARATIONS
Over the counter: Available as tincture and as fresh or dried leaves, seeds, stems, and roots.

At home:
Tea: Steep 1 to 2 tsp dried leaves or roots per cup of boiling water for 5 to 10 minutes in a closed container. Drink up to 3 cups a day.

Nutrition and diet: Eat raw green leaves as a breath freshener.

SIDE EFFECTS
None expected.

SPECIAL INFORMATION
WARNING: Pregnant and nursing women should not take parsley juice or oil in medicinal doses. Eating a few sprigs served as garnish will probably not cause any harm.

WARNING: If you use this herb frequently as a medicine, you should also eat foods high in potassium, such as bananas, because diuretics deplete the body of potassium.

➤ Do not give medicinal doses to children younger than two years old.

➤ Only experienced field botanists should pick wild parsley, because of its resemblance to toxic plants.

Passionflower
Passiflora incarnata

Because of its purported calming effect on the central nervous system, herbalists use passionflower as a sedative, a digestive aid, and a pain reliever.

■ TARGET AILMENTS
Take internally for insomnia, anxiety, neuralgia, shingles, persistent hiccups, asthma, and to aid withdrawal from addictive disorders.

PREPARATIONS
Over the counter: Available in commercial homeopathic or herbal remedies and as dried or fresh leaves, capsules, and tincture.

At home:
Tea: Steep 2 tsp dried herb per cup of boiling water for 15 minutes. For insomnia, drink 1 cup in the evening.

Tincture: 1 dropperful in warm water, up to four times a day, for anxiety in adults and in children weighing more than 100 pounds. For smaller children, consult a trained practitioner for dosages and give only under medical supervision.

SIDE EFFECTS
Not serious: Gastric upset, diarrhea. Discontinue and call your doctor.

Serious: May cause sleepiness; do not take during the day if you operate heavy machinery or drive.

SPECIAL INFORMATION
➤ Always use passionflower under medical supervision.

➤ Use only professionally prepared remedies; another species, *Passiflora caerulea,* contains cyanide.

➤ Do not take if you are pregnant.

➤ Use low-strength preparations for adults over 65 or children between two and 12 years old. Do not give to children under two years of age.

POSSIBLE INTERACTIONS
Use caution when combining with prescription sedatives.

The 75 Most Effective Herbs

Pau d'Arco
Tabebuia impetiginosa

Pau d'arco is the name of both a tree and a medicinal extract from the tree's bark or heartwood. The extract is believed to be effective against bacterial, fungal, viral, and parasitic infections, and is also considered to be an anti-inflammatory agent. It is thought to destroy microorganisms by increasing the supply of oxygen to cells. For centuries before modern science isolated some 20 of its chemical ingredients, pau d'arco was used as a folk remedy. The pau d'arco tree, also called the trumpet tree, is native to Central and South America and the West Indies. It can reach a height of 125 feet.

■ **TARGET AILMENTS**
Take internally for bacterial, fungal, viral, and parasitic infections; indigestion.

PREPARATIONS
Over the counter: Pau d'arco is available as capsules, tincture, and dried bark.
At home:
Decoction: Boil 1 tbsp bark in 2 to 3 cups water for 10 to 15 minutes. Drink 2 to 8 cups a day.

SIDE EFFECTS
None expected.

Peppermint
Mentha piperita

Peppermint plants have stems with a purplish cast; long, serrated leaves; and a familiar minty aroma. This common, pleasant-tasting herb has been used as a remedy for indigestion since the time of the pharaohs of ancient Egypt. Menthol, the principal active ingredient, stimulates the stomach lining, thereby reducing the amount of time food spends in the stomach. It also relaxes the muscles of the digestive system.

■ **TARGET AILMENTS**
Take internally for cramps, stomach pain, gas, nausea associated with migraine headaches, morning sickness, travel sickness, insomnia, anxiety, fever, colds, flu.
Apply externally for itching and inflammation.

PREPARATIONS
Over the counter: Available as commercial tea, tincture, and fresh or dried leaves and flowers.
At home:
Tea: Drink commercial brands or steep 1 to 2 heaping tsp dried herb per cup of boiling water for 10 minutes. Drink up to 3 cups a day.
Bath: Fill a cloth bag with several handfuls of dried or fresh herb and let hot water run over it.

SIDE EFFECTS
None expected.

SPECIAL INFORMATION
WARNING: Do not ingest pure menthol or pure peppermint; these substances are extremely toxic.
➤ Give only very dilute preparations to children younger than two and only under a doctor's supervision.
➤ Pregnant women with morning sickness should use a dilute tea rather than a more potent infusion. Peppermint should not be used by women who have a history of miscarriage.

Polygonum
Polygonum multiflorum (root)

Polygonum, which is also known as fleeceflower root and frequently called fo-ti by practitioners, is prescribed in Chinese medicine for a wide variety of disorders ranging from signs of premature aging to symptoms of malaria.

■ **TARGET AILMENTS**
Take internally for dizziness and blurred vision; insomnia; prematurely gray hair; nocturnal emission; vaginal discharge; carbuncles, sores, abscesses, scrofula, goiter, and neck lumps; constipation; sore knees and back; malaria (chronic only, not the acute stages).

PREPARATIONS
Polygonum is available at Chinese pharmacies, Asian markets, and some Western health food stores. It can also be found in pill form.

Combinations: With lycium fruit, psorolea fruit, and cuscuta, it is prescribed for sore knees and back, dizziness, and premature aging. A preparation containing polygonum, scrophularia, and forsythia fruit is prescribed for scrofula, abscesses, and other swellings. A combination with Asian ginseng, dong quai, and tangerine peel is recommended for chronic malarial symptoms. For information on dosages and additional preparations, check with a Chinese medicine practitioner.

SIDE EFFECTS
Not serious: May cause flushing of face, diarrhea, and gastric distress.

SPECIAL INFORMATION
➤ The herb is not prescribed for patients with phlegm or diarrhea.

POSSIBLE INTERACTIONS
Some traditional sources suggest that you should not take this herb with onions, chives, or garlic.

CONTINUED

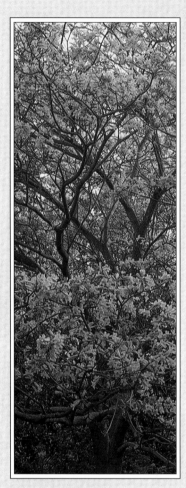

Pau d'Arco

Psyllium
Plantago psyllium

Psyllium, whose seeds, rich in fiber, make a safe, bulk-forming laxative, has long been used to treat constipation, diarrhea, hemorrhoids, and urinary problems. Because the herb absorbs excess fluid in the intestinal tract and increases stool volume, both diarrhea and constipation can be treated.

■ TARGET AILMENTS
Take internally for constipation, hemorrhoidal irritation, diarrhea.

PREPARATIONS
Over the counter: Available as whole seeds, ground or powdered seeds, and in various commercial bulk-forming laxative preparations.
At home:
Drink: Mix 1 tsp ground seeds or powder in 1 cup cool liquid. Drink 2 to 3 cups a day.
Seeds: Take 1 tsp seeds with water at mealtimes.

SIDE EFFECTS
Not serious: Psyllium can cause allergic reactions in people who have allergies to dust or grasses. Call your doctor if bothersome.
Serious: Severe allergic reactions are rare; if you have difficulty breathing, seek emergency help.

SPECIAL INFORMATION
WARNING: To prevent intestinal blockage when taking psyllium as a laxative, you must drink 8 to 10 glasses of water throughout the day.
❧ Start using this herb gradually to allow your body to adjust to the increase in fiber.
❧ Do not give this herb to children younger than two years of age. Consult your pediatrician if your infant or child is constipated.
❧ If you are pregnant you should avoid psyllium and all laxatives, because they stimulate the lower pelvis near the uterus.

Red Clover
Trifolium pratense

The medicinal parts of this perennial are the red or purple ball-shaped flowers. Herbalists prescribe red clover for skin ailments, indigestion, and coughs. It is an anti-inflammatory agent and, as an expectorant, helps remove excess mucus from the lungs. In addition, the herb appears to act like the female hormone estrogen; it is believed to help women with menopausal symptoms.

■ TARGET AILMENTS
Take internally for coughs, bronchitis, whooping cough, indigestion, menopausal symptoms.
Use internally and externally for skin problems such as eczema and psoriasis.

PREPARATIONS
Over the counter: Red clover is available in dried bulk and tincture.
At home:
Tea: Steep 1 to 3 tsp dried flower tops in 1 cup boiling water for 15 minutes. Drink up to 3 cups daily.
Compress: Soak a clean cloth in the infusion and apply to the skin.

SIDE EFFECTS
Serious: Discontinue use if you experience stomachaches or diarrhea.

SPECIAL INFORMATION
WARNING: Do not use red clover if you are pregnant, because of its estrogen-like behavior.
WARNING: Avoid the herb if you have estrogen-dependent cancer or a history of heart disease, stroke, or thrombophlebitis.
❧ If you are taking birth-control pills, consult your doctor before using red clover.
❧ Do not give the herb to children under two. Older children and people over 65 should start with a low dose and increase as needed.

The 75 Most Effective Herbs

Red Raspberry
Rubus idaeus

The berry of this biennial bush is commonly used in desserts, but herbalists value the leaves. These have high concentrations of tannin, a chemical that herbalists believe is effective in treating diarrhea, nausea, vomiting, and morning sickness in pregnancy. It is also thought that tannin, an astringent substance, helps prevent miscarriages and, during labor, checks hemorrhaging, strengthens contractions, and reduces labor pains; you should not, however, use red raspberry for this purpose at home. Red raspberry leaves are included in several herbal pregnancy formulas sold in the U.S. The herb is also used as a gargle for sore throats.

■ TARGET AILMENTS
Take internally for morning sickness, threatened miscarriage, problems arising during labor, diarrhea, mouth ulcers, bleeding gums.

PREPARATIONS
Over the counter: Available as dried leaves or berries and as tincture.
At home:
Infusion: Use 1 to 2 tsp dried leaves or berries per cup of boiling water. Steep for 10 to 15 minutes. Drink cold and as desired. During pregnancy, steep ½ oz dried leaves with 1 pt boiling water for 3 to 5 minutes and drink warm, 1 pt per day. For children, dilute with more water.

SIDE EFFECTS
Not serious: May cause stomach upset or diarrhea if you exceed the recommended dose.

SPECIAL INFORMATION
- Pregnant women should take red raspberry only with the consent and under the supervision of a physician.
- Animal tests suggest that red raspberry may reduce levels of glucose (blood sugar) and hence may help in the management of diabetes.

Rosemary
Rosmarinus officinalis

Herbalists believe the leaves of rosemary stimulate the circulatory and nervous systems and serve as an antidepressant. The leaves are thought to contain antispasmodic chemicals that relax the smooth muscle lining of the digestive tract and also are used to treat muscle pain. Rosemary has antibacterial and antifungal properties.

■ TARGET AILMENTS
Take internally for indigestion, upper respiratory tract infections that require a decongestant, tension, muscle pain, sprains, rheumatism, neuralgia.
Apply externally, as an antiseptic, for skin infections.

PREPARATIONS
Over the counter: Available as dried bulk, tincture, and two types of oil, one for internal use and the other for external application.
At home:
Tea: Use 1 tsp crushed leaves per cup of boiling water. Steep 15 minutes. To settle the stomach or clear a stuffy nose, drink 3 cups a day. For children younger than two, dilute the infusion with more water.

SIDE EFFECTS
Not serious: Rosemary oil for internal use may cause mild stomach, kidney, and intestinal irritation, even in small doses. If you experience any of these discomforts, consult your physician.
Serious: Rosemary oil, taken internally in large amounts, can be poisonous. Keep to the prescribed dosage.

SPECIAL INFORMATION
WARNING: Do not confuse rosemary oil for internal use with that for external use.. Never ingest the latter.
- Do not use if you are pregnant.

Sage
Salvia officinalis

The scientific name of sage, Salvia, derives from the Latin for "to save," which underscores the herb's early reputation as a cure-all. Modern herbalists believe sage contains an aromatic oil that reduces excessive perspiration and night sweats. Sage has antiseptic and astringent properties. It is also used to aid digestion, cleanse wounds, and stem lactation in nursing mothers.

■ TARGET AILMENTS
Take internally for indigestion, gas, nausea, and to stem lactation or reduce the night sweats of menopause.
Apply externally for bacterial infections in wounds; insect bites.

PREPARATIONS
Over the counter: Available as tincture, tea, and dried or fresh leaves.
At home:
Tea: Steep 2 to 3 tsp leaves per cup of boiling water for 10 minutes. Drink 3 cups a day or use as a wash for infected wounds.
Compress: Soak a clean cloth in the infusion and apply to insect bites.
Fresh: Apply fresh sage leaves to minor cuts or scrapes before washing and bandaging.

SIDE EFFECTS
Not serious: Drinking the tea may inflame the lips and mouth lining.

SPECIAL INFORMATION
WARNING: Sage contains the toxic chemical thujone, which can lead to convulsions if taken in high doses. However, the heat of cooking or preparing an infusion reduces toxicity. Sage oil should not be ingested.
- Do not take if you are pregnant or nursing, or if you have epilepsy.
- Use dilute preparations for children under 12 and adults over 65.

CONTINUED

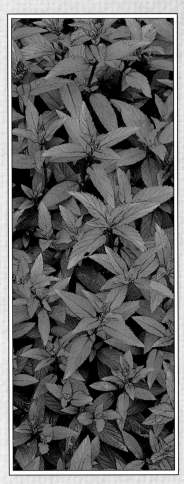

Peppermint

Saw Palmetto
Serenoa repens

An extract made from the berries of this shrub is used to treat and strengthen the male reproductive system. It is particularly recommended for benign prostatic hyperplasia, or enlargement of the prostate gland. Common among men over 50, the condition is thought to be caused by an accumulation of a testosterone derivative called dihydrotestosterone, which saw palmetto appears to block the production of. The herb has also been used as an expectorant, diuretic, tonic, antiseptic, sedative, and digestive aid.

■ TARGET AILMENTS
Take internally for benign prostatic hyperplasia; nasal congestion; asthma and bronchitis; coughs due to colds; sore throats; sinus ailments.

PREPARATIONS
Over the counter: Available as fresh or dried berries and in powder or capsule form. Gel capsules are preferable to tea or tincture.
At home:
Infusion: Steep ½ to 1 tsp fresh berries per cup of boiling water for 10 minutes. Drink 6 oz, two or three times a day.
Decoction: Add ½ to 1 tsp dried berries to 1 cup water, bring to a boil, and simmer for 5 minutes. Drink three times daily.
Tincture: Drink 15 to 60 drops in water two or three times daily.

SIDE EFFECTS
None expected.

SPECIAL INFORMATION
WARNING: Do not substitute saw palmetto for medical treatment. Because the symptoms of prostate enlargement and prostate cancer are similar, men should see a doctor when they have symptoms such as urine retention, dribbling, and passage of blood in the urine.

Skullcap
Scutellaria baicalensis

Chinese herbalists prescribe the root of skullcap for a wide range of disorders.

■ TARGET AILMENTS
Take internally for diarrhea, dysentery; upper respiratory infections with fever; urinary tract infections, jaundice, hepatitis; tension, irritability, headache, insomnia, epileptic and other seizures; red face or eyes; coughing up or vomiting blood, nosebleeds, blood in the stool; abdominal pain and vaginal bleeding, threatened miscarriage, PMS.

PREPARATIONS
Available in bulk from Chinese pharmacies, Asian markets, and Western health food stores. The herb can also be obtained as pills. The root is usually decocted, but it can be fried dry for use in pregnancy and to treat diarrhea and infections of the urinary tract, or cooked in wine for upper respiratory infections and redness of the face and eyes.

Combinations: A mixture with coptis is prescribed for high fever and irritability. Skullcap root mixed with anemarrhena is thought to alleviate chronic coughs. For further information on preparations and doses, consult a Chinese medicine practitioner.

SIDE EFFECTS
None expected.

SPECIAL INFORMATION
❧ Before using skullcap to treat diarrhea or the problems of pregnancy, check with a Chinese medicine practitioner.

POSSIBLE INTERACTIONS
Some sources in traditional Chinese medicine suggest that skullcap counteracts the effects of moutan and veratrum.

The 75 Most Effective Herbs

Skullcap
Scutellaria lateriflora

Skullcap's leaves and blue flowers are used in many over-the-counter herbal sleep remedies. Some researchers report that skullcap calms the nervous system. Chinese medicine physicians use it to treat hepatitis. In the United States, however, skullcap is considered controversial and even useless by many medical authorities, at least partly because of its early—and unearned—reputation for curing rabies, for which it garnered the now archaic name of mad dog weed. Its current name comes from a caplike appendage on the upper lip of the flower.

■ TARGET AILMENTS
Take internally for nervous tension; headaches, muscle aches, and symptoms of PMS aggravated or caused by stress; insomnia; convulsions; drug or alcohol withdrawal.

PREPARATIONS
Over the counter: Available as prepared tea, tincture, dried leaves, or capsules.
At home:
Tea: Pour 1 cup boiling water over 2 tsp dried leaves and steep for 10 to 15 minutes; drink this amount up to three times daily.
Tincture: Take ½ to 1 tsp per 8-oz glass of warm water.

SIDE EFFECTS
Not serious: Stomach upset or diarrhea. Reduce intake or stop using it.

SPECIAL INFORMATION
WARNING: Skullcap may cause drowsiness. Do not operate a car or heavy machinery after taking it.
WARNING: Taking large amounts of the tincture may cause confusion, giddiness, twitching, and possibly convulsions.
✒ Skullcap in medicinal amounts should be used only under professional supervision.

Slippery Elm
Ulmus fulva

The U.S. Food and Drug Administration calls slippery elm a good demulcent, or soothing agent. Herbalists recommend its use externally to ease wounds and skin problems, and internally to soothe sore throats, coughing, and diarrhea and other gastrointestinal disorders. Slippery elm's active ingredient is found in the white inner bark, whose mucilaginous cells expand into a spongy mass when mixed with water.

■ TARGET AILMENTS
Apply externally for wounds, cuts, abrasions.
Take internally for coughing, sore throats, digestive complaints.
Use externally and internally for gynecological problems.

PREPARATIONS
Over the counter: Available in health food stores as capsules, tea, powder.
At home:
Poultice: For wounds that have been thoroughly cleansed with soap and water, moisten powdered bark with enough water to make a paste; apply to wound and allow to dry. This forms a natural bandage that delivers soothing agents to the wound.
Tea: Add 2 tsp powder to a cup of boiling water; simmer for 15 minutes. Drink up to 3 cups a day for throat, digestive, and gynecological problems.
Food: Mix slippery elm powder with water or milk until it has the consistency of a thin porridge.

SPECIAL INFORMATION
✒ Consult your doctor if you do not improve significantly within two weeks.
✒ Some people may be allergic to the powdered bark; if so, discontinue use. Consult your doctor before taking larger-than-recommended doses.

Spearmint
Mentha spicata

Spearmint, used since ancient times to promote digestion, heal wounds, and relieve colds and congestion, is prescribed by herbalists today for digestive ills, colds, insomnia, and itching and inflammation. The crushed or boiled leaves release carvone, a chemical similar to but milder than the menthol found in peppermint. Many herbalists prescribe spearmint and peppermint interchangeably, although the latter is considered more potent.

■ TARGET AILMENTS
Take internally for upset stomach, stomach spasms, flatulence, heartburn, stomach cramps, morning sickness during pregnancy; nasal, sinus, and chest congestion; colds; headache; sore throat or mouth.
Take internally and apply externally for muscle pains, external infections, chapped hands.

PREPARATIONS
Over the counter: Available as capsules, prepared tea, fresh or dried leaves, tincture, oil.
At home:
Tea: Boil 1 to 2 tsp dried herb or several fresh leaves per cup of water; steep 10 minutes. Drink up to 3 cups a day.
Tincture: Add ¼ to 1 tsp to an 8-oz glass of water and drink up to three glasses a day.
Herbal bath: Fill a cloth bag with a few handfuls of dried or fresh spearmint leaves and add to running bathwater.

SIDE EFFECTS
None expected.

SPECIAL INFORMATION
✒ Spearmint oil (carvone) may cause stomach upset if ingested. It is recommended for external use only.
✒ For children under two, dilute tea or tincture with water.

CONTINUED

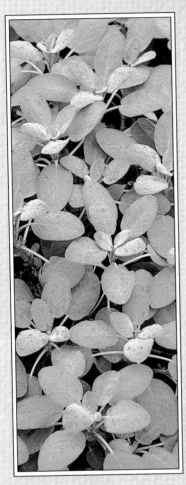

Sage

St.-John's-Wort
Hypericum perforatum

For centuries herbalists have used the blood red flowers of St-John's-wort to heal wounds and treat depression.

■ TARGET AILMENTS
Use externally for wounds (cuts, abrasions, burns); scar tissue.
Take internally in consultation with an herbalist or a doctor for depression.

PREPARATIONS
Over the counter: Available as dried leaves and flowers, tincture, extract, oil, ointment, capsules, and prepared tea.
At home:
Tea: Add 1 to 2 tsp dried herb to 1 cup boiling water; steep for 15 minutes. Drink up to 3 cups a day.
Oil: Use a commercial preparation, or soak the flowers in almond or olive oil until the oil turns bright red.
Ointment: Use a commercial preparation, or warm the leaves in hot petroleum jelly or a mixture of beeswax and almond oil.
Fresh: Apply crushed leaves and flowers to cleansed wounds.
Tincture: Add ¼ to 1 tsp to an 8-oz glass of water and drink daily.

SIDE EFFECTS
Serious: High blood pressure, headaches, stiff neck, nausea, and vomiting. Can exacerbate sunburn in the fair-skinned.

SPECIAL INFORMATION
🍃 Consult a doctor or an herbalist before using St.-John's-wort.

POSSIBLE INTERACTIONS
WARNING: Avoid the amino acids tryptophan and tyrosine; amphetamines; asthma inhalants; beer, coffee, wine; chocolate, fava beans, salami, smoked or pickled foods, and yogurt; cold or hay fever medicines; diet pills; narcotics; nasal decongestants.

Tangerine Peel
Citrus reticulata

Sometimes called mandarin orange peel, this herb is prescribed for digestive disorders. Practitioners of Chinese medicine believe that the peel gets better as it ages. The best samples of the fruit are thin skinned, pliable, oily, and fragrant.

■ TARGET AILMENTS
Take internally for indigestion, gas; a feeling of fullness in the abdomen; nausea; loose stools; phlegm.

PREPARATIONS
Available at Asian food markets, Chinese pharmacies, and Western health food stores. Also available as pills.

Combinations: In a preparation with Asian ginseng, tangerine peel is used as a digestive stimulant. Chinese herbalists prescribe a mixture of tangerine peel, ripe bitter orange, and aucklandia for abdominal distention and pain. And a preparation containing tangerine peel and pinellia root is used to treat an excess of phlegm together with a stifling feeling in the chest that makes deep breathing difficult. For further information on appropriate preparations and doses, check with an herbal practitioner.

SIDE EFFECTS
None expected.

SPECIAL INFORMATION
🍃 Do not use this herb if you have a dry cough or an excessively red tongue, or if you are spitting up blood.
🍃 Herbalists use the red part of tangerine peel (when dried, some parts are orange and others red) to control vomiting and belching.
🍃 Chinese practitioners also prescribe young, or green, tangerine peel for breast and side pain and for hernia pain.

The 75 Most Effective Herbs

Tea Tree Oil
Melaleuca spp.

The first Europeans to reach Australia made tea from the leaves of what then became known as the tea tree, which should not be confused with the common tea plant. For centuries before the Europeans arrived, native Australians were using the leaves of this tree as an antiseptic. Eventually the Europeans learned to use the leaves' volatile oil to treat cuts, abrasions, burns, insect bites, and other minor skin ailments. Modern studies show that the strong germicidal activity of tea tree oil is caused primarily by a single ingredient, terpineol. The oil, which smells like nutmeg, is extracted from the leaves by steam distillation. During World War II, tea tree oil was added to machine oils to reduce infections in the hands of workers during metal fabrication. The oils of some species of Melaleuca may irritate the skin and are not used.

■ TARGET AILMENTS
Apply externally for cuts, abrasions, insect bites, teenage acne, fungal infections such as athlete's foot, and other skin ailments. Use as a douche for minor vaginal infections.

PREPARATIONS
Over the counter: Available as oil and also as an additive to health and beauty products such as toothpaste, soap, and shampoo. Tea tree oil is also used in flea shampoos.
At home:
Apply fresh leaves directly to wounds.

SIDE EFFECTS
Not serious: Local skin and vaginal irritation may develop in sensitive individuals. Let your doctor know if the irritation persists.

SPECIAL INFORMATION
⋆ People with sensitive skin should dilute tea tree oil with a bland oil, such as vegetable oil.

Turmeric
Curcuma longa

Turmeric root, a main ingredient in Indian curries, is also used in Ayurvedic and Chinese medicine and by Western herbalists to treat a variety of ailments.

■ TARGET AILMENTS
Chinese:
Take internally for shoulder pain, menstrual cramps, pain after childbirth, menstrual irregularity.
Apply externally for infections of the skin.
Western:
Take internally for digestive disorders, fever, chest congestion, menstrual irregularity, arthritis pain.
Apply externally for pain and swelling caused by trauma.

PREPARATIONS
Over the counter: Available as powdered root, capsules, liquid extract.
At home:
Chinese:
Combinations: Turmeric is mixed with cinnamon twig and astragalus for shoulder pain; with cinnamon bark for menstrual cramps and pain after childbirth; with dong quai for menstrual irregularity. The herb is mixed with sesame or salad oil and applied externally to swollen areas.
Western:
Decoction: Steep 1 tsp turmeric powder in 1 cup milk for 15 to 20 minutes. Drink up to 3 cups a day.

SIDE EFFECTS
Not serious: Heartburn or upset stomach. Discontinue and consult your practitioner.

SPECIAL INFORMATION
⋆ If you are pregnant, trying to conceive or have fertility problems, or have a blood-clotting disorder, consult your practitioner before using.
⋆ Use low-strength preparations for children, or adults over 65. Do not give to children under two.

Usnea
Usnea spp.

Usnea, or larch moss, refers to a group of lichens, plants made up of algae and fungi that grow together interdependently. Usnea is found hanging from the larch and many other trees in the Northern Hemisphere. The active ingredient, usnic acid, seems to have an antibiotic effect against the Gram-positive class of bacteria, which includes Streptococcus. It may also be effective against some fungi and protozoans. Usnea is believed to work by disrupting the cell metabolism of bacteria and other simple organisms, though it does not damage human cells. Herbalists consider it an immune system stimulant and a muscle relaxant.

■ TARGET AILMENTS
Take internally for colds, influenza, sore throats, respiratory infections; gastrointestinal irritations.
Apply externally for skin ulcers and fungal infections such as athlete's foot; use as a douche for vaginal infections and urinary tract infections such as urethritis or cystitis.

PREPARATIONS
Over the counter: Available in bulk, powder, or tincture.
At home:
Tea: Steep 2 to 3 tsp dried lichen or 1 to 2 tsp powder in 1 cup boiling water. Take three times daily.

SIDE EFFECTS
Not serious: If digestive disorders arise, reduce dosage. Call your doctor if these symptoms persist.

SPECIAL INFORMATION
WARNING: Pregnant women should avoid using this herb because it may stimulate uterine contractions.
⋆ Dilute tincture before ingesting; high concentrations may cause digestive problems.
⋆ Do not use for more than three consecutive weeks.

CONTINUED

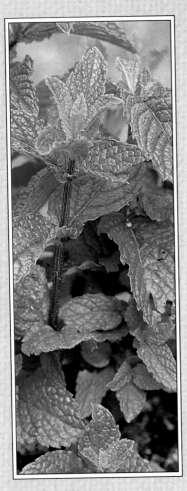

Spearmint

Uva Ursi
Arctostaphylos uva-ursi

Uva ursi, prescribed by herbalists for urinary problems, is also used to treat minor wounds. Its leaves contain arbutin, which is converted in the urinary tract to the antiseptic hydroquinone.

■ TARGET AILMENTS
Take internally for mild urinary tract infections, such as urethritis and cystitis; high blood pressure; menstrual bloating.
Apply externally for skin problems such as cuts and abrasions.

PREPARATIONS
Over the counter: Available as dried leaves; as a tincture; and as a tea, alone or in combination with other ingredients.
At home:
Tea: Simmer for 5 to 10 minutes; let stand for 12 to 24 hours. To counteract the effect of the tannin content, add peppermint or chamomile. Drink 3 cups a day.
Compress: Make a tea; strain; soak a pad in the tea and apply.

SIDE EFFECTS
Not serious: Taking uva ursi may produce dark green urine; this is harmless. The herb's high tannin content may cause stomach upset.
Serious: A 1949 study involving very high doses of hydroquinone reported tinnitus, nausea, and convulsions. Prescribed doses of the whole herb are considered safe; in case of side effects, discontinue taking until you contact your doctor.

SPECIAL INFORMATION
🍂 Uva ursi works only in an alkaline environment; avoid acidic foods and vitamin C when taking.
🍂 Because hydroquinone is toxic in high doses, use uva ursi only in recommended amounts.
🍂 Do not use if you are pregnant; it may stimulate uterine contractions.

Valerian
Valeriana officinalis

Valerian root has been used for more than a thousand years for its calming qualities, and recent research has confirmed its efficacy and safety as a mild tranquilizer and sleep aid. Valerian hastens the onset of sleep, improves sleep quality, and reduces nighttime awakenings. Unlike barbiturates or benzodiazepines, prescribed amounts leave no morning grogginess and do not interfere with the vivid dreaming sleep known as REM sleep. It is not habit forming and produces no withdrawal symptoms when discontinued.

■ TARGET AILMENTS
Take internally for insomnia, anxiety, nervousness, headache, intestinal pains, menstrual cramps.

PREPARATIONS
Over the counter: Available dried or as capsules, tincture, and teas.
At home:
Tea: Steep 2 tsp dried, chopped root in 1 cup boiling water. Let stand 8 to 12 hours. Drink 1 cup before bed.

SIDE EFFECTS
Not serious: A mild headache or upset stomach may develop. Reduce dosage. Tell your doctor if it persists.
Serious: More severe headache, restlessness, nausea, morning grogginess, or blurred vision may be caused by using too much valerian. Contact your doctor, who will probably tell you to take less or to stop using the herb.

SPECIAL INFORMATION
🍂 Do not take valerian with conventional tranquilizers or sedatives, because of possible additive effects.
🍂 Paradoxically, valerian may produce excitability in some people.
🍂 Be careful about driving until you know how the herb affects you.

The 75 Most Effective Herbs

White Willow
Salix alba

White willow is a source of salicin, a precursor of aspirin. Though all parts of the plant contain some salicin, the best source is the mature bark. As do other salicin-producing plants, white willow also reduces fever and inflammation. Besides salicin, willow bark contains other compounds that the body metabolizes to salicylic acid. For this reason it acts more slowly and over a longer period of time than aspirin does.

■ TARGET AILMENTS
Take internally for gout, minor muscle strains, menstrual cramps, headache, fever, aches and pains, pain and inflammation of arthritis.
Apply externally for sores, burns; pain and inflammation of arthritis.

PREPARATIONS
Over the counter: Available as tea, tincture, dried bark, and capsules.
At home:
Tea: Steep 1 to 2 tsp powdered bark in 1 cup boiling water for 8 hours; strain. Drink up to 3 cups daily. Honey and lemon improve taste.

SIDE EFFECTS
Not serious: Upset stomach, nausea, or tinnitus may result. Lower the dosage or discontinue. Call your doctor if symptoms persist.

SPECIAL INFORMATION
WARNING: Children under 16 should not use white willow if they have a cold, flu, or other viral illness. Using salicylates may cause Reye's syndrome, a potentially fatal condition.
↣ Individuals with ulcers or other stomach problems should use white willow with caution.

POSSIBLE INTERACTIONS
Do not mix white willow with other salicylates, such as aspirin or wintergreen oil, because of the potential for additive side effects.

Wild Yam
Dioscorea villosa

Used during the 18th and 19th centuries as a remedy for menstrual pain and complications associated with childbearing, wild yam is a perennial vine that entwines itself around fences and bushes. It is recognized by a slender reddish brown stem and drooping yellow flowers that bloom in summer. Wild yam extract, taken from the root, contains an alkaloid substance that relaxes the muscles of the entire abdominal region. Consequently, it is prescribed to alleviate menstrual cramps and to relieve the nausea and muscle tension associated with pregnancy. Wild yam also contains steroidal saponins, believed to act as anti-inflammatory agents and used to lessen the swelling of rheumatoid arthritis.

■ TARGET AILMENTS
Take internally for morning sickness, nausea of pregnancy, menstrual cramps, urinary tract disorders, intestinal colic, rheumatoid arthritis.

PREPARATIONS
Over the counter: Available as dried root, tincture, or capsules.
At home:
Tea: Boil 1 oz wild yam root with 1 cup water for 15 to 20 minutes. Drink three times daily.
Combinations: For intestinal colic, wild yam is combined with calamus, chamomile, and ginger. Rheumatoid arthritis is treated with a mix of wild yam and black cohosh. Herbalists use a combination of wild yam and cramp bark for menstrual cramps.

SPECIAL INFORMATION
↣ Herbalists sometimes prescribe wild yam for its alleged progesterone-like properties for women undergoing menopause; the effectiveness of this treatment, however, is debated. Consult a practitioner before using wild yam as a progesterone supplement.

Yarrow
Achillea millefolium

Yarrow has been used to heal wounds since ancient times. Modern investigation has revealed many chemicals in this herb that have pain-relieving and anti-inflammatory effects. The leaves, stems, and flower tops contain more than 10 active ingredients, including salicylic acid, menthol, and camphor. Two major constituents, achilletin and achilleine, are thought to help blood coagulate, while thujone (also found in chamomile) has mild sedative properties. Because yarrow may have diuretic properties, it is sometimes used to treat menstrual bloating and high blood pressure. The somewhat bitter taste of yarrow tea can be relieved by adding sweeteners. A naturalized perennial from Eurasia, yarrow is widely planted in flower and herb gardens. The herb is found growing wild in most areas of the United States.

■ TARGET AILMENTS
Take internally for fever, digestive disorders, menstrual cramps, anxiety, insomnia, high blood pressure.
Apply externally for minor wounds, bleeding. Use as a douche for vaginal irritations.

PREPARATIONS
Over the counter: Available as dried herb or tea.
At home:
Tea: Steep 1 to 2 tsp dried herb in 1 cup boiling water for 10 to 15 minutes. Drink up to 3 cups a day.

SIDE EFFECTS
Not serious: Yarrow may produce a rash or diarrhea. Stop using the herb and consult your doctor.

SPECIAL INFORMATION
↣ If you are allergic to ragweed, you may develop a rash from ingesting yarrow.

■

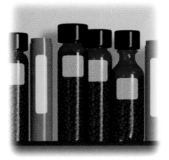

Target Ailments

■ Allergies

■ Arthritis

■ Asthma

■ Athletic Injuries

■ Bladder Infections

■ Chronic Fatigue Syndrome

■ Common Cold

■ Diarrhea

■ Earache

■ Fever and Chills

■ Flu

■ Food Poisoning

■ Hay Fever

■ Headache

■ Hemorrhoids

■ Insomnia

■ Menstrual Problems

■ Motion Sickness

■ Pneumonia

■ Premenstrual Syndrome

■ Sore Throat

See Common Ailments, beginning on page 194.

Homeopathy

Homeopathy is a method of healing based on the idea that like cures like; that is, that substances causing specific symptoms in a healthy person can cure these symptoms in someone who is sick. Also called the law of similars, this principle gives homeopathy its name: "homeo" for similar, "pathy" for disease. The remedies are prepared from plant, mineral, and animal extracts that are highly diluted in a specific way that makes toxicity impossible and, paradoxically, increases their potential to cure.

Homeopathic treatment, in its principles and procedures, is unlike any other system of medicinal care. Although a few conventional therapies, such as allergy desensitization and immunization, involve the use of "similars" to some degree, modern medicine relies almost exclusively on counteracting substances; laxatives, for example, are medications that work to counteract constipation.

Origins

Modern homeopathy was founded in the 1790s by a German physician named Samuel Hahnemann. Unhappy with existing medical techniques, Hahnemann experimented with small doses of substances known to cure specific diseases. Just as he had suspected, when given to healthy people these substances induced symptoms of the very diseases they were used to treat. In time, Hahnemann developed a method of preparing remedies by diluting small quantities of herbs, minerals, and animal extracts in a water-alcohol solution. The results convinced him that using increasingly smaller amounts of a substance in dilution not only eliminated unwanted side effects but actually boosted the remedy's potency. To unlock these curative powers, though, the solution had to be shaken vigorously. He called his method of preparing remedies potentizing, believing that shaking, or "succussing," the substances released their stores of vital energy.

Hahnemann was not the first to theorize that cures could be fashioned from the causes of disease. In the fifth century BC, the Greek physician Hippocrates described a system of healing by "similars"; this notion of fighting illness with like substances contrasted

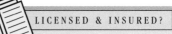

LICENSED & INSURED?

Licensing varies from state to state for homeopathic practitioners, most of whom have prior medical training, such as a degree in medicine, osteopathy, or naturopathic medicine. The pharmaceuticals they prescribe are recognized and regulated by the FDA. Although many homeopathy products can be purchased over the counter, those offered for treating serious conditions must be dispensed under the supervision of a licensed practitioner.

Homeopathy

with the more orthodox practice of healing by "contraries," or antidotes. Over time, medical practitioners came to rely almost exclusively on contraries, deriving treatments from substances that reverse or work against the actions of particular diseases. Yet the principle of similars persisted in folk medicine for hundreds of years, providing the groundwork for Hahnemann's revolutionary methods.

Testing the Remedies

Most homeopathic remedies have undergone "provings," or medical trials in which healthy individuals are given doses of undiluted or slightly diluted substances known to cause illnesses. During each test, researchers note the subjects' mental, emotional, and physical changes, which together paint a full picture of the symptoms brought on by a given substance. Responses have been recorded over the years in the materia medica, a master reference collection that gives homeopaths a basis for deciding which remedy is best suited for a patient with a particular set of symptoms.

What It's Good For

Used for a wide range of conditions, homeopathy is especially effective for noncritical ailments and for those that do not involve severe structural damage or organ destruction. It is also appropriate for diseases for which no effective conventional treatment is available, such as viral illnesses and multiple sclerosis; for ailments that require continuous use of drugs (allergies, arthritis, and digestive problems, for example); and for behavioral and emotional disorders.

Although not every remedy has undergone conventional double-blind drug testing, clinical trials have shown a positive effect for a number of conditions, including hay fever, flu, acute childhood diarrhea, asthma, rheumatoid arthritis, and pain, as well as cardiovascular, respiratory, and gastrointestinal diseases. Further research is being conducted in the United States (under the auspices of the National Institutes of Health) and in a number of other countries.

Preparations/Techniques

Remedies come in a variety of forms, including tablets, powders, wafers, and liquids in an alcohol base. Recently, over-the-counter combination remedies have become available for common ailments. These products, labeled according to the name of the ailment, allow self-treatment of such minor conditions as insomnia, flu, sore throat, and headache.

The specific dilution of a remedy is the ratio of active substance to inactive base. Ratios containing an x indicate that the remedy consists of 1 part mother tincture (concentrated extract) mixed with 9 parts alcohol base; ratios containing a c consist of 1 part mother tincture and 99 parts base. Further dilutions are represented

CAUTION

Although homeopathic remedies are too highly diluted to cause toxicity from overdose, taking them for too long a time can cause your symptoms to worsen, and taking ones that are inappropriate for you may cause new symptoms to appear.

CONTINUED

Homeopathy CONTINUED

by a number preceding the *x* or *c*. For example, a remedy labeled 30c has first been mixed 1 part to 99; then, 1 part of the resulting mixture is diluted again with 99 parts of the base, and this process is repeated for a total of 30 times. Modern over-the-counter remedies usually have dilution ratios ranging from 1x to 30c; remedies restricted to professional use generally range from 200c to 1,000,000c.

When taking homeopathic remedies in tablet form, be careful not to touch them. Instead, pour the tablets into the bottle cap, then tip them directly onto or under your tongue. If you spill any tablets, throw them away. Practitioners recommend that the mouth be clean of flavors 15 minutes before and after taking a remedy. Avoid strong flavors and aromas—such as mint, camphor, coffee, and heavily scented perfumes—for the duration of the treatment.

Visiting a Professional

For chronic problems, most practitioners practice "constitutional" homeopathy, which is based on the idea that the patient's constitution must be considered along with the disease itself. Acute, or short-term, conditions are usually treated with remedies specific to the illness. Typically, the practitioner takes an extensive medical history of the patient, notes the physical and psychological symptoms, then prescribes a single remedy. If this prescription does not have the desired effect, the homeopath performs another analysis and gives a second prescription. Symptom analysis is the key to success; consequently, two patients suffering from the same disorder but displaying different symptoms may receive different prescriptions.

If the correct remedy has been prescribed, healing may begin immediately or within a few days or weeks. When it does, stop taking the remedy, and start again only if your symptoms return. In some cases a prescription will cause what's known as an aggravation, or a temporary worsening of your symptoms. This is usually an indication that the remedy is going to work. Stop taking it and wait for the positive effect.

Wellness

Homeopathic practitioners often provide constitutional treatments—regimens based on personal and family medical histories—to patients who are not sick but want to maintain or improve their general health.

What the Critics Say

Critics argue that some homeopathic remedies are so diluted they no longer contain even a single molecule of the original healing substance. Many homeopathic remedies have been proved effective in clinical trials, but opponents attribute any therapeutic success to the placebo effect. The idea that a substance can cure by releasing energy, say skeptics, puts homeopathy in the realm of metaphysics. ■

FOR MORE INFO

Following is a list of organizations you can contact to learn more about homeopathy:

National Center for Homeopathy
801 North Fairfax Street, #306
Alexandria, VA 22314
(703) 548-7790

International Foundation for Homeopathy
PO Box 7
Edmonds, WA 98020
(206) 776-4147

The 30 Most Effective Homeopathic Remedies

Aconite • *Aconitum napellus*

Aconite grows throughout the mountainous regions of Europe, Russia, and central Asia, producing clusters of bluish violet flowers that hang from the stem like monks' cowls, giving the plant its common name, monkshood. Highly toxic, aconite was the preferred poison of the ancient Greeks. Administered in very small doses, it produces mental and physical restlessness and tissue inflammation. Homeopathic physicians prescribe *Aconite* for those patients whose symptoms resemble the effects of the poison—who seem distressed or fearful and complain of thirst and unbearable aches and pains that accompany their illnesses.

For homeopathic use, the whole plant—except the root, which is the most poisonous part—is gathered while in full bloom and pounded to a pulp. Juice is pressed from the pulp and mixed with alcohol, then diluted to nontoxic levels.

TARGET AILMENTS

Angina, arrhythmia, anxiety induced by sudden shock, arthritis, asthma, bronchitis, colds and flu, croup, fevers with rapid onset and chills that may be accompanied by restlessness or thirst, eye inflammations with burning pain and sensitivity to light, laryngitis, sore throat, middle ear infections, toothaches with a sensitivity to cold water.

Allium cepa • *Allium cepa*

Cultivated worldwide, *Allium cepa,* otherwise known as red onion, has been used in folk medicine for centuries. This common garden vegetable has been applied to the skin in poultices for acne, arthritis, and congestion, and used internally to clear worms from the intestines. Modern-day herbalists find onion useful for treating conditions as varied as earaches, hemorrhoids, and high blood pressure. Homeopathic practitioners consider *Allium cepa* a remedy for conditions that are accompanied by the same symptoms as those brought on by exposure to red onions—watering eyes and a burning, runny nose.

For the homeopathic preparation, red onions are harvested in midsummer. The bulbs are pounded to a pulp and then mixed with water and alcohol through several stages of extreme dilution.

TARGET AILMENTS

Colds with sinus congestion that shifts from side to side in the head; coughs that cause a ripping, tearing pain in the throat; watery and inflamed eyes, hay fever; neuralgic pains; earaches.

Apis • *Apis mellifica*

The medicinal value of *Apis,* the scientific name for the honeybee, may date back to ancient Egypt, where bees were a symbol of power, wealth, and health. Egyptian doctors revered honey over all other healing substances, and extensive methods of beekeeping were already in practice in 4000 BC. It is not the honey but the bee itself, however, that is used in homeopathic medicine.

This remedy is made from the body of the honeybee; it is used to treat those patients whose ailments are accompanied by symptoms similar to the results of a bee sting, such as redness and swelling, and also patients who express behavior considered beelike, such as restlessness or irritability. To prepare this remedy, the entire live honeybee is crushed and highly diluted by mixing it into a water-and-alcohol base.

TARGET AILMENTS

Bites and stings, especially those that burn, itch, or swell; conjunctivitis; edema (accumulation of fluids in body tissues) and conditions of general swelling such as hives and food allergies; headaches that include sudden, stabbing pains; red, swollen joints; mumps.

CONTINUED

The 30 Most Effective Homeopathic Remedies

Arnica • *Arnica montana*

Arnica, sometimes called mountain daisy, grows wild across the higher elevations of Europe, northern Asia, and parts of the United States. Mountain climbers in the Alps have traditionally chewed arnica after a long day's hike to relieve muscle aches. Homeopathic practitioners prescribe *Arnica* for bruises, sprains, strains, and other types of accidents that are sudden and may induce shock. The flowers, leaves, stem, and root of arnica are crushed to a pulp and soaked in alcohol before undergoing the homeopathic dilution process, which renders the substance nontoxic.

TARGET AILMENTS

Blood blisters; broken bones, sprains, strains, and other sudden injuries with swelling, tenderness, and pain where post-trauma shock is a threat; bruises; sore and swollen joints, as in rheumatism; head pain; toothache and pain from dental work; groin strain.

Arsenicum album • *Arsenicum album*

This remedy, also called *Ars alb* by homeopathic practitioners, is an extremely dilute form of arsenic, a metallic poison derived from the chemical element of the same name. Weak preparations of arsenic have had a history of medicinal use; but slow accumulation of the element in body tissues can cause chronic poisoning, leading to gastrointestinal disorders, nausea, dehydration, and even paralysis and death. In step with the homeopathic theory that like cures like, *Ars alb* is preferred by practitioners to treat patients with various digestive complaints that are accompanied by signs of dehydration and burning pains, the same symptoms that are induced by arsenic.

In its homeopathic form, arsenic is separated from other metals like iron, cobalt, and nickel by baking at high temperatures. The extracted powder is then finely ground and weakened by mixing successively greater amounts of lactose (milk sugar) with the poison.

TARGET AILMENTS

Angina; anxiety disorders and panic attacks; asthma; hay fever; burns that form blisters; chronic skin problems; high fevers accompanied by chills; recurrent headaches; dry, hacking coughs; colds accompanied by excessive, watery nasal discharge and frequent sneezing; colitis, indigestion, food poisoning, Crohn's disease; influenza; insomnia; exhaustion from an illness coupled with restlessness.

Belladonna • *Belladonna*

Belladonna, a highly toxic plant also known as deadly nightshade, grows wild across Europe, producing yellow flowers in July and dark red berries in late summer. Its name, meaning "beautiful woman" in Italian, dates from the Renaissance, when ladies of Italy dilated their pupils with belladonna eye drops for a doe-eyed appearance. Belladonna poisoning brings on a range of symptoms, including a dry mouth and hot, flushed skin, nausea, convulsive movements, and delirium. Homeopathic practitioners prescribe *Belladonna* for illnesses that are accompanied by these same symptoms. All parts of the belladonna plant are gathered for use in the homeopathic remedy. The plant is crushed and pressed, and the extracted juice is mixed with alcohol in an extremely dilute preparation.

TARGET AILMENTS

Common cold, flu, sore throat, painful earache, high fever with chills but with no thirst, acute inflammatory arthritis, acute bursitis, gallstones, colic, measles, mumps, acute diverticulitis, neuralgia, sunstroke, acutely inflamed varicose veins, painful toothache, painful menstrual periods, teething pains, breastfeeding complications.

The 30 Most Effective Homeopathic Remedies

Bryonia · *Bryonia alba*

Bryonia, or wild hops, is a creeping vine commonly found along hedgerows and in forests across southern Europe. Its medicinal value was known to the Greeks, who used the root as a purgative and may have given the plant its name, derived from *bryo*, meaning "to thrust or sprout," a reference to how quickly the vine grows. Accidental ingestion of the root can cause tissue inflammation, severe vomiting, and diarrhea violent enough to cause death. Homeopathic physicians prescribe their dilute solutions of *Bryonia* for illnesses that are accompanied by similar symptoms. The homeopathic remedy is prepared from the root, which is harvested in early spring. An extract pressed from the root pulp is mixed with alcohol into an extremely dilute solution.

TARGET AILMENTS

Arthritis with sharp, sticking pains; backaches centered in the small of the back; bursitis; colds accompanied by chest congestion; painful coughs; sore throat with pain upon swallowing; influenza; severe headaches worsened by light, sound, or motion; dizziness; nausea, vomiting, constipation, gastritis, acute diverticulitis, stomach flu; inflammation during breast-feeding.

Calcarea carbonica · *Calcarea carbonica*

Calcarea carbonica, or calcium carbonate, is a source of calcium, one of the most abundant natural elements in the human body. Essential to cell structure and bone strength, calcium comes from many materials, including chalk, coral, and limestone. Perhaps as a reflection of its body-building properties, *Calcarea carbonica*, also called *Calc carb*, is used by homeopathic physicians for conditions that are accompanied by symptoms of exhaustion, depression, and anxiety. Calcium carbonate prepared for homeopathic use is ground from oyster shells and used at full strength.

TARGET AILMENTS

Lower-back pain, broken bones, sprains, muscle cramps, constipation, chronic ear infections, eye inflammations, headaches, insomnia, eczema, allergies, teething problems, gastritis, gallstones, childhood diarrhea, menstrual problems, asthma, palpitations, arthritis.

Cantharis · *Cantharis*

Popularly known as Spanish fly, cantharis is actually a beetle found in southern France and Spain. It produces an irritant so caustic that the skin will blister if exposed to it.

Cantharis has had a long career in medicine and has been used for all manner of disorders. In high concentrations the irritant can be toxic, prompting abdominal cramps and burning pains in the throat and stomach, vomiting of blood, diarrhea, kidney damage, convulsions, coma, and death. Homeopaths prescribe *Cantharis* for patients whose ailments are coupled with symptoms like those of cantharis poisoning.

According to homeopathic tradition, the beetles are collected at daybreak, when they are still sluggish from the cool of the night, and heated in the steam of boiling vinegar until dead. The beetles are then crushed and mixed with successively greater amounts of milk sugar, a pharmaceutical process called trituration. The resulting powder is highly dilute.

TARGET AILMENTS

Bladder infections or cystitis, with a constant desire to urinate accompanied by blood and pain during urination; sunburns, scalds, and blistering second-degree burns.

CONTINUED

The 30 Most Effective Homeopathic Remedies

Chamomilla • *Chamomilla*

Chamomilla is made from the flowering German chamomile plant common in Europe. The whole plant is crushed, and its juices are mixed with equal parts of alcohol, then succussed. In homeopathy *Chamomilla* is considered to work best for people who are extremely sensitive to pain, irritable, impatient, and implacable. *Chamomilla* patients sweat easily and are sensitive to wind and chills. *Chamomilla* is most often given to children who work themselves into violent temper tantrums.

TARGET AILMENTS

Irritability; toothaches aggravated by cold air and warm food; painful menstrual periods with severe cramping and a feeling of anger or restlessness; extremely painful earaches; teething pain, especially if the child is irritable; difficulty getting to sleep.

Ferrum phosphoricum • *Ferrum phosphoricum*

Ferrum phosphoricum, also called ferrum phos or iron phosphate, is a mineral compound of iron and phosphorus. Both elements are present in the body independently; iron aids the exchange of oxygen in the blood, and phosphorus contributes to bone and muscle health. Ferrum phos is derived from mixing solutions of iron sulfate, phosphate, and sodium acetate. The resulting iron phosphate is ground with large quantities of lactose (milk sugar) to render it nontoxic. Homeopathic practitioners consider *Ferrum phos* good for patients who suffer from conditions accompanied by low energy and anemia.

TARGET AILMENTS

Tickling, hacking coughs with chest pain, headaches, fevers that begin slowly, ear infections, incontinence, rheumatic joints, early menstrual periods accompanied by headaches, anemia, fatigue, nosebleeds, sore throat, vomiting, diarrhea, palpitations.

Gelsemium • *Gelsemium sempervirens*

Sometimes called yellow jasmine, gelsemium is not really part of the jasmine family but is related to the plants ignatia and nux vomica. A climbing vine with trumpetlike yellow flowers, it is common in the woods and coastal shoreline of the southern United States. Taken in large doses, gelsemium causes paralysis of the motor nerves, impairing physical and mental functions like vision, balance, thought, and movement; ultimately, poisoning causes convulsions and death. Homeopathic physicians prescribe dilute solutions of gelsemium for ailments that are accompanied by symptoms like those of gelsemium poisoning. In its homeopathic form *Gelsemium* is prepared from the fresh root, which is chopped, soaked in alcohol, strained, and diluted to the desired, highly dilute potencies.

TARGET AILMENTS

Anxiety; flu with aches, chills, and exhaustion; headache beginning in the back of the head and moving forward; measles; sore throat; fever with chills that move up and down the spine, although the patient may not feel cold.

The 30 Most Effective Homeopathic Remedies

Hepar sulphuris • *Hepar sulphuris calcareum*

The flaky inner layer of oyster shells provides the calcium used in this homeopathic remedy, also called *Hepar sulph* and commonly known as calcium sulfide. Once an antidote for mercury poisoning, *Hepar sulphuris* is now used by homeopathic physicians to treat patients with conditions that tend to be infected, often producing pus. These disorders are accompanied by symptoms that include mental and physical hypersensitivity and an intolerance of pain and cold.

Finely ground oyster shell and sulfur are mixed together and then heated in an airtight container. The resulting powder is dissolved in hot hydrochloric acid, then combined with lactose (milk sugar) in a pharmaceutical process of dilution called trituration.

TARGET AILMENTS

Abscesses that are swollen and painful but have not yet opened; colds, sore throat, and earache; inflamed cuts and wounds that may be taking longer than normal to heal; aching joints; fits of coughing with chest pain, hoarseness, asthma, emphysema, croup; genital herpes; constipation.

Hypericum • *Hypericum perforatum*

Also known as St.-John's-wort, hypericum grows in woodlands across Europe, Asia, and the United States, blooming with a profusion of yellow flowers from June to September. The flowers, if bruised, bleed a reddish juice. The dark green leaves of the plant are dotted with oil-producing pores. According to ancient healing wisdom, because hypericum seemed to resemble skin, with its pores and its simulation of bleeding on injury, it was considered ideal for all manner of flesh wounds. *(See St.-John's-wort, page 100.)* In homeopathy *Hypericum* is often prescribed for bodily injuries, among other conditions, but it is selected for the soothing effect it is said to have on injured nerves rather than for any traditional reason.

For homeopathic use the entire plant is harvested in summer, when its yellow flowers are in full bloom. It is pounded to a pulp and soaked in an alcohol solution before being weakened to the desired potencies through a vigorous dilution process.

TARGET AILMENTS

Backaches centered along the lower spine that may include shooting pains; bites and stings from animals and insects, especially when they have become inflamed or include nerve damage; cuts and wounds in nerve-rich parts of the body, like the fingers and lips, caused by accidents or surgery.

Ignatia • *Ignatia amara*

The beans of this plant, sometimes called St. Ignatius bean, are in fact seeds from the fruit of a small tree native to China and the Philippines. Spanish missionaries in the Philippines were introduced to the seeds by the locals, who wore them as amulets to ward off disease. Small doses of the seed can produce mild but unpleasant symptoms of poisoning, including increased salivation, pounding headache, cramps, giddiness, twitching, and trembling; large doses can be fatal. Homeopaths may prescribe *Ignatia,* a dilute solution of the seed, for ailments that include symptoms like those associated with mild poisoning.

For the homeopathic preparation, the seeds are collected and ground to a powder, then mixed with alcohol. When the powder is saturated, the mixture is strained and diluted until it becomes a nontoxic substance.

TARGET AILMENTS

Anxiety; dry, tickling coughs; a sore throat that feels like there is a lump in it; painful tension headaches; indigestion; insomnia; irritable bowel syndrome; painful hemorrhoids; effects of grief, shock, or disappointment, or depression where the patient tends to sigh frequently.

CONTINUED

The 30 Most Effective Homeopathic Remedies

Ipecac • *Ipecacuanha*

The *ipecacuanha* shrub, native to Central and South America, was named by Portuguese colonists, who called it "roadside sick-making plant" in recognition of its ability to induce vomiting. Varying dosages of its root can produce a variety of symptoms, including mild appetite stimulation, sweating, expectoration, vomiting, gastritis, inflammation of the lungs, and cardiac failure. Other health disorders can display symptoms similar to those of mild ipecac poisoning, and it is these symptoms that homeopathic practitioners hope to counteract when they prescribe *Ipecac.*

The homeopathic remedy is made from the root, the most potent part of the plant. The root is dried and then ground into a coarse powder, which is diluted either in milk sugar to be used as a dry substance or in a water-and-alcohol base. Both preparations are weakened to a nontoxic level.

TARGET AILMENTS

Persistent nausea, vomiting, motion sickness; menstrual problems; asthma; dry, irritating cough accompanied by wheezing; diarrhea; flu with nausea; colic; gastroenteritis.

Kali bichromicum • *Kali bichromicum*

Kali bichromicum is often called potassium bichromate; it is a chemical compound that may be acquired from chromium iron ore or by processing potassium chromate with one of a number of strong acids. A highly corrosive substance, it is used primarily in textile dyeing, in the staining of wood, and as a component in electric batteries. It is also a very powerful poison. Homeopathic practitioners believe *Kali bichromicum* works best for conditions that are accompanied by the symptom of pain in a distinct spot, where the ache is easily located with a fingertip.

For homeopathic use this caustic chemical, also called *Kali bi,* is diluted to nontoxic levels with large amounts of milk sugar, a pharmaceutical process called trituration.

TARGET AILMENTS

Acute bronchitis, colds in which there is a thick mucus discharge and a heavy cough that produces pain in the chest, croup, sinusitis and resulting headaches, indigestion, pains in the joints.

Lachesis • *Lachesis*

The South American bushmaster snake grows to a length of seven feet and kills its prey, both animal and human, by constriction or by injection of its highly poisonous venom, known as lachesis, from which this homeopathic remedy is derived. Small doses of the venom can destroy red blood cells and impair the clotting of blood. Larger amounts of lachesis poison the heart. Homeopathic practitioners believe that the conditions best treated with *Lachesis* are those accompanied by symptoms similar to the ones induced by the venom. To prepare the homeopathic remedy, venom is extracted from the snake and diluted in large quantities of lactose (milk sugar).

TARGET AILMENTS

Choking coughs, croup, a constricted feeling in the throat, earaches that are worse during swallowing, left-sided sore throats, indigestion, throbbing headaches, especially those that appear during menopause, insomnia, hot flashes, heart arrhythmias, hemorrhoids, sciatica.

The 30 Most Effective Homeopathic Remedies

Ledum • *Ledum palustre*

Ledum, sometimes called marsh tea, can be found in bogs across northern Europe, Canada, and the United States. The herb has an antiseptic smell, and its upper branches are covered with a coat of tiny brown hairs. These may have given ledum its name; in Greek, *ledos* means "woolly robe." Once used in Scandinavia for insect control, ledum has also served as a tea substitute and replaced hops in beer, although overconsumption has resulted in dizziness and a splitting headache—even before the hangover. Homeopathic practitioners consider dilute doses of *Ledum* helpful for conditions that may be accompanied by signs of infection or inflammation.

The homeopathic remedy is prepared from the whole plant, which is gathered, dried, and crushed to a powder. This is diluted to nontoxic levels in a water-and-alcohol mix.

TARGET AILMENTS

Animal bites or insect stings, bruises that have already discolored the skin, deep cuts or puncture wounds where there is danger of infection, gout, aching joints.

Lycopodium • *Lycopodium clavatum*

Lycopodium, also known as club moss, grows in pastures and woodlands throughout Great Britain, northern Europe, and North America. Its spores contain a highly flammable pollen that was once used in fireworks and other pyrotechnics. Powder made from its ground-up spores has been used for internal complaints like diarrhea and dysentery since the 17th century. Homeopathic physicians use dilute doses of *Lycopodium* for complaints that are accompanied by symptoms of digestive upset, ailments that seem to develop on the right side of the body, a strong desire for sweets, anxiety, and symptoms that worsen in the early evening. To create the homeopathic remedy, pollen is extracted from the spores and diluted with milk sugar.

TARGET AILMENTS

Backache with stiffness and soreness in the lower back, bedwetting, colds with stuffy nose, constipation, coughs with mucus, cystitis, headache with throbbing pain, gout, indigestion accompanied by abdominal cramps, gas, heartburn, joint pain, sciatica, right-sided sore throat, eczema.

Mercurius vivus • *Mercurius vivus*

One of the metallic chemical elements, mercury, also called quicksilver, was known in ancient Chinese and Hindu civilizations and has had a long history of medicinal use. Ingesting certain mercury compounds can cause increased perspiration and salivation; and so in ancient medicine mercury was used, along with bloodletting and purging, as a means of ridding the body of impurities. Undilute mercury is toxic, however, and severe symptoms of mercury poisoning may include nausea, inflammation of the digestive tract, and kidney failure.

Homeopathic practitioners prescribe *Merc viv,* as the homeopathic preparation of mercury is sometimes called, for conditions accompanied by symptoms of shaking, hot and cold sweats, and restlessness. *Merc viv* is made from the chemical element mercury by dilution with large quantities of milk sugar.

TARGET AILMENTS

Abscesses, especially dental or glandular; backache with burning, shooting pains in the lower back; chickenpox; colds with an exceptionally runny nose and pain in the nostrils; cystitis with slow urination; painful diarrhea; influenza; earache with discharge of pus; eye inflammation; indigestion; mouth ulcers; burning sore throat; toothache with increased salivation.

CONTINUED

The 30 Most Effective Homeopathic Remedies

Natrum muriaticum • *Natrum muriaticum*

Natrum muriaticum is simply salt, or sodium chloride, a substance present in the natural world in quantities greater than any other except water. Essential to life and health, salt has been valued in human commerce throughout history. Roman soldiers were given a stipend, called a *salarium*, which they used to buy salt; from this we get the word *salary*. Homeopaths prescribe dilute solutions of *Nat mur*, as they call it, for conditions that are coupled with symptoms of extreme thirst, emotional sensitivity, and a strong desire for salt.

   Nat mur is prepared by adding pure sodium chloride to boiling water. Once the salt has dissolved, the solution is filtered and crystallized by evaporation. The final product is diluted in water to the desired potency.

TARGET AILMENTS

Backaches that are relieved by firm pressure; cold sores, especially in the corners of the mouth; colds with sneezing, watery eyes, and runny nose; constipation; fevers accompanied by weakness and chills; genital herpes; eczema; anemia; hay fever; migraine headaches; menstrual irregularity; indigestion; depression caused by grief, with a desire to be alone.

Nux vomica • *Nux vomica*

Nux vomica, also known as poison nut, is a remedy made from the seeds of an evergreen tree indigenous to parts of India, Thailand, China, and Australia. The seeds contain strychnine and have a bitter, unpleasant taste. Small doses of the seed stimulate the appetite, while somewhat larger doses decrease the appetite and cause motor dysfunction, including stiffness in the arms and legs and a staggering walk. Toxic doses can cause convulsions and death. *Nux vomica* is prescribed by homeopaths for ailments that occur from overindulgence in food, coffee, or alcohol, usually accompanied by irritability. To prepare the homeopathic remedy, poison-nut seeds are ground to a powder and then diluted with milk sugar to the desired potency.

TARGET AILMENTS

Colic and stomach cramps from overeating, colds with sneezing and a stuffy nose, constipation, cystitis, headache with dizziness, fevers with chills, gas and gas pains, hangovers, indigestion, insomnia, irritable bowel syndrome, nausea, menstrual cramps with a heavy flow, sinusitis, stomach flu, vomiting from overeating or eating rich foods.

Phosphorus • *Phosphorus*

The chemical element phosphorus can be found in the cellular fluid of all living tissue. Phosphorus plays a vital role in the activity of the body's cells, most importantly in the transfer of genetic information. Many phosphorus compounds are used commercially in toothpaste, fertilizer, and laundry detergent. Phosphorus poisoning causes irritation of the mucous membranes and inflammation of tissue; over time, it can destroy bone. As a homeopathic remedy, minute doses are prescribed by practitioners for conditions accompanied by symptoms of fatigue and nervousness with a tendency to bleed easily and an unquenchable thirst for cold water. Pure phosphorus is diluted in large quantities of milk sugar to prepare the homeopathic remedy.

TARGET AILMENTS

Bronchitis, pneumonia, coughs with congestion and burning pains in the chest, visual problems resulting from eyestrain, gastritis, nosebleeds, indigestion accompanied by vomiting or pain, stomach ulcers, kidney infections, nasal polyps, hepatitis, anemia, hemorrhages, diarrhea, menstrual problems.

The 30 Most Effective Homeopathic Remedies

Pulsatilla • *Pulsatilla nigricans*

Common in the meadowlands of northern and central Europe, the pulsatilla, or windflower, contains a caustic substance, and chewing the plant may cause blisters in the mouth and throat. Homeopathic physicians often prescribe *Pulsatilla* to patients with conditions accompanied by a thick yellow or white discharge. For homeopathic use the plant is collected when in full bloom and pounded to a pulp. The pulp is steeped in an alcohol-and-water solution and then strained and diluted.

TARGET AILMENTS

Bedwetting, breast infections, chickenpox, coughs, headaches, eye inflammation, fever with chills, hay fever, incontinence, indigestion, aching joints that improve with movement and cold compresses, urethritis in men, late menstrual periods, otitis media, sciatica, sinusitis, varicose veins, depression.

Rhus toxicodendron • *Rhus toxicodendron*

This vinelike shrub, also known as poison ivy, grows throughout North America and is well known for the itchy red rash its oil can cause on the skin. The medicinal history of its leaves and stalk began in the late 18th century, when it was used to treat conditions such as paralysis and rheumatism. The effects of its undilute form can range from a rash to nausea, fever, delirium, swollen glands, and ulcers in the oral cavity. For this reason homeopathic practitioners use *Rhus toxicodendron,* or *Rhus tox,* as it is also called, to treat conditions that may be accompanied by fever, restlessness, and swollen glands.

Rhus tox is prepared from plants gathered at night, when the oil is said to be in its most potent state. The leaves and stalks are pounded to a pulp and mixed with alcohol, then strained and diluted.

TARGET AILMENTS

Arthritis with stiffness that is worse in the morning and better with motion; backache with stiffness along the spine; bursitis; carpal tunnel syndrome; eye inflammation with swelling, itching, and sticky matter; genital herpes; hamstring injury; influenza with painful joints; headaches; hives that itch, sting, and intensify after scratching; joint and back pains from overexertion; impetigo; poison ivy; sprains with stiffness; toothaches.

Ruta • *Ruta graveolens*

Native to southern Europe, ruta spread across the continent in the wake of the Romans, who valued it for its medicinal properties. *Ruta* comes from the Greek *reuo,* meaning "to set free," an allusion to its historical popularity as a cure for numerous complaints, including headaches, coughs, and croup. Through centuries of use, this small shrub, sometimes called rue or rue bitterwort, has spread to herb gardens worldwide.

In large doses, ruta has toxic properties, but homeopathic physicians prescribe minute doses to treat conditions or injuries that may be accompanied by symptoms of weakness or a bruised sensation. The plant is collected just before blossoming; it is pounded to a pulp and pressed for its juice, which is then diluted in a water-and-alcohol base.

TARGET AILMENTS

Carpal tunnel syndrome, eyestrain caused by overwork and accompanied by heat and pain, sciatica, groin strain, sprains with pain and a bruised sensation, tennis elbow, injuries of tendons and cartilage.

CONTINUED

The 30 Most Effective Homeopathic Remedies

Sepia • Sepia

The cuttlefish is a soft-bodied mollusk with eight arms that is closely related to the squid and octopus; it propels itself by squirting jets of water from special organs in its body. When threatened, it releases spurts of dark ink called sepia that cloud the water and camouflage its retreat. Sepia has been used for artistic purposes, although its ingestion, such as when a painter licks the brush, can bring about unpleasant side effects. Homeopathic physicians prescribe *Sepia* to patients with conditions whose symptoms include apathy, moodiness, and weakness. The cuttlefish ink is collected for the homeopathic preparation and diluted with large quantities of milk sugar for final use.

TARGET AILMENTS

Backaches and weakness in the small of the back; violent fits of coughing; cold sores and fever blisters around the mouth; exhaustion; genital herpes; hair loss; gas; headaches with throbbing pain; sinusitis; urinary incontinence; menopausal hot flashes; menstrual cramps with intense, bearing-down pain; nausea resulting from motion sickness or during pregnancy; brown spots on the skin.

Silica • Silica

Silica, also called flint, is a mineral that is present in the human body in only trace amounts but is vital to the development of bones, the flexibility of cartilage, and the health of the skin and connective tissues. Many industrial operations rely on silica, including the manufacture of concrete, paper, glass, and enamelware. Flint's medicinal use is limited to homeopathy. Minute doses are prescribed for patients with conditions accompanied by excessive sweating, weakness, and extreme sensitivity to cold. For homeopathic use silica powder is mixed with sodium carbonate through a pharmaceutical process of dry substance dilution.

TARGET AILMENTS

Athlete's foot, constipation, wounds that have been inflamed by foreign matter, earache with decreased hearing and a stopped-up sensation, fingernails that have white spots and split easily, headaches beginning in the back of the head and spreading forward to the eyes, abscesses, swollen glands in the neck, gum infections, hemorrhoids, breast cysts.

Sulphur • Sulphur

The chemical element sulphur, or more commonly, "sulfur," is present in all living tissue. It was known to ancient societies, and in the Bible it is called brimstone. Among the various conditions to which it has been applied as a medication for some 2,000 years are skin disorders such as scabies. Commercially, sulfur is used in the production of dyes, fungicides, and gunpowder. Homeopathic physicians may prescribe dilute doses of the remedy *Sulphur* to treat conditions accompanied by irritability, intense itching, burning pains, and offensive odors. The homeopathic remedy is made from pure sulfur powder that is diluted with either milk sugar or a water-and-alcohol solution.

TARGET AILMENTS

Asthma that is worse at night and is accompanied by rattling mucus, cough with chest pain, morning diarrhea, eye inflammation, bursitis, headaches with burning pain, indigestion, joint pain, anal itching with redness, burning vaginal discharge, eczema with intense itching and burning.

$\mathcal{H}$ydrotherapy

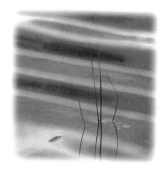

Hydrotherapy, which literally means water therapy, encompasses a variety of therapeutic uses of water. As either ice, liquid, or steam, water may relieve the symptoms of numerous types of infections, acute and chronic pain, circulatory problems, and more. External hydrotherapy treatments typically involve applications of hot or cold water (or the alternation of both) to the skin. Internal treatments consist of water taken internally as a cleansing agent.

Treatments range from the homey footbath to sophisticated physical therapy in a hospital pool, and can include wraps, sprays, and douches, as well as the use of steam rooms, saunas, and hot and cold baths. In general, the aim is to stimulate an immune response or to detoxify the body by changing body temperature.

Origins

Using water as a source of healing is a concept as old as civilization itself. In its modern form, hydrotherapy came to the United States from Germany, where the 19th-century passion for spas and water treatments influenced such healers as the Austrian peasant Vincenz Priessnitz, the founder of hydrotherapy; and Father Sebastian Kneipp, the originator of "Kneipp's cure," which employed forms of hydrotherapy. By the turn of the century, the term "water cure" had become a catchall phrase for many forms of natural healing. Ultimately, hydrotherapy became one of the key treatments of naturopathy *(pages 141-143),* and today, outside the home, it is practiced primarily by naturopathic doctors and physical therapists.

What It's Good For

Hydrotherapy has a wide range of applications, but it is particularly useful for treating muscle and joint pain and inflammation, burns and frostbite, fevers, sinusitis, headaches, the upper respiratory tract, indigestion, pelvic pain, and stress. In pools and whirlpool baths, hydrotherapy treatment is also used to strengthen limbs after injury. Internal hydrotherapy can ease digestive problems and help detoxify the blood.

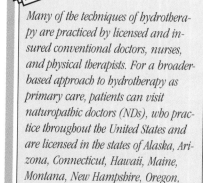

LICENSED & INSURED?

Many of the techniques of hydrotherapy are practiced by licensed and insured conventional doctors, nurses, and physical therapists. For a broader-based approach to hydrotherapy as primary care, patients can visit naturopathic doctors (NDs), who practice throughout the United States and are licensed in the states of Alaska, Arizona, Connecticut, Hawaii, Maine, Montana, New Hampshire, Oregon, Utah, Vermont, and Washington. Some, but not all, insurance plans cover treatments from NDs.

Target Ailments

- Arthritis
- Athletic Injuries
- Bursitis
- Circulatory Problems
- Common Cold
- Fever and Chills
- Headache
- Hemorrhoids
- Indigestion
- Muscle Cramps
- Pain, Chronic
- Rashes and Skin Problems
- Sinusitis
- Stress
- Tendinitis
- Varicose Veins

See Common Ailments, beginning on page 194.

CONTINUED

Hydrotherapy CONTINUED

CAUTION

Pregnant women, as well as those with diabetes, atherosclerosis, or a decreased sensitivity to hot and cold, should consult a doctor before using any heat therapies. When using hot water or hot packs, you should always test the temperature first to make sure it won't burn. Avoid using the microwave for heating: It can result in irregular hot and cold spots.

FOR MORE INFO

Following is a list of organizations you can contact to learn more about hydrotherapy:

National College of Naturopathic Medicine
11231 SE Market Street
Portland, OR 97216
(503) 255-4860

Bastyr University of Natural Health Sciences
14500 Juanita Drive, NE
Bothell, WA 98011
(206) 523-9585

Southwest College of Naturopathic Medicine
2140 East Broadway Road
Tempe, AZ 85251
(602) 858-9100

Uchee Pines Lifestyle Center
30 Uchee Pines Road, Box 75
Seale, AL 36875
Phone: (334) 855-4764

Preparations/Techniques

External hydrotherapy relies primarily on the effects of water temperature—hot, neutral, cold, or alternating hot and cold—to produce its effects. Hot water soothes and relaxes while stimulating the immune system. Neutral or body-temperature baths are also soothing, particularly for people with stress and insomnia. Cold water discourages inflammation and fever, while the contrast of hot and cold can improve circulation and reduce congestion.

A practitioner might recommend treatments either at a facility with the right kinds of pools and whirlpool tubs, or at home. Some treatments should take place under the watchful eye of a trained physician or therapist—hyperthermia, for example, which is a fever-inducing therapy for patients fighting viruses and infections. Paraplegics, those suffering from burns and frostbite, and anyone with diminished sensation also need to work with therapists if they are being treated in baths.

However, many of the treatments of hydrotherapy can easily be done at home. A simple example is the cold compress. For an inflamed joint or a feverish headache, take a terry cloth washcloth, wring it out in ice water, and apply it to the afflicted area. As the cloth warms up, chill it down again and repeat.

To improve immune function and for general stimulation, a hydrotherapist might suggest immediately following a hot shower with a cold one. Or if a handheld hose or sprayer is available, you can hook up the sprayer to a faucet after a hot shower and spray (or ask a friend to spray) cold water along both sides of the spine.

Hydrotherapists may also recommend adding therapeutic herbs and oils to the bath. Among them could be chamomile to soothe the skin, oatmeal for hives or sunburn, or ginger for relaxation. *(See Herbal Therapies, pages 70-73).*

Wellness

Proponents of hydrotherapy believe that a healthy body maintains a certain internal balance. In order to keep this stability, it must constantly adjust to environmental influences such as heat, cold, food and water, and clothing. Water therapies enhance and reinforce the body's reaction to these external influences, helping it to stay well.

What the Critics Say

Most forms of external hydrotherapy—whirlpool baths, cold compresses, and the like—are widely accepted by the medical establishment. Internal hydrotherapy, particularly the use of enemas and colonic irrigation, comes in for more criticism, however. Critics say that such methods have little scientific justification and that they can actually spread infection if not carefully applied. ■

Light Therapy

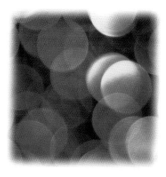

S imply put, light therapy is the use of natural or artificial light to promote healing. Specific techniques differ primarily in the type of light involved. Full-spectrum light therapy consists of regular exposure to controlled amounts of either natural sunlight or artificial light that contains all wavelengths of light, from infrared to ultraviolet. Bright light therapy involves exposure to nonultraviolet white light in levels that match the amount of natural sunlight found outdoors shortly after sunrise or before sunset. In cold laser therapy, small beams of low-intensity laser light are applied directly to the skin. Colored light therapy focuses different colored lights on the skin.

The Importance of Light

Recent research indicates that for the body to be healthy, it must receive adequate exposure to the full and balanced spectrum of light found in natural sunlight. Adequate light is especially needed for the regulation of circadian rhythms, the daily internal pacemakers that govern a host of biological functions in humans, from hormone production to patterns of sleeping and waking. In healthy people, these rhythms run in regular cycles, reset each morning by the light of the rising sun. If the rhythms become disturbed for any reason, health problems can result.

Origins

Sunlight has been used for healing throughout history. The ancient Greek physician Hippocrates prescribed sunlight for certain disorders, often sending his patients to recuperate in roofless buildings. During the Middle Ages, red light was a popular treatment for smallpox. The windows of sickrooms were covered with red curtains, and patients were wrapped in red sheets. Doctors started using bright light therapy for seasonal affective disorder and other ailments beginning in the 1980s.

What It's Good For

Full-spectrum light therapy is used to treat various ailments, including high blood pressure, rashes and skin problems, depression, insomnia, PMS, migraines, jaundice in newborns, and jet lag. Bright light therapy has been shown to be highly effective in treating seasonal affective disorder (SAD), a form of depression that strikes

Target Ailments

- Arthritis
- Carpal Tunnel Syndrome
- Depression
- Headache
- High Blood Pressure
- Insomnia
- Menstrual Problems
- Pain, Chronic
- Premenstrual Syndrome
- Rashes and Skin Problems
- Seasonal Affective Disorder
- Stress
- Tendinitis

See Common Ailments, beginning on page 194.

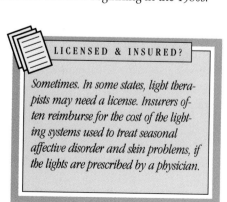

LICENSED & INSURED?

Sometimes. In some states, light therapists may need a license. Insurers often reimburse for the cost of the lighting systems used to treat seasonal affective disorder and skin problems, if the lights are prescribed by a physician.

119

CONTINUED

Light Therapy CONTINUED

CAUTION

If you have glaucoma, cataracts, retinal detachment, or other eye problems, check with your eye doctor before undergoing light therapy. If you have a rash and fever, obtain a professional diagnosis to rule out infections such as measles or chickenpox. Ultraviolet light therapy may cause premature aging of the skin and increase your risk of skin cancer.

FOR MORE INFO
Following is a list of organizations you can contact to learn more about light therapy:

Dinshaw Health Society
PO Box 707
Malaga, NJ 08328
(609) 692-4686
(information on color therapy)

Institute for Frontier Science
7711-D McCallum Street
Philadelphia, PA 19118
e-mail: 101471.1777@compuserve.com
(information on laser therapy)

Society for Light Treatment and Biological Rhythms
10200 West 44th Avenue, Suite 304
Wheat Ridge, CO 80033-2840
(303) 424-3697
e-mail: sltbr@resourcenter.com
(Researches light therapy for the treatment of SAD, sleep disorders, and related conditions. Send $7 for a light therapy information packet.)

people during winter, when days are short. Bright light therapy is also used to treat bulimia, irregular menstrual cycles, and sleep disorders. Cold laser therapy is used primarily to relieve chronic pain and help heal wounds, but it is also a part of laser acupuncture, a form of acupuncture that addresses a variety of health concerns. Colored light therapy is used for depression, sleep problems, chronic pain, stress, menstrual problems, arthritis, tendinitis, sore throat, and hives and insect bites.

Preparations/Techniques

Most light therapy can be self-administered, either by spending more time outdoors or by purchasing special therapeutic lights and then following the directions that come with them. Full-spectrum light therapy is accomplished indoors by installing full-spectrum lighting in place of incandescent and fluorescent lighting, which lacks the complete balanced spectrum of sunlight. Bright light therapy requires that you sit near a light box, usually for about 30 minutes, early in the morning from late fall through early spring. Cold lasers are held over the affected area of the body for specified lengths of time, generally no more than a few minutes. The treatment is then repeated once or twice a day for several days or until the condition improves. Some forms of colored light therapy also involve directing small beams of light, usually red, over the area of the body that needs healing. Another method involves bathing the body with colored light from filtered floodlights.

Visiting a Professional

You may find it useful to consult a knowledgeable healthcare professional about applying some forms of light therapy to your particular health concern. Before using bright light therapy for the treatment of SAD, you should see a healthcare professional skilled in the diagnosis and treatment of that illness. Ultraviolet light therapy treatments for dermatitis, psoriasis, and other skin problems should be administered only by a professional.

Wellness

People who use light therapy report that it reduces stress and relaxes and rejuvenates the body, thus contributing to an overall feeling of physical and mental well-being. Research has also shown that exposure to full-spectrum and bright light helps promote wellness by keeping the body's biological rhythms synchronized.

What the Critics Say

Although the use of light therapy for the treatment of seasonal affective disorder and skin problems is widely accepted, other forms of light therapy have not undergone rigorous scientific studies. ■

Massage

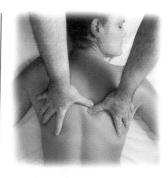

Massage therapy, defined as the systematic manipulation of the soft tissues, relieves sore muscles and promotes relaxation. It is usually performed with various standard hand strokes, but sometimes pressure is applied with other parts of the body, such as the forearm, elbow, or foot.

The general purposes of massage are to reduce tension, improve circulation, aid in the healing of soft-tissue injuries, control pain, and promote overall well-being. Massage can gently stretch tissues, increase range of motion, and reduce some types of edema (swelling). It can also help lower blood pressure and heart rate and improve respiration. Researchers believe massage helps the brain make endorphins, chemicals that act as natural painkillers—which perhaps explains why recipients feel better and more tranquil after a massage.

The Nature of Touch

Touching is, of course, an integral part of massage, and it may play a significant role in massage's therapeutic effects. Studies have found that animals that are touched grow faster and that infants who are not touched develop more slowly, physically and psychologically, than those who are. Touch can convey the therapeutic emotions of caring and concern. Some massage therapists believe that touch can create trust and openness and help release blocked emotions.

Origins

One of the earliest forms of healing, massage was mentioned in Chinese medical texts 4,000 years ago. It has been advocated in Western societies since the Greek physician Hippocrates, in the fourth century BC, referred to a technique called rubbing. In ancient Rome, Julius Caesar is said to have had himself pinched all over every day to treat his neuralgia.

At the beginning of the 19th century, a Swedish gymnastics instructor and fencing master, Pehr Henrik Ling, cured himself of an elbow ailment with percussion strokes (tapping

LICENSED & INSURED?

Twenty-four states and some localities currently license massage therapy. Licensing laws are pending in additional states. Most states require 500 or more hours of education from a recognized school program as well as an examination. In 1992, the National Certification Examination in Therapeutic Massage and Bodywork was inaugurated, and states are gradually adopting it as their test. Massage is covered by some insurance companies.

Target Ailments

■ Arthritis

■ Asthma

■ Athletic Injuries

■ Back Problems

■ Carpal Tunnel Syndrome

■ Chronic Fatigue Syndrome

■ Constipation

■ Depression

■ Headache

■ Heartburn

■ Immune Problems

■ Insomnia

■ Irritable Bowel Syndrome

■ Multiple Sclerosis

■ Muscle Cramps

■ Neuralgia

■ Pain, Chronic

■ Premenstrual Syndrome

■ Stomach Ulcers

■ Tendinitis

■ TMJ Syndrome

See Common Ailments, beginning on page 194.

CONTINUED

Massage CONTINUED

CAUTION

Consult a physician if you are considering massage therapy and have had an injury or a chronic illness such as heart or kidney disease. You should not use massage if you have an infection, inflammation, or cancer that could spread throughout the body or if you have a blood clot. Massage is not appropriate for some cases of edema because it can encourage more bleeding and swelling. If you have a nerve injury, you might find pressure on the skin painful. Do not use massage on your abdomen if you have high blood pressure or a peptic ulcer, and avoid massaging burned areas until they are healed.

movements). He subsequently developed a method of healing that became known as Swedish massage. This therapy, which was based on the then-emerging science of physiology, came to the United States in the mid-19th century. Interest dwindled, however, when healthcare in the United States took a technological turn in the early 1900s and didn't pick up again until the alternative healthcare movement gained momentum in the 1970s.

What It's Good For

Massage is recommended for countless injuries and ailments. Well-designed studies have proved the benefits of particular methods of massage to treat pain, nausea, muscle spasm, and soft-tissue problems, as well as anxiety, depression, insomnia, and emotional stress. Massage helps premature infants gain weight and develop motor skills, and it helps elderly people relax. Researchers believe it also may improve immune system response. Many studies are under way to evaluate massage therapy further, including research on its effects in infants exposed to HIV, children with asthma, adolescents with eating disorders, adults with hypertension, and patients recovering from surgery.

Massage can also aid people who cannot use their muscles actively because of injury, illness, or paralysis. Although it cannot substitute for the normal muscular activity that rids the muscles of toxic products, massage can help the process when a person is unable to be normally active.

Preparations/Techniques

There are approximately 100 different methods of massage therapy, about 80 of them born in the period of revival since the mid-1970s. A simple classification includes traditional European methods, contemporary Western methods, energetic manual techniques, and Oriental manual techniques.

The traditional European methods are based on longstanding Western concepts of anatomy and physiology. They use the five kinds of soft-tissue manipulation—effleurage, petrissage, friction, percussion, and vibration and jostling (the basic Swedish massage strokes)—illustrated in the Gallery of Massage Techniques that begins on page 124.

Contemporary Western methods add to the traditional techniques more recent knowledge of the effects of massage on the nervous system, posture, movement, and emotion. Also included in contemporary methods are techniques such as Rolfing and the Alexander and Feldenkrais methods *(see Bodywork, pages 47-56)* that are said to integrate the body in relationship to gravity.

Energetic and Oriental manual techniques use pressure and manipulation to assess, evaluate, and balance the energy system said to surround and infuse the

Massage

human body. Polarity therapy *(page 64)* and therapeutic touch *(page 55)* are energetic techniques. Oriental methods include shiatsu and acupressure *(pages 16-17)*.

Visiting a Professional

You can find a qualified massage therapist through a physician's recommendation, a friend's advice (make sure the therapist is nationally certified or state-licensed), or by contacting one of the organizations listed below, right. On your first visit, the massage therapist should ask about your medical history and current state of health in order to tailor the therapy to your particular problems.

You will probably need to disrobe completely or partially, depending on the areas to be worked on. The therapist will position you comfortably on a massage table and provide a sheet or large towel to drape over the areas of your body that are not being massaged. During your session, pay attention to your reactions and speak up if an area is painful or tender to the touch.

Doing It Yourself

If you are planning to practice massage with a partner, start with a few of the basic strokes and begin lightly, adding deeper strokes gradually. Wear loose clothing, remove your watch and rings, and keep your fingernails short to avoid scratching. Wash your hands thoroughly before beginning. Although shiatsu is done on the floor on a pad or futon, massage is best performed on a massage table. Keep the lighting gentle for optimum relaxation, and keep the room warm.

While massaging, keep your hands on your partner as much as possible, breaking contact gently and slowly to change areas. If your partner's muscles tighten, the pressure may be either too severe, causing discomfort, or too light, causing a tickling sensation. Do not massage directly a very tender area or the exact site of an injury. Put your body weight behind the pressure, rather than using your hands and arms alone, and keep your hands as relaxed as possible.

Wellness

The ability of massage to reduce stress and tension, tone muscles, and enhance well-being makes it a useful part of a regular health maintenance program. Athletes often use massage to prepare muscles for strenuous activity or to recover after activity.

What the Critics Say

Some conventional practitioners worry that ill or injured people may seek massage in place of required medical treatment; however, certified massage therapists are usually knowledgeable about the need for conventional treatment. As with any therapy, patients should be wary of any extreme or quick-cure claims. ■

FOR MORE INFO
Following is a list of organizations you can contact to learn more about massage therapy:

American Massage Therapy Association
820 Davis Street, Suite 100
Evanston, IL 60201
(847) 864-0123

National Certification Board for Therapeutic Massage and Bodywork
8201 Greensboro Drive, Suite 300
McLean, VA 22102
(703) 610-9015

Gallery of Massage Techniques

Effleurage

Massage of most areas of the body begins and ends with effleurage, a slow, rhythmic, gliding stroke performed with the fingertips, palms, thumbs, knuckles, or whole hand. Generally, effleurage moves from the extremities toward the heart—from wrist to shoulder, for example. An exception is the nerve stroke, which does not affect blood flow and is done in the direction opposite to a preceding series of effleurage strokes.

Start lightly and gradually work deeper. You may end your massage of each area with the nerve stroke, which is particularly soothing. The broad surface of the back is ideal for practicing the variations of effleurage pictured here. Keep your hands relaxed; tense, rigid hands have less sensitivity and don't feel as good to your partner.

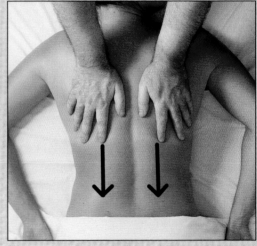

Basic Effleurage • Position your hands close together, with your thumbs an inch or two apart. Stroke downward, keeping your hands in firm and full contact with your partner's body until you reach the top of the pelvic bone.

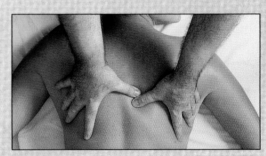

Adjacent Thumb • Place one thumb next to the other and glide down the back. Most of the pressure should be applied by your thumbs.

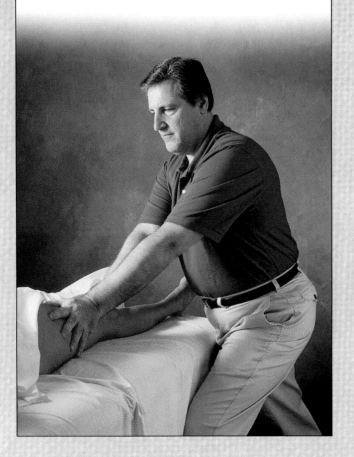

Posture • Align your body properly to prevent fatigue and strain. Use the entire weight of your upper body, rather than your hands alone, for pressure; the lower body should balance and support. In general, face the direction in which your hands are moving.

Gallery of Massage Techniques

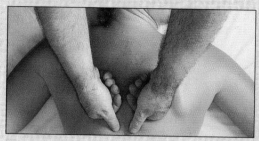

Loose Fist • *Work large muscles with a loose fist, making contact with the area of the fingers between the second and third joints. Glide down the back.*

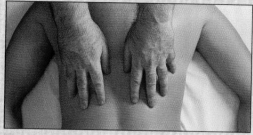

Nerve Stroke • *While barely touching the skin, drag your fingertips up the back, moving in the reverse direction from previous effleurage strokes.*

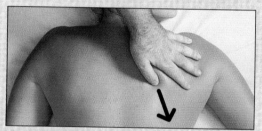

One Thumb • *For a deeper stroke, use one thumb to glide deeply along smaller muscles. Use a little more pressure to contact muscles that lie underneath the superficial layers of muscle.*

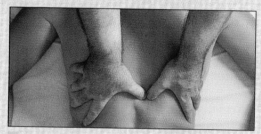

Joined Thumb • *Place your thumbs along the erector muscles next to the spine. Starting just below the base of the neck, slide your thumbs down, using more pressure than with previous strokes.*

Petrissage

A more complex technique, petrissage works specific muscle groups, usually where tissue is easily grasped. It can be performed deeply or superficially. Deep petrissage helps promote circulation and can counteract muscle tightness or degeneration. Alternately tighten and loosen your hands, fingers, or thumbs as you pick up and release muscles. Variations include rolling, heel of palm, and compression. Note the change in musculature as you go from tendons and ligaments toward the center of a muscle, which can usually withstand more pressure.

Hand on Hand • *Use this stroke on the abdomen. Place the fingers of your top hand over the bottom hand for support. Ask your partner to bend her knees. Proceed clockwise in a circle, exerting even pressure.*

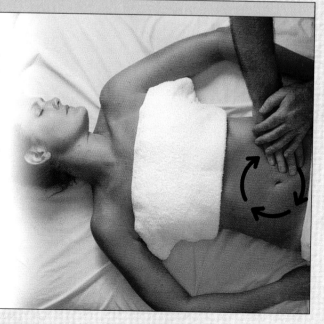

CONTINUED

Gallery of Massage Techniques

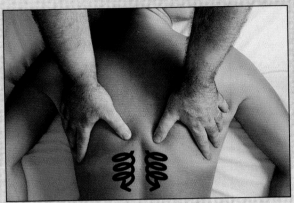

Spiral • *Pressing with both thumbs while making a sweeping motion, spiral down the back, using a counterclockwise motion with the left thumb and a clockwise motion with the right thumb. Go from the base of the neck to the waist.*

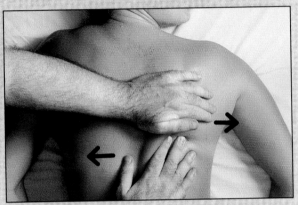

Rolling • *Slide your hand firmly back and forth across your partner's back. Push with the heel of one hand, and pull/lift the skin with the fingers of the other. Note how this stroke wrings the tissues between your two hands.*

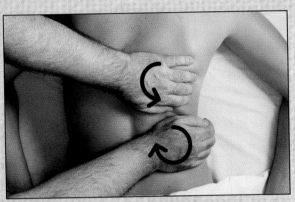

Heel of Palm • *Place the heels of your palms next to your partner's spine. Alternately rotating your palms in opposite directions, push the muscle gently away from the spine as you work down the back, so the muscle is kneaded but not pinched.*

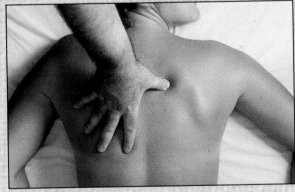

Direct Pressure • *For trigger points (which feel like small marbles), for knots of muscle tension, or to execute shiatsu techniques, press with the pad of your thumb or finger straight into the tissue. Hold for five to 15 seconds or until you feel the tension release.*

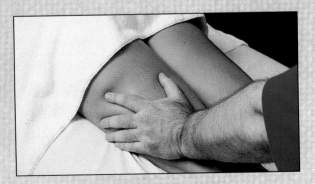

Compression • *Place one palm flat with the fingers relaxed. Pump your hand up and down rhythmically, directing the pressure toward the bone underneath, then releasing the pressure. Do not use this technique on joints.*

Friction

Friction is often used in areas around joints. As in petrissage, you move muscle or other soft tissue away from bone. But in friction, the fingers or thumbs move over the underlying structures without sliding on the surface of the skin where the fingers or thumbs touch.

Because they have a relatively poor blood supply, tendons and ligaments tend to heal slowly, particularly during vigorous activities, sometimes resulting in "overuse" syndromes. Friction increases circulation and helps restore range of motion; it is a mainstay of sports massage, where it is referred to as cross-fiber stroking. Use your fingertips and thumbs to perform friction; lighten pressure if your partner experiences discomfort. Friction should not be used on an area that has been injured within the past 24 to 48 hours.

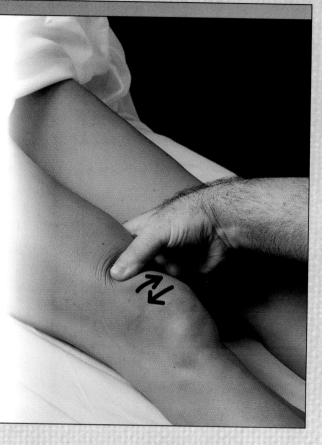

■ **Cross-Fiber** • Pressing down, slide the thumb across the grain of the muscle (perpendicular to the muscle fiber) in a rhythmic motion. Keep your thumb on the same spot on the skin surface. You may feel the muscle fibers moving under your thumb.

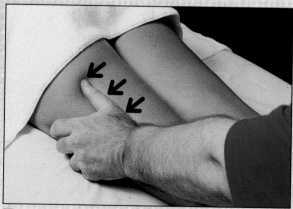

■ **Broad Cross-Fiber Stroking** • Place your hand on the center of the back of the leg. While applying pressure with the outside edge of your thumb and palm, stroke across the grain of the muscle of the entire outer leg. Switch hands, and repeat on the inner portion of the leg.

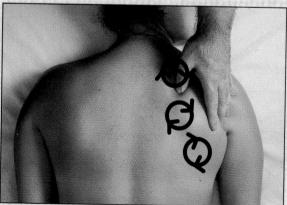

■ **Circular Friction** • Locate the ropelike tissues that join the shoulder blade to the back. Using your hand for balance, place your thumb on the tissues and rotate it in small circles. Move down a bit, repeat the motion, and continue until the entire area is covered.

CONTINUED

Percussion

Percussion strokes, also called tapotement (French for tapping), are alternate drumming hand movements performed on broad areas of the body, particularly the back. This stroke is clearly beneficial for increasing surface blood circulation, and it can help loosen phlegm and make it easier to expectorate it from the lungs.

When done properly, percussion is stimulating rather than painful or harsh. Keep your hands and wrists relaxed and elbows flexed. Strike the skin with alternating hands, moving rapidly over the surface you are working on. You should strike firmly but never so hard that you cause pain. Because even light percussion may cause discomfort to internal organs, do not apply it on the lower abdomen, the lower back near the kidneys, or directly on the spine.

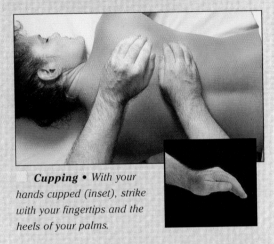

Cupping • With your hands cupped (inset), strike with your fingertips and the heels of your palms.

Beating • Form a loose fist (inset) and strike gently with the outside surface. Beating works best on the fleshier areas of the body, such as the back, waist, and thighs.

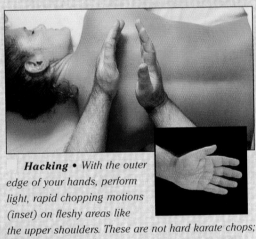

Hacking • With the outer edge of your hands, perform light, rapid chopping motions (inset) on fleshy areas like the upper shoulders. These are not hard karate chops; keep your hands relaxed with your fingers slightly separated.

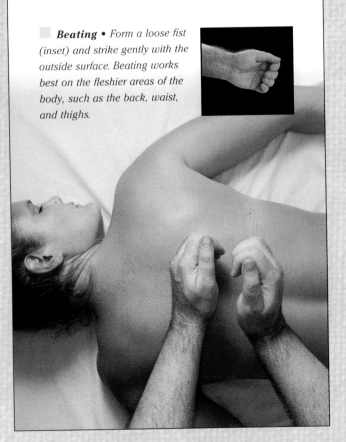

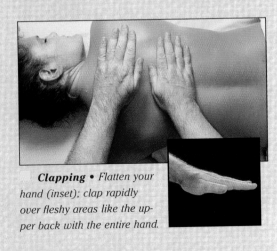

Clapping • Flatten your hand (inset); clap rapidly over fleshy areas like the upper back with the entire hand.

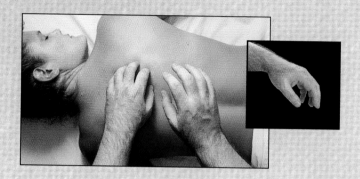

 Tapping • *Strike with the fingertips (inset), alternating your hands quickly. Unlike other percussion strokes, tapping may be helpful on bony areas such as the shoulder blades or scalp.*

Vibration and Jostling

Like percussion, these techniques either stimulate or relax body tissue. The strokes are particularly effective on the limbs and fleshy areas. Vibration does not proceed in any specific direction; jostling works up and down a muscle.

Vibration requires a rapid contraction and relaxation of your own muscles, which sets up a vibratory wave that is transmitted to your partner through your hands. (Some professional massage therapists use mechanical vibrators for this effect.) One form of joint mobilization is a variation of vibration that uses larger motions to work the joints.

Jostling, which is not as strenuous, is used in sports massage, especially to treat sore muscles. If your partner's muscles tense up during massage, interrupt your sequence and relax the muscle area by jostling it for five or 10 seconds. You can insert jostling into a massage as often as you want.

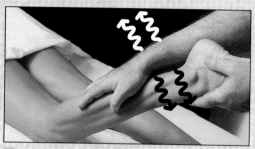

Jostling • *Place your hands on your partner's calf and shake back and forth, progressing along the muscle.*

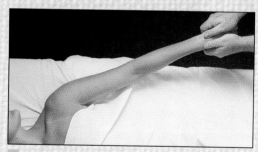

Joint Mobilization • *Grasp your partner's hand firmly between your hands. Move far enough away so that your partner's arm is fully extended, and shake the arm with a wavelike motion while pulling away slightly from the joint.*

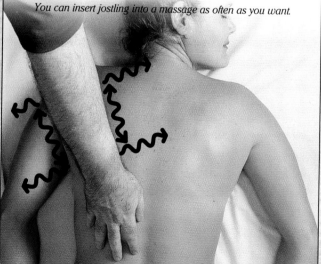

Vibration • *With your fingertips lightly touching your partner, tense all the muscles in your arm repeatedly, creating a trembling motion (left). The vibration you create in your arm is transferred through your fingers to the area being worked on.*

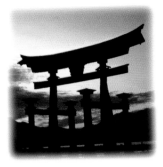

Target Ailments

- Back Problems
- Cancer
- Chronic Fatigue Syndrome
- Depression
- Diabetes
- Headache
- Heart Problems
- High Blood Pressure
- Immune Problems
- Incontinence
- Insomnia
- Irritable Bowel Syndrome
- Menopause
- Menstrual Problems
- Pain, Chronic
- Seasonal Affective Disorder
- Stress
- TMJ Syndrome

See Common Ailments, beginning on page 194.

Mind/Body Medicine

C lose your eyes and imagine holding a freshly cut, bright yellow lemon in your hand. Imagine raising it to your mouth and biting into the tart pulp. The saliva now flooding your mouth is evidence of the powerful connection between the thoughts in your mind and the physical processes of your body.

Western science has long viewed the mind and the body as separate entities. Using increasingly sophisticated drugs and surgical techniques, physicians have focused on the body while almost wholly ignoring the mind's role in illness and healing. Yet the mind appears to have enormous influence on the progress of disease: Studies suggest that people's opinions about the state of their own health can dramatically affect their chances of developing a serious disease later in life.

Mind/body medicine seeks to explore connections between the tangible body and the intangible mind, and to use these linkages to improve physical as well as mental health. The techniques are not so much treatments as they are processes that help people learn how to influence their physical reactions. A common goal among the various mind/body techniques is relaxation, an important weapon in the modern battle against stress-related disease.

Stress and Relaxation

The body reacts to stressful situations—sudden danger, for example—by releasing chemicals that produce a number of physical effects, such as an increase in heart rate, blood pressure, and muscle tension. Chronic or long-term stress can take a serious toll. It suppresses immune system activity and can lead to insomnia, anxiety, high blood pressure, depression, and possibly even cancer. Fortunately, the body has a recuperative reaction that can reverse many of the harmful effects of chronic stress: relaxation. Mind/body medicine is the quest to invoke the relaxation response and strengthen the body in pursuit of good health.

Mind/body techniques cannot replace conventional treatment, especially in the case of serious or chronic ailments, but they can be extremely useful as complementary therapies. Low in risk and cost, easy to learn, and adaptable to individual tastes, these methods can be combined and practiced in a number of ways. They can be used in conjunction with conventional or other alternative therapies to control the symptoms of disease or the side effects of certain treatments, or they can be practiced on a regular basis to promote and maintain overall health. And because they involve the active participation of the patient, mind/body techniques help foster a sense of control and self-reliance that in itself can be of significant therapeutic value.

Mind/Body Medicine

The Power of the Patient

Medical science generally has not accepted mind/body medicine, perhaps because thoughts do not lend themselves readily to scientific testing methods. However, a number of mind/body therapies—meditation, guided imagery, and prayer, for example—have been used successfully by traditional healers for hundreds of years. Even today, many physicians who do not embrace mind/body concepts acknowledge the influence the mind can have on disease. Some medical schools, in fact, teach the importance of a good bedside manner, realizing that what the patient believes about an illness—and also what the patient thinks the *doctor* believes—can change the course of the disease. The placebo effect is another familiar example of the curative power of belief: Convinced that a given medicine will bring relief, the patient actually does improve, even though the pills contain nothing but sugar.

The effectiveness of mind/body medicine depends largely on the level of patient commitment, as well as on the strength of one's belief that positive thinking can translate into better health. For these techniques to work, you must have realistic expectations and guidance from a competent, experienced therapist. Finding such a person may take some work, but the effort could pay off in long-term health benefits.

What the Critics Say

Despite evidence that the mind can and does play a role in healing, a number of healthcare professionals—even some who accept the general premise—remain skeptical of mind/body techniques. Some think that the benefits are limited, that patients will become frustrated if a technique does not produce significant improvements right away, or that patients will rely solely on mind/body techniques when other types of medical care are warranted. Many conventional doctors, for example, are concerned that patients using mind/body techniques will neglect to get proper, proven treatment for serious illnesses such as cancer, heart disease, or diabetes. While mind/body methods are themselves safe and can often help people recover from disease, using them as substitutes for a doctor's care can delay necessary treatment and lead to serious problems.

Mind/body techniques also have come under attack because of possible dangers of receiving treatment from practitioners who are unlicensed or poorly qualified: For some of these therapies, practitioners are not required to pass a state examination or get special training. This, say critics, opens the way for unscrupulous practitioners to take a patient's money and offer nothing in return but false hopes. And while proponents point to numerous studies showing that thoughts and deeply held beliefs can have a tremendous effect on one's health, some skeptics argue that the claims of mind/body medicine are not supported by scientific research.

CONTINUED

Biofeedback

In biofeedback, sensors on the body pick up electrical signals from the muscles or brain and pass them along to a computer, which translates the pulses into images or sounds. The patient watches or listens to these processed signals and, with the help of a therapist, develops ways to affect their rate or intensity. Eventually, the patient learns to exercise conscious control over normally unconscious bodily processes, such as blood pressure and heart rate.

What It's Good For • Biofeedback is used in many areas of medicine. It is especially helpful in the treatment of ailments that are caused or exacerbated by stress or anxiety, such as stress-induced hypertension and headaches. Many physical therapists use biofeedback to reeducate weak or overactive muscles, as well as to treat nerve damage and temporomandibular joint (TMJ) syndrome. Biofeedback may also be used to help reduce the frequency of epileptic seizures.

- **Headaches:** The American Medical Association sanctions biofeedback training for the treatment of certain types of headaches.
- **Raynaud's syndrome:** Thermal, or temperature regulation, biofeedback is a successful therapy for this disorder, which causes cold feet and hands due to constricted blood vessels.
- **Attention deficit disorder:** One promising new form of biofeedback aims to teach people with this disorder how to normalize brain waves associated with concentration, attention, and hyperactivity.
- **Diabetes:** Biofeedback training in relaxation techniques may help diabetics gain better metabolic control and learn to manage stress; stress can contribute to increased blood sugar levels in some people with the disease.

Visiting a Professional
Biofeedback is best learned with the help of a healthcare professional who has experience using its techniques to treat your condition. Learning to access and then control the body's functions usually takes at least eight to 10 visits. Consult your healthcare provider for a referral, or contact a national biofeedback society for more information.

LICENSED & INSURED?

Many biofeedback therapists are licensed physicians or other healthcare professionals who have received training in these techniques. Practitioners are certified by the Biofeedback Certification Institute of America, which also sets standards. Many insurance companies reimburse patients for biofeedback training provided by a licensed healthcare provider.

CAUTION

If you use a pacemaker or other implanted electrical aid or if you have a serious heart disorder, check with your physician before using a biofeedback device that measures the output of the sweat glands. These devices use a tiny amount of electricity, and although no problems have been reported with their use, several biofeedback organizations recommend this precaution.

FOR MORE INFO
Following is a list of organizations you can contact to learn more about biofeedback:

**Society for the Study
of Neuronal Regulation**
4600 Post Oak Place, Suite 301
Houston, TX 77027
(713) 552-0091
fax: (713) 552-0752
e-mail: ssnr@primenet.com

**Association for Applied
Psychophysiology and Biofeedback**
10200 West 44th Ave., Suite 304
Wheat Ridge, CO 80033-2840
(800) 477-8892
fax: (303) 422-8894

**Biofeedback Certification
Institute of America**
10200 West 44th Ave., Suite 304
Wheat Ridge, CO 80033-2840
(303) 420-2902
fax: (303) 422-3394

Mind/Body Medicine

Guided Imagery

Guided imagery is a technique that uses the mind's ability to imagine sights, sounds, movements, and other sensory experiences as a means to induce specific physical reactions in the body or to encourage changes in a patient's emotional outlook. Buddhists have used mental images to promote healing since the 13th century or earlier, and many shamanistic traditions around the world include the power of imagery. The technique can be used in many ways and can be adapted to suit different personalities; what doesn't work for one person might be the perfect therapy for another.

What It's Good For • Just as lying on a warm beach, listening to the ocean waves, and feeling the warm sunshine can have a relaxing effect on your body, so can visualizing such a scene in your mind. Similarly, imagining your immune cells as a conquering army or a swarm of victorious hunters may actually boost the cells' activity and, at the same time, promote a sense of self-reliance that further improves the functioning of your immune system. Simply relaxing and allowing images to take shape in your mind may give you insight into a symptom or ailment, and perhaps even suggest ideas about how to cope with it.

Guided imagery can have a profound influence on physical as well as psychological conditions. Studies of the brain indicate that merely imagining a certain activity stimulates the same regions of the cerebral cortex as actually experiencing the activity. This suggests that guided imagery has the potential to bring about positive physiological changes in the body, allowing a patient to exercise conscious control over such vital functions as heart rate, brain-wave rhythms, and blood glucose levels.

A number of natural childbirth groups rely on a type of preparatory guided imagery called mental rehearsal, in which women imagine going through delivery before the actual event. Mental rehearsal is also frequently used by patients as a way to relieve anxiety before surgery. This sort of preview can reduce pain and side effects, and even shorten recovery time.

■ **Immune problems:** A number of studies show improvement in

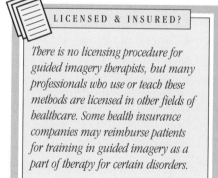

LICENSED & INSURED?

There is no licensing procedure for guided imagery therapists, but many professionals who use or teach these methods are licensed in other fields of healthcare. Some health insurance companies may reimburse patients for training in guided imagery as a part of therapy for certain disorders.

CAUTION

Guided imagery and hypnosis can be used as diagnostic tools in certain kinds of emotional therapy, sometimes involving the recovery of so-called repressed memories. In a number of cases, however, these memories, though seemingly quite real to both patient and therapist at the time of recovery, have been found to be false. This is an area where it pays to be careful and move slowly.

CONTINUED

some immune reactions following imagery training. Sometimes guided imagery is combined with other mind/body techniques to boost the effectiveness of the immune system.

- **Cancer:** Guided imagery is often used by cancer patients in an effort to mobilize their immune system against the disease. There is no direct evidence that imagery alone can improve the prognosis, but people often report that imagery makes them better able to cope with cancer. Studies have shown that imagery can also ease nausea and promote weight gain in cancer patients undergoing treatments that interfere with their eating habits.
- **Irritable bowel syndrome:** Using guided imagery to visualize a soothing scene or activity can help relieve the symptoms of IBS.
- **Asthma:** Guided imagery may help asthma patients relax and assume better control of their breathing.

Preparations/Techniques • Guided imagery can be used actively— as when a cancer patient imagines immune cells attacking malignant cells—or receptively, allowing the mind to form images that might shed light on a particular ailment or condition. Techniques for both approaches can be learned on your own from a book or an audiotape, or under the guidance of a trained therapist.

Taking the time to concentrate on observing the world around you helps your mind create more convincing images. Clarity is important for healing, because the more vivid the image, the more "real" it seems and the greater its effect on the nervous system. While conjuring "pictures" is perhaps the easiest form of imagery, it is also possible—and equally relaxing—to imagine soothing sounds, sensations of touch, and smells. For chronic conditions, guided imagery is most beneficial when practiced for 15 or 20 minutes once or twice every day. You may want to keep a journal of your sessions and your symptoms to help you evaluate the results. Guided imagery for relaxation can be used regularly or on the spur of the moment—to handle a tense situation or cope with sudden pain, for example.

Visiting a Professional • Many kinds of therapists use guided imagery, and some teach individuals or groups how to continue its use on their own. It may take several sessions with a professional and some time working on your own before you notice results. Ask your healthcare provider for a referral to a therapist, or contact the Academy for Guided Imagery *(see For More Info, left)*.

Wellness • Guided imagery can help you picture well-being or success in any number of endeavors. Using imagery to take minivacations throughout the day can keep you relaxed and help prevent or tone down the stress response.

FOR MORE INFO
Following is a list of organizations you can contact to learn more about guided imagery:

The Academy for Guided Imagery
PO Box 2070
Mill Valley, CA 94942
(800) 726-2070
fax: (415) 389-9342

**The Institute of
Transpersonal Psychology**
744 San Antonio Road
Palo Alto, CA 94303
(415) 493-4430
fax: (415) 493-6835

Mind/Body Medicine

Hypnotherapy

Healers have used hypnotism to induce trance states in patients since ancient times. Although the practice has largely fallen out of favor among mainstream physicians, over the last few decades a number of healthcare practitioners in various fields have begun to harness the power of hypnotherapy to treat an array of conditions.

What It's Good For

Hypnotherapy aims to induce a state of focused concentration, described as neither sleep nor wakefulness, during which a willing subject is open and responsive to suggestion. (An unwilling subject cannot be hypnotized.) Hypnotherapy is most effective when used to treat ailments involving stress or anxiety. There are also reports of success with hypnotherapy in helping people break bad habits, such as bedwetting in children, or establish good ones.

- **Skin problems:** Hypnotherapy has been used successfully to treat warts and ichthyosis (fish skin disease), a severe genetic disorder.
- **Pain:** Some doctors, dentists, and childbirth attendants use hypnotherapy to counteract the fear and anxiety that can heighten pain, complicate healing, and slow labor in pregnant women. Clinical trials also show that hypnotherapy can help burn patients deal more effectively with pain.
- **Hemophilia:** Research shows that hypnotherapy may help reduce bleeding in people with this disorder, which interferes with the blood's ability to form clots.
- **Anxiety:** Hypnotherapy can help people overcome certain phobias, including stage fright, or cope with distressing situations such as hospitalization.

Visiting a Professional

A trained therapist can guide you through the steps of hypnosis or teach you how to perform the techniques yourself. Ask your healthcare provider for a referral to a qualified therapist, or contact a national organization *(far right)*.

Wellness

Hypnosis is thought to bring about physiological changes similar to those induced by other relaxation techniques. It also offers the same potential for increased overall well-being and helps prevent or reduce the intensity of the stress response.

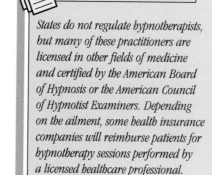

LICENSED & INSURED?

States do not regulate hypnotherapists, but many of these practitioners are licensed in other fields of medicine and certified by the American Board of Hypnosis or the American Council of Hypnotist Examiners. Depending on the ailment, some health insurance companies will reimburse patients for hypnotherapy sessions performed by a licensed healthcare professional.

CAUTION

Hypnotic suggestions can be very powerful. Before undergoing hypnotherapy, make sure that your practitioner is qualified and has experience in treating your particular condition.

FOR MORE INFO

Following is a list of organizations you can contact to learn more about hypnotherapy:

American Council of Hypnotist Examiners
1147 East Broadway, Suite 340
Glendale, CA 91205
(818) 242-5378
fax: (818) 247-9379

American Society of Clinical Hypnosis
2200 East Devon Ave., Suite 291
Des Plaines, IL 60018
(847) 297-3317
fax: (847) 297-7309

Milton H. Erickson Foundation
3606 North 24th Street
Phoenix, AZ 85016
(602) 956-6196
fax: (602) 956-0519

CONTINUED

Mind/Body Medicine CONTINUED

Meditation

Many cultures throughout the world have recognized the calming, therapeutic effect of quiet contemplation. Most types of meditation practiced today, however, come from ancient Eastern or other religious traditions. Almost all of these methods share a few simple steps: Students are instructed to sit quietly, usually with eyes closed, and focus the mind on a single thought, allowing all other thoughts to float away. Some forms are more active or complex, meant to be performed while walking or chanting, for example.

One of the most famous methods is transcendental meditation, or TM, a simplified variation of ancient yoga that was brought to the United States by Maharishi Mahesh Yogi in the 1960s. Another type is known as the relaxation response (pages 138-139). A traditional Buddhist method called vipassana, or mindfulness meditation, has been practiced in the East for 2,500 years but only recently become known to the Western world. Students of mindfulness meditation are taught simply to focus on the present moment. The goal is to face and accept all aspects of life, thereby achieving a deeper sense of balance that contributes to overall well-being.

■ *What It's Good For* • Meditation is commonly thought of as a spiritual endeavor, but it has frequently demonstrated physical effects as well. Most forms of meditation promote regular quiet relaxation, which in itself can help alleviate symptoms of stress-related ailments ranging from headaches to high blood pressure.

■ **Chronic pain:** Use of TM or mindfulness meditation has been shown to reduce the suffering associated with chronic pain, possibly by helping people examine and sort out the negative thoughts commonly generated during intense discomfort.

■ **High blood pressure:** Studies have shown a decrease in blood pressure among regular practitioners of TM. This evidence is so persuasive that cardiologists sometimes recommend meditation to their patients to help lower stress-related hypertension.

■ **Stress:** TM has been used in treating posttraumatic stress disor-

LICENSED & INSURED?

There are no licensing procedures for teachers of meditation, although sometimes the technique is taught in affiliation with a hospital, clinic, or medical practice. Under certain circumstances, some health insurance providers cover the costs of training in meditation techniques.

Mind/Body Medicine

der. Recent studies suggest a connection between meditation and a decrease in the levels of harmful stress-induced chemicals in the brain. Mindfulness meditation has been shown to reduce anxiety, depression, and other symptoms associated with chronic stress.

- **Panic disorders:** Mindfulness meditation can help people prone to panic attacks control their breathing and reactions, thereby forestalling full attacks.
- **Headaches:** The relaxation achieved through meditation can help reduce or eliminate headaches brought on by stress or muscle tension.
- **Respiratory problems:** For some patients with emphysema, asthma, or other lung ailments, mindfulness meditation can reduce the frequency and severity of attacks of breathlessness.

Preparations/Techniques • Meditation seems simple, but learning to stop the usual stream of conscious thoughts flowing through your mind takes practice. First, you must find a quiet place with as few distractions as possible. Sit quietly in a comfortable position, preferably with your back straight. Focus your mind on your breath or on a silently repeated sound, word, or phrase (called a mantra), or on a stationary object such as a flower or candle flame. If other thoughts intrude, take notice of them, but then let them go and return your focus to the phrase or object. Gently refocus as many times as necessary. Practice this for 15 to 20 minutes twice a day; meditating at the same time every day helps reinforce the habit.

For mindfulness meditation, begin the same way, using a single point of concentration to achieve calm. When thoughts or feelings surface, observe them without intention or judgment; don't try to decide if your thoughts are right or wrong, just be aware of them. The goal of this form of meditation is acceptance of the reality of the moment. For a technique known as the body scan, performed while seated or lying down, concentrate on moving your attention through your body, taking note of any sensations or impressions as you go along.

Although it is possible to learn to meditate on your own with the help of instruction books or courses on audiotape or videotape, it is best to begin with a qualified instructor. Classes and retreats in the various methods are widely available; many people, in fact, find that the support of others in a group setting provides the motivation necessary for developing the proper meditation skills.

Wellness • Many who practice meditation say that the relaxation and focus provided by regular sessions positively affects every aspect of life. Mindfulness meditation, in particular, appears to foster a sense of connection that promotes general good health and may actually bring about beneficial changes in specific areas of the body, including the cardiovascular system.

FOR MORE INFO
Following is a list of organizations you can contact to learn more about meditation:

Institute for Noetic Sciences
475 Gate Five Road, Suite 300
Sausalito, CA 94965
(415) 331-5650
fax: (415) 331-5673

Insight Meditation Society
1230 Pleasant Street
Barre, MA 01005
(508) 355-4378
fax: (508) 355-6398

Vipassana Meditation Center
PO Box 24
Shelbourne Falls, MA 01370
(413) 625-2160

CONTINUED

Mind/Body Medicine CONTINUED

Relaxation Techniques

CAUTION

Relaxation methods can reduce your need for certain medications. Whatever technique you decide to use, keep your healthcare provider informed so he or she can make any necessary adjustments in dosage.

In the late 1960s, Harvard cardiologist Herbert Benson became intrigued by the incidence of high blood pressure in patients who were under stress. While researching this phenomenon, he noticed that blood pressure levels were lower in people who meditated than in those who didn't. Eventually, he identified a mechanism in the body that helps reduce stress. This mechanism, which Benson called the relaxation response, can be invoked in a number of ways. Yoga (pages 182-183), t'ai chi (pages 172-173), and qigong (pages 165-166), for example, are excellent techniques for promoting relaxation and reducing stress. Others include the relaxation methods listed below in "Preparations/Techniques." These simple techniques can be used virtually anywhere at any time, and most of them need no special training, just practice.

■ *What It's Good For* • Relaxation is the goal of mind/body medicine because it helps reduce the negative effects of stress, which has been linked to many serious and chronic diseases, including cancer, heart disease, and depression. Summoning the relaxation response also lowers the respiration rate and relaxes muscle tension. One researcher found that regular use of relaxation techniques makes the body less responsive throughout the day to the effects of norepinephrine, a stress hormone that increases blood pressure and heart rate. Relaxation training may also be helpful after surgery or other medical procedures: Research suggests that using these techniques may speed healing, reduce bleeding and other complications, decrease pain and reliance on medications, and perhaps allow a quicker return to full function.

■ **Insomnia:** Learning to evoke the relaxation response can help many people with chronic insomnia improve their ability to fall asleep. A technique referred to as progressive muscle relaxation (opposite) is a particularly beneficial way to promote deep, all-body relaxation and to overcome sleeplessness.

LICENSED & INSURED?

Relaxation therapists are not licensed as such, but a number of medical professionals who are licensed in other fields—physicians, psychologists, and social workers, for example—offer training in these techniques, as do many hospitals and clinics. In some cases health insurance companies cover the costs of relaxation therapy for certain conditions. Check with your therapist or insurance carrier.

Mind/Body Medicine

- **Premenstrual syndrome:** Symptoms of PMS were significantly reduced in women who practiced relaxation techniques twice a day for three months.
- **Immune problems:** Studies show an increase in immune cell activity after relaxation training.
- **High blood pressure:** Relaxation techniques are very effective in lowering elevated blood pressure in cases of stress-related hypertension.
- **Infertility:** Stress can interfere with the normal hormonal cycle of the reproductive process in women, sometimes resulting in infertility. In one study, a group of women thought to be infertile participated in relaxation training, and a third of them became pregnant. Relaxation techniques can also help alleviate the stress associated with the experience of infertility or its treatment.

Preparations/Techniques • Herbert Benson suggests the following technique for triggering the relaxation response: Sit comfortably in a place with minimal distractions. Close your eyes and relax your muscles. Breathe naturally; as you exhale, silently repeat a word or phrase you have chosen that has meaning to you—this is your "focus word." Many people use "peace" or "love," a short prayer, or the name of a religious figure as a focus word. Remain passive; when other thoughts intrude, let them go and return to your focus word. Continue to concentrate for 10 to 20 minutes, then open your eyes and sit quietly for a moment before you get up. Practice this technique once or twice a day.

Another method, which is called progressive muscle relaxation, involves concentrating on each muscle group in the body, one at a time, and moving progressively from one end of the body to the other. Inhale and clench your muscles for five seconds, then exhale and relax. Repeat for each area of your body until your entire body is relaxed.

A technique called autogenic training combines relaxation with self-hypnosis and guided imagery. Autogenic training involves the repetition of meaningful phrases to yourself while focusing on a sense of heaviness and warmth in the limbs, breathing calmly, and keeping the muscles limp and relaxed.

A number of relaxation techniques, including yoga and moving meditation, focus on the breath. Deep breathing can release tension and speed delivery of oxygen to the body and relax the nervous system. Breathing exercises can be done anywhere at any time and are easily combined with most other relaxation methods.

Wellness • Habitual use of relaxation techniques rests and recharges the body, thereby strengthening it against daily or unusual stress. Quieting the mind may also promote greater concentration and receptivity to information, suggesting that relaxation techniques can foster good health and boost overall well-being.

FOR MORE INFO

Contact the following organization to learn more about relaxation techniques:

The Mind/Body Medical Institute
Deaconess Hospital
1 Deaconess Road
Boston, MA 02215

CONTINUED

Mind/Body Medicine CONTINUED

Spiritual Healing and Prayer

Almost every culture, society, and religious tradition throughout history has acknowledged the healing power of faith and prayer.

■ *What It's Good For* • Religious belief and prayer bring comfort, hope, and relaxation to the faithful of all backgrounds. Studies have shown that regular spiritual observance, prayer, and religious ritual are beneficial to overall health.

- **Heart problems:** In one study showing the power of intercessory prayer, a group of heart patients for whom strangers had secretly prayed were found to have fewer complications than another group of patients who did not receive the prayers of others.
- **Addiction:** Many treatment programs use the concept of a "higher power" to help people refrain from substance abuse or other bad habits.
- **Terminal illness:** Spirituality and religion help dying patients cope with the prospect of death, especially as they search for meaning in their lives and in their suffering.

■ *Preparations/Techniques* • People of various faiths pray in different ways, and the style of prayer can differ vastly even among people who attend the same place of worship. Believers do not need a deity to pray, nor does prayer require words; certain feelings, such as compassion, and even silent contemplation of the infinite are also considered types of prayer. For some, it may be best to surrender health problems to a higher power and trust in the outcome, rather than to pray for a specific result.

■ *Wellness* • Spiritual belief can help people transcend sickness or pain and achieve a sense of health and well-being. To experience the healing effects of spirituality does not require religious adherence, though religious commitment can have positive effects. Rather, it demands nothing more than an ability to love, to forgive, and to seek meaning and purpose beyond the circumstances of the moment. ■

LICENSED & INSURED?

Spiritual healers are not licensed as such, but a number of licensed medical professionals use prayer, therapeutic touch, or related techniques in conjunction with other treatments. While insurance companies may provide coverage for the services of these licensed professionals, spiritual therapy itself is usually not covered. On the other hand, the healthcare services of practitioners of Christian Science, a church that rejects all medical methods and teaches that only religious belief can overcome illness, are covered by some insurance companies.

FOR MORE INFO

Following is a list of organizations you can contact to learn more about spiritual healing:

National Institute for Healthcare Research
6110 Executive Blvd., Suite 908
Rockville, MD 20852
(301) 984-7162
fax: (301) 984-8143

Center for Mind-Body Medicine
5225 Connecticut Ave. NW, Suite 414
Washington, DC 20015
(202) 966-7338
fax: (202) 966-2589

The Interfaith Health Program
The Carter Center
One Copenhill
Atlanta, GA 30307
(404) 614-3757
fax: (404) 420-5158

Naturopathic Medicine

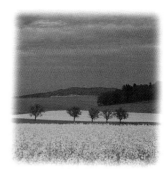

Naturopathic medicine aims to provide holistic, or whole-body, healthcare by drawing from numerous traditional healing systems. At its core is the idea of vis medicatrix naturae—the healing power of nature. Naturopathic doctors believe that the body naturally strives for health and that the physician's role is to support the body's efforts. To achieve this, naturopathic physicians follow seven basic principles: Help nature heal, do no harm, find the underlying cause, treat the whole person, encourage prevention, recognize wellness, and act as a teacher.

A naturopathic doctor, or ND, may pay considerable attention to a patient's lifestyle, since naturopathic theory holds that physical, psychological, and even spiritual elements can all contribute to disease. In treating patients the naturopathic practitioner might use a number of alternative therapies, including homeopathy, herbal remedies, Chinese medicine, spinal manipulation, nutrition, hydrotherapy, massage, and exercise.

Origins

Although its origins trace to ancient times, naturopathy as a modern system of healing began in 1902, when German immigrant Benedict Lust founded the American School of Naturopathy in New York City. Having been cured of a debilitating condition by hydrotherapy, Lust became convinced that "nature cures" were the best approach to wellness. His school grew rapidly, and by 1919 the American Naturopathic Association, also founded by Lust, was incorporated in 19 states. The movement flourished in the twenties and thirties, with thousands of practitioners attending national conventions and naturopathic journals and books gaining a growing

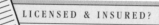

LICENSED & INSURED?

At present naturopathic doctors are licensed to practice in 11 states: Alaska, Arizona, Connecticut, Hawaii, Maine, Montana, New Hampshire, Oregon, Utah, Vermont, and Washington. They have a legal right to practice in the District of Columbia and Idaho, and the majority of other states allow them to practice in limited ways. Naturopathic practice is regulated by state law, which dictates the therapies and prescriptive rights of NDs. Naturopathic doctors are eligible for malpractice insurance.

Some, but not all, insurance plans cover care by a naturopathic physician. In most cases the NDs are viewed as primary, preventive-care doctors within physician provider plans. Patients who are under the care of conventional physicians or HMOs will rarely be referred to naturopaths, however, unless they specifically request such a referral.

Target Ailments

■ Allergies

■ Arthritis

■ Asthma

■ Back Problems

■ Cholesterol Problems

■ Constipation

■ Depression

■ Headache

■ Heartburn

■ High Blood Pressure

■ Insomnia

■ Menstrual Problems

■ Nausea

■ Pain, Chronic

■ Stress

See Common Ailments, beginning on page 194.

CONTINUED

audience. By the 1990s many of naturopathy's practices regarding diet, exercise, and lifestyle had become accepted by the wider medical community.

What It's Good For

Because of its emphasis on whole-body health, and with its wide range of techniques, naturopathy may be used for almost all basic healthcare. Patients visit naturopathic doctors for preventive care or for alternative therapies when conventional approaches have been unsatisfactory. Naturopathic physicians have reported success with conditions such as chronic infections, fatigue, and menstrual and menopausal problems. Diseases that are strongly affected by lifestyle and environment are among those most commonly treated by naturopaths. In a typical case of high blood pressure, for example, an ND might suggest a multifaceted approach involving changed diet, vitamin and mineral supplements, herbal medicines, and lifestyle modifications. For an arthritis sufferer, the primary treatments could include diet, homeopathic medicines, acupuncture, hydrotherapy, and massage. Naturopathic doctors also provide counseling for emotional and mental problems, such as depression and anxiety.

Visiting a Professional

Naturopathic doctors are usually office-based primary-care providers. Their approaches and treatments depend on their background and philosophy. Some stick to a strict "natural" regimen of diet, detoxification, and hydrotherapy; others may differ from conventional doctors only in using herbal medicines instead of synthetic drugs. Some naturopathic doctors specialize in a particular form of alternative medicine such as homeopathy or acupuncture; others are generalists.

A first visit might take an hour,

OF SPECIAL INTEREST

Educational Background

In states without licensing requirements, the naturopathic doctor's credentials may vary, although most will maintain an active license in one of the states that allow it. Most NDs licensed in recent years will have a degree from one of the three accredited naturopathic schools in the U.S.: National College of Naturopathic Medicine, Bastyr University, or the Southwest College of Naturopathic Medicine and Health Sciences. These physicians have undergone conventional premed training, followed by four years of graduate school. Their studies include standard subjects—anatomy, histology, pharmacology, pathology, and the like—as well as naturopathic philosophy, Chinese medicine, nutrition, hydrotherapy, and other alternative therapies. After learning standard diagnostic procedures, they will have worked with a licensed naturopath in a clinical setting before gaining an ND degree themselves.

Naturopathic Medicine

during which the doctor conducts a standard physical exam, possibly including conventional laboratory tests and radiology. In addition, the physician will spend considerable time taking a patient history, assessing every aspect of the person's lifestyle, including diet, exercise, stress, and mental, emotional, and spiritual issues.

After the initial evaluation, doctor and patient work together to establish a treatment program. Because naturopathy emphasizes noninvasive therapies, the doctor will probably suggest ways the patient can change disease-promoting habits, help set realistic, progressive goals, and identify the causes of unhealthy behavior.

If the patient has a specific complaint, the doctor may prescribe any one of many natural treatments or a combination of those treatments. These could include nutrition, homeopathic remedies, massage, botanical medicines, physical medicine (bodywork), hydrotherapy, acupuncture, or psychological and family counseling. Depending on state law, the naturopath may also prescribe conventional drugs, give vaccinations, or perform outpatient surgery. In general, though, the aim of naturopathy is not only to cure a particular ailment but also to aid the body in sustaining lifelong good health.

Wellness

Wellness is what naturopathic medicine is all about. Naturopathic physicians believe that the body has an innate intelligence that strives for health; the role of both patient and doctor is to work with the body to help it promote its own well-being. Health, therefore, is more than the absence of disease; it is a vital state that needs encouragement and the proper environment. These physicians point out, for instance, that the substantial decline in deaths from heart attacks in recent decades is due not to improved coronary surgery but to public education regarding nutrition, exercise, and stress. In naturopathy, doctor and patient together will not only correct imbalances and states of disease but also plan a lifelong course of diet, exercise, and mental attitude that is designed to support the body's natural processes and fend off chronic disease and the debilitation normally associated with aging.

What the Critics Say

Many members of the conventional medical establishment criticize naturopathy as being overly vague, too dependent on nutritional counseling and untested herbal remedies, and not subject to the scientific methods of experimentation and peer review. They say that the placebo effect is responsible for many of naturopathy's positive results. Because most states do not provide licensing for naturopathic doctors, critics also point out that almost anyone can get a mail-order naturopathy degree. Accredited NDs also acknowledge this danger and are attempting to persuade the government to establish standards for naturopathic physicians in all states. ∎

FOR MORE INFO

Following is a list of organizations you can contact to learn more about naturopathy:

American Association of Naturopathic Physicians
2366 Eastlake Avenue East, Suite 322
Seattle, WA 98102
(206) 323-7610

National College of Naturopathic Medicine
11231 SE Market Street
Portland, OR 97216
(503) 255-4860

Bastyr University
14500 Juanita Drive, NE
Bothell, WA 98011
(206) 523-9585

Southwest College of Naturopathic Medicine and Health Sciences
2140 East Broadway, Suite 703
Tempe, AZ 85251
(602) 858-9100

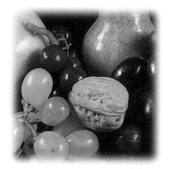

$\mathcal{N}$utrition and Diet

E ating a balanced diet is a major factor in a healthy lifestyle. Your body requires more than 40 nutrients for energy, growth, and tissue maintenance. Water, as the most plentiful component in the body, is also crucial to survival. It is the medium for bodily fluids, and it transports nutrients into cells and carries waste products and toxins out.

Conventional and alternative practitioners alike acknowledge the importance of a healthful diet. Alternative practitioners, however, place more emphasis on dietary intervention in some conditions where conventional medicine would turn first to drugs or even surgery. Treatment of atherosclerosis, for example, may take the form of an extremely low-fat diet with a program of meditation, exercise, and support-group therapy.

Basic Nutrition

Carbohydrates, proteins, and fats—macronutrients or "energy nutrients"—provide fuel in the form of calories. Carbohydrates, the body's main energy source, are divided into two types: Simple carbohydrates are sugars, such as cane sugar and molasses; complex carbohydrates include starches, such as those found in potatoes and whole grains.

Proteins support tissue growth and repair, and help produce antibodies, hormones, and enzymes, which are essential for all the body's chemical reactions. Protein sources include meat, fish, dairy products, poultry, dried beans, nuts, and eggs.

Dietary fat protects internal organs, provides energy, insulates against cold, and helps the body absorb certain vitamins. There are three kinds of fats: saturated, found in meat, dairy products, and coconut oil; monounsaturated, in canola, olive, and peanut oils; and polyunsaturated, in corn, cottonseed, safflower, sesame, soybean, and sunflower oils.

Your diet also supplies the important micronutrients we call vitamins and minerals. They are needed only in trace amounts, but the absence or deficiency of just one can cause major illness. With a few exceptions, the body does not manufacture micronutrients and so must obtain them from food.

Thirteen vitamins and some twenty minerals are considered essential for health. The Food and Nutrition Board of the National Research Council, National Academy of Sciences, has determined a recommended dietary allowance (RDA)—an appropriate range of intake with built-in margins to allow for variations in individual needs. Essential nutrients that do not yet have RDAs are assigned a safe and adequate daily intake or an estimated minimum daily requirement (EMDR). *(See pages 152-162 for information on specific vitamins and minerals.)*

Nutrition and Diet

Your body also needs dietary fiber, the indigestible part of plant foods. A high-fiber diet reduces the risks of various gastrointestinal problems, promotes cardiovascular health, and may help decrease the risk of breast cancer and colon cancer.

Diet Planning

In general, Americans eat more fat, protein, cholesterol, sugar, and salt than they need. Official diet guidelines, established jointly by the U.S. Departments of Agriculture and Health and Human Services, include some basic recommendations:

- **Eat a variety of foods.** This will help ensure that you get the calories, protein, fiber, vitamins, minerals, and other nutrients you need.
- **Control your weight.** Keep within recommended weight limits for your age, sex, and build.
- **Eat a low-fat, low-cholesterol diet.** Ideally, no more than 30 percent of your daily calories should come from fat, and no more than 10 percent should come from saturated fat.
- **Eat plenty of vegetables, fruits, and grains.** More than half of your daily calories should come from carbohydrates, rich in nutrients and low in fats; 80 percent of those calories should be from complex carbohydrates.
- **Eat sugar and salt in moderation.** Sugar is high in calories and promotes tooth decay. Too much salt may increase the risk of developing high blood pressure. Prepared foods are notoriously high in salt or other forms of sodium, so check labels.
- **If you drink alcohol, do so in moderation.** Alcohol

CONTINUED

Nutrition and Diet CONTINUED

provides calories but no nutrients, and too much is harmful. However, some studies indicate that moderate consumption of red wine may actually lower the risk of heart disease. "Moderation" generally means one drink a day for women or two drinks for men.

Nutritional Supplements

If you consistently eat a well-balanced diet of fresh fruits, vegetables, grains, and some animal protein, you probably don't require a nutritional supplement. Multinutrient supplements offer insurance for those times when eating well is a challenge—and can be indispensable during pregnancy or when you are ill, injured, or under great mental or physical strain.

Generally, vitamins and minerals are recommended for daily use as a preventive measure. Supplements do, however, figure in the dietary recommendations of many therapies. Orthomolecular medicine, a form of nutrient therapy, uses combinations of vitamins, minerals, and amino acids normally found in the body to treat specific conditions such as asthma, heart disease, depression, and schizophrenia. Such therapy can also be used to maintain general good health.

Taking vitamins or minerals in excess can upset the natural balance of nutrients. The fat-soluble vitamins—A, D, E, and K—can be retained in your body and may be toxic in high amounts. The rest are water soluble and are unlikely to be toxic; excess amounts are excreted in the urine. Always take supplements in moderation; they are safe in doses at or below RDAs, but higher doses may be harmful and should be taken only under the guidance of a doctor or a registered dietitian.

Supplement doses are measured by weight in milligrams (mg), or thousandths of a gram; in micrograms (mcg), or millionths of a gram; or in a universal standard known as international units (IU).

Food Allergies and Sensitivities

Some people cannot tolerate certain foods or food additives; the most common culprits include dairy products, soybeans, peanuts, wheat, eggs, and shellfish. Allergic reactions can be very severe, even causing death, whereas sensitivities can cause troublesome symptoms such as rashes or bloating. Food intolerance may even be a factor in hyperactivity and many chronic diseases such as rheumatoid arthritis.

An elimination diet can help you pin down what food or foods are causing the reaction, and banning the offenders from your diet is one way to deal with this problem. A controversial method called desensitizing aims to train the body to accept foods it would otherwise not tolerate. One fairly common intolerance, that for milk sugar, can be addressed by adding a specific enzyme to the diet or by limiting the intake of dairy products to those, such as yogurt, that are more easily digested.

Nutrition and Diet

The Food Guide Pyramid—developed on the advice of nutritional scientists—makes healthy eating easier by showing how much of each type of food you should eat for good nutrition. Each of the groups provides some of the nutrients you need each day; no one group provides them all. Variety within and among groups is key.

The foundation of the pyramid is grain-based foods, which provide complex carbohydrates, vitamins, minerals, and fiber. On the next level are fruits and vegetables, which are rich in vitamins, minerals, and fiber but low in fat. The next two groups are critical sources of protein, calcium, iron, zinc, and other nutrients, but many of these foods are also high in fat and cholesterol. Fats, oils, and sweets occupy the tip of the pyramid and should be eaten sparingly.

The pyramid suggests a range of daily servings for each group. Your actual needs depend on your daily caloric requirements. Experts recommend about 1,600 calories for older adults and sedentary women; 2,200 calories for children, teenage girls, active women, and sedentary men; and 2,800 calories for teenage boys, active men, and very active women.

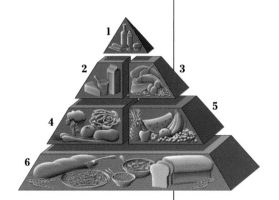

1 Fats, Oils, & Sweets Group
USE SPARINGLY
One teaspoon of butter, oil, or margarine is a single serving.

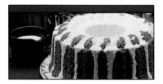

2 Milk, Yogurt, & Cheese Group
2-3 SERVINGS
One serving equals 1 cup of milk or yogurt, 1½ oz of natural cheese, or 2 oz of processed cheese.

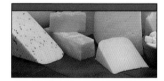

3 Meat, Poultry, Fish, Dried Beans, Eggs, & Nuts Group   2-3 SERVINGS
One serving is 2 to 3 oz of cooked lean meat, poultry, or fish. An ounce of meat equals one egg or ½ cup cooked dried beans.

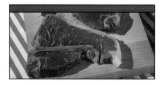

4 Vegetable Group
3-5 SERVINGS
One serving equals 1 cup of raw leafy greens, ½ cup of other vegetables, or ¾ cup of vegetable juice.

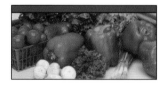

5 Fruit Group
2-4 SERVINGS
One serving from the fruit group is equal to one apple, orange, or banana; ½ cup of chopped, cooked, or canned fruit; or ¾ cup of fruit juice.

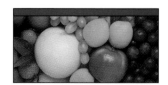

6 Bread, Cereal, Rice, & Pasta Group
6-11 SERVINGS
One serving equals one slice of bread; half a bun, bagel, or muffin; 1 oz of dry cereal; or ½ cup of cooked cereal, rice, or pasta.

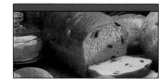

CONTINUED

Nutrition and Diet CONTINUED

B elow and on the following pages are descriptions of four diets, two of which (Asian and Mediterranean) are based on the traditional eating habits of certain cultures. All four plans are reported to have specific health benefits and may be recommended to help treat or prevent specific ailments.

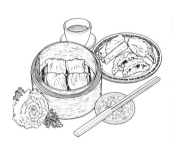

Asian Diet

People in Japan, Korea, Southeast Asia, and China have traditionally eaten a diet largely composed of rice, soybean products, and fresh vegetables, with little meat or dairy products. This diet is low in fat and high in complex carbohydrates.

What It's Good For

Besides generally avoiding saturated fats, the traditional Asian diet promotes good health in other ways.

- **Cancer:** Rice, a staple of the Asian diet, is high in protease inhibitors, substances believed to retard cancer. High consumption of rice is linked to low rates of some cancers, including colon, breast, and prostate. Soybeans also contain protease inhibitors; a study showed that consumption of one bowl a day of miso (soybean paste) soup lowered risk of stomach cancer by almost a third.

  Sea vegetables are also included in the Japanese diet, and they appear to have anticancer properties as well. Oriental green tea exhibits antimutagenic properties and lowers rates of stomach cancer in people who drink it regularly.

- **Atherosclerosis:** Regular consumption of soy foods confers many health benefits, including lower blood cholesterol levels and less risk of atherosclerosis.

Preparations/Techniques

A diet based on Asian practices would include lots of rice—especially steamed—and soybean foods, commonly tofu and miso; fresh vegetables and seaweed, steamed or stir-fried; fresh fruit; moderate amounts of fish; and very little red meat or other animal products, including dairy products. Important seasonings are garlic, ginger, and soy sauce.

What the Critics Say

As with all diets that minimize animal proteins, a wide variety of foods and attention to menu planning are essential.

Nutrition and Diet

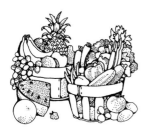

Macrobiotic Diet

From the Greek words for "long" and "life," the macrobiotic diet is based on a system taught by Japanese educator and philosopher George Ohsawa in the early 20th century. The diet eliminates all animal products except a small amount of fish, and emphasizes whole grains and cooked vegetables. Foods are described as *yin* (contractive) or *yang* (expansive), with a balance sought between the two. Foods that are excessively one or the other are excluded.

What It's Good For

Studies suggest that this diet's emphasis on whole grains and vegetables, and its elimination of processed foods, may have healthful effects on the body.

- **Heart disease:** Low in fat and high in complex carbohydrates and fiber, the macrobiotic diet promotes cardiovascular health.
- **Cancer:** There is evidence that a macrobiotic diet may lower the risk of breast cancer, and indeed the diet includes foods, such as soybean products and sea vegetables, that contain cancer-fighting compounds. Use of a macrobiotic diet to help treat cancer is, however, controversial *(see What the Critics Say, below)*.

Preparations/Techniques

A macrobiotic diet prescribes deriving about 50 percent of the diet from whole cereal grains; 20 to 30 percent from vegetables; 5 to 10 percent from beans and sea vegetables; and 5 to 10 percent from soups. Occasional foods include fish—white-meat fish such as flounder and sole are recommended—fruits, and nuts.

Foods to be avoided include potatoes, peppers, meat products, eggs, warm drinks, hot spices, and any refined, mass-produced, or artificially treated food.

What the Critics Say

While a low-fat, high-carbohydrate diet is widely considered healthful, some experts worry that a strict macrobiotic diet does not have enough variety, especially for children and pregnant women. Iron, calcium, and some vitamins are particular concerns on such a limited diet. Extremely restrictive versions that rely almost solely on grains could be dangerously low in protein and other nutrients for anyone.

Research is being conducted to determine the effect of macrobiotic food on the progress of some cancers. However, even some of those who support the diet and its avoidance of processed foods and saturated fats caution that there is so far no good evidence that any diet alone can cure disease.

CONTINUED

Nutrition and Diet CONTINUED

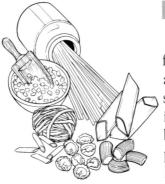

Mediterranean Diet

The populations of 15 countries on three different continents live near the Mediterranean Sea, and despite variations from culture to culture, they share a remarkably similar traditional diet. Staples include grains, potatoes, pasta, legumes, vegetables, garlic, and olive oil. Sweets and most animal products are limited. Some fish is consumed, mostly of the oily varieties, such as mullet and tuna.

What It's Good For

Quantities of complex carbohydrates and fresh vegetables align this diet with the Food Guide Pyramid's recommendations.

- **Heart disease:** The Mediterranean diet is quite high in fat, but it is mostly monounsaturated fat from olive oil, which has been shown to reduce the "bad" kind of cholesterol (low-density lipoprotein, or LDL) without lowering the amount of "good" cholesterol (high-density lipoprotein, or HDL) in the body—and so may help protect against heart disease.

  Omega-3 fatty acids present in oily fish seem to help lower blood cholesterol levels, and the vitamins and beta carotene present in brightly colored vegetables can protect the body against heart disease. Large amounts of garlic may be effective in lowering blood pressure.

  Mediterranean cultures traditionally consume red wine with meals. Some studies indicate that moderate consumption of red wine may help reduce the risk of heart disease for certain individuals.

- **Diabetes:** A high level of monounsaturated fats in the diet has been shown to help control blood sugar levels in the adult-onset type of diabetes.

- **Cancer:** The diet's emphasis on complex carbohydrates may help protect against colon cancer.

Preparations/Techniques

Specifics of the Mediterranean diet vary from culture to culture, and recipes are widely available. Two simple ways to get some of the benefits of this diet are to substitute olive oil for other fats, and to add more vegetables and garlic to your meals.

What the Critics Say

Olive oil is not a cure-all; you still must ensure enough variety in your diet to get all the nutrients you need.

Nutrition and Diet

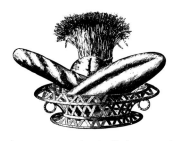

Vegetarian Diet

Many cultures have a longstanding tradition of avoiding the consumption of some or all animal products. The several forms of vegetarianism are among the most popular alternatives to a standard diet in the U.S. today. Some people believe that humans are physically better suited to digesting grains, beans, vegetables, and fruits than meat and other animal products; others avoid meat for philosophical or ecological reasons. In general, vegetarians enjoy a diet lower in fat and higher in complex carbohydrates than one with a lot of red meat and other animal products

What It's Good For

Cutting your fat intake from animal products can be beneficial in many ways.

- **Heart disease:** Lower amounts of saturated fats and higher intake of polyunsaturated fats and fiber may help lower blood pressure and prevent heart disease.
- **Digestive disorders:** Higher consumption of fiber-rich foods may help vegetarians avoid diverticular disease and colon cancer.

Preparations/Techniques

Vegans eat no animal foods at all. Lactovegetarians consume dairy products but no eggs or meat. Lacto-ovo-vegetarians eat eggs and milk products but no meat. Others exclude only red meat; some also abstain from either poultry or fish.

Take care to get enough variety to ensure proper nutrition. Protein is available from beans, grains, and some vegetables. Vitamin B_{12} is a special worry on a vegetarian diet because there is no good plant source—supplements are necessary. Other micronutrients to be concerned about are vitamin D (available from egg yolks, fortified milk, or adequate sunshine); calcium (milk, fortified soybean milk, and dark green vegetables except spinach and chard); riboflavin (dark green vegetables, legumes, and whole grains); and iron (use iron cookware, eat soybeans, and ensure a plentiful intake of foods containing ascorbic acid to boost absorption of iron).

What the Critics Say

Nutrition experts generally warn pregnant or lactating women to be very careful to assure adequate nutrition on this diet. Also, there is concern for children; rapid growth requires plenty of protein and adequate amounts of several micronutrients that can be in short supply in a totally vegetarian diet. A dietitian or nutritionist can help safeguard your well-being. For most adults who make wise food choices, vegetarianism can supply a healthful diet. ■

The 32 Most Common Vitamins and Minerals

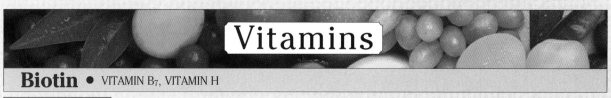

Vitamins

Biotin • VITAMIN B₇, VITAMIN H

EMDR:
30 mcg to 100 mcg

Along with other B vitamins, biotin helps convert food to energy and is required for the synthesis of carbohydrates, proteins, and fatty acids. Biotin is especially important for maintaining the health of hair, skin, and nails.

Among the types of food that are good dietary sources of biotin are cheese, kidneys, salmon, soybeans, sunflower seeds, nuts, broccoli, and sweet potatoes. Biotin deficiency is rare, and supplements are unnecessary. People can become biotin deficient through long-term use of antibiotics or by regularly eating raw egg whites, which contain avidin, a protein that blocks the body's absorption of biotin.

Because breast milk contains little biotin, infants who are breast-fed can suffer biotin deficiency, although this is uncommon. Signs of biotin deficiency include a scaly, oily skin rash; hair loss; nausea; vomiting; muscle pain; loss of appetite; a red, inflamed tongue; and fatigue. Research has not revealed a toxic level for biotin. ∎

Folic Acid • VITAMIN B₉

RDA:
Men: 200 mcg
Women: 180 mcg
Women of childbearing age: 400 mcg

Healthy hair, skin, nails, nerves, mucous membranes, and blood all depend on folic acid—sometimes called vitamin B₉, folacin, or folate. A critical component of RNA and DNA—the genetic material that controls the growth and repair of all cells—folic acid supports immune function and may help deter atherosclerosis as well as some cancers of the mucous membranes.

Sources of folic acid include liver, kidneys, avocados, beans, beets, celery, eggs, fish, green leafy vegetables, nuts, seeds, peas, orange juice, and vitamin-fortified breakfast cereals. A healthy diet should provide adequate folic acid, but the need increases during pregnancy, with injury, with some diseases—especially cancer—and with long-term use of drugs such as aspirin and oral contraceptives. Supplements taken during pregnancy may help deter the birth defects spina bifida and cleft palate. For this reason, experts now recommend that all women of childbearing age consume 400 mcg daily. High doses of folic acid are not toxic but may mask the symptoms of vitamin B₁₂ deficiency. Therefore, it's best to increase folic acid intake through diet or a multivitamin that contains a low dose of folic acid, rather than through individual supplements, which have to be prescribed by a doctor.

Extreme vitamin B₉ deficiency may cause megaloblastic anemia, a disease characterized by red blood cells that are too few in number and malformed. Symptoms include pallor; fatigue; loss of appetite; insomnia; diarrhea; and a red, inflamed tongue. Those who are most susceptible to folic acid deficiency include alcoholics, people with gastrointestinal diseases, adolescents who subsist mainly on junk food, women taking oral contraceptives, and pregnant women who are not taking supplements. ∎

Niacin • VITAMIN B₃

RDA:
Men: 19 mg
Women: 15 mg
Pregnant women: 17 mg

Niacin contributes to more than 50 vital bodily processes: It helps convert food into energy; build red blood cells; synthesize hormones, steroids, and fatty acids; maintain the skin, nerves, and blood vessels; support the gastrointestinal tract; stabilize mental health; and detoxify certain drugs and chemicals in the body. In addition, it helps insulin regulate blood sugar levels. Niacin is also a powerful drug, capable of lowering blood cholesterol and triglycerides, dilating blood vessels to improve circulation, and alleviating depression, insomnia, and hyperactivity.

Niacin-rich foods include liver, poultry, lean meats, fish, nuts, peanut butter, and enriched flour. If you get enough protein, you are probably getting enough niacin. If adequate vitamin B₆ is present, the body can also produce niacin from the amino acid tryptophan, found in milk, eggs, and cheese. Signs of niacin deficiency include indigestion, diarrhea,

The 32 Most Common Vitamins and Minerals

muscle weakness, appetite loss, dermatitis made worse by sunlight, mouth sores, an inflamed tongue, headaches, irritability, anxiety, and depression. Pregnant or breast-feeding women, the elderly, alcoholics, and people with hyperthyroidism are most likely to be niacin deficient. Extreme deficiency results in pellagra, characterized by diarrhea, dermatitis, and mental illness. Pellagra was common until the discovery that niacin was a cure; the disease is now virtually nonexistent in the U.S. thanks to niacin-enriched flour and other foods. Multivitamin supplements can raise niacin levels safely. Vitamin B_3 is toxic in high amounts, so take megadoses only under a doctor's supervision. Nausea, which often prevents further intake, is the first symptom; continued overuse may cause a rash, itchy skin, and liver damage. ■

Vitamin A ● BETA CAROTENE, RETINOL

RDA:
Men: 5,000 IU
(or 3 mg beta carotene)
Women: 4,000 IU
(or 2.4 mg beta carotene)

The first vitamin ever discovered, vitamin A is essential for good vision—especially in dim light—and for healthy skin, hair, and mucous membranes of the nose, throat, respiratory system, and digestive system. This vitamin is also necessary for the proper development of bones and teeth. It stimulates wound healing and is used to treat some skin disorders. Beta carotene, the precursor to vitamin A, is a carotenoid, a type of pigment found in plants. Your skin stores beta carotene and your body metabolizes it to produce vitamin A as needed. Excess beta carotene, along with other carotenoids, acts as an antioxidant and supports immune function, so it increases your resistance to infection; it may help prevent some cancers and vision problems such as night blindness. Beta carotene may also help lower cholesterol levels and reduce the risk of heart disease.

Vitamin A is present in orange and yellow vegetables and fruits; dark green leafy vegetables such as mustard greens and kale; whole milk, cream, and butter; and organ meats. Because it is fat soluble, vitamin A is stored in the body for a long time, and supplements are generally not recommended. Too much vitamin A can cause headaches, vision problems, nausea, vomiting, dry and flaking skin, or an enlarged liver or spleen. Other names for vitamin A are retinol, retinene, retinoic acid, and retinyl palmitate. ■

Vitamin B Complex

RDA:
See individual
vitamin entries

As its name implies, vitamin B complex is a combination, or mixture, of eight essential vitamins. Although each is chemically distinct, the B vitamins coexist in many of the same foods and often work together to bolster metabolism, maintain healthy skin and muscle tone, enhance immune and nervous system function, and promote cell growth and division—including that of the red blood cells that help prevent anemia.

Foods rich in B-complex vitamins include liver and other organ meats, fish, poultry, brewer's yeast, eggs, beans and peas, dark green leafy vegetables, whole-grain cereals, and dairy products. B vitamins, which are water soluble, are dispersed throughout the body and must be replenished daily; any excess is excreted in urine. People susceptible to vitamin B deficiency include pregnant women, nursing mothers, vegetarians, alcoholics, "sugarholics," the elderly, and people who have malabsorption conditions or who take certain antibiotics over a long period of time; the symptoms include oily and scaly skin, upset stomach, headaches, anxiety, moodiness, and heart arrhythmias. A deficiency of one B vitamin usually means that intake of all B vitamins is low. If your doctor suggests you need more B vitamins, take a daily multivitamin or B-complex supplement rather than individual B-vitamin supplements. Most B vitamins are nontoxic unless taken in excessively large amounts. ■

Vitamin B₁ ● THIAMINE

RDA:
Men: 1.5 mg
Women: 1.1 mg

Thiamine, sometimes called the energy vitamin because it is needed to metabolize carbohydrates, fats, and proteins, helps convert excess glucose into stored fat. Vitamin B_1 also ensures proper nerve-impulse transmission and contributes to maintaining normal appetite, muscle tone, and mental health. In the 1930s thiamine was discovered to be the cure for the crippling and potentially fatal disease beriberi.

CONTINUED

The 32 Most Common Vitamins and Minerals

Now that rice, flour, and bread are generally enriched with thiamine, beriberi is relatively rare.

A diet that regularly includes lean pork, milk, whole grains, peas, beans, peanuts, or soybeans generally provides enough thiamine. Athletes, laborers, pregnant women, and others who burn lots of energy may require more than the adult RDA of thiamine. Mild deficiency may cause fatigue, loss of appetite, nausea, moodiness, confusion, anemia, and possibly heart arrhythmias. Alcohol suppresses thiamine absorption; for this reason and because of typically poor diets, alcoholics are likely to be deficient in thiamine and other nutrients. To increase thiamine levels, try changing your diet or taking a multivitamin rather than thiamine supplements. Large doses up to 100 mg of thiamine may alleviate itching from insect bites; otherwise, megasupplements are not known to be either harmful or helpful. ∎

Vitamin B₂ ● RIBOFLAVIN

RDA:
Men: 1.7 mg
Women: 1.3 mg
Pregnant women:
1.6 mg

Like other members of the vitamin B complex, riboflavin helps produce energy from carbohydrates, fats, and proteins. Riboflavin also promotes healthy skin, hair, nails, and mucous membranes; aids the production of red blood cells, corticosteroids, and thyroid hormones; and is required for the proper function of the nerves, eyes, and adrenal glands. It is often used to treat acne, anemia, cataracts, and depression.

A well-balanced diet provides most people with adequate riboflavin, although athletes and others who need a great deal of energy may require more than the RDA. Lean organ meats, enriched bread and flour, cheese, yogurt, eggs, almonds, soybean products such as tofu, and green leafy vegetables—especially broccoli—are good sources. Store these foods in the dark, because vitamin B₂ breaks down in sunlight. Alcoholics and elderly people are susceptible to riboflavin deficiency: The signs include oily, scaly skin rash; sores, especially on the lips and corners of the mouth; a swollen, red, painful tongue; sensitivity to light; and burning or red, itchy eyes. Although vitamin B₂ supplements are available, they provide far more riboflavin than anyone needs. Diet changes are better, or take a multivitamin supplement. It is best to take the supplements with food, which increases their absorption tremendously compared with tablets alone. ∎

Vitamin B₅ ● PANTOTHENIC ACID

EMDR:
4 mg to 7 mg

The Greek term *pan* in *pantothenic acid* means "everywhere," indicating this vitamin's abundance. Along with other B vitamins, pantothenic acid is required for converting food to energy; building red blood cells; making bile; and synthesizing fats, adrenal gland steroids, antibodies, and acetylcholine and other neurotransmitters—chemicals that permit nerve transmission. Pantothenic acid in dexpanthenol lotions and creams relieves the pain of burns, cuts, and abrasions; reduces skin inflammation; and speeds the healing of wounds.

Vitamin B₅ is abundant in organ meats, dark turkey meat, salmon, wheat bran, brewer's yeast, brown rice, lentils, nuts, beans, corn, peas, sweet potatoes, and eggs. Excess pantothenic acid may cause diarrhea. A deficiency in this vitamin does not seem to occur naturally in humans and is likely only with extreme starvation. A pantothenic acid supplement, calcium pantothenate, is available. ∎

Vitamin B₆ ● PYRIDOXINE

RDA:
Men: 2 mg
Women: 1.6 mg
Pregnant women:
2.2 mg

Vitamin B₆ encompasses a family of compounds that includes pyridoxine, pyridoxamine, and pyridoxal. This vitamin supports immune function, transmission of nerve impulses (especially in the brain), energy metabolism, and synthesis of red blood cells. Prescribed as a drug, it can sometimes alleviate carpal tunnel syndrome, infant seizures, and PMS.

A healthy diet provides enough vitamin B₆ for most people. Brown rice, lean meats, poultry, fish, bananas, avocados, whole grains, corn, and nuts are rich in vitamin B₆. People most likely to be at risk for vitamin B₆ deficiency include anyone with a malabsorption problem such as lactose intolerance or celiac disease; diabetic or elderly people; and

The 32 Most Common Vitamins and Minerals

women who are pregnant, nursing, or taking oral contraceptives. Severe deficiency is rare. Mild deficiency may cause acne and inflamed skin, insomnia, muscle weakness, nausea, irritability, depression, and fatigue. A daily multivitamin supplement is usually recommended to boost low vitamin B_6 levels. Taking too much or too little vitamin B_6 can impair nerve function and mental health. If high levels (2,000 mg to 5,000 mg) are taken for several months, vitamin B_6 can become habit forming and may induce sleepiness as well as tingling, numb hands and feet. These symptoms will most likely disappear when the vitamin B_6 intake is reduced, and there is usually no permanent damage. ■

Vitamin B_{12} • COBALAMIN

RDA:
Adults: 2 mcg
Pregnant women: 2.2 mcg

The largest and most complex family of the B vitamins, Vitamin B_{12} includes several chemical compounds known as cobalamins. Cyanocobalamin, the stablest form, is the one most likely to be found in supplements. Like other B vitamins, B_{12} is important for converting fats, carbohydrates, and protein into energy, and assisting in the synthesis of red blood cells. It is critical for producing the genetic materials RNA and DNA, as well as myelin, a fatty substance that forms a protective sheath around nerves. Unlike other B vitamins, vitamin B_{12} needs several hours to be absorbed in the digestive tract. Excess vitamin B_{12} is excreted in urine, even though a backup supply can be stored for several years in the liver.

Vitamin B_{12} is not produced by plants but is supplied through animal products such as organ meats, fish, eggs, and dairy products. Dietary deficiency is uncommon and is usually limited to alcoholics, strict vegetarians, and pregnant or nursing women—who should take supplements. More often, deficiency stems from an inability to absorb the vitamin, a problem that may occur for years before symptoms show; it tends to affect the elderly, those who have had stomach surgery, or people who have a disease of malabsorption, such as colitis.

Lack of calcium, vitamin B_6, or iron may also interfere with the normal absorption of B_{12}. Signs of vitamin B_{12} deficiency include a sore tongue, weakness, weight loss, body odor, back pains, and tingling arms and legs. Severe deficiency leads to pernicious anemia, causing fatigue, a tendency to bleed, lemon yellow pallor, abdominal pain, stiff arms and legs, irritability, and depression.

Without treatment, pernicious anemia can lead to permanent nerve damage and possibly death; the disease can be controlled, although not cured, with regular B_{12} injections. Vitamin B_{12} is considered nontoxic, even when taken at several times the RDA. ■

Vitamin C • ASCORBIC ACID

RDA:
Adults: 60 mg
Pregnant women: 70 mg

Vitamin C is well known for its ability to prevent and treat scurvy, a disease that causes swollen and bleeding gums, aching bones and muscles, and in some cases even death. It is also essential to the healing of wounds, burns, bruises, and broken bones because collagen, the substance that constitutes the body's connective tissue, depends on vitamin C for its production. As a powerful antioxidant and immune system booster, vitamin C may alleviate the pain of rheumatoid arthritis, protect against atherosclerosis and heart disease, and help prevent some forms of cancer; and has the reputed potential capacity (yet unproved) to prevent the common cold. More than the RDA may be needed under conditions of physical or emotional stress.

Sources of vitamin C include citrus fruits, rose hips, bell peppers, strawberries, broccoli, cantaloupes, tomatoes, and leafy greens. Vitamin C breaks down faster than any other vitamin, so it is best to eat fruits and vegetables when fresh and to cook them minimally or not at all. Slight vitamin C deficiency is rather common, although severe deficiencies are rare in the United States today. Symptoms of deficiency include weight loss, fatigue, bleeding gums, easy bruising, reduced resistance to colds and other infections, and slow healing of wounds and fractures.

Because it is water soluble, excess vitamin C is excreted in the urine, so large amounts of it may usually be taken without fear of toxicity. Doses larger than 1,000 mg a day have been suggested for preventing cancer, infections such as the common cold, and other ailments. In some people, large doses may induce such side effects as nausea, diarrhea, reduced selenium and copper absorption, excessive iron absorption, increased kidney stone formation, and a false-positive reaction to diabetes tests. ■

CONTINUED

The 32 Most Common Vitamins and Minerals

Vitamin D • CHOLECALCIFEROL, ERGOCALCIFEROL

RDA:
Adults:
200 IU (5 mcg)
**Children, adolescents,
and pregnant women:**
400 IU (10 mcg)

Vitamin D not only promotes healthy bones and teeth by regulating the absorption and balance of calcium and phosphorus, but also fosters normal muscle contraction and nerve function. Vitamin D prevents rickets, a disease of calcium-deprived bone that results in bowlegs, knock-knees, and other bone defects. Vitamin D supplements may help treat psoriasis and slow or even reverse some cancers, such as myeloid leukemia.

Fatty fish such as herring, salmon, and tuna, followed by dairy products, are the richest natural sources of this nutrient. Few other foods naturally contain vitamin D, but 10 minutes in midday summer sun enables the body to produce about 200 IU of it. Milk, breakfast cereals, and infant formulas are fortified with vitamin D. In adults, vitamin D deficiency can cause nervousness and diarrhea, insomnia, muscle twitches, and bone weakening, and it may worsen osteoporosis. Too much vitamin D raises the calcium level in the blood, which in turn may induce headaches, nausea, loss of appetite, excessive thirst, muscle weakness, and even heart, liver, or kidney damage as calcium deposits accumulate in soft tissue. Vitamin D is fat soluble; excess amounts of it are stored in the body. Because of its potentially toxic effects, vitamin D should not be taken in supplements of more than 400 IU daily unless prescribed by a doctor. ∎

Vitamin E

RDA:
Women: 12 IU (8 mg)
**Men and pregnant
or nursing women:**
15 IU (10 mg)

Vitamin E encompasses a family of compounds called tocopherols, of which alpha-tocopherol is the most common. It is required for proper function of the immune system, endocrine system, and sex glands. As a potent antioxidant, it prevents unstable molecules known as free radicals from damaging cells and tissues. In this capacity, vitamin E deters atherosclerosis, accelerates wound healing, protects lung tissue from inhaled pollutants, and may reduce risk of heart disease and prevent premature aging of skin. Researchers suspect that vitamin E has other beneficial effects ranging from preventing cancer and cataracts to alleviating rheumatoid arthritis and a skin disorder associated with lupus.

Most people get enough vitamin E through their diet and don't need supplements. Vegetable oils, nuts, dark green leafy vegetables, organ meats, seafood, eggs, and avocados are rich food sources. Symptoms of vitamin E deficiency, such as fluid retention and hemolytic anemia, are rare in adults but are sometimes seen in premature infants. Because of its many suggested therapeutic roles, vitamin E is popular as an oral supplement and an ingredient of skin-care products. Although it is fat soluble, vitamin E is considered nontoxic because it does no harm except in extremely high doses. ∎

Vitamin K • MENADIONE, PHYTONADIONE

RDA:
Men: 80 mcg
Women: 65 mcg

Vitamin K is needed in a small but critical amount to form certain proteins essential mainly for blood clotting but also for kidney function and bone metabolism. Vitamin K exists in two natural forms that require some dietary fat for absorption.

Bacteria living in the intestines produce about half the body's needs; the rest comes from diet. Good food sources include spinach, cabbage, broccoli, turnip greens, or other leafy vegetables; beef liver; green tea; cheese; and oats. Vitamin K deficiency is extremely rare in adults but may occur in newborns until their intestinal bacteria begin producing the vitamin. To enhance blood-clotting ability in a newborn, the mother may take vitamin K supplements before delivery, and infants usually receive them after birth. Otherwise, supplements are neither necessary nor recommended. Megadoses higher than 500 mcg can be toxic or cause an allergic reaction and must be prescribed by a doctor. Large doses of vitamin E may interfere with vitamin K's blood-clotting effects. ∎

The 32 Most Common Vitamins and Minerals

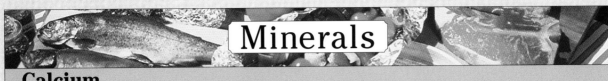

Minerals

Calcium

RDA:
Adults: 800 mg
Pregnant women and young adults: 1,200 mg

Calcium, the most abundant mineral in the body, is essential for the growth and maintenance of bones and teeth. It enables muscles, including the heart, to contract; it is essential for normal blood clotting, proper nerve-impulse transmission, and connective-tissue maintenance. It helps keep blood pressure normal and may reduce the risk of heart disease; taken with vitamin D, it may help lessen the risk of colorectal cancer. It helps prevent rickets in children and osteoporosis in adults.

Good sources include dairy products, dark green leafy vegetables, sardines, salmon, and almonds. Calcium is needed in varying amounts by different people. Too much calcium can lead to constipation and to calcium deposits in soft tissue, causing damage to the heart, liver, or kidneys. For calcium to be properly absorbed, the body must have sufficient levels of vitamin D and of hydrochloric acid in the stomach and a balance of other minerals, including magnesium and phosphorus. A sedentary lifestyle and consuming too much alcohol, dietary fiber, and fat can interfere with calcium absorption; too much protein and caffeine results in calcium being excreted in urine. Supplemental calcium is available in many forms; the form that is best absorbed by the body is calcium citrate-malate. ∎

Chloride

EMDR:
Adults: 750 mg

A natural salt of the mineral chlorine, chloride works with sodium and potassium to help maintain the proper distribution and pH of all bodily fluids and to encourage healthy nerve and muscle function. Independently, chloride contributes to digestion and waste elimination. It is a key component of hydrochloric acid, one of the gastric juices that digest food.

A diet of unprocessed natural foods provides more than enough chloride for human health. Just a pinch of table salt contains about 250 mg, one-third of the EMDR. Chloride deficiency is extremely rare and is usually due to illness. Excessive vomiting can reduce the stomach's chloride level, upsetting its pH balance and causing sweating, diarrhea, loss of appetite, slow and shallow breathing, listlessness, and muscle cramps. Although toxic in large amounts, excess chloride is excreted in urine, preventing potentially dangerous accumulation. ∎

Chromium

EMDR:
Adults: 50 mcg
to 200 mcg

As a component of a natural substance called glucose tolerance factor, chromium works with insulin to regulate the body's use of sugar and is essential to fatty-acid metabolism. Its contribution to metabolism makes chromium a helpful supplement in weight-loss programs. Additional evidence suggests that chromium may help deter atherosclerosis and reduce risk of cardiovascular disease. Inadequate chromium can result in alcohol intolerance, elevate blood sugar levels, and possibly induce diabetes-like symptoms such as tingling in the extremities and reduced muscle coordination.

Trace amounts of chromium are found in many foods, including brewer's yeast, liver, lean meats, poultry, molasses, whole grains, eggs, and cheese. Chromium is not absorbed well, so the body must take in far more than it actually uses. Most people do not get enough dietary chromium, and some may benefit from a multinutrient supplement, such as chromium citrate or chromium picolinate. Supplemental chromium may be used to treat some cases of adult-onset diabetes, to reduce insulin requirements of some diabetic children, and to relieve symptoms of hypoglycemia. Taken regularly in supplements greater than 1,000 mcg, however, chromium inhibits insulin's activity and can be toxic. ∎

CONTINUED

The 32 Most Common Vitamins and Minerals

Cobalt

RDA/EMDR:
Not established

The mineral cobalt is a constituent of cobalamin (vitamin B_{12}). Cobalt helps form red blood cells and maintain nerve tissue. Consuming large amounts of inorganic cobalt stimulates growth of the thyroid gland and may lead to the overproduction of red blood cells, a disorder known as polycythemia.

To be biologically useful, cobalt must be obtained from foods such as liver, kidneys, milk, oysters, clams, or sea vegetables, or from vitamin B_{12} supplements. Inorganic cobalt has no nutritional value but is sometimes added to beer as an antifoaming agent. ∎

Copper

EMDR:
Adults: 1.5 mg to 3 mg

Copper is indispensable to human health. Its many functions include the following: helping to form hemoglobin in the blood; facilitating the absorption and use of iron so that red blood cells can transport oxygen to tissues; assisting in the regulation of blood pressure and heart rate; strengthening blood vessels, bones, tendons, and nerves; promoting fertility; and ensuring normal skin and hair pigmentation. Some evidence suggests that copper helps prevent cardiovascular problems such as high blood pressure and heart arrhythmias and that it may help treat arthritis and scoliosis. Copper may also protect tissue from damage by free radicals, support the body's immune function, and contribute to preventing cancer.

Most adults get enough copper from a normal, varied diet. Seafood and organ meats are the richest sources; blackstrap molasses, nuts, seeds, green vegetables, black pepper, cocoa, and water passed through copper pipes also contain significant quantities. Supplemental copper should be taken only on a doctor's advice. Common supplemental forms are copper aspartate, copper citrate, and copper picolinate. Excess calcium and zinc will interfere with copper absorption, but a true copper deficiency is rare and tends to be limited to people either with certain inherited diseases that inhibit copper absorption, such as albinism, or with acquired malabsorption ailments, such as Crohn's disease and celiac disease. The deficiency may also occur in infants who are not breast-fed and in some premature babies. Symptoms of copper deficiency include brittle, discolored hair; skeletal defects; anemia; high blood pressure; heart arrhythmias; and infertility. Taking more than 10 mg of copper daily can bring on nausea, vomiting, muscle pain, and stomachaches. Women who are pregnant or taking birth-control pills are susceptible to excess blood levels of copper. Some research suggests that high levels of copper and iron may play a role in hyperactivity and autism. ∎

Fluoride

EMDR:
Adults: 1.5 mg to 4 mg

Fluoride, a natural form of the mineral fluorine, is required for healthy teeth and bones. It helps form the tough enamel that protects the teeth from decay and cavities, and increases bone strength and stability. Since the 1950s, many U.S. cities have added fluoride to municipal drinking water at a ratio of about 1 part per million (ppm), or 1 mg per liter. Many believe this practice is responsible for the 40 to 70 percent reduction in tooth decay that dentists have since observed. Fluoride's decay-reducing effects are strongest if children are exposed to the mineral while their teeth are forming. Fluoride toothpaste is helpful, but it is not nearly as effective as regularly ingested fluoride.

Fluoridated water provides most individuals with at least 1 mg of fluoride per day; other dietary sources are dried seaweed, seafood—especially sardines and salmon—cheese, meat, and tea. Nursing babies and children who do not regularly drink fluoridated water should be given supplements, but only as prescribed by a dentist or doctor, because excess fluoride can have adverse effects: At levels of 2 ppm to 8 ppm, the teeth may soften and discolor; at over 8 ppm, fluoride toxicity can depress growth, harden ligaments and tendons, make bones brittle, and induce degeneration of major body systems; 50 ppm may cause fatal poisoning. The low fluoride levels in fluoridated drinking water, however, pose no harmful effects to health. ∎

The 32 Most Common Vitamins and Minerals

Iodine

> **RDA:**
> **Adults:** 150 mcg
> **Pregnant women:**
> 175 mcg

Iodine was one of the first minerals recognized as essential to human health. For centuries, it has been known to prevent and treat goiter—enlargement of the thyroid gland. As part of several thyroid hormones, iodine strongly influences nutrient metabolism; nerve and muscle function; skin, hair, tooth, and nail condition; and physical and mental development. Iodine may also help convert beta carotene into vitamin A.

Kelp, seafood, and vegetables grown in iodine-rich soils are good sources of this mineral. More than half of all the salt consumed in the U.S. is iodized, supplying sufficient iodine in a regular diet. Supplements are usually unnecessary, but pregnant women should take in enough iodine for themselves and their babies to prevent potential mental retardation or cretinism, a form of dwarfism in infants. Iodine deficiency is now uncommon; besides goiter, its effects include weight gain, hair loss, listlessness, insomnia, and some forms of mental retardation. Most excess iodine is excreted, but extremely high intake may cause nervousness, hyperactivity, headache, rashes, a metallic taste in the mouth, and goiter—in this case due to thyroid hyperactivity. ■

Iron

> **RDA:**
> **Adults:** 10 mg
> **Premenopausal women:** 15 mg
> **Pregnant women:**
> 30 mg

Iron is found in hemoglobin, the protein in red blood cells that transports oxygen from the lungs to body tissues. It is also a component of myoglobin, a protein that provides extra fuel to muscles during exertion.

Dietary iron exists in two forms: heme iron, found in red meat, chicken, seafood, and other animal products; and nonheme iron, found in dark green vegetables, whole grains, nuts, dried fruit, and other plant foods. Many flour-based food products are fortified with iron. Heme iron is easier to absorb, but eating foods containing nonheme iron along with foods that have heme iron or vitamin C will maximize iron absorption.

Coffee, tea, soy-based foods, antacids, and tetracycline inhibit iron absorption, as do excessive amounts of calcium, zinc, and manganese. Lack of iron deprives body tissues of oxygen and may cause iron deficiency anemia; warning signs include fatigue, paleness, dizziness, sensitivity to cold, listlessness, irritability, poor concentration, and heart palpitations. Because iron strengthens immune function, iron deficiency also may increase susceptibility to infection. Women need more iron before menopause than after, because menstruation causes iron loss each month. People who have special iron intake needs include menstruating or pregnant women, children under two years of age, vegetarians, anyone with bleeding conditions such as hemorrhoids or bleeding stomach ulcers, and anyone taking the medications listed above.

On a doctor's recommendation, adults can augment their iron intake by means of a multinutrient supplement; straight iron supplements should be taken only under a doctor's supervision. Excess iron inhibits absorption of phosphorus, interferes with immune function, and may increase your risk of developing cancer, cirrhosis, or heart attack. Symptoms of iron toxicity include diarrhea, vomiting, headache, dizziness, fatigue, stomach cramps, and weak pulse. Though uncommon, severe iron poisoning can result in coma, heart failure, and death. Children should never be given adult iron supplements, which can easily poison them. If your pediatrician recommends an iron supplement, make sure it is a specific, child-formulated variety. ■

Magnesium

> **RDA:**
> **Men:** 350 mg
> **Women:** 280 mg
> **Pregnant women:**
> 320 mg

Magnesium contributes to health in many ways. Along with calcium and phosphorus, it is a main constituent of bone. A proper balance of calcium and magnesium is essential for healthy bones and teeth, reduces the risk of developing osteoporosis, and may minimize the effects of existing osteoporosis. Calcium and magnesium also help regulate muscle activity: While calcium stimulates contraction, magnesium induces relaxation. Magnesium is essential for metabolism—converting food to energy—and for building proteins. Adequate blood levels of magnesium protect the body from cardiovascular disease, heart arrhythmias, and possibly, stroke due to blood clotting in the brain.

CONTINUED

The 32 Most Common Vitamins and Minerals

On average, people get enough (or nearly enough) magnesium in their diet. Fish, green leafy vegetables, milk, nuts, seeds, and whole grains are good sources. Many over-the-counter antacids, laxatives, and analgesics contain magnesium, but these medications should not be used as magnesium supplements. A multinutrient supplement is a relatively safe way to augment your magnesium intake. Take specific magnesium supplements only under a doctor's supervision. Of the supplemental forms, magnesium citrate-malate is the easiest to absorb, while magnesium glycinate is the least likely to cause diarrhea at high doses.

The body's need for magnesium increases with stress or illness. Administered as a supplement, magnesium may successfully treat insomnia, muscle cramps, premenstrual syndrome, and cardiovascular problems including high blood pressure, angina due to coronary artery spasm, and leg pain and cramping due to insufficient blood flow. Studies indicate that giving magnesium immediately to a heart attack patient greatly increases the chance of survival.

The body processes magnesium efficiently; the kidneys conserve it as needed and excrete any excess, so both severe deficiency and toxicity are rare. These conditions are dangerous when they do occur, however. Magnesium deficiency may cause nausea, listlessness, muscle weakness, tremor, disorientation, and heart palpitations. Toxicity can induce diarrhea, fatigue, muscle weakness, and in extreme cases, severely depressed heart rate and blood pressure, shallow breathing, loss of reflexes, coma, and possibly death. People who abuse laxatives or experience kidney failure are the most vulnerable to magnesium poisoning. ∎

Manganese

EMDR:
2.5 mg to 5 mg

Manganese is essential for the proper formation and maintenance of bone, cartilage, and connective tissue; it contributes to the synthesis of proteins and genetic material; it helps produce energy from foods; it acts as an antioxidant; and it assists in normal blood clotting.

Most people get enough manganese through their diet alone; for example, a breakfast consisting of orange juice, a 1-oz serving of bran cereal, and a banana provides just over 2.5 mg of manganese. Other food sources include brown rice, nuts, seeds, wheat germ, beans, whole grains, peas, and strawberries. Manganese citrate, a supplement, may help repair damaged tendons and ligaments. Excess dietary manganese is not considered toxic, and manganese deficiency is extremely rare. ∎

Molybdenum

EMDR:
Adults: 75 mcg
to 250 mcg

The obscure mineral molybdenum is an enzyme component. It helps generate energy, process waste for excretion, mobilize stored iron for the body's use, and detoxify sulfites—chemicals used as food preservatives. As such, molybdenum is essential to normal development, particularly of the nervous system. It is also a component of tooth enamel and may help prevent tooth decay.

Molybdenum is present in peas, beans, cereals, pastas, leafy vegetables, yeast, milk, and organ meats. People generally get enough through diet; deficiency is virtually nonexistent. Toxicity is also rare. Molybdenum is available in supplement form as molybdenum picolinate; however, prolonged intake of more than 10 mg daily can cause gout-like symptoms such as joint pain and swelling. ∎

Phosphorus

RDA:
Adults over 25 years old: 800 mg
Young adults and pregnant women:
1,200 mg

Phosphorus is the second most plentiful mineral in the body and is found in every cell. Like calcium, phosphorus is essential for bone formation and maintenance; more than 75 percent of the body's phosphorus is contained in bones and teeth. Phosphorus stimulates muscle contraction and contributes to tissue growth and repair, energy production, nerve-impulse transmission, and heart and kidney function.

Phosphorus exists to some degree in nearly all foods, especially meats, poultry, eggs, fish, nuts, dairy products,

The 32 Most Common Vitamins and Minerals

whole grains, and soft drinks. Deficiency is rare—most people take in far more phosphorus than they need—but may be induced by long-term use of antacids or anticonvulsant drugs that contain aluminum hydroxide. Symptoms of phosphorus deficiency include general weakness, loss of appetite, bone pain, and increased susceptibility to bone fracture. Excess phosphorus in the bloodstream promotes calcium loss, which may weaken bones. Extreme phosphorus toxicity is rare, except in the event of kidney disease. ■

Potassium

EMDR:
Adults: 2,000 mg

Potassium is the third most abundant mineral in the body. It works closely with sodium and chloride to maintain fluid distribution and pH balance and to augment nerve-impulse transmission, muscle contraction, and regulation of heartbeat and blood pressure. It is also required for protein synthesis, carbohydrate metabolism, and insulin secretion by the pancreas. Studies suggest that people who regularly eat potassium-rich foods are less likely to develop atherosclerosis, heart disease, and high blood pressure, or to die of a stroke.

Dietary sources include lean meats, raw vegetables, fruits—especially citrus fruits, bananas, and avocados—and potatoes. Many Americans may get only marginal amounts of potassium, but supplements, such as potassium aspartate, are best taken only under a doctor's guidance. Marginal potassium deficiency causes no symptoms but may increase the risk of developing high blood pressure or aggravate existing heart disease. More severe deficiency can result in nausea, diarrhea, muscle cramps and muscle weakness, poor reflexes, poor concentration, heart arrhythmias, and rarely, death due to heart failure. Acute potassium toxicity may have similar effects, including possible heart failure. However, acute toxicity is rarely linked to diet and tends to occur only in the event of kidney failure. ■

Selenium

RDA:
Men: 70 mcg
Women: 55 mcg
Pregnant women:
65 mcg

An antioxidant, selenium protects cells and tissues from damage wrought by free radicals. Because its antioxidant effects complement those of vitamin E, the two are said to potentiate, or reinforce, each other. Selenium also supports immune function and neutralizes certain poisonous substances such as cadmium, mercury, and arsenic that may be ingested or inhaled. Although its full therapeutic value is unknown, adequate selenium levels may help combat arthritis, deter heart disease, and prevent cancer.

Whole grains, asparagus, garlic, eggs, and mushrooms are typically good sources, as are lean meats and seafood. Very little selenium is required for good health, and most people get adequate amounts through diet alone. High-dose supplements such as selenium citrate and selenium picolinate should be taken only if prescribed by a doctor. Selenium can be toxic in extremely high doses, causing hair loss, nail problems, accelerated tooth decay, and swelling of the fingers, among other symptoms. Some multinutrients contain selenium, but always in small, safe amounts. ■

Sodium

EMDR:
Adults: 500 mg

All bodily fluids—including blood, tears, and perspiration—contain the mineral sodium. Together with potassium and chloride, sodium maintains fluid distribution and pH balance; with potassium, sodium also helps control muscle contraction and nerve function.

Most of the sodium in the American diet is from table salt. Among many other sources are processed foods, soft drinks, meats, shellfish, condiments, snack foods, food additives, and over-the-counter laxatives. Americans generally consume far too much sodium. A single teaspoon of salt contains 2,000 mg—four times the daily minimum—but average daily consumption in the United States ranges from 3,000 mg to 7,000 mg.

Keeping sodium intake within reasonable limits is critical to maintaining long-term health. When sodium levels are persistently elevated, the body loses potassium and retains water, making blood pressure rise. Adopting a low-sodium

CONTINUED

The 32 Most Common Vitamins and Minerals

diet can reduce high blood pressure and correct a potassium deficiency. Overexertion, particularly in the hot sun, can induce temporary sodium deficiency, which is characterized by nausea, dehydration, muscle cramps, and other symptoms of heatstroke and exhaustion. Drinking several glasses of water with a pinch of salt added replaces the sodium and eases the symptoms. ∎

Sulfur

RDA/EMDR:
Not established

Accounting for some 10 percent of the body's mineral content, sulfur is part of every cell, especially in the protein-rich tissues of hair, nails, muscle, and skin. It assists in metabolism as a part of vitamin B_1, biotin, and vitamin B_5; helps regulate blood sugar levels as a constituent of insulin; and helps regulate blood clotting. Sulfur is also known to convert some toxic substances into nontoxic ones that can then be excreted, and therefore is used to treat poisoning from aluminum, cadmium, lead, and mercury.

Any diet that provides sufficient protein is also providing adequate sulfur. Meat, fish, poultry, eggs, dairy products, peas, and beans are rich in both nutrients. Neither sulfur deficiency nor toxicity occurs naturally in humans. Inorganic sulfur ingested in large amounts can be harmful, but excess organic sulfur from food is readily excreted. ∎

Vanadium

RDA/EMDR:
Not established

Vanadium is a trace mineral whose role in nutrition is uncertain but possibly essential. Evidence suggests that it lowers blood sugar levels in some people and inhibits tumor development, perhaps protecting against diabetes and some cancers. It also may contribute to cholesterol metabolism and hormone production. Vanadium exists in whole grains, nuts, root vegetables, liver, fish, and vegetable oils. Because symptoms of its deficiency are unknown, it is assumed that humans need only a small amount, which diet apparently provides. ∎

Zinc

RDA:
Adults: 15 mg
Pregnant women:
30 mg

The mineral zinc is integral to the synthesis of RNA and DNA, the genetic material that controls cell growth, division, and function. In various proteins, enzymes, hormones, and hormonelike substances called prostaglandins, zinc contributes to many bodily processes, including bone development and growth; cell respiration; energy metabolism; wound healing; the liver's ability to remove toxic substances such as alcohol from the body; immune function; and the regulation of heart rate and blood pressure. An adequate zinc intake enhances the ability to taste, promotes healthy skin and hair, enhances reproductive functions, and may improve short-term memory and attention span. As an anti-inflammatory agent, zinc is sometimes used to treat acne, rheumatoid arthritis, and prostatitis. Taking supplemental zinc may boost resistance to infection, especially in the elderly, and stimulate wound healing.

Zinc is most easily obtained from lean meat and seafood, but it is also found in eggs, soybeans, peanuts, wheat bran, cheese, oysters, and other foods. Many American diets are slightly low in zinc. Young children, pregnant women, vegetarians, and elderly people are the most susceptible to zinc deficiency. Loss of taste is usually the first warning; other symptoms are hair loss or discoloration, white streaks on the nails, dermatitis, loss of appetite, fatigue, and poor healing of wounds. In children, zinc deficiency can retard growth and stunt sexual development in boys. On the other hand, ingesting extreme amounts of zinc daily can impair immune function and cause nausea, headaches, vomiting, dehydration, stomachaches, poor muscle coordination, fatigue, and possibly kidney failure. Experts recommend increasing zinc levels by increasing the zinc-rich foods in your diet or by taking a multinutrient supplement that includes zinc chelate, zinc picolinate, or zinc aspartate, the three most easily absorbed forms. If zinc is used for more than three to six months to treat a chronic condition, it is essential to consult a nutritionist to avoid creating a mineral imbalance. Zinc ointment, which contains zinc oxide, is the most common topical form, and is useful for treating skin disorders, burns, and other wounds. ∎

$\mathcal{O}$steopathy

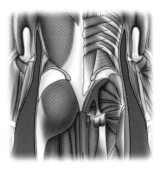

O steopathic medicine is a system of healing and health maintenance that focuses on the musculoskeletal system in order to improve the overall functioning of the body. To restore structural balance and thus help a patient regain health, an osteopathic physician will combine manipulation of the joints and soft tissues with instruction in proper posture, body mechanics, and exercise. Because osteopathic care is holistic, or targeted to the whole person, the doctor also considers psychological factors, lifestyle, and diet in addressing an illness or developing a plan for maintaining health.

Origins

Manipulation of muscles and joints was used to treat illness as far back as the days of the pharaohs of ancient Egypt. But the specific techniques and theoretical underpinnings of osteopathy were not developed until the late 19th century, by an American physician named Andrew Taylor Still. After losing three of his children to a spinal meningitis epidemic in 1864, Still became disillusioned with conventional medicine—particularly the use of drugs—and began a personal search for a better way of treating disease and restoring health. He eventually concluded that the entire body had to be considered when treating an illness and that the musculoskeletal system played a central role in both health and disease.

What It's Good For

Founded as it is on holistic principles, osteopathic medicine is used to diagnose and treat virtually all types of ailments, from viral infections to sports injuries; the list at right is a representative sample of conditions treated by osteopathic physicians. As well as employing techniques specific to osteopathy, practitioners incorporate both conventional and other therapies into their care of patients. For example, osteopathic physicians are licensed to prescribe antibiotics and other drugs, to deliver and care for babies, and to perform surgery, including brain and heart surgery.

LICENSED & INSURED?

YES! *Osteopathic physicians must complete four years of medical training at an accredited college of osteopathic medicine, followed by a one-year internship in primary care (family practice, internal medicine, pediatrics, or obstetrics and gynecology). Many also complete a residency in one of 120 medical specialties, ranging from dermatology to neurosurgery. Osteopathic physicians are licensed in all 50 states as full physicians and are authorized to prescribe medication and to practice the specialties for which they are qualified. Insurance coverage is the same as for MDs.*

Target Ailments

- Arthritis
- Asthma
- Athletic Injuries
- Back Problems
- Bronchitis
- Bursitis
- Carpal Tunnel Syndrome
- Constipation
- Earache
- Endometriosis
- Flu
- Headache
- Hearing Problems
- Heartburn
- Hemorrhoids
- Menstrual Problems
- Muscle Cramps
- Pain, Chronic
- Prostate Problems
- Sinusitis
- Varicose Veins

See Common Ailments, beginning on page 194.

CONTINUED

Osteopathy <small>CONTINUED</small>

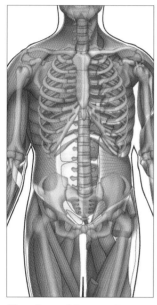

Muscle and bone *• In oste-opathic medicine, both diag-nosis and treatment involve manipulation of the muscles, bones, and joints of the mus-culoskeletal system.*

FOR MORE INFO
Following is a list of organizations you can contact to learn more about osteopathy:

American Osteopathic Association
142 East Ontario Street
Chicago, IL 60611
(800) 621-1773
e-mail: www.am.osteo.assn.org

The American Academy of Osteopathy
3500 DePauw Boulevard, Suite 1080
Indianapolis, IN 46268-1139
(317) 879-1881

Preparations/Techniques

What sets osteopathic medicine apart from other healing approaches is its use of a diagnostic and treatment system known as osteopathic manipulative ther-apy, or OMT. Literally a hands-on approach to medical care, OMT involves various forms of massage, muscle pressure, and joint realignment. The purposes of ma-nipulation are threefold: to relieve tension in the affected muscles and ligaments and to restore them to their proper position; to improve circulation and stimulate the nervous system; and to improve body mechanics, such as posture. Osteopathic manipulative therapy is thus designed to treat the underlying mechanical dys-function that is presumed to be causing or contributing to a disease, rather than simply the disease itself.

Visiting a Professional

When you visit an osteopathic physician, you will receive a complete physi-cal exam, including, if your condition warrants it, standard blood tests, urine tests, and imaging techniques such as x-rays. Your osteopathic physician will also give you a so-called structural exam, which begins with an assessment of your posture, spine, and balance. The various muscles, tendons, and ligaments of your body will be gently pressed for indications of tenderness, tension, and weakness. Your joints will also be examined to discover whether their movement is restricted or causes pain. If a structural abnormality is found to be the source of your illness or injury, your physician will then apply the techniques of osteopathic manipula-tive therapy to treat the problem. It is possible that more than one treatment ses-sion will be recommended.

Wellness

Osteopathic medicine has always emphasized preventive medicine. At the core of its philosophy is the belief that the body is inherently capable of healing itself. Osteopathic physicians thus work closely with their patients to help them develop healthier lifestyles. Preventive techniques recommended by osteopathic practitioners vary, but may include nutritional counseling, acupressure, medicinal herbs, yoga, and other forms of alternative medicine.

What the Critics Say

Although once ridiculed and shunned by conventional practitioners, osteo-pathic medicine has gained considerable favor from the medical mainstream in re-cent years, primarily because of its holistic approach to treatment and its emphasis on prevention of illness and maintenance of a healthy lifestyle. ■

$\mathcal{Q}$igong

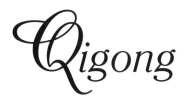

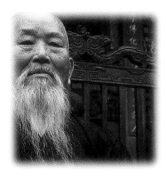

Q | igong ("chee-goong") is an ancient Chinese discipline that uses breathing exercises, movement, and meditation to balance and strengthen the body's vital energy (chi, sometimes spelled "qi"). Several of the martial arts, including t'ai chi (pages 172-173) and kung fu, are derived from qigong, but qigong itself is oriented more toward healing and less toward self-defense than these related practices.

Qigong, meaning "energy cultivation," is intended to manipulate two forms of energy: internal chi and external chi. Internal chi can be developed by the repetition of qigong's ritual exercises and by meditation, a practice that is believed to balance the body's energies and promote internal wellness. Some qigong masters are said to be able to emit external chi, energy transmitted from one person to another for healing purposes.

Target Ailments

■ Back Problems

■ Carpal Tunnel Syndrome

■ Circulatory Problems

■ Depression

■ Hay Fever

■ High Blood Pressure

■ Insomnia

■ Menopause

■ Neuralgia

■ Pain, Chronic

■ TMJ Syndrome

See Common Ailments, beginning on page 194.

Origins

Like many other forms of Chinese medicine, qigong dates back thousands of years. The modern practice of strengthening chi through ritual exercise and meditation contains strands of Buddhist, Taoist, and Confucian philosophy developed over millennia. The Buddhist approach concentrates on freeing the self through awareness; the Taoist focuses on connection with the natural world; and the Confucian philosophy is more concerned with the place of the individual in society. Together they form the balance of inner and outer awareness that marks qigong today.

During China's Cultural Revolution in the 1960s and 1970s qigong was banned, but it later became clear that the discipline had millions of proponents in its native country. By the 1990s qigong was gaining popularity in the West as well.

What It's Good For

Qigong's supporters say that the practice can greatly improve overall health and even help cure a wide variety of ailments. In the years since the Cultural Revolution, China has hosted a number of medical conferences devoted to the healing effects of qigong. Papers presented at these meetings claim beneficial effects for ailments ranging from allergies and asthma to diabetes, hypertension, liver disorders, and even paralysis and cancer. In more serious diseases, patients usually employ qigong along with conventional medical care to speed recovery and alleviate pain.

Preparations/Techniques

Those wishing to practice qigong should begin by studying with a teacher. The exercises are deceptively simple and need to be performed over and over again under

CONTINUED

Qigong CONTINUED

the guidance of an expert before the student begins to feel their effects. There are literally thousands of qigong exercises, but the techniques can be divided into standing, sitting, lying, and walking. Students may stand with legs apart and breathe from the diaphragm in a particular pattern while performing ritual movements with arms and legs; or they may sit and roll objects between their palms to stimulate energy points. Walking may be slow and regular, or more random and free. Students may also practice meditation techniques, focusing the mind on an energy point while counting breaths.

Between classes (which are taken once or twice a week), students go through the movements every day for about 30 minutes, morning and evening. Those who have particular medical problems may practice movements specific to their ailments for longer daily periods.

Some patients want to take the next step and visit a qigong master to experience the reputed healing power of external chi. These masters, more commonly found in China than in the United States, believe that energy emitted from their hands passes into the patient's body, helping it to balance its own chi and heal its ailments. Such a master might touch or press specific "chi points" on the body, or might pass his or her hands several inches above the body. Even these masters, however, will encourage patients to learn to develop internal chi so that they can take charge of their own health.

Wellness

Qigong, say its supporters, is a way of life. When practiced every day, it is supposed to boost chi circulation and enhance overall health. Although people do turn to it for specific ailments, it is most properly used as a daily approach to wellness.

What the Critics Say

Because the medical research on qigong's health benefits is almost entirely Chinese, and critics claim that much of it does not conform to Western scientific standards, the Western medical establishment does not give much credence to qigong's reputed cures. The concept of external chi comes in for special criticism as being unlikely and unscientific. As with any form of medicine, conventional doctors urge the public to be extremely cautious of any practitioner making claims for "miracle cures." ∎

FOR MORE INFO

Following is a list of organizations you can contact to learn more about qigong:

Qigong Institute
East West Academy of Healing Arts
450 Sutter Place, Suite 2104
San Francisco, CA 94108
(415) 788-2227
fax: (415) 788-2242

World Natural Medicine Foundation
College of Medical Qi Gong
9904 106 Street
Edmonton, AB T5K 1C4 Canada
(403) 424-2231
fax: (403) 424-8520

LICENSED & INSURED?

Although some practitioners of qigong may have licenses in other specialties, such as acupuncture, qigong itself is not subject to licensing, and only in rare cases has it been covered by insurance companies.

ℛeflexology

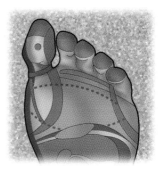

R eflexology involves the manipulation of specific areas on the feet—and sometimes on the hands or limbs—with the goal of bringing the body into homeostasis, or balance. According to reflexologists, distinct regions of the feet correspond to particular organs or body systems. Stimulating the appropriate region with a thumb or finger is intended to eliminate energy blockages thought to produce pain or disease in the associated structures. The arrangement of reflexology areas on the feet mirrors the organization of the body, to the extent that organs on the right side of the body are represented on the right foot, and so with the left.

Origins

The precise beginnings of reflexology are obscure, but the practice seems to have its roots in ancient Egypt as well as in Chinese medicine *(pages 57-60),* with its belief in energy pathways and body zones. Around 1900, American physician William Fitzgerald, who had worked with European practitioners, introduced foot reflexology and the related practice of hand reflexology into the United States. These therapies were then described in such books as *Stories the Feet Can Tell,* written by Eunice Ingham in 1938.

What It's Good For

The overall goal of reflexology is to balance the body's vital energies and thus promote overall health. Reflexologists maintain that their therapy helps improve blood supply, normalize overactive or underactive glands, unblock nerve impulses, and relieve stress. Although prevention, rather than cure, is the primary aim of reflexology, practitioners use it to relieve a wide variety of ailments, including headaches, sinus problems, constipation, and insomnia.

Preparations/Techniques

Patients who want to try reflexology can visit a certified reflexologist for treatment. However, most people can also perform reflexology at home after studying the reflex areas and the techniques for working them.

Reflexologists divide the body into 10 longitudinal zones running from the head to the soles of the feet. By working a particular zone on the foot, proponents claim, you are affecting an organ within the corresponding zone in the upper body. The foot is further subdivided into specific reflex areas that relate to particular organs and structures, such as the eyes, liver, and kidneys. Reflexologists recognize nearly 30 areas on the sole of each foot *(see the illustration on page 169).*

Reflexology features techniques that can be performed either by yourself or by

Target Ailments

- Anemia
- Arthritis
- Back Problems
- Carpal Tunnel Syndrome
- Constipation
- Gout
- Hay Fever
- High Blood Pressure
- Ménière's Disease
- Motion Sickness
- Premenstrual Syndrome
- Stress
- Thyroid Problems

See Common Ailments, beginning on page 194.

CONTINUED

Reflexology CONTINUED

a partner. The basic thumb technique uses the inside edge of the thumb pad (the side away from the fingers) to "walk" along reflex areas; walking consists of a forward, creeping movement, with the first joint of the thumb bending and unbending slightly as the digit inches ahead. The finger technique uses the same walking motion but with the edge of the index finger next to the thumb. When working an area, one hand should work and the other should hold the foot in a comfortable position with the sole flat and the toes straight. As they work each reflex area, reflexologists feel for tension or minute grainy spots, or "crystals," beneath the skin, believing that these are signs of blockages or pain in the relevant part of the body. The thumb and finger techniques aim to remove the tension and these crystals.

Some reflexologists also teach that the hands and other so-called referral areas can be worked in the same way. In hand reflexology, the thumb of one hand works the palm of the other; the index finger works the areas between the fingers and the V between the thumb and the index finger of the opposite hand. Referral areas are places on the body thought to have an anatomical similarity to the afflicted area. For instance, the elbow would be the referral area for the knee, the wrist for the ankle. If a patient sprained a right ankle, a reflexologist might work the right wrist in addition to, or in place of, the corresponding area on the foot.

Wellness

Reflexologists view their therapy as preventive maintenance: Daily practice of its techniques, they say, can keep the body running smoothly. Like the ancient physicians who went before them, reflexologists believe that a person who pursues wellness by balancing the body's energies and relaxing stress and tension will rarely fall sick.

What the Critics Say

Many conventional medical practitioners dismiss reflexology as an example of "magical thinking"—the belief that objects can be influenced simply by thinking about them. Skeptics also point out that reflexologists have not established any scientific basis for asserting that the feet or hands are connected in a therapeutic way with other parts of the body. To some critics, in fact, reflexology treatments are nothing more than glorified foot massages. Proponents, however, maintain that the health benefits of reflexology are extensive and well documented. ∎

LICENSED & INSURED?

Reflexology is not recognized as a valid treatment by the medical establishment, and therefore reflexologists are unlikely to be licensed or insured. However, practitioners who have completed formal instruction in reflexology may be certified by the International Institute of Reflexology.

FOR MORE INFO

Following is a list of organizations you can contact to learn more about reflexology:

**International Institute
of Reflexology**
PO Box 12642
St. Petersburg, FL 33733
(813) 343-4811

Reflexology Research
PO Box 35820
Station D
Albuquerque, NM 87176
(505) 344-9392

Reflexology

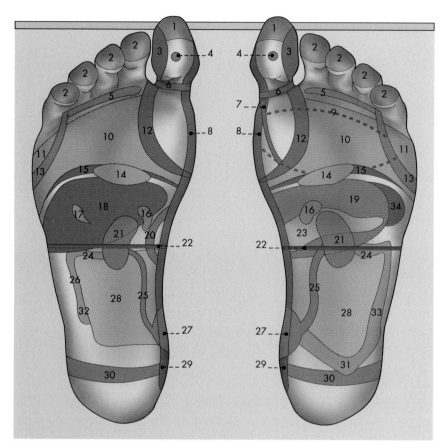

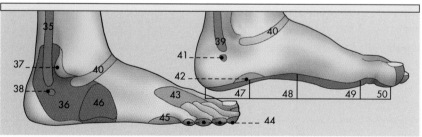

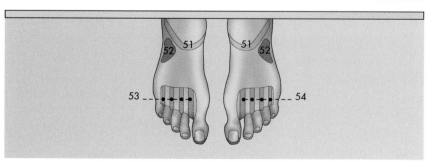

REFLEXOLOGY AREAS

Right and Left Bottom
1. Brain
2. Sinus, Head, Brain
3. Side, Neck
4. Pituitary, Pineal
5. Eyes, Ears
6. Throat, Neck, Thyroid
7. Esophagus
8. Thymus
9. Heart
10. Lung, Breast
11. Arm
12. Thyroid, Bronchi
13. Shoulder
14. Solar Plexus
15. Diaphragm
16. Adrenal Glands
17. Gallbladder
18. Liver
19. Stomach
20. Duodenum
21. Kidneys
22. Waistline
23. Pancreas
24. Transverse Colon
25. Ureter Tubes
26. Ascending Colon
27. Bladder
28. Small Intestine
29. Sacrum, Coccyx
30. Sciatic
31. Sigmoid Colon
32. Ileocecal Valve, Appendix
33. Descending Colon
34. Spleen

Right Outside, Left Inside
35. Sciatic
36. Pelvic Area
37. Hip, Back, Sciatic
38. Ovary, Testicle
39. Prostate, Uterus, Rectum, Sciatic
40. Lymph, Groin, Fallopian Tube
41. Uterus, Prostate
42. Bladder
43. Breast, Lung
44. Sinus, Head, Brain
45. Arm, Shoulder
46. Lower Back
47. Sacrum, Coccyx
48. Lumbar
49. Thoracic
50. Cervical

Right and Left Top
51. Lymph, Groin, Fallopian Tube
52. Knee, Leg, Hip, Lower Back
53. Chest, Lung, Breast, Back
54. Chest, Lung, Breast, Back, Heart

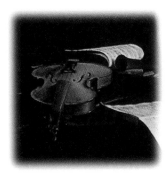

Target Ailments

■ Cancer

■ Chronic Fatigue Syndrome

■ Depression

■ Headache

■ Heart Problems

■ High Blood Pressure

■ Immune Problems

■ Insomnia

■ Irritable Bowel Syndrome

■ Menopause

■ Pain, Chronic

■ Premenstrual Syndrome

■ Stomach Ulcers

■ Stress

See Common Ailments, beginning on page 194.

Sound Therapy

Using sound to soothe is as natural as singing a lullaby to a cranky baby. This notion has developed into the complex system of healing known as sound therapy, the two major elements of which are the related practices of music therapy and sound healing. Both approaches are designed to foster physical, psychological, and social health. In music therapy, patients listen to or perform music—anything from Mozart to rhythmic drumming—with the goal of addressing specific problems or ailments. In sound healing, a practitioner projects nonmusical sound directly onto a part of the patient's body, a technique based on the belief that the body contains its own interlocking system of vibrations that can be brought into balance by sound waves.

Music and Sound

Music therapy is as eclectic as music itself, encompassing both classical and popular forms, ancient folk music, and even pure percussion. Those who have apparently benefited include a diverse array as well: people with chronic pain, autistic children and adults, Alzheimer's sufferers, and patients undergoing surgery. Depending on the ailment, therapists may ask patients to listen to music, perform it, move to its rhythms, or react to the memories it might evoke.

Sound healing, in contrast, uses the physical vibrations of sound waves to promote health. Many different methods exist, based on different theories about the inner workings of the body. One sound healer might train the patient to project nonverbal sounds inward to balance the body's energy fields. Another might use a tuning fork or a computerized sound generator, held near the body, to restore the normal vibration of systems and organs. Others might "read" the patient's body or energy by singing a series of tones and detecting areas of resistance, or they might ask patients to listen to a specific range of tones in order to restore frequencies missing from the patient's life.

Origins

Some forms of sound healing are ancient, such as the use of Tibetan

---

LICENSED & INSURED?

A music therapist must hold a degree in music therapy, complete an internship, and pass a national examination in order to be board certified by the Certification Board for Music Therapists. The United States currently has more than 80 degree-granting programs. There are no established certification or licensing procedures for other kinds of sound healers.

Music therapy is usually not covered by health insurance, but some insurers will reimburse for treatment for specific conditions.

Sound Therapy

singing bowls, sacred instruments said to produce healing sounds. Others, especially those that use computerized equipment, developed only recently. Music therapy dates from the 1940s, when music was used to rehabilitate soldiers returning from war.

What It's Good For

Music therapists and sound healers alike seek to improve health and reduce dysfunction, heal emotional and psychological disorders, and enhance creativity, energy, and brain function. Music therapy has been shown to ease headaches, improve gait in stroke patients, enhance memory among those with Alzheimer's disease, encourage learning in children with autism or learning disabilities, and ease anxiety and pain during surgery and labor. Sound healing addresses similar problems, including chronic pain and stress, with a particular emphasis on physical functioning, body alignment, and energy balancing.

Preparations/Techniques

Informal music therapy can be as easy as playing upbeat tunes when energy is low. Seriously ill patients and their families often gain comfort from listening to music together. Soothing music can augment guided imagery, or visualization, techniques, strengthening the relaxation response. *(See Mind/Body Medicine, pages 133-134.)* Music therapists work in many kinds of treatment facilities and schools, and in private practice. Some specialize in areas such as stroke recovery, pain management, or mental health. Consult with a board-certified music therapist for information on the application of music therapy in particular health issues.

Some kinds of sound healing can be learned and practiced anywhere; others require tapes or other special equipment. Sound healers from many backgrounds use different methods to analyze conditions and promote healing. Some offer therapeutic sessions; others teach methods that can be used independently.

Wellness

Music can promote relaxation and reduce stress. Advocates of sound healing assert that regular use of sound can bolster energy and empower the body's self-healing mechanisms.

What the Critics Say

Although music therapy is well supported by scientific study, there is little scientific evidence to support many claims of sound healers. These practices are often based on longstanding non-Western approaches to health such as Chinese or Ayurvedic medicine. Critics urge caution when deciding to use an unconventional therapy. Ask potential healers about their training, methods, and experience. ■

FOR MORE INFO
Following is a list of organizations you can contact to learn more about sound therapy:

National Association for Music Therapy
8455 Colesville Road, Suite 1000
Silver Spring, MD 20910
(301) 589-3300
e-mail: info@namt.com
(can provide list of music therapists by area and informational brochures)

Institute for Music, Health, and Education
3010 Hennepin Avenue South, #269
Minneapolis, MN 55408
(800) 490-4968
e-mail: imhemn@pressenter.com
(offers training in sound-healing techniques)

Sound Healers Association
PO Box 2240
Boulder, CO 80306
(303) 443-8181
(can provide a directory of members)

Sound Healers Colloquium
219 Grant Road
Newmarket, NH 03857
(distributes books and tapes on sound healing)

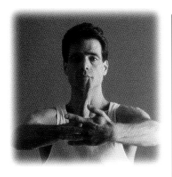

Target Ailments

- Arthritis
- Back Problems
- Bronchitis
- Cholesterol Problems
- Depression
- Gas and Gas Pains
- Hay Fever
- Headache
- Insomnia
- Neuralgia
- Osteoporosis
- Pain, Chronic
- Stress
- Tendinitis

See Common Ailments, beginning on page 194.

T'ai Chi

T'ai chi ch'uan—*commonly known as t'ai chi—is an ancient Chinese practice that combines martial arts, exercise, and meditation in one graceful, slow-motion art. Every morning in parks across Asia, and increasingly in America and Europe as well, practitioners of t'ai chi perform what appears to be a trancelike, controlled dance. This dance is in fact a combination of t'ai chi "forms"—ritual movements intended to promote the flow of internal energy, increase self-awareness, and strengthen and relax the body.*

Though often considered more a martial art than a therapeutic technique, t'ai chi provides many health benefits, including improved strength, flexibility, and relaxation. The ritual movements are meant to move the body's energy (chi—sometimes spelled "qi") to its natural center, called the tan t'ien, about two inches below the navel. The energy is then said to circulate throughout the body, correcting existing conditions and preventing illness.

Origins

T'ai chi's roots reach down thousands of years to the origins of Eastern philosophy itself. Many of its principles are found in the *Tao Tê Ching,* traditionally written by the sage Lao-tzu (604-531 BC). Taoist philosophy holds that *tao*—"the way"—is the force that gives shape and energy to all things, and that to understand tao one must understand one's place in the natural world. Chinese physicians and martial artists alike incorporated Taoist and then Buddhist views into their practices, developing ritual exercises that mimicked the natural movements of animals such as the horse, the tiger, and the crane.

By the 19th century, the modern forms of t'ai chi were brought to Beijing, where they quickly became popular. Chinese immigrants then took the art to America. In recent years t'ai chi has gained a considerable following in the United States.

What It's Good For

Advocates of t'ai chi discourage its use as a remedy for specific ills. Instead, they say, the art is intended to

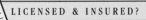

LICENSED & INSURED?

T'ai chi is not a medical art but a martial one. Although some of its teachers may also have specialties in Chinese therapies such as acupuncture, in general those who teach t'ai chi will have varying credentials and will not be licensed. Experts advise students to check their teacher's credentials as they would with any provider of services: Ask for the teacher's background and experience, visit a class, and talk to students.

T'ai Chi

correct imbalances in one's life and to strengthen inner energy, so that those who practice it feel calm, harmonious, and invigorated. The positive effects of this slow, intense exercise include improved muscle strength, particularly in the lower body, better flexibility, better posture and balance, and relaxation. Proponents say the exercise may also prevent sleeplessness, backache, and the pain of arthritis. Because it is slow and can be practiced so as not to stress joints, t'ai chi is good exercise for children and the elderly. In fact, older people are among its devoutest followers.

Preparations/Techniques

Newcomers to t'ai chi are advised to study the art with an experienced teacher. Classes can be found through local YMCAs, health clubs, Taoist centers, and in the yellow pages under "Martial Arts." A class might begin with meditation and warm-ups, proceed to work on specific forms, and end with a cooldown. The slow, lissome movements look deceptively easy; in fact, they require serious concentration and control, and participants will work up a sweat. Progress takes time. Although some of the forms can be learned in a few weeks, students typically need one or two years to achieve the state of relaxed alertness and control of detail that t'ai chi requires.

Students should attend class at least once a week and then practice at home every day. The movements require only a modest amount of flat, open space. Many people like to practice in the morning, when they are alert and fresh, or in the evening, as a way to unwind after a stressful day. Experts recommend exercising in the open air, if possible; the fresh air and tranquillity are conducive to a peaceful state of mind, and some advocates feel that energy travels more freely in a natural setting.

T'ai chi forms are combinations of stances that flow continuously into one another. "Short forms" might have as few as 24 postures; a "long form" would have up to 88. The following eight pages show basic stances that might be used in a 30-movement short form.

Wellness

T'ai chi, like other Chinese arts, is devoted to wellness. Incorporating physical, mental, and spiritual exercise, t'ai chi's mission is to invigorate both body and mind and clear the flow of energy. In that way, proponents claim, t'ai chi practitioners can live into old age strong and free of disease.

What the Critics Say

The concept of chi—energy flowing through channels in the body—is not accepted by everyone. Critics note that there is no scientific evidence for such an energy flow. But even critics acknowledge that t'ai chi exercises are unlikely to do harm—and, like any exercise, quite probably do some good. ∎

FOR MORE INFO
Following is a list of organizations you can contact to learn more about t'ai chi:

Qigong Institute
East West Academy
of Healing Arts
450 Sutter Place, Suite 2104
San Francisco, CA 94108
(415) 788-2227
fax: (415) 788-2242

Taoist T'ai chi Society of USA
1060 Bannock Street
Denver, CO 80204
(303) 623-5163
fax: (303) 623-7908

Gallery of T'ai Chi Positions

Learning a "Form"

Mastering t'ai chi requires a knowledgeable teacher, who will instruct you in what are known as t'ai chi forms—a series of movements and positions that are performed in sequence, without stopping. The images here and on the following pages depict stances that might be components of a short form; they represent key transitional moments in the continuous flow through the various positions. Whenever you perform t'ai chi, stay relaxed, yet alert; note the position of your hands and feet, and keep your back straight. With a teacher's guidance and everyday practice, you may begin to experience the long-term health benefits that t'ai chi can provide.

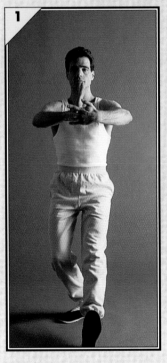

Salutation to the Buddha

Start out standing erect. Turn your right foot out 45 degrees and sink down slightly on your right leg. Shift all your weight onto that leg and extend your left leg, flexing your foot and crossing your hands in front of your chest.

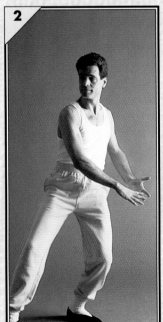

Grasp Bird's Tail

Step back onto your left foot, turning it out, then move your hands to waist level as you shift your weight onto your left leg.

Gallery of T'ai Chi Positions

3

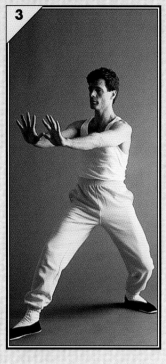

Grasp Bird's Tail

■ Swing your arms to the right and press forward, shifting some of your weight onto your right leg.

4

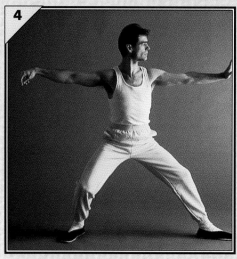

Single Whip

■ Pivot left, shifting your weight to your right leg, bringing your left foot around, and opening your arms.

5

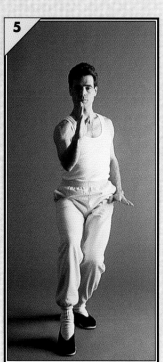

White Crane Spreads Its Wings

■ Step forward, leading with your right leg. Align your right hand, elbow, knee, and toes.

6

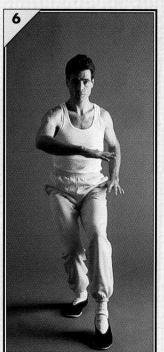

White Crane Spreads Its Wings

■ Slide your left foot forward and move your right arm so that it is parallel to the floor.

CONTINUED

Gallery of T'ai Chi Positions

7

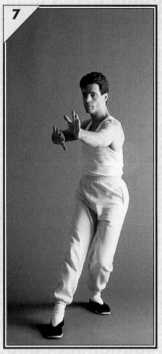

Brush, Knee, Twist, Step

■ Step back onto your left foot as you raise your left hand and twist to the right.

8

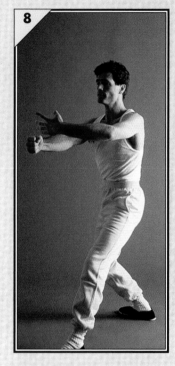

Parry, Punch

■ Step back onto your right foot, and change the position of your hands as shown.

9

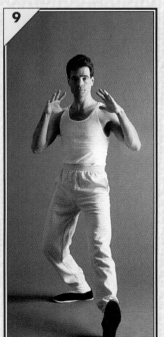

Closing

■ Parry with your left arm and punch with your right. Rock back onto your right leg and bring your arms up.

10

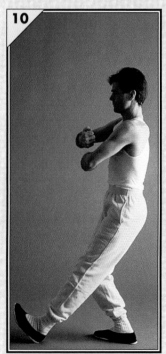

Embracing Tiger

■ Pivot 90 degrees to the right, crossing your arms in front of you.

Gallery of T'ai Chi Positions

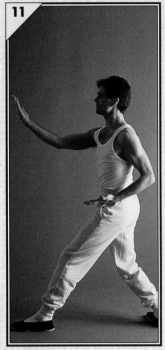

11

Fist under Elbow

Slide forward, dropping your left hand to waist level and extending your right hand.

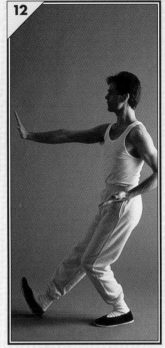

12

Repulse Monkey

Step back with your left foot and straighten your right leg and arm.

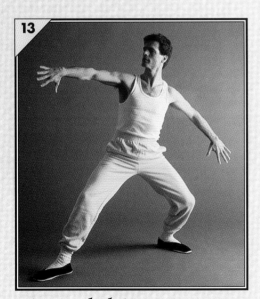

13

Diagonal Flying

Pivot on your left foot, and step out with your right, opening your arms.

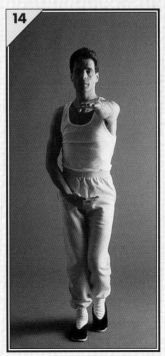

14

Raise Left Hand

Come forward, shifting your weight to your right leg, and extend your left arm.

CONTINUED

Gallery of T'ai Chi Positions

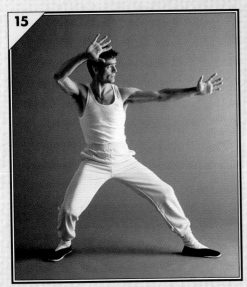

15

Fan through the Arms

▪ Pivot and step out with your left foot, moving your right hand up to your temple.

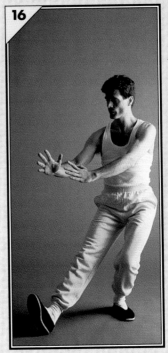

16

Green Dragon Dropping Water

▪ Pivot right, changing the position of your legs and arms as shown.

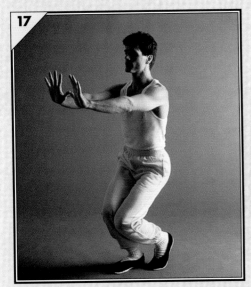

17

Step Up and Push

▪ Step up, with knees bent, and push out with hands flexed.

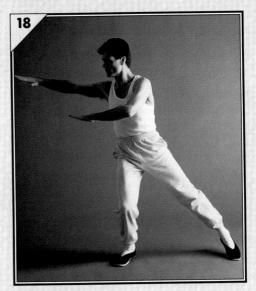

18

Cloud Hands

▪ Pivot right, and extend your left leg out as your arms and torso rotate right.

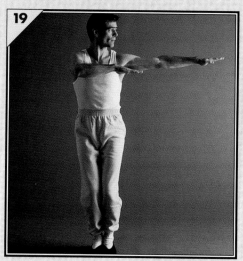

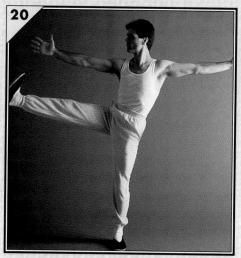

Cloud Hands

■ *Rotate to the left as you bring your feet together and move your arms as shown.*

Separation of Legs

■ *Rotate right, then left, four times, ending in a Single Whip (step 4). Rotate your torso right and kick your right leg straight out as you open your arms.*

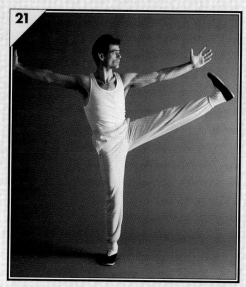

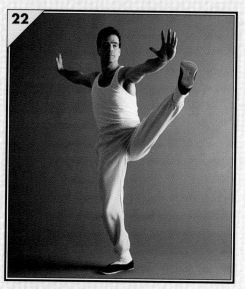

Separation of Legs

■ *Shift your weight to your right leg and kick with your left.*

Separation of Legs

■ *Lower your leg almost to the floor, turn your right foot out, and kick again with your left leg.*

CONTINUED

Gallery of T'ai Chi Positions

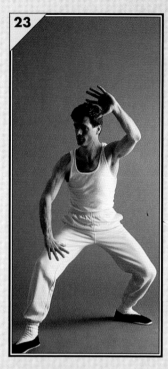

Wind Blowing Lotus

■ Drop your left leg back, shift your weight onto it, and parry high and low with your arms.

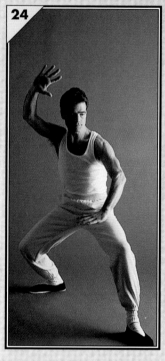

Wind Blowing Lotus

■ Pivot on your left foot and switch the position of your hands.

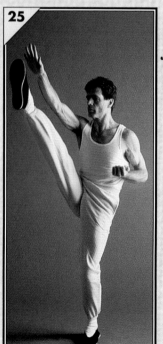

Double Jump Kick

■ Pivot on your right foot, jump onto the left, and kick your right leg—without straining—toward your extended right arm.

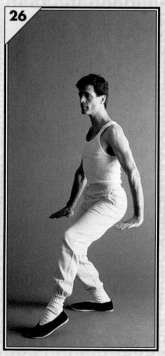

Step Back, Hands to the Side

■ Step back on your right leg, drop your arms, then shift backward onto your left foot.

Gallery of T'ai Chi Positions

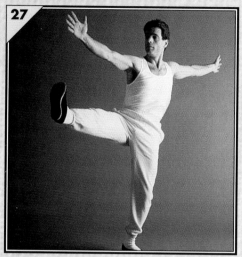

Kick with the Sole

Pivot on your left foot until you complete a full circle, coming around to stand on your left leg, and kick with your right.

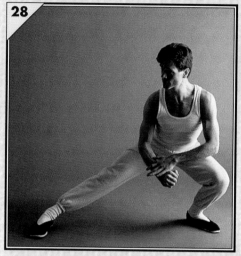

Clap Opponent with Fist

Drop down on your left leg, keeping your right leg straight and your feet parallel; cover your right wrist with your left palm.

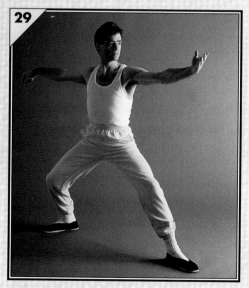

Diagonal Single Whip

Swing your right leg back while you open your arms.

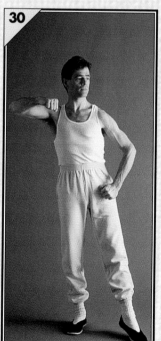

Parting of Wild Horse's Mane

Step forward, moving your fists to your chest and hip.

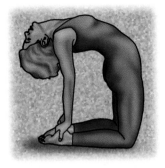

Target Ailments

■ Asthma

■ Athletic Injuries

■ Back Problems

■ Cancer

■ Chronic Fatigue Syndrome

■ Depression

■ Diabetes

■ Headache

■ Heart Problems

■ High Blood Pressure

■ Indigestion

■ Irritable Bowel Syndrome

■ Menstrual Problems

■ Mononucleosis

■ Pain, Chronic

■ Premenstrual Syndrome

■ Sore Throat

■ Stress

See Common Ailments, beginning on page 194.

Yoga

*Y*oga is an ancient philosophy of life developed in India over the course of thousands of years. The word "yoga" is derived from the Sanskrit "yuj," which means union. Practitioners of yoga believe that by following its precepts, which include ethical principles, dietary restrictions, and physical exercise, they can unite—or bring into equilibrium—the mind, the body, and the spirit. According to yoga teaching, physical illness is a sign that these elements are out of balance.

There are many different forms of yoga. Hatha-yoga, widely practiced in the West, consists of a series of body positions and movements, known as asanas, and breathing exercises, called pranayama. Many Western practitioners also include relaxation and meditation in their daily yoga routine.

Origins

No one knows exactly when people in India began practicing yoga, but small stone carvings of figures in yogic postures, thought to be more than 5,000 years old, have been excavated in the Indus Valley. In the third century BC, the sage Patanjali wrote the Yoga Sutras, verses that describe eight steps to spiritual enlightenment. The postures and breathing techniques in the Yoga Sutras form the foundation of the modern practice of hatha-yoga.

What It's Good For

Yoga is thought to be a powerful health enhancer, helping the body become stronger and more resilient against disease and injuries. The postures stretch and strengthen muscles, massage internal organs, relax nerves, and increase blood circulation. Because yoga can work every muscle, nerve, and gland in the body, it is used to treat and prevent a wide array of conditions and illnesses.

■ **Athletic injuries.** Athletes from long-distance runners to professional football players use yoga stretches to keep the body agile and the muscles injury free.

■ **Back problems.** Because yoga postures flex, tone, and strengthen muscles, they are often prescribed for chronic back problems.

■ **Heart problems.** Studies have shown that performing yoga can

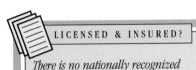

LICENSED & INSURED?

There is no nationally recognized standard for the certification of yoga instructors. Although some organizations grant certification, their requirements vary widely. Health insurance companies in several states offer discounts on yoga classes.

Yoga

help the heart work more efficiently. It can also aid in lowering blood pressure and cholesterol levels.

■ **Stress.** Regular yoga practice has been found to reduce feelings of anxiety, anger, fatigue, and depression.

Preparations/Techniques

Yoga can be performed with an instructor or alone. Experts recommend that you set aside at least half an hour each day, preferably in the morning or late evening, primarily because the postures should be done on an empty stomach. Choose a clean, warm area with a level floor. Wear loose clothing.

Begin with a few minutes of deep breathing to draw energy and oxygen into your body and help calm your mind. Follow with a few warmup exercises, then practice the postures you have chosen for that day's session *(see pages 184-193 for recommended postures)*. Go slowly and gently; no posture should cause extreme or increased pain. End each session with the Corpse pose *(page 186)* and five to 10 minutes of relaxation.

Visiting a Professional

To find an instructor, check the phone book to see if your community has a yoga center. Yoga classes are also offered in many health clubs, hospitals, and community centers. When choosing a yoga teacher for class or individual instruction, find one who practices yoga daily and who studies regularly with a teacher of his or her own. Your teacher should also be knowledgeable about major muscle groups and body systems and should tailor yoga techniques to your individual capability.

Wellness

Daily yoga practice offers a gentle and effective way of achieving good health and staying well. Practitioners believe that because yoga calms the mind as well as the body, it can prevent many chronic stress-related diseases and conditions.

What the Critics Say

Although acknowledging yoga's many beneficial effects, critics worry that people will injure themselves by jumping into yoga too enthusiastically and attempting advanced postures for which they have not adequately prepared their body. They are also concerned that people will use yoga instead of, rather than as a complement to, conventional medicine for serious conditions such as cancer and diabetes. Most yoga experts share these concerns and stress that beginners should start with easy postures and gradually work toward more difficult ones. They also advise people with preexisting conditions to check with their doctor before trying any postures. ■

CAUTION

Some of the more advanced, upside-down yoga postures, such as headstands, can be dangerous for people with high blood pressure or eye problems. Pregnant women should avoid postures that compress or strain the abdomen or back.

FOR MORE INFO

Following is a list of organizations you can contact to learn more about yoga:

The American Yoga Association
513 South Orange Avenue
Sarasota, FL 34236-7598
(800) 226-5859
e-mail: AmYogaAssn@aol.com

International Association of Yoga Therapists
20 Sunnyside Avenue
Suite A243
Mill Valley, CA 94941
(415) 868-1147
e-mail: IAYT@yoganet.com

Alternative Therapies

Gallery of Yoga Positions

Abdominal Massage

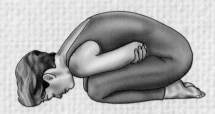

■ *Kneel upright and fold your arms, placing your left fist on the right side of your belly and your right hand over your left elbow. Bend at the hips and lower your forehead toward the floor. Raise your torso slowly, then switch arm positions and repeat.*

Boat

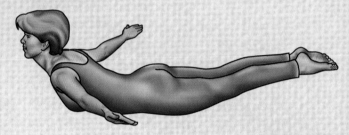

■ *Lie on your stomach with your arms at your sides and lift your head, chest, arms, and legs off the floor. Stretch and hold your arms behind you, then relax back onto the floor.*

Bow

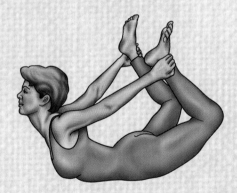

■ *Lie on your stomach and grasp both ankles. While inhaling, squeeze your buttocks and slowly raise your head, chest, and thighs off the floor, pressing your ankles outward. Exhale and breathe slowly, then release.*

Bridge

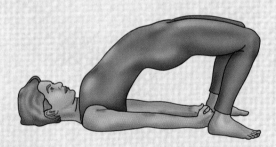

■ *Lie on your back, knees bent, palms on the floor. Tense your buttocks and slowly raise your pelvis. Clasp your hands, arching as you press your shoulders to the floor. Hold this position, then unclasp your hands and slowly lower your pelvis to the floor.*

C

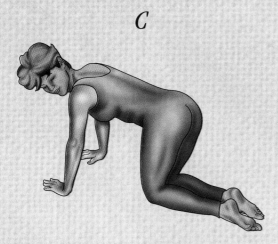

■ On your hands and knees, exhale and swing your head and buttocks as far to the left as you can. Inhale as you slowly straighten your back, and then do the same movement to the right.

Camel

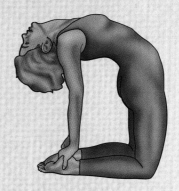

■ From an upright kneeling position, bend your head backward. Exhale and arch your back, placing your right hand on your right heel, your left hand on your left heel. Then slowly straighten up, breathing evenly. Relax, sit back on your heels, and lift your head.

Cat

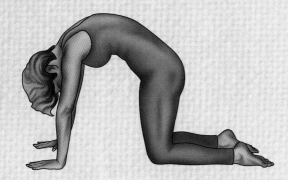

■ On your hands and knees, exhale as you arch your back, stretching your shoulder, neck, and back muscles. Inhale and bring your back to the horizontal.

Child

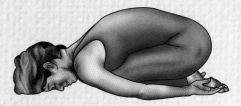

■ Sit on your heels, knees together. With your arms at your sides, palms up, bend from the hips and extend your upper body over your knees, bringing your forehead toward the floor. Then slowly sit up.

CONTINUED

Gallery of Yoga Positions

Cobra

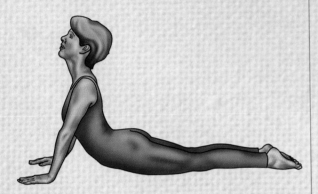

■ Place both forearms on the floor, elbows directly under your shoulders. Slowly straighten your arms and arch your back until your abdomen is off the ground. Relax and slowly uncurl, lowering your torso back to the floor.

Cobra (Half)

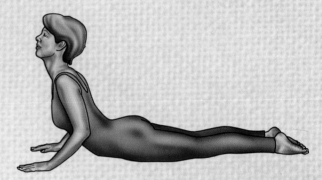

■ Begin as you would for the Cobra. Press your pelvis and palms against the floor to raise your chest. Keep your arms bent as you arch your back, stopping just before your navel comes off the floor. Lower your torso to release.

Corpse

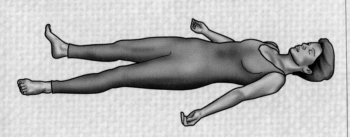

■ Lie on your back, with your feet about 18 inches apart and turned out slightly. Place your hands about 6 inches from your hips, palms up. Close your eyes and breathe deeply.

Dog

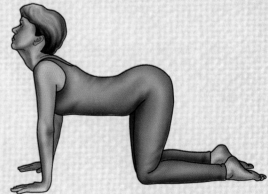

■ While on your hands and knees, inhale as you dip your back, bringing your head and buttocks up. Exhale as you return your back to the horizontal.

Gallery of Yoga Positions

Downward Dog

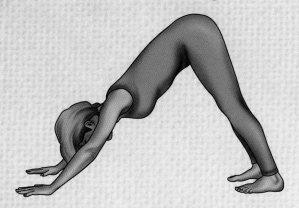

■ Get on your hands and knees. Inhale and raise your pelvis to form an inverted V, with knees slightly bent. Press your palms and heels against the floor as you breathe deeply. Hold for 20 to 30 seconds. Exhale as you return to the starting position.

Half-Moon

■ Inhale and clasp your hands over your head. Exhale and stretch to the left, pushing out your right hip. Breathe deeply, keeping your shoulders and hips in the same plane. Inhale and return to the center. Repeat on the right side.

Hand and Thumb Squeeze

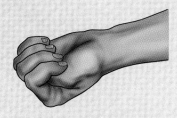

■ To loosen finger joints, curl your fingers into a fist around your thumb and gently squeeze. Then release slowly. Do this 10 times with each hand.

Head to Knee

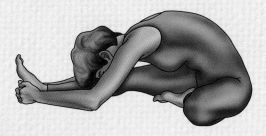

■ Sit with your right leg out, the sole of your left foot against your right thigh. Raise your arms overhead, then bend forward from the hips and clasp your right foot with both hands, pressing your forehead to your knee. Release and repeat on the other side.

CONTINUED

Gallery of Yoga Positions

Hero

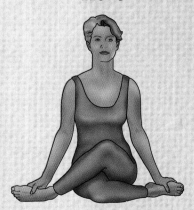

■ While on hands and knees, cross your left knee in front of your right knee. Keep your knees in place as you sit back between your heels. With your back straight, place your palms on the soles of your feet, then slowly release. Repeat on the other side.

Knee Down Twist

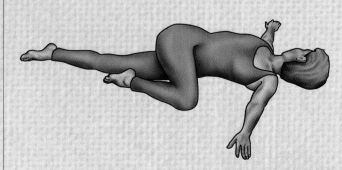

■ Lie on your back with your arms out. Inhale and place your right foot on your left knee. Exhale, then turn your head to the right and bring your right knee toward the floor to your left (above). Release slowly, then repeat on the other side.

Locust (Full)

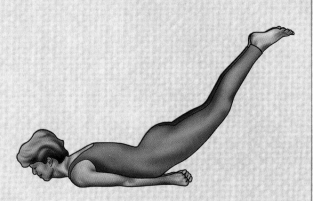

■ Lie on your stomach, arms under your body. Squeeze your buttocks as you press down with your arms. Raise your legs, keeping them straight as you press outward through the toes and heels. Slowly lower legs to release.

Locust (Half)

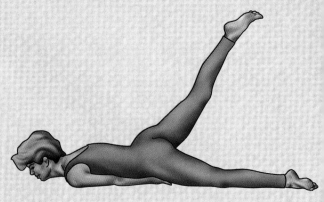

■ While on your stomach, put your arms under your body. Squeeze your buttocks as you press down with your arms. Raise your right leg, keeping it straight as you press outward through the toes and heel. Release slowly and do the same with the left leg.

Gallery of Yoga Positions

Lotus (Half)

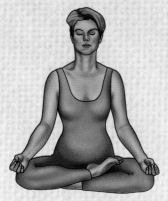

■ Sit with your legs in a V, spine straight. Bend one leg and bring the foot close to your body. Bend the other leg and place the foot high on the opposite thigh. Ideally, your knees should touch the floor. (For full Lotus, place each foot on the opposite thigh.)

Mountain

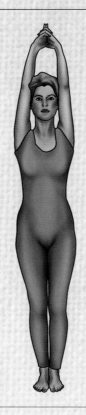

■ Stand with your feet together. Inhale and raise your arms straight out from your sides, then join them over your head. To release, exhale and slowly lower your arms.

Pigeon

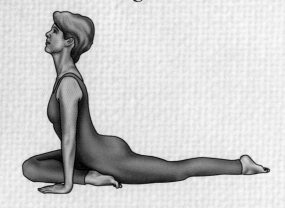

■ From a kneeling position, slide your left leg straight behind you and place your right knee between your hands. Inhale and stretch up through your torso while arching your back slightly. Release, then repeat on the other side.

Plow

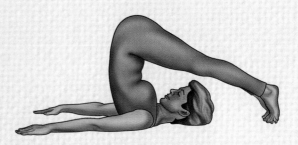

■ While on your back, inhale and raise both legs, using your hands to support your hips. Exhale as you try to touch the floor behind you with your toes. Stretch out your arms on the floor, then place your hands back on your hips and slowly lower your legs.

CONTINUED

Gallery of Yoga Positions

Posterior Stretch

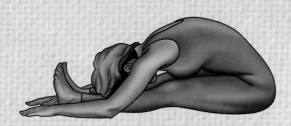

■ Sit with legs extended and feet together. Raise your arms overhead, then bend forward from the hips and place your hands on your ankles or on the floor beside your feet. Move your head as close to your toes as possible. Slowly raise your torso as you inhale.

Rag Doll

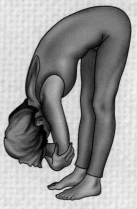

■ Standing with arms at your sides, exhale and bend forward from the hips, letting the top of your head drop toward the floor. Cup your elbows in your palms and breathe deeply. Slowly stand up, bringing your head up last.

Seated Angle

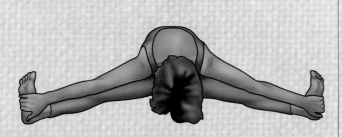

■ Sit with your legs in a V. Raise your arms over your head. Bending from the hips, extend your arms and grab your legs or feet. Move your head toward the floor. Release by lifting your arms back over your head, then slowly raise your torso.

Shoulder Crunch

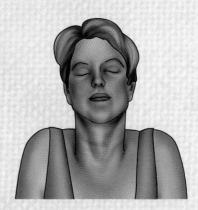

■ Straighten your back and relax your neck. Slowly lift your right shoulder, then lower it. Repeat with your left shoulder. Lift both shoulders together and slowly bring them down.

Shoulder Stand

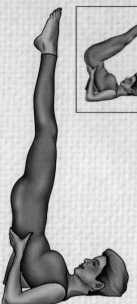

■ *Lie on your back, hands at your sides. Lift both legs until they are at a right angle to your back. Supporting your hips with hands, inhale and extend your legs at the angle shown (inset) for the Half Shoulder Stand. Extend back and legs vertically for the full position (left). Slowly lower legs to release.*

Sphinx

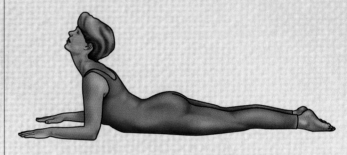

■ *Lie on your stomach and place both forearms on the floor, palms down and elbows directly under your shoulders. Push your chest away from the floor as far as comfortably possible and look upward slightly. Lower your torso to release.*

Spider

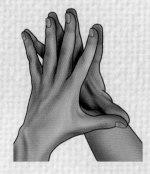
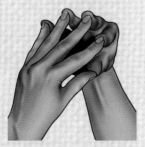

■ *Press your fingertips together firmly, holding your palms two to three inches apart. Then push your palms toward each other (above, left) and with your fingertips still together move them apart (above, right). Relax, then repeat the push-up motion.*

Spinal Twist

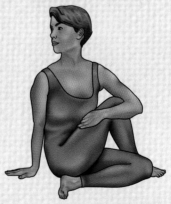

■ *While sitting, place your right foot outside of the left knee. Grasp your right knee with your left arm and place your right hand on the floor behind you. Inhale, then exhale as you twist your torso slowly as far as you can to the right. Repeat on the other side.*

CONTINUED

Gallery of Yoga Positions

Standing Angle

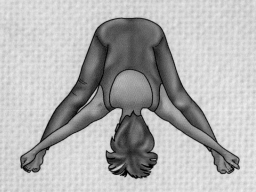

■ *Inhale and step wide to your right with arms out-stretched. Exhaling, bend forward at the hips and grasp your feet, moving the top of your head toward the floor. Rise slowly, keeping your back straight.*

Standing Yoga Mudra

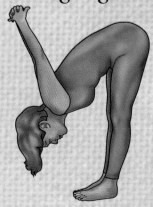

■ *Stand with your arms at your sides. Inhale, raise your arms in front of you, then exhale and sweep them behind your back, squeezing the shoulder blades. Inter-lace your fingers and bend forward as you lift your arms. Raise your torso and drop your arms to release.*

Tree

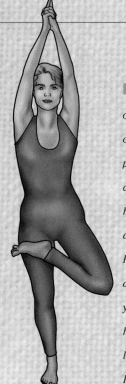

■ *Use your hands to lift one foot to the top of the opposite thigh. Place your palms together at heart level and raise your hands over-head; point the index fingers and interlace the others. Press your bent knee down and back without tilting your pelvis. Bring your hands back down to heart level and lower your leg. Repeat on the other side.*

Triangle

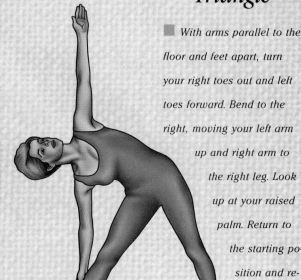

■ *With arms parallel to the floor and feet apart, turn your right toes out and left toes forward. Bend to the right, moving your left arm up and right arm to the right leg. Look up at your raised palm. Return to the starting po-sition and re-peat on the other side.*

Gallery of Yoga Positions

Upward Dog

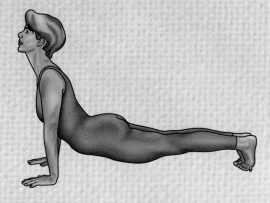

■ Lie facedown, palms at chest level and elbows close to the body. Spread your fingers, keeping the index fingers forward. Using your hands and toes, lift your torso, hips, and knees off the floor, arching your back slightly. Return to the starting position.

Warrior 1

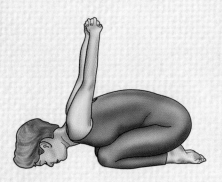

■ Raise your arms overhead, palms together. Lunge forward with your right foot, keeping the knee directly above the ankle. Press your left heel down and left hip forward. Arch your back slightly. Step forward and lower your arms to release. Repeat on the other side.

Warrior 2

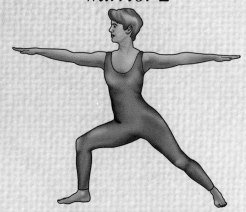

■ With arms parallel to the floor and feet apart, turn your right toes out and left toes forward. Bend your right knee and bring it above your right ankle, keeping your hips forward. Look over your right hand. Return to the starting position, then repeat on the opposite side.

Yoga Mudra

■ Sit on your heels, knees together, then follow the arm motion and stretch for Standing Yoga Mudra. Move your forehead to the floor and stretch your arms overhead. Breathe deeply, then exhale, bringing your arms back down. Inhale and slowly raise your torso.

Common Ailments

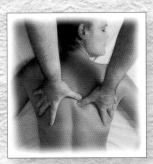

Alternative therapies are used with varying degrees of success to treat virtually every known medical condition. Depending on the type and severity of the disorder, the benefits range from complete cures to relief of symptoms such as pain, dizziness, and nausea. In many cases, alternative remedies are used alone or in combination with other techniques to complement or boost the effectiveness of conventional treatments. It is important to note, however, that while many ailments can be treated effectively with alternative therapies, some disorders require the care of a conventional medical doctor. Listed here are more than 80 ailments—some of them minor and merely annoying, others chronic and potentially life threatening—for which various forms of alternative medicine have proved to be beneficial in one way or another.

For the most part, the ailments in this section are listed individually by name in alphabetical order. In a few cases, however, similar or related disorders have been grouped under a single heading. "Athletic Injuries," for example, contains information about a number of common sports-related complaints, from ligament sprains and muscle strains to bone fractures and joint dislocations. Various skin disorders, including psoriasis, dermatitis, and skin cancer, are discussed in "Rashes and Skin Problems." Conditions that cause persistent discomfort in the back, joints, neck, and other areas of the body are covered in the entry labeled "Pain, Chronic." Information about heart disease, heart arrhythmias, pericardial disease, and other disorders affecting the body's blood pump can be found under "Heart Problems." If you have trouble locating an ailment entry, you should be able to find it easily in the index.

Each entry begins with a general overview of the ailment, briefly touching on such aspects as its cause or causes, how it affects the body, and the prospects for recovery. Following the introduction is a section entitled Treatment Options, which is a detailed list of alternative therapies that may be useful in caring for the condition; information on convention-al medical care is included as necessary. Here you'll find specific infor-mation and suggestions that will help you decide which alternative av-enue to pursue. (Bold italic type indicates a cross reference to the lists of herbs, homeopathic remedies, and other natural remedies in the Alterna-tive Therapies section of the book.) Techniques discussed under the heading Home Remedies are simple but effective ways you can treat the ailment yourself using materials you have around the house or can easily obtain. The section headed Prevention suggests steps you can take to lessen your chances of a recurrence of the condition or of developing it in the first place.

A permanent fixture at the beginning of each entry is the Symptoms box, a summary of the ailment's characteristic warning signs. Immediate-ly below it is the Call Your Doctor If box, which describes symptoms that are serious enough to warrant the attention of a physician or, in some cases, a trip to the emergency room. Important warnings about the dis-ease or its treatment appear in a Caution box, located in the bottom left corner of the opening page. Other boxes placed throughout the entry shed additional light on the ailment, separating fact from myth, explain-ing important new findings, or pointing out other matters of interest. Many entries also feature drawings that show affected areas of the body (sometimes revealing the ailment's damage-causing mechanism), or that give step-by-step instructions on how to perform certain therapeutic tech-niques, such as acupressure or yoga.

As it turns out, not every alternative therapy is appropriate for every individual. You'll find that some work better for you than others; or you may discover that a combination of techniques—say, herbal therapy and yoga—produces the most-effective results. The best way to learn which approach is best suited to you and your condition is to consult your healthcare practitioner. And never hesitate to consult a physician if circumstances warrant. ■

A

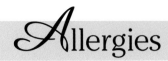

Allergies

Symptoms

- Sneezing, wheezing, nasal congestion, and coughing indicate asthma, or drug or respiratory allergies.

- Itchy eyes, mouth, and throat are symptoms of respiratory allergies.

- Stomachache, frequent indigestion, and heartburn are signs of food sensitivities.

- Irritated, itchy, reddening, or swelling skin is associated with drug, food, and insect-sting allergies.

- Stiffness, pain, and swelling of joints may indicate food or drug allergies.

- Fatigue or feeling run-down, difficulty concentrating, emotional upset or irritability, or difficulty sleeping may be associated with food allergies or seasonal allergies such as hay fever.

Call Your Doctor If

- you have violent stomach cramps, vomiting, bloating, or diarrhea; this could point to a serious food or other allergic reaction or food poisoning.

- breathing becomes extremely difficult or painful; you may be experiencing an asthma episode, another serious allergic reaction, or a heart attack. Get emergency medical treatment.

- you suddenly develop skin welts accompanied by intense flushing and itching; your heart may also be beating rapidly. These symptoms may indicate the onset of anaphylactic shock, an extremely serious allergic reaction *(box, opposite)*. Get emergency medical treatment. *(See also Shock in Essential First Aid, page 378.)*

T he term *"allergy"* applies to an abnormal reaction by your immune system to a substance that is usually safe. Allergies come in many forms and range from mildly bothersome to life threatening.

The immune system protects the body from foreign substances—known as antigens—by producing antibodies and other chemicals to fight them. Usually, the immune system ignores benign substances, such as food, and fights only dangerous ones, such as bacteria. A person develops an allergic reaction when the immune system cannot tell the good from the bad and releases a type of chemical called histamine to attack the harmless substance as if it were a threat. Histamine produces many of the symptoms associated with allergies. Allergens, or substances that may trigger allergic reactions, range from pollen to pet dander to penicillin.

Most allergic reactions are not serious, but some, such as anaphylaxis, can be fatal (see box, below, right). Only a few allergies can be cured outright, but the symptoms can be relieved. If your allergy is severe, it is vital that you visit a conventional medical doctor and get immediate treatment on an emergency basis.

Treatment Options

Since allergies can be hard to diagnose and are in many cases incurable, alternative remedies for them have become quite popular. But for severe allergies, or for emergencies, you must see a conventional physician. Blood tests can detect food allergies.

Aromatherapy
To relieve nasal congestion, try mixing 1 drop each of the oils of **lavender** (*Lavandula angustifolia*) and **niaouli** (*Melaleuca viridiflora*), and 1 tsp of a carrier oil such as sweet almond or sunflower; massage into the skin around your sinuses once a day. **Eucalyptus globulus** (*E. globulus*) and **peppermint** (*Mentha piperita*) oils also act as decongestants; dab on a handkerchief and inhale.

Chinese Medicine
Chinese herbalists use the mixture *Bi Yan Pian* for allergies with a runny nose, as well as a commercially prepared mixture of herbs, found in many natural food stores, called Hayfever. Acupuncture, too, may be helpful; consult a qualified practitioner.

*A*llergies

Herbal Therapies

Infusions of **chamomile** *(Matricaria recutita)*, elder *(Sambucus nigra)* flower, **eyebright** *(Euphrasia officinalis)*, **garlic** *(Allium sativum)*, goldenrod *(Solidago virgaurea)*, **nettle** *(Urtica dioica)*, and **yarrow** *(Achillea millefolium)* have antimucus and anti-inflammatory effects. Some herbs, such as nettles, may cause an allergic reaction; use with caution.

Ginger tea can help reduce sinus inflammation. Simmer 2 tsp chopped or grated **ginger** *(Zingiber officinale)* in 2 cups water for 20 minutes. Breathe in the steam for five to seven minutes; repeat several times each day, until your symptoms subside.

Homeopathy

For a runny nose, itchy throat, and sneezing, a practitioner might suggest **Arsenicum album** (12c) or *Sabadilla* (30c); for chronic thick mucus, **Pulsatilla** (12c); for a runny nose, sore upper lip, and itchy eyes, **Allium cepa** (12c); for hives, allergic swelling—including painful joints, or allergic reactions to bee stings—**Apis** (12c); for indigestion with stuffiness and runny nose, **Nux vomica** (30c).

Nutrition and Diet

Vitamin C and bioflavonoids (found in the white pith of citrus fruits) act as natural antihistamines, so you should increase your citrus intake or take 1,000 mg of vitamin C three times daily. **Vitamins A**

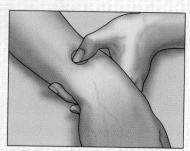

Acupressure

Triple Warmer 5 • *Use this point to help fortify the immune system. Center your thumb on the top of your forearm, two thumb widths from the wrist joint, and press firmly. Repeat on the other arm.*

and **B complex** appear to stimulate the immune system. Products made with bee pollen and royal jelly may alleviate or eliminate respiratory symptoms but should not be taken if you are allergic to bee stings. For food allergies, read labels carefully and make sure you know what foods to avoid.

Avoid all stimulants, such as caffeinated beverages and white sugar, and decaffeinated drinks; these substances can overstimulate the immune system, making allergies worse.

Prevention

Respiratory allergies: Install a high-efficiency air cleaner to help remove pollen and mold spores, and use an air conditioner in your home and car during warm seasons to keep pollen out; regularly clean damp areas with bleach to kill molds. Consider hiring a special cleaning service to rid furniture and upholstery of dust mites. Isolate (or, if you can stand it, get rid of) your pets and keep them outside as much as possible. Regular baths for your pet will help reduce dander.

Food allergies: Avoid foods that are highly allergenic, such as dairy products, wheat, corn, soybean, and citrus fruits. Instead of dairy products, try tofu-based foods. Always check food labels for additives that are known allergens, such as yellow food dye no. 5 and gum arabic. ∎

OF SPECIAL INTEREST

What Triggers Anaphylactic Shock?

The most dangerous of allergic reactions is anaphylaxis, or anaphylactic shock, which begins within minutes after exposure and advances quickly. Although any allergen can trigger anaphylactic shock, the most common are insect stings, foods such as shellfish and nuts, and injections of certain drugs. Standard emergency treatment includes an injection of epinephrine to open airways and blood vessels; in severe cases, cardiopulmonary resuscitation (CPR) may be needed (see Shock, page 378).

Anemia
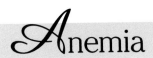

Symptoms

- Weakness, fatigue, and a general feeling of malaise; you may be mildly anemic.

- Your lips look bluish, your skin is pasty or yellowish, and your gums, nail beds, eyelid linings, or palm creases are pale; you are almost certainly anemic.

- In addition to feeling weak and tired, you are frequently out of breath, faint, or dizzy; you may have severe anemia.

- Your tongue burns; you may have vitamin B_{12} anemia.

- Your tongue feels unusually slick and you experience movement or balance problems, tingling in the extremities, confusion, depression, or memory loss; you may have pernicious anemia.

- Other possible symptoms: headache, insomnia, decreased appetite, poor concentration, and an irregular heartbeat.

Call Your Doctor If

- you have the symptoms of pernicious anemia; this disorder can damage the spinal cord.

- you have been taking iron supplements and experience symptoms such as vomiting, bloody diarrhea, fever, jaundice, lethargy, or seizures; you may be suffering from iron overload, which can be life threatening, especially in children.

A nemia, in which body tissues are deprived of oxygen, is caused by a reduction in the number of circulating red blood cells or by inadequate amounts of the essential protein hemoglobin. The severity can range from mild to life threatening. Anemia can occur if large amounts of blood are lost or if something interferes with the production of red blood cells or accelerates their destruction. Because hemoglobin is the main component of red blood cells and the carrier for oxygen molecules, anemia also occurs if the hemoglobin supply is insufficient or if the hemoglobin itself is dysfunctional.

More than 400 forms of anemia have been identified. The disorder may arise from a number of underlying conditions, some of which may be hereditary, but in many cases poor diet is to blame. Iron deficiency anemia, the leading form, occurs when the body does not store enough iron, the chief raw material of hemoglobin. The only way to know what kind of anemia you have is to ask your doctor to run tests on a sample of your blood.

Treatment Options

Some remedies treat anemia by promoting better circulation, others by increasing *iron* absorption, stimulating digestion, or adjusting the diet to include more iron- or vitamin-rich foods.

Herbal Therapies

In the history of folk medicine, bitter substances have always been thought to stimulate digestion and thereby promote the absorption of valuable nutrients. The bitter herb gentian *(Gentiana lutea)* is a popular remedy in Europe for a number of nutritionally based ailments, including anemia. Gentian can be brewed into a tea or ingested in the form of a commercially available alcoholic extract. **Dandelion** *(Taraxacum officinale)* is also thought to benefit people with anemia, simply because it is rich in vitamins and minerals. Other iron-rich herbs include **parsley** *(Petroselinum crispum)* and **nettle** *(Urtica dioica)*.

In traditional Chinese medicine, anemia is a condition known as deficient blood. Treatment might involve acupuncture and herbal therapies. Research suggests that **Asian ginseng** *(Panax ginseng)* is useful as a general tonic to counteract

Anemia

anemia-induced fatigue. **Dong quai** *(Angelica sinensis),* another Asian herb used medicinally for thousands of years, is a blood tonic. For anemic patients who have a gray cast, a Chinese herbalist might recommend a combination of dong quai and **Chinese foxglove root** *(Rehmannia glutinosa).* For patients with a stark white complexion, the remedy might be a mixture of ginseng and **astragalus** *(Astragalus membranaceus).* After diagnosing a person with anemia, a Chinese medicine practitioner might recommend the following herbal formulas: *Ba Zhen Wan* (Eight Treasure Pills) or *Shi Quan Da Bu Wan* (Ten Complete Great Tonifying Pills).

■ Homeopathy

Consult a professional homeopath for an evaluation that will determine which substances are most suitable for treating your type of anemia.

■ Nutrition and Diet

Adjusting your diet is the easiest, most healthful, and longest-lasting way to combat any anemia linked to nutritional deficiency. A vast array of foods can boost your iron count, including enriched breads and cereals, rice, potatoes, carrots, broccoli, tomatoes, dried beans, blackstrap molasses, lean red meat, liver, poultry, dried fruits, almonds, and shellfish. Research indicates that iron from animal sources is absorbed more readily than plant iron. Evidence also suggests that **vitamin C** and **copper** help the body absorb iron.

If you're low on **folic acid,** a key player in red blood cell production, step up your consumption of citrus fruits, mushrooms, dark green vegetables, liver, eggs, milk, and bulking agents like wheat germ and brewer's yeast. Also, pumpkin is an excellent source of folate, which is the **vitamin B complex** component of folic acid. Keep in mind that folic acid is destroyed by heat and light, so fruits and vegetables should be eaten fresh and cooked as little as possible.

Vegetarians are at risk for **vitamin B_{12}** anemia because this vitamin is found only in animal products and in some fermented foods. If you are a vegetarian, you need to include in your diet dairy products and eggs or fermented foods such as miso and tofu, or take a daily supplement of B_{12}.

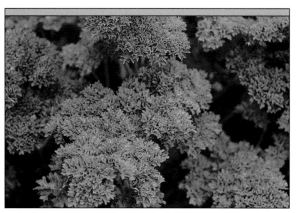

Parsley • *A versatile and nutritious herb, parsley is a good natural source of iron and thus can be useful in treating iron deficiency anemia. Parsley is also rich in vitamin C, which promotes iron absorption in the body.*

Home Remedies

- Keep track of the foods you eat and find out whether they are rich in iron, folic acid, or vitamin B_{12}. You might be surprised to learn that some of the foods you eat are preventing the absorption of needed nutrients.
- Don't drink caffeinated or decaffeinated tea, coffee, or cola with meals; caffeine inhibits iron absorption, as does the tannin in black tea. The acids in decaffeinated beverages can also be a problem. You should, however, drink citrus juices, because they are rich in vitamin C, which promotes iron absorption.
- Consider taking a daily multivitamin. Be sure to consult a doctor or nutritionist before taking iron supplements; excess amounts of iron in your system can be harmful.

Prevention

- Avoid excessive consumption of alcohol. Chronic drinking can undermine proper nutrition and interfere with the digestive system's ability to absorb folic acid, necessary for the production of red blood cells.
- Take a daily multivitamin to maintain a healthful balance of vitamins and minerals. ■

Angina
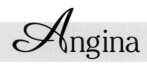

Symptoms

■ Pain that is crushing, constricting, strangling, suffocating, sharp, or burning; it is normally felt in the chest but may also occur in peripheral areas such as the arm, jaw, or abdomen. Location and specific sensations vary from person to person but are usually consistent from one attack to the next.

■ Chest pain that occurs with exertion and then recedes with rest.

■ Weakness, sweating, shortness of breath, anxiety, palpitations, nausea, or lightheadedness—symptoms that may or may not be associated with a heart attack.

Call Your Doctor If

■ an attack lasts more than 15 minutes; this may be a heart attack. Call 911 or your emergency number now.

■ you think this may be your first angina attack; find out for sure.

■ your attacks have become more intense, frequent, prolonged, and unpredictable; these are signs of unstable angina.

Acupressure

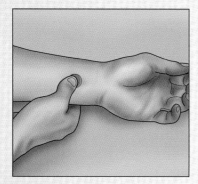

Pericardium 6 • *To help calm nerves and reduce feelings of uneasiness, press Pericardium 6. Place your thumb in the center of your inner wrist, two finger widths from the wrist crease and between the two bones of the forearm. Press firmly for one minute, three to five times; repeat on other arm.*

Angina is the heart's way of saying it is not getting enough oxygen, usually because coronary arteries—those that supply blood to the heart—are blocked or narrowed. Angina is often confused with indigestion because the tight, burning sensations are similar. It can also be misinterpreted as a heart attack; the pain may be similar but does not last as long—usually no more than five minutes.

Of the many types of angina, stable (or classical) angina—triggered by exertion and receding with rest—is the most common. Another type, unstable angina, occurs unpredictably, even during rest, and should be interpreted as a warning sign of serious heart trouble.

Treatment Options

Always consult a doctor if you think you have angina. The therapies below may help relieve symptoms or prevent attacks, but they should be considered as complements to—rather than substitutes for—conventional medical care.

■ Ayurvedic Medicine
An Ayurvedic mixture of herbs and minerals known as *Abana* has been shown to reduce the frequency and severity of angina attacks. *Abana* comes in tablet form, and the initial dosage for adults is typically two tablets two or three times daily, then one tablet two or three times daily for maintenance. Consult a practitioner for the specific dosage.

■ Chelation Therapy
Although controversial, chelation therapy, which involves injecting the chemical EDTA into the bloodstream, has been sought by many angina sufferers. Advocates claim that it is safer and cheaper than many conventional treatments—and just as effective. Critics insist that it undergo more rigorous scientific scrutiny before joining the ranks of standard treatment for clogged arteries. If you decide to try this therapy, seek a practitioner certified by one of the major American chelation societies.

■ Exercise
Gentle aerobic exercise is very beneficial for angina patients. Build stamina gradually, and exercise inside during cold weather.

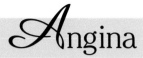ngina

■ Herbal Therapy

Hawthorn *(Crataegus laevigata)* is an excellent long-term tonic for angina because it simultaneously dilates coronary arteries and calms the heart. It is often an ingredient in herbal treatments that a traditional Chinese medicine practitioner or a naturopathic doctor might prescribe for angina.

■ Homeopathy

For immediate relief during an acute attack, *Cactus grandiflorus* (30c) is recommended. Cactus may bring relief if during an attack your chest feels like it's bound with an iron band. *Latrodectus mactans* is prescribed for difficult breathing with pain radiating down the left arm. *Naja tripudians* is used for anxiety and coldness with pains radiating up into the neck or shoulder. Among the long-term remedies that might be prescribed are **Nux vomica** and **Arsenicum album.**

■ Mind/Body Medicine

If you have trouble controlling your emotions or stress levels, you must learn to relax. Many types of relaxation techniques—from biofeedback to yoga—can help. Choose a method you like and stick with it; the effectiveness of relaxation techniques varies from person to person and improves with time.

■ Nutrition and Diet

The principal goals of nutritional therapy for angina are to improve blood flow to the heart and to boost the energy metabolism of the heart so that it requires less oxygen. The main way to improve blood flow is to control atherosclerosis, and consuming less saturated fat and cholesterol is a critical first step. To improve energy metabolism, be sure to get enough **magnesium** in your diet or as part of a multivitamin supplement.

Home Remedies

- Certain air pollutants, particularly carbon monoxide, are known to aggravate angina. To avoid carbon monoxide, steer clear of tobacco smoke and stay inside on heavy smog days.
- Avoid alcohol or drink only sparingly while on angina medication because of possible adverse reactions.
- Spend at least an hour digesting meals; exertion after eating can cause angina attacks.
- An aspirin every other day, with your doctor's permission, can reduce the risk of heart attack associated with angina.
- Do not take birth-control pills if you have angina: Estrogens are associated with increased risk of blood clots.

Prevention

- Adopt a low-fat, low-cholesterol diet that will help keep arteries free of fatty deposits.
- Exercise! People who exercise are less likely to develop atherosclerosis.
- If you smoke, quit. ■

Areas of Anginal Pain

Anginal pain can be distributed throughout the upper body in any of the following areas (shown below, left), including the center and left part of the chest, the neck, and inside the left arm (purple). Pain may also develop in the jaw (green), right chest and arm (pink), and between the navel and breastbone (yellow); the shoulders may be affected as well. In some cases, pain occurs between the shoulder blades (purple area below).

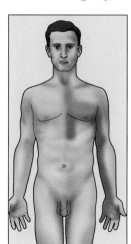

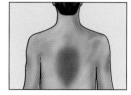

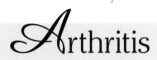rthritis

Symptoms

- Pain and progressive stiffness without noticeable swelling, chills, or fever during normal activities probably indicate the gradual onset of osteoarthritis.

- Painful swelling, inflammation, and stiffness in the arms, legs, wrists, or fingers in the same joints on both sides of the body, especially on awakening, may be signs of rheumatoid arthritis.

- Fever, joint inflammation, tenderness, and sharp pain, sometimes accompanied by chills and associated with an injury or another illness, may indicate infectious arthritis.

- In children, intermittent fever, loss of appetite, weight loss, anemia, or blotchy rash on the arms and legs may signal juvenile rheumatoid arthritis.

Call Your Doctor If

- the pain and stiffness come on quickly, whether from an injury or an unknown cause; you may be experiencing the onset of rheumatoid arthritis.

- the pain is accompanied by fever; you may have infectious arthritis.

- you notice pain and stiffness in your arms, legs, or back after sitting for short periods or after a night's sleep; you may be developing osteoarthritis or another arthritic condition.

- a child develops pain or a rash on armpits, knees, wrists, and ankles, or has fever swings, poor appetite, and weight loss; the child may have juvenile rheumatoid arthritis.

*A*lthough the term is applied to a wide variety of disorders, arthritis strictly means the inflammation of a joint, whether as the result of a disease, an infection, a genetic defect, or some other cause.

Major Types of Arthritis

Rheumatoid arthritis, also called rheumatism or synovitis, tends to affect people over the age of 40 and women two to three times as frequently as men. It is characterized by inflammation and pain in the hands—especially the knuckles and second joints—as well as in the arms, legs, and feet, and by general fatigue and sleeplessness. It can also cause systemic damage to other parts of the body, including the heart, lungs, eyes, nerves, and muscles. Rheumatoid arthritis in older people may eventually cause the hands and feet to become gnarled and misshapen as muscles weaken, tendons shrink, and the ends of bones become abnormally enlarged.

Juvenile rheumatoid arthritis, or Still's disease, is characterized by chronic fever and anemia. It can also affect the heart, lungs, eyes, and nervous system. Arthritic episodes in children younger than five can last for several weeks and may recur, although the symptoms tend to be less severe in recurrent attacks. Most affected children recover from the disease fully with no ill effects.

Infectious arthritis refers to various ailments that affect larger arm and leg joints as well as the fingers or toes. Arthritic infection is usually a complication of an injury or of another disease and is much less common than arthritic conditions that come on with age.

Osteoarthritis, or degenerative joint disease, refers to the pain and inflammation that can result from the systematic loss of bone tissue in the joints. It is the most common form of arthritis, particularly in the elderly. In osteoarthritis, the protective cartilage at the ends of bones in joints—especially in the spine and legs—gradually wears away. The inner bone surfaces become exposed and rub together. In some cases, bony spurs develop on the edges of joints, causing damage to muscles and nerves, pain, deformity, and difficulty in movement.

Although the mechanism of osteoarthritis is unknown, some people appear to have a genetic

Arthritis

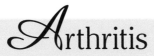

predisposition to degenerative bone disorders. In rare cases, congenital bone deformation appears at an early age. Misuse of anabolic steroids, which are popular among some athletes, can also bring on early osteoarthritic degeneration.

In many people the onset of osteoarthritis is gradual and is not seriously debilitating, although it can change the shape and size of bones. In other people, bony growths and gnarled joints may cause painful muscle inflammation or nerve damage, along with changes in posture and mobility.

Treatment Options

Sometimes arthritic damage can be slowed or stopped, but in most cases the damage continues as the disease runs its course, regardless of the use of drugs or other therapies. Because medical science has not found any full cures for the various kinds of arthritis, many people turn to alternative treatments to ease their pain and disability. While the effectiveness of few alternative approaches can be substantiated, research indicates that some of these methods, such as meditation, self-hypnosis, guided imagery, and relaxation techniques, can play a significant role in treating arthritic ailments.

■ **Acupressure and Acupuncture**
Some arthritis patients find that these therapies, administered by a trained practitioner, offer effective relief from the pain of rheumatoid arthritis or osteoarthritis for several weeks or months.

Joint Degeneration

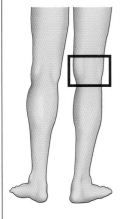

In a healthy joint, *a tough, rubbery tissue called cartilage cushions the ends of the bones at contact points. A thin membrane called the synovium lines the entire joint cavity and secretes synovial fluid to lubricate the joint.*

In rheumatoid arthritis, *the synovial membrane becomes thickened and inflamed. The inflammation causes cartilage to break down at the pivot point of the joint, while excess synovial fluid causes the cavity to swell.*

Osteoarthritis—*also called wear-and-tear arthritis—results from gradual deterioration of cartilage in the joint after years of use. Without the protective cartilage, the bones begin to rub together, creating friction and pain.*

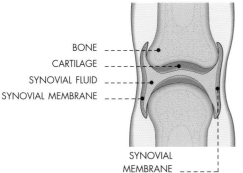

BONE
CARTILAGE
SYNOVIAL FLUID
SYNOVIAL MEMBRANE

SYNOVIAL MEMBRANE

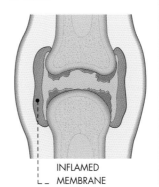

INFLAMED MEMBRANE

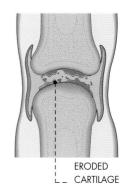

ERODED CARTILAGE

CONTINUED

*A*rthritis

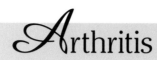

Bodywork

Soft-tissue massage around affected joints or compassionate touching can have a comforting effect on those who suffer from arthritis. Manipulation by a therapist constitutes passive exercise for people unable to perform vigorous exercise. Besides making a patient feel better physically, sympathetically administered touch therapy can help soothe the emotional effects of chronic illness. Further, studies suggest that relieving stress and tension has a positive influence on the body's hormonal balance.

Chiropractic

A chiropractor may manipulate the spine and other arthritic joints very carefully to relieve pain and help reestablish normal use. A program for arthritis may also include exercise, physiotherapy, and nutritional interventions.

Yoga

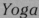

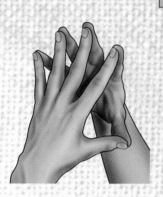

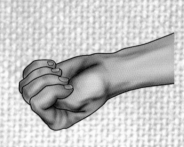

Spider • *To loosen the joints of the hand, use this exercise. Press your fingertips together firmly, palms two to three inches apart. Push your palms toward each other while keeping your fingertips touching. Do this 20 times.*

Hand and Thumb Squeeze • *Use this exercise to ease stiff finger joints. Curl your fingers into a fist around your thumb. Gently squeeze, then slowly release. Do this 10 times with each hand.*

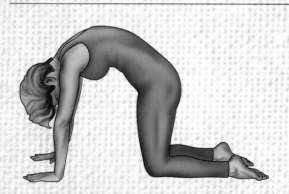

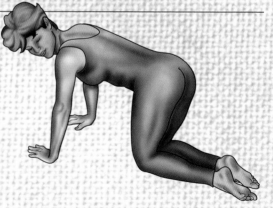

Dog and Cat • *These exercises help stretch your hips and back. On your hands and knees in the Table position, inhale as you lower your back and lift your head and buttocks (Dog). Then exhale as you arch your back and drop your head and buttocks (Cat). Repeat nine times.*

C • *Do this exercise on your hands and knees. Exhale and swing your head and buttocks as far to the left as you can. Breathe deeply as you hold this position for 10 seconds; exhale as you slowly straighten your back. Repeat to the right. Do this 10 times.*

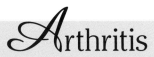Arthritis

Flower Remedy

To help relieve inflammation, apply **Rescue Remedy** cream, a Bach flower remedy, to the inflamed or painful area three to four times a day.

Herbal Therapies

Among the various remedies herbalists recommend to relieve pain is a 5-ml tincture made from 2 parts willow *(Salix* spp.) bark and 1 part each of **black cohosh** *(Cimicifuga racemosa)* and **nettle** *(Urtica dioica),* taken three times a day. To relieve muscle tension, rub a tincture of **lobelia** *(Lobelia inflata)* and cramp bark *(Viburnum opulus)* on the affected area. The Chinese herbal formula *Du Huo Ji Sheng Wan* is useful for some types of arthritis.

Homeopathy

For chronic osteoarthritis and rheumatoid arthritis, constitutional remedies may be prescribed after consultation with a trained homeopathic practitioner. Homeopathic remedies to relieve immediate pain and joint stiffness may include **Rhus toxicodendron** or **Bryonia.**

Hydrotherapy

Swimming or other water exercise, preferably in a heated pool, can improve joint movement and muscle strength; the water helps support the body and reduce the stress of gravity.

Massage

Massage can soothe pain, relax stiff muscles, and reduce the swelling that accompanies arthritis. Massage and gentle stretching help maintain a joint's range of motion.

Nutrition and Diet

Avoiding specific foods can stop arthritic symptoms associated with allergies, especially allergies to grains, nuts, meats, eggs, and dairy products. Use trial and error, preferably under the supervision of an allergist.

Avoid caffeinated and decaffeinated beverages and sugary foods, which tighten the tendons and cause blood vessels to constrict; this increases pain and decreases flexibility.

Some practitioners recommend cutting out plants in the nightshade family: tomato, potato, eggplant, and pepper. They believe the alkaloids in these foods inhibit formation of the collagen that makes up cartilage. Be patient—it may take up to six months before you see an improvement. Once you determine that these foods do affect you, eat them only occasionally. If your symptoms don't improve after six months, then nightshades aren't a factor in your arthritis.

Low-fat, low-protein vegetarian diets may ease the discomfort of rheumatoid arthritis. Good results are reported from eliminating partially hydrogenated fats and polyunsaturated vegetable oils and supplementing the diet with flax oil, sardines, and other oily fish as a source of omega-3 fatty acids.

Vitamin therapy may relieve certain arthritic symptoms. Beta carotene **(vitamin A)** has an antioxidant effect on cells, neutralizing destructive molecules called free radicals. **Vitamins C, B_6,** and **E,** as well as **zinc,** are thought to enhance collagen production and the repair of connective tissue. Vitamin C may also be advised for people taking aspirin, which depletes the body's vitamin C balance. **Niacin** (vitamin B_3) may also be helpful, although excessive use may aggravate liver problems. Always take vitamin supplements under professional guidance, since overdoses of some vitamin compounds can have side effects or undesirable interactions with drugs.

Some therapists recommend cherries or dark red berries to stimulate the production of collagen, essential to cartilage repair. The nutritional supplement glucosamine sulfate may also help.

Home Remedies

Heat and rest—traditional remedies for arthritic pain—are very effective in the short term for most people. Weight control is important, especially when arthritis strikes the lower back and legs.

If arthritic pain comes on unexpectedly, supplement an over-the-counter painkiller with dry heat from a heating pad or moist heat in the form of a hot bath or a hot-water bottle wrapped in a towel. However, do not use heat if you have infectious arthritis. For all types of arthritis, regular exercise is important to keep the joints mobile. ∎

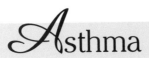 Asthma

Symptoms

- Restlessness or insomnia.

- Increasing, but relatively painless, tightness in chest.

- Mild to moderate shortness of breath.

- When breathing, a wheezing or whistling sound that can range from faint to clearly audible.

- Coughing, sometimes accompanied by phlegm.

Call Your Doctor If

- you or another person is experiencing an episode of asthma for the first time; asthma is a chronic condition and can be quite serious if not treated properly.

- the prescribed asthma medicine does not work in the time it is supposed to; you need a new prescription, or you may be suffering from a severe episode.

- you or the person with asthma has a suffocating feeling, making it difficult to talk; nostrils flare, the skin between the ribs appears sucked in, and the lips or the skin under the nails looks grayish or bluish. These are all signs of extreme oxygen deprivation. Get immediate emergency treatment.

Yoga

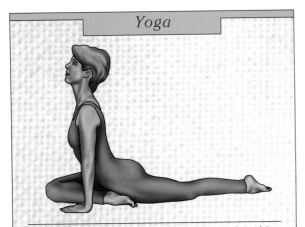

Pigeon • *This yoga position may enhance breathing. From a kneeling position, slide your left leg straight behind you and place your right knee between your hands. Inhale and stretch up through your torso while arching your back slightly. Hold for 20 or 30 seconds, breathing deeply. Repeat with the other leg.*

*A*sthma is a chronic respiratory disease that, like bronchitis and emphysema, causes a tightening of the chest and difficulty in breathing. In the case of asthma, however, these symptoms are not always present. They come in episodes set off by various environmental or emotional triggers, such as pollen, animal dander, tobacco smoke, and stress. Episodes can be brought on by a variety of factors working alone or in combination. Allergies are the primary offenders. Some people with asthma experience only mild and infrequent attacks; for them the condition is an occasional inconvenience. For others, episodes can be frequent and serious, requiring emergency medical treatment. If you have asthma, you should seek the help of a doctor before trying alternative therapies.

Treatment Options

Many people have reported success with alternative asthma treatments, but even advocates recommend these methods only as complements to conventional therapies. Once diagnosed, asthma should be monitored by a physician; serious episodes require conventional medical attention.

Acupuncture
Medical studies suggest that acupuncture may help alleviate asthma symptoms. The procedure should be carried out only by a licensed acupuncturist.

Aromatherapy
Essential oils such as **eucalyptus globulus** (*E. globulus*), aniseed (*Pimpinella anisum*), **lavender** (*Lavandula angustifolia*), pine (*Pinus sylvestris*), and **rosemary** (*Rosmarinus officinalis*) may help ease breathing and relieve nasal congestion. Inhaled through the nose, a few drops of one of the oils or a mixture of several dabbed on a handkerchief or tissue can help ease breathing during a mild episode of asthma. If you feel congested at other times (not during an episode), mix a few drops of essential oil in a sink full of hot water, cover your head with a towel, and inhale the fragrant steam through your nose. Use caution with essential oils if you have not used them before; in some circumstances they can precipitate an attack. Try applying them topically first before inhaling.

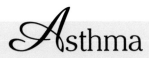 Asthma

■ Herbal Therapies

Elecampane *(Inula helenium),* a root that acts as a soothing expectorant, may help clear the body of excess mucus. To prepare an infusion, shred the root to yield 1 tsp and add a full cup of cold water; let the infusion stand for 10 hours, then strain and drink it hot three times daily. An infusion made from **mullein** *(Verbascum thapsus)* is recommended for soothing the mucous membranes, especially during nighttime episodes.

One formula recommended by practitioners of Chinese medicine is cinnamon twig decoction. Mix 9 grams cinnamon *(Cinnamomum cassia)* twigs, 9 grams white peony root, 9 grams **ginger** *(Zingiber officinale),* 6 grams Chinese licorice *(Glycyrrhiza uralensis),* and 12 pieces Chinese dates; steep the mixture in cold water, then bring to a boil. Drink it hot.

■ Homeopathy

A number of homeopathic remedies are available for treating asthma symptoms. Following are just a few: To help calm restlessness and anxiety, take **Arsenicum album** (30c) as required. For symptoms that worsen at night or during cold weather, or that come on very suddenly, take **Aconite** (6c) as required. For symptoms exacerbated by dampness, take *Natrum sulphuricum* (6c) as required. For more remedies, consult a licensed homeopathic or naturopathic physician.

■ Reflexology

Working the reflexology areas corresponding to the lungs, chest, diaphragm, and adrenals may help relieve an attack. See the diagram on page 169 for information on the location of these areas.

■ Yoga

Yoga can help you learn to breathe deeply and to relax, thereby helping you deal more effectively with stress, a common trigger for asthma.

Prevention

- Learn to identify your triggers: Keep a diary detailing all the environmental and emotional factors that affect you every day over the course of several months. When you have an

Asthmatic Airways

Air travels down the trachea and into the lungs through branching tubes called bronchioles, which normally are lined with a thin mucous membrane. For people with asthma, certain conditions or inhaled substances can act as triggers, prompting the release of chemicals that cause the bronchioles to constrict and produce excess mucus. The clogged airways trap air and make breathing difficult.

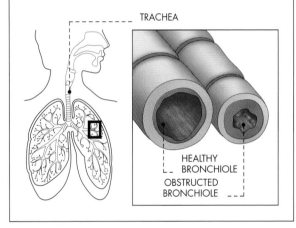

TRACHEA

HEALTHY BRONCHIOLE
OBSTRUCTED BRONCHIOLE

asthma attack, go back to your diary to see which factor, or combination of factors, might have contributed to it.

- Avoid foods and drinks that have high concentrations of sulfites, such as beer, wine, wine vinegar, instant tea, grape juice, lemon juice, grapes, fresh shrimp, pizza dough, dried fruits (such as apricots and apples), canned vegetables, instant potatoes, corn syrup, fruit topping, molasses, and foods found in salad bars. Some nutritionists recommend that you also steer clear of foods that cause excess mucus production, such as milk.

- A daily dose of **B-complex vitamins** (50 to 100 mg) and **magnesium** (400 to 600 mg) may help reduce the frequency and severity of asthma episodes. ■

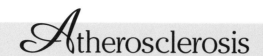

Atherosclerosis

Symptoms

In its early stages, atherosclerosis has no obvious symptoms. Damaged or partially blocked blood vessels may cause one or more of the following:

■ Dull, crampy pain in your buttock, thigh, and calf muscles during exertion. This may be a sign of atherosclerosis in the pelvic region or leg.

■ Sudden onset of localized paralysis, tingling, or numbness in a limb; partial vision or speech loss. These symptoms may indicate cerebral atherosclerosis, which can lead to stroke.

■ Angina, a feeling of tightness or heavy pressure in the chest. This may signal atherosclerosis in the coronary arteries.

Call Your Doctor If

■ you experience angina pain for the first time, or angina attacks progress from predictable to unstable. Either event is a serious condition that needs immediate medical attention.

■ you have discolored or ulcerated skin on your legs and sudden sharp pains in the legs or feet when you are at rest. This may indicate severe atherosclerosis and possibly a circulatory blockage that requires treatment by a doctor to prevent gangrene.

■ you notice unexplained loss of balance, coordination, speech, or vision. Any such loss indicates a temporary halt in the flow of blood to the brain, a situation that can result in stroke if left unattended. See your doctor right away.

A therosclerosis is an inflammatory disease that results in scarring of the artery walls, primarily from long-term buildup of fatty deposits and calcifications. Atherosclerosis is one of the most common cardiovascular diseases. Depending on the location and degree of arterial damage, atherosclerosis can lead to kidney problems, high blood pressure, stroke, and other life-threatening conditions. The disease tends to target the aorta—the body's largest artery, which leads from the heart—and arteries leading to the brain, lower limbs, and kidneys. Blockage occurring in the coronary arteries is called coronary heart disease; complications include angina, arrhythmia, and heart attack.

Treatment Options

Since diet and lifestyle are significant factors in both the development and the prevention of atherosclerosis, alternative therapies offer a range of choices to keep the ailment at bay.

■ Ayurvedic Medicine
Ayurvedic therapy combines diet, herbal remedies, relaxation, and exercise. Consult a specialist for a comprehensive program of treatment.

■ Herbal Therapies
Herbal remedies to combat atherosclerosis are typically intended to reduce existing plaques (calcified deposits) or to improve blood vessel integrity so plaques are less likely to form. **Hawthorn** *(Crataegus laevigata)* is considered one of the best plaque fighters because of its reputation for strengthening arteries. Its flowers, leaves, and berries can be brewed as tea, and it is also available in extract and tincture form.

A number of Chinese herbs are recommended for atherosclerosis, including the commonly used herb **notoginseng** *(Panax notoginseng)* **root;** the Chinese name is *tien chi.* Consult a practitioner of Chinese medicine for exact mixtures and dosages.

■ Homeopathy
Various long-term remedies may be prescribed by a licensed homeopath for treating atherosclerosis. Diagnosis and prescriptions will vary according to the practitioner's evaluation of the patient.

$\mathcal{A}$therosclerosis

Mind/Body Medicine

Since stress is believed to accelerate the rate at which atherosclerosis develops, therapeutic relaxation techniques may help prevent or retard its progress. A number of approaches can help you relax, including yoga, meditation, guided imagery, and biofeedback.

Nutrition and Diet

Diet and lifestyle changes, if started early and maintained aggressively, may be enough to prevent or even reverse atherosclerosis. First, your diet should be not only low in cholesterol and saturated fat but high in antioxidants, which neutralize free radicals believed to aggravate tissue damage. The key antioxidants are *vitamins E* and *C,* and *selenium,* which can be toxic in high dosages. Be careful about taking any vitamin indiscriminately, however: Too much *vitamin D,* for example, may actually accelerate calcification of arterial plaques. To be safe, seek advice from a doctor or nutritionist.

Some evidence suggests that garlic *(Allium sativum),* eaten in large quantities, deters oxidation of cholesterol. Grape-skin extracts and gugulipid *(Commiphora mukul),* an herb from southern India, are reputed to reduce plaque deposits. Alfalfa *(Medicago sativa)* and bromelain, a pineapple enzyme, are also reported to have reduced plaque

buildup in animals, and they may work on humans.

Numerous studies over the past 30 years have indicated that moderate alcohol consumption—a glass or two of wine a day—may protect against atherosclerosis and coronary artery disease. Red wine is thought to be particularly beneficial. One study suggests that flavonoids in grape skins, which give red wine its color and flavor, inhibit buildup of fatty deposits.

Prevention

Atherosclerosis develops when genetic predispositions meet known risk factors head-on. If you have a family history of atherosclerosis, the prudent course of action is to accept what you cannot change and change what you can.

- Adopt a low-fat, high-fiber diet. Take extra pains to avoid foods high in saturated fat and cholesterol.
- If you smoke, quit.
- If your blood pressure is high, get it down. *(See High Blood Pressure.)*
- Get moderate exercise—a 30-minute walk, swim, or bicycle ride—several times a week, and daily if possible.
- Find a relaxation program that you enjoy and incorporate it into your daily routine. ∎

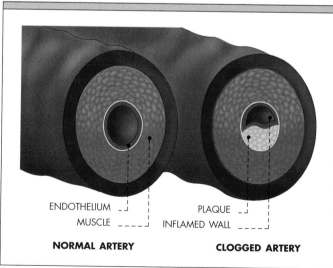

ENDOTHELIUM
MUSCLE

PLAQUE
INFLAMED WALL

NORMAL ARTERY　　　**CLOGGED ARTERY**

Blockage in the Arteries

Inside a normal artery, a layer of muscle surrounds the endothelium, the smooth inner lining through which blood flows (far left). In some people the endothelium can develop streaks or bumps of fat deposits. Over time, continued accumulation of fatty deposits results in inflammation of the artery wall. Eventually, a hard, calcified plaque can develop that may obstruct blood flow (left).

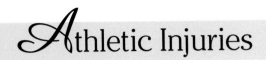thletic Injuries

Symptoms

- Pain, discomfort, restricted movement, tenderness, and possible swelling may be indicative of some form of muscle or ligament injury, such as a sprain or strain.

- Pain, swelling, tenderness, and deformity may indicate a fracture.

- Pain, restricted movement, misshapen appearance, and swelling in a joint are symptoms of a dislocation.

- Localized pain just below the kneecap may be a sign of patellar tendinitis. In adolescents, the condition may indicate Osgood-Schlatter disease if accompanied by swelling.

- Pain in the elbow, often accompanied by tenderness in the inner or outer portion of the elbow and forearm, and possibly a weak and painful grasp, may be an indication of epicondylitis.

Call Your Doctor If

- your muscles gradually become weak for no apparent reason; you may have a neurological problem or another disorder of immediate concern.

- you experience chronic muscle cramps. Although most often benign, this may be a sign of serious problems such as blood clotting, restricted blood flow, or nerve damage.

- you think your swelling or puffiness is caused by a fracture, dislocation, ligament or muscle tear, or cartilage damage. If not treated by a physician in a timely manner, the affected area could suffer permanent damage.

*E*very family has seen its share of injuries tracing to athletic endeavors or, ironically, the pursuit of physical fitness. For the most part, athletic injuries are a result of stress put on bones or muscles. Most common are injuries to soft tissue—muscles, tendons, and ligaments.

A dislocation occurs when two bones are jolted apart at a joint and is often accompanied by a ligament tear in the joint. The pain is caused by the severe stretching of soft tissues.

A fracture is either simple (closed)—in which the broken bone remains beneath the skin surface and does minimal damage to surrounding tissues—or compound (open), in which the bone protrudes through the skin. The ankle, hand, wrist, and collarbone are common sites of fracture.

INJURIES TO THE UPPER BODY

Shoulder injuries are common in sports that require throwing motions or intense contact. Dislocations are most common in the shoulder joint. Acromioclavicular joint (AC) separation occurs when the ligaments that support the collarbone are torn as a result of sudden impact on the side of the shoulder or on an outstretched arm. The rotator cuff is where four muscles meet and attach to the humerus; overuse of the shoulder, perhaps as a result of sports that require overhead motion like that in a tennis serve, may inflame or tear tendons in the area, causing rotator cuff tendinitis.

Epicondylitis affects the elbow and typically occurs in sports requiring frequent wrist manipulation and forearm rotation. The lateral (affecting the outer elbow) form is tennis elbow. Medial epicondylitis, caused by repetitive arm motion, as in pitching a baseball, involves the inner elbow.

The sudden tearing of muscle fibers that may occur after excessive athletic activity and the consequent accumulation of fluid in the muscle that causes pain, tenderness, and local swelling characterize a charley horse.

INJURIES TO THE LOWER BODY

Lower back injuries, such as muscle tears, are common in sports that involve a lot of bending. The

Athletic Injuries

high velocity and full-contact nature of hockey and football frequently cause neck and spine injuries, such as a herniated disk, in which an intervertebral disk protrudes from the spinal column.

Intense leg movement, including twisting and spreading, may tear the adductor muscle, causing groin strain. This muscle connects the leg with the pubic bone.

The knees are involved in some of the most common lower body injuries. Continual jumping may result in tearing of the tendon just below the kneecap (patella), causing patellar tendinitis, or jumper's knee. The knees may also suffer from other injuries, such as tears of the meniscus, a piece of cartilage in the knee joint between the femur and tibia.

Increased interest in jogging and cross training has resulted in a parallel rise in leg injuries, including shin splints, tendinitis, and stress fractures, especially in the tibia or fibula bones. If continually exposed to stress from prolonged standing, running, or walking, a stress fracture may result in a larger fracture.

The foot often falls victim to injury because it must support the weight of the entire body. Plantar fasciitis often affects inexperienced runners, caus-

---

Common Sports Injuries

The highlighted areas below show some of the sites of common injuries sustained from sports or other physical activity. The best way to prevent an athletic injury is to be in good physical condition and to stretch for several minutes before and after exercising. Never attempt to "play through" pain—doing so may cause more-extensive injury and lengthen the time needed for complete healing.

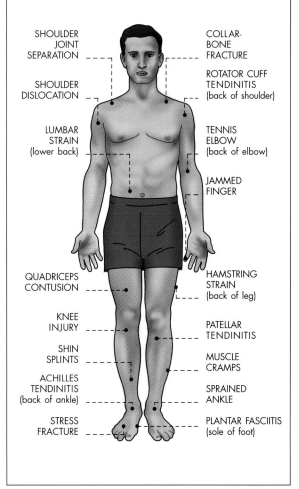

SHOULDER JOINT SEPARATION

SHOULDER DISLOCATION

LUMBAR STRAIN (lower back)

COLLAR-BONE FRACTURE

ROTATOR CUFF TENDINITIS (back of shoulder)

TENNIS ELBOW (back of elbow)

JAMMED FINGER

QUADRICEPS CONTUSION

KNEE INJURY

SHIN SPLINTS

ACHILLES TENDINITIS (back of ankle)

STRESS FRACTURE

HAMSTRING STRAIN (back of leg)

PATELLAR TENDINITIS

MUSCLE CRAMPS

SPRAINED ANKLE

PLANTAR FASCIITIS (sole of foot)

OF SPECIAL INTEREST

Growing Pains

Osgood-Schlatter disease is a condition associated with sudden growth spurts in adolescence (usually in boys ages 10 to 14). It is characterized by pain and swelling below the kneecap, where the patellar tendon attaches to the shinbone. The quadriceps muscle, located at the front of the thigh, continually pulls on the affected tendon, causing the disorder. Osgood-Schlatter disease persists for six months to a year and usually clears up completely without treatment. However, as long as your child suffers from symptoms, activities such as running, jumping, and squatting should be kept to a minimum, if not eliminated completely.

CONTINUED

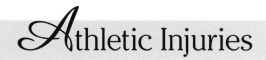
ing pain along the inner heel and along the arch of the foot, sometimes accompanied by stiffness and numbness in the heel. A similar problem, march fracture, develops in the bones of the foot when extreme stress (as in running) is continually placed on the ball of the foot.

Treatment Options

Most minor soft-tissue injuries are best treated with RICE: rest, ice, compression, and elevation. The following alternative therapies can help alleviate the pain and other symptoms of an athletic injury, but severe injuries require a doctor's care.

Acupuncture

Administered by a professional, acupuncture may be helpful in treating athletic injuries and soothing the body after strenuous training. It has been shown to reduce pain and swelling, and it may also speed recovery of injured muscles, tendons, and ligaments. For best results, acupuncture should be performed as soon as possible after injury occurs.

Bodywork

Administered by a professional, the Alexander technique, Rolfing, and the Feldenkrais method may be useful, particularly when the problem involves body structure or movement patterns.

Chinese Medicine

Various combinations of Chinese herbs, tailored to the individual's condition, can be used to treat athletic injuries. Herbal liniments often recommended by practitioners include *Tieh Ta Yao Gin* (Traumatic Injury Medicine) and *Zheng Gu Shui*.

Homeopathy

Arnica (12c) may be taken every 10 minutes for one to two hours, until the shock of injury passes, and then every eight hours until the pain is gone. Taken every eight to 12 hours for up to three days, *Ruta* (12c) may aid healing after a dislocation or any tendon or ligament injury. The symptoms of any muscle strain or sprain may be eased with *Rhus toxicodendron* (12c), taken three times a day for as long as a week. For joint pain, including tennis elbow, or discomfort associated with excessive use of the wrist, a homeopath might recommend *Calcarea carbonica.*

Hydrotherapy

Water is the perfect place for athletes recovering from injuries to work out. Aquatic movement provides muscle resistance without straining joints.

Lifestyle

Heat and stretching exercises before vigorous physical activity can loosen joints and soft tissue, thereby helping to prevent injury. Various types of braces and supports worn during exercise can protect joints and soft tissue and stabilize an uncomfortable joint or tendon. To avoid ankle injuries, always wear appropriate shoes with ample protection and support.

Massage

Massage can be extremely helpful in the treatment of acute traumatic injuries as well as those brought on by chronic overuse. Besides relieving aches and pains, massage shortens the recovery time after working out and helps prevent injuries. It also promotes flexibility, especially when used with stretching exercises. For serious athletes, massage helps the body cope with the wear and tear of training.

OF SPECIAL INTEREST

Child Sports Injuries: What Parents Should Know

Each year during the high-school football season there are an estimated one million injuries; wrestling, soccer, and basketball also carry a high risk of injury.

Children are at a higher risk of injury than adult athletes because those playing together may be at vastly different weights, stages of development, and strengths. To help prevent injury, try to ensure that participants in a group are at a similar level of physical development.

$\mathscr{A}$thletic Injuries

Hamstring Stretch

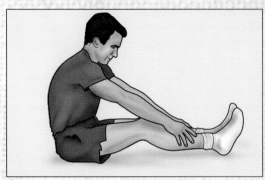

1 *Sit on the floor with your legs extended and slightly bent at the knees. Keeping your back as straight as possible, slowly bend from the hips and reach down your legs as far as you can without forcing the stretch. Hold in place for 15 seconds.*

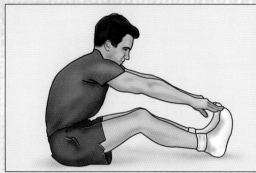

2 *Without changing your position, reach toward your feet and try to touch your toes with your fingertips. Hold this position for 15 seconds, then slowly relax the stretch and sit back. Rest for 10 seconds, then repeat the exercise. Do eight to 10 times.*

Treat a charley horse by kneading the affected area; rub in the direction of the muscle fibers.

Nutrition and Diet

Many experts advise athletes to maintain a high-carbohydrate, low-fat diet to increase energy levels and promote muscle strength.

Taken orally or topically, ***vitamin E*** may guard against muscle damage during exercise. ***Magnesium*** helps maintain muscle flexibility, which lessens susceptibility to injury.

For bone fractures, ***vitamin B complex*** and ***zinc*** may help. Nutritionists sometimes recommend supplemental use of ***calcium*** and ***potassium*** for maintenance of good musculoskeletal health.

Avoid sugar and stimulants such as caffeinated and decaffeinated beverages, particularly before exercising. Stimulants tighten muscles, increasing the risk of injury.

Home Remedies

- Replacing fluids lost through perspiration with a carbohydrate-electrolyte sports drink helps prevent cramping.
- Ice packs reduce swelling; a bag of frozen vegetables can be a makeshift ice pack. Do not use chemical cold packs, since they are much colder than water packs. Place a damp towel around your pack so that it is not directly on your skin.
- A warm compress may relieve muscle pain, especially before massage and stretching.
- To relieve cramping, elevate the affected area to direct blood flow toward the heart.
- If muscles are sore the day after a tough workout, soak in a hot tub and rest the area.

Prevention

Before you begin a sport or exercise routine, have a physical exam. This advice is particularly appropriate if you are over the age of 40.

Sports injuries usually result when the muscles are poorly conditioned. You should have a 10-minute warmup session—running in place or doing jumping jacks—before an athletic activity to increase your body temperature and diminish chances of muscle injury. Stretching after your workout will prevent soreness the next day.

Engage in your sport or exercise at least three times a week to maintain proper conditioning. ■

Back Problems

Symptoms

■ Persistent aching or stiffness anywhere along your spine, from the base of the neck to the hips.

■ Sharp, localized pain in the neck, upper back, or lower back, especially after lifting heavy objects or engaging in other strenuous activity.

■ Chronic ache in the middle or lower back, especially after sitting or standing for extended periods.

Call Your Doctor If

■ you feel numbness, tingling, or loss of control in your arms or legs; you may have damaged your spinal cord.

■ the pain in your back extends downward along the back of the leg; you may be suffering from sciatica.

■ the pain increases when you cough or bend forward at the waist; this may be the sign of a herniated disk.

■ the pain is accompanied by fever; you may have a bacterial infection.

■ you have dull pain in one area of your spine when lying in or getting out of bed, especially if you are over the age of 50; you may be suffering from osteoarthritis (see Arthritis).

B *ack problems are the most common physical complaints among American adults. Non-specific back pain is a leading cause of lost job time, to say nothing of the time and money spent in search of relief. And it's all because of one characteristic that makes us different from other animals: our upright posture. Many people spend their days sitting at desks, at work stations, or in cars and trucks. Those who walk a lot or do physical labor develop good muscle tone in their backs and legs. But people who sit most of the day either lose or don't develop that muscle tone, and their backs are the first place to show it.*

Treatment Options

Alternative therapies can be directed toward relieving the immediate discomfort of a back problem as well as conditioning and strengthening the body to prevent recurrence.

■ Acupressure
To relieve lower back pain, apply 60 seconds of thumb pressure on either side of the spine just above the top of the pelvic bone, then massage at this point, as well as at the hip and knee joints.

■ Acupuncture
Therapy involves inserting needles into points in specific muscles and on the ear to relieve blockages in the energy channels associated with back pain. Acute problems can be relieved in one to four sessions, while chronic pain problems typically require 12 or more treatments.

■ Bodywork
The Alexander technique and the Feldenkrais method are useful for corrective whole-body alignment, which can relieve chronic tension and stress.

■ Chiropractic
Traditional chiropractic therapy relies on spinal manipulation to correct subluxations, or misaligned vertebrae, which may be responsible for problems anywhere along the spine. By helping restore motion to poorly functioning vertebrae, chiropractic therapy diminishes the accompanying pain and muscle spasm.

Back Problems

■ Herbal Therapies

For general pain relief, drink infusions of **white willow** *(Salix alba)* or vervain *(Verbena officinalis).* For inflammation, try teas brewed from cimicifuga *(Cimicifuga foetida),* **yarrow** *(Achillea millefolium),* cramp bark *(Viburnum opulus),* or white willow. **Valerian** *(Valeriana officinalis)* is particularly recommended as a muscle relaxant and sedative.

■ Homeopathy

Over-the-counter remedies reported to help non-specific back problems include **Arnica** for bruised or sore muscles, **Bryonia** and **Rhus toxicodendron** for sharp pain that gets worse when you move, and **Ruta** for persistent backache.

■ Massage

Muscles that parallel the spine and support it often go into spasms during attacks of back pain. Massage can reduce pain by relaxing these muscles.

■ Mind/Body Medicine

Biofeedback therapy is reported to help those suffering from back pain. Special electronic instruments monitor the electrical activity of the muscles, and patients learn via feedback signals how to decrease the tension or pain in their muscles.

■ Osteopathy

Osteopathic treatment is likely to combine drug therapy with spinal manipulation or traction, followed by physical therapy and exercise. More and more doctors and physical therapists are using spinal manipulation as part of back-pain therapy.

■ Yoga

Yoga postures done in a gentle way are very helpful in relaxing and stretching tense and painful muscles in the back that can lead to back problems.

Prevention

The most important preventive measure for lower back pain is practicing good posture. But it's also wise to stretch out your back if you've been sitting or standing for an hour. Analyze your posture by standing with your heels against a wall. Your

Where It Hurts

Back pain can have many causes. Pain caused by osteoarthritis (1) can occur anywhere along the spine. The larger back muscles can be affected by fibrositis (2). Pain in the loin area on either side of the spine

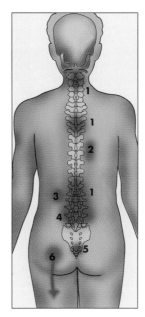

may indicate a kidney infection (3). Damage to spinal disks, joints, ligaments, or muscles can result in lower-back pain (4). A fall or other injury can cause pain in the coccyx (5). Pain radiating from the buttock down the back or outside of the leg may be sciatica (6).

calves, buttocks, shoulders, and the back of your head should touch the wall, and you should be able to slip your hand behind the small of your back. Then step forward and stand normally: If your posture changes, correct it right away. If you stand for long periods at work, wear flat shoes with good arch support and get a box or step about six inches high to rest one foot on from time to time.

Your sitting posture may be even more important. A good chair bottom supports your hips but doesn't touch the backs of your knees. Your chair back should be set at an angle of about 10 degrees and should cradle the small of your back comfortably; if necessary, use a wedge-shaped cushion or lumbar pad. Your feet should rest flat on the floor. Your forearms should rest on your desk or work surface with your elbows almost at a right angle. ■

$\mathscr{B}$ladder Infections

Symptoms

■ A burning sensation when urinating; this is the most common sign of a bladder infection, but any pain or difficulty in urination may also indicate the condition.

■ Frequent urge to urinate.

■ Urine with a strong, foul odor.

■ Heaviness or cramping in the lower abdomen.

■ In the elderly: lethargy, incontinence, mental confusion.

In severe cases, these symptoms may be accompanied by fever and chills, abdominal pain, or blood in the urine. These symptoms could signal a kidney infection. See below.

Call Your Doctor If

■ the burning sensation persists for more than 24 hours after you begin trying self-help treatments. Untreated, bladder infections can lead to more serious conditions.

■ painful urination is accompanied by vomiting, fever, chills, bloody urine, or abdominal or back pain; it may indicate potentially life-threatening kidney disease, a kidney infection, a bladder or kidney tumor, or a prostate infection. Seek medical help immediately.

■ the burning is accompanied by a discharge from the vagina or penis, a sign of sexually transmitted disease, pelvic inflammatory disease (PID), or other serious infection. See your doctor without delay.

■ you experience any persistent pain or difficulty with urination; this may also be a sign of sexually transmitted disease, a vaginal infection, a kidney stone, enlargement of the prostate *(see Prostate Problems)*, or a bladder or prostate tumor. See your doctor without delay.

Bladder infections—generally termed cystitis, which means inflammation of the bladder—are common in women and very rare in men. In fact, about half of all women get at least one bladder infection at some time in their lives. The reason may be that women have a shorter urethra, the tube that carries urine from the bladder. This relatively short passageway—only about an inch and a half long—makes it easier for bacteria to migrate into the bladder. Also, the opening to a woman's urethra lies close to both the vagina and the anus, giving bacteria from those areas access to the urinary tract. Bladder infections are not serious if treated promptly. But recurrences are common in susceptible people and can lead to kidney infections, which are more serious and may result in permanent kidney damage.

Treatment Options

If begun promptly at the first hint of burning during urination, alternative remedies can be successful in getting rid of a bladder infection. But if these methods do not bring relief within 24 hours, you should call your doctor for antibiotic treatment. Consult with your doctor if you wish to continue with alternative methods while on the antibiotics, to speed up the recovery process.

■ Acupuncture
Acupuncture treatment may help prevent recurrences of bladder infections. Consult a professional acupuncturist.

■ Aromatherapy
Hot sitz baths can help relieve the symptoms of a bladder infection. Adding certain pungent herbal oils to the bathwater creates a soothing, fragrant steam that aromatherapists believe makes the treatment particularly effective. Try putting in a few drops of the essential oils of juniper berry, *eucalyptus globulus (E. globulus)*, sandalwood, pine, parsley, cedarwood, *German chamomile (Matricaria recutita)*, or cajuput.

You can also try a massage oil made with 1 oz vegetable oil and 5 drops each of any combination of the herbs above. Massage daily, rubbing the oil over your lower back, abdomen, stomach, and hips.

ℬladder Infections

◼ Chiropractic

Adjusting the bones and joints around the pelvis can act to strengthen the bladder muscles, helping to ward off recurrences of the infection. An osteopath can also provide this treatment.

◼ Herbal Therapies

Some herbs have been found useful in both clearing up bladder infections and easing the burning that accompanies them. Perhaps the best known is cranberry, which, recent scientific studies show, has a remarkable ability to combat bladder and other urinary tract infections.

Another herb useful in treating bladder infections is **nettle** (Urtica dioica), which has anti-inflammatory properties. Mix 1 tsp dried, crushed nettle leaves or root in 1 cup boiling water. Allow the infusion to cool, then drink 1 tbsp every hour or two—up to 1 cup a day.

The evergreen shrub **uva ursi** (Arctostaphylos uva-ursi), or bearberry, which acts as a diuretic and an anti-inflammatory medication, has a long history as a folk remedy for bladder infections. Soak fresh leaves in brandy or other liquor for a few hours, then add to boiling water—about 1 tsp leaves per cup of water. If you have dried leaves, you can boil them directly in the water without a preliminary alcohol soak. Do not use uva ursi more than one week.

Women who are prone to bladder infections after sexual activity can help prevent recurrences by washing their perineal area with a medicinal solution of the herb **goldenseal** (Hydrastis canadensis) before and after intercourse. Mix 2 tsp of the herb per cup of water, bring to a boil, and simmer for 15 minutes. Cool to room temperature before using.

◼ Homeopathy

- If the urge to urinate is very strong and the burning is intense, **Cantharis.**
- If you experience painful cramping with urination or your urine is very dark or bloody, *Mercurius corrosivus.*
- For women whose infections are brought on by sexual contact, *Staphysagria.*

Take these remedies every hour until symptoms disappear. If you experience no relief after 24 hours, seek professional help.

◼ Nutrition and Diet

Drinking plenty of fluids to keep you urinating frequently and to flush out your urinary tract thoroughly is one of the most effective means of combating a bladder infection—whatever its cause. However, you should avoid beverages that might irritate the urinary tract and aggravate the burning. Culprits include alcohol, coffee, black tea, chocolate milk, carbonated beverages, and citrus juices. Until clear of the infection, you should also avoid potentially irritating foods such as citrus fruits, tomatoes, vinegar, sugar, chocolate, artificial sweeteners, and heavily spiced dishes. Wait 10 days after the burning is gone before reintroducing these foods and drinks—one at a time—into your diet.

Prevention

- Practice good bathroom hygiene. Clean the anal area thoroughly after a bowel movement. Women should wipe from front to back to avoid spreading fecal bacteria to the urethra.
- Urinate as soon as possible when you feel the urge, and make sure you empty your bladder completely each time.
- Drink plenty of liquids, particularly water and cranberry juice, which contains a substance that inhibits the growth of certain bacteria.

Women:

- Empty your bladder as soon as possible after intercourse to wash out any bacteria that may have been pushed into the urethra.
- Avoid using perfumed soaps, bubble baths, scented douches, and vaginal deodorants. These products contain substances that can irritate the urethra and make it more vulnerable to infection.
- If you use a diaphragm for birth control, make sure it fits properly, and don't leave it in place for too long. If you have recurring urinary tract infections, consider switching birth-control methods. ◼

*B*reast Problems

Symptoms

■ Pain or a feeling of fullness in one or both breasts, most likely caused by premenstrual swelling.

■ Pain accompanied by redness and warmth or a discharge from the nipple; this may indicate an infection. Discharge can also signal a benign growth or breast cancer.

■ A lump that is movable and feels unattached to the chest wall; you may have a cyst or a fibroadenoma.

■ A lump that is hard, is not movable, or feels attached to the chest wall, with or without pain, perhaps with dimpling or puckering of the breast; this may be a sign of breast cancer.

Call Your Doctor If

■ you notice any kind of new or unusual lump in your breasts, especially one that remains throughout your menstrual cycle. Although most lumps are harmless, in rare instances they may signal infection or cancer. Have your doctor check any lump.

*T*he female breast changes with puberty, with the monthly menstrual cycle, and with pregnancy; it also continues to change with age. Most changes in your breast are perfectly normal and are no cause for concern. However, you may experience any of several conditions that require medical attention. Chief among these are breast pain and masses or lumps.

Starting at puberty, you should examine your breasts every month so that you become familiar with their structure and can detect any abnormalities. Premenstrual changes can cause thickening that disappears after the period, so it is best to check your breasts about a week after your period. If you are no longer menstruating, examine your breasts monthly on a day you will remember, such as the day corresponding to your birthday.

BREAST PAIN

Breast pain can have many causes, including the normal swelling of breast tissue during the menstrual cycle. This swelling is due to hormonal changes, including increases in estrogen and progesterone, that bring more fluid into the breasts. Other causes include infection or injury; growths, including cancer; and perhaps diet. Cysts may pro-

How to Check Your Breasts

Check your breasts monthly, seven to 10 days after your menstrual period ends (it's easiest in the shower, using soap to smooth your skin). Look for dimpling, then try either the spiral or the grid method at right, using light pressure to check for lumps near the surface and firm pressure to explore deeper tissues. Squeeze each nipple gently; if there is any discharge—especially if it is bloody —consult your doctor.

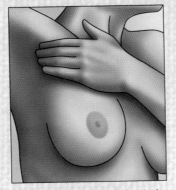

With either method, *begin by raising your arm and always use the flat of your fingers. To feel for any tiny lumps near the surface, apply light pressure by barely depressing your skin.*

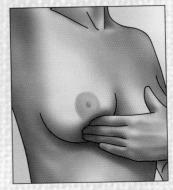

To apply firm pressure, *press deeply into the tissue, again using the flat surface of your fingers. Be aware of any sensitive areas, unusual lumps, or thickened tissue.*

Breast Problems

duce pain, but breast cancer rarely does (although pain does not rule out the possibility of cancer).

Treatment Options

Herbal Therapy

Evening primrose *(Oenothera biennis)* oil, although not approved in the United States for treating breast pain, is used in Europe and has proved effective. You can take a 500-mg capsule three times a day, every day if necessary.

Nutrition and Diet

Vitamin E effectively relieves breast pain. How it does this is unclear, but researchers do know that this vitamin affects blood clotting; if you are taking a blood thinner, consult your doctor before taking any vitamin E. Alternative practitioners sometimes recommend dosages up to 1,200 IU a day, but many women find relief with only 400 IU a day.

To prevent and treat monthly swelling of the breasts, maintain a healthy weight and eat a balanced diet. Because fat in the diet is associated with estrogen production, you can reduce your estrogen levels by eating a low-fat diet. Salt can con-

tribute to fluid retention; restrict your salt intake near your period. For some women, eliminating caffeine and substances called methylxanthines (found in chocolate and tea) can alleviate the pain.

Home Remedies

For pain relief, try applying a warm castor-oil pack to your breast. Saturate a flannel cloth with high-grade castor oil, put it on the breast, and cover it with plastic wrap and a towel; apply heat to the pack with a heating pad or hot-water bottle for 20 to 30 minutes. Wear a bra, even 24 hours a day, to reduce breast movement until the tenderness passes.

LUMPS

Breast lumps come in many forms, including cysts (benign fluid-filled sacs), adenomas (tumors that are sometimes associated with cancer), and papillomas (growths that can occur in the nipple area).

Treatment Options

Alternative medicine emphasizes prevention to manage breast problems. Diet and nutritional supplements are the first line of defense.

Herbal Therapy

Evening primrose *(Oenothera biennis)* oil—500 mg two or three times a day—may be helpful in reducing breast lumps.

Nutrition and Diet

Although no studies have proved that diet causes breast tumors, some do suggest a relationship. Many practitioners of alternative medicine urge eliminating caffeine. They also advise taking 400 to 1,200 IU of *vitamin E,* plus no more than 150 mcg a day of *selenium.* CAUTION: Selenium can be toxic in higher doses; you should use it only under the supervision of your healthcare practitioner. ■

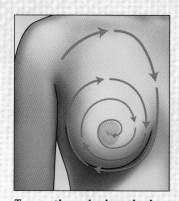

To use the spiral method, *begin at the top of your breast near your armpit and follow the pattern illustrated above. Apply light pressure first, then repeat using firm pressure.*

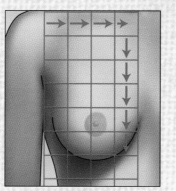

To use the grid method, *imagine the pattern of squares above, and follow the direction indicated by the arrows. Make a tiny spiral in each square, using first light pressure, then firm.*

*B*ronchitis

Symptoms

Acute Bronchitis:

- Hacking cough.

- Yellow, white, or green phlegm, usually appearing 24 to 48 hours after a cough.

- Fever, chills.

- Soreness and tightness in chest.

- Some pain below breastbone during deep breathing.

Chronic Bronchitis:

- Persistent cough producing yellow, white, or green phlegm (for at least three months of the year, and for more than two consecutive years).

- Wheezing, some breathlessness.

Call Your Doctor If

- your cough is so persistent or severe that it interferes with sleep or daily activities; you could be damaging sensitive air sacs in your lungs.

- your symptoms last more than a week, and your mucus becomes darker, thicker, or increases in volume; most likely, you have an infection requiring antibiotics.

- you display symptoms of acute bronchitis and have chronic lung or heart problems or are infected with the virus that causes AIDS; respiratory infections can leave you vulnerable to more serious lung diseases, such as pneumonia.

- you have great difficulty breathing. This symptom, sometimes mistakenly associated with bronchitis, could signal asthma, emphysema, tuberculosis, heart disease, a serious allergic reaction, or cancer.

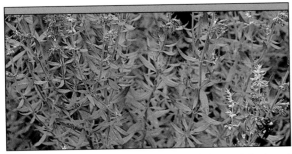

Hyssop • *To treat cases of acute bronchitis, an infusion of the herb hyssop (Hyssopus officinalis) may encourage sweating (thus lowering fever) and lessen inflammation.*

Bronchitis is an upper respiratory disease in which the mucous membrane in the upper bronchial passages becomes inflamed. As the membrane swells and grows thicker, it narrows or shuts off the tiny airways in the lungs, resulting in coughing spells accompanied by thick phlegm and breathlessness. The disease comes in two forms: acute and chronic.

Acute bronchitis sometimes accompanies an upper respiratory infection that may be either viral or bacterial. If you are otherwise in good health, the mucous membrane will return to normal after you've recovered from the initial infection, which usually lasts for several days.

Chronic bronchitis, like the lung disease emphysema, is a serious long-term disorder that requires regular medical treatment. People who have chronic bronchitis tend to be obese and lead sedentary lives, and most are heavy smokers; they typically have emphysema as well.

Treatment Options

Although acute bronchitis can often be treated effectively without a physician, you will need to see a doctor for a prescription of antibiotics if the underlying infection is bacterial. You may also benefit from a prescription cough syrup. If you suffer from chronic bronchitis, you are at risk of developing cardiovascular problems as well as more serious lung diseases and infections, so you should be monitored by a doctor.

Alternative therapies can help to ease some of the symptoms of acute and chronic bronchitis, but keep in mind that they do not always cure infections.

Aromatherapy

Essential oils such as **eucalyptus globulus** (*E. globulus*), hyssop (*Hyssopus officinalis*), aniseed (*Pimpinella anisum*), **lavender** (*Lavandula angustifolia*), pine (*Pinus sylvestris*), and **rosemary** (*Rosmarinus officinalis*) may help ease breathing and relieve nasal congestion. Inhaling deeply through your nose, breathe the aroma from a few drops of one or more of these oils dabbed on a handkerchief, or sniff directly from the bottle. Try mixing a few drops of essential oil in a sink full of hot water; cover your head with a towel and breathe in the fragrant steam.

Bronchitis

The Bronchial Tubes

Air flows down the windpipe and into the lungs through branching conduits called the bronchial tubes, or bronchioles, which normally are lined with only a thin mucous membrane. In bronchitis, however, this membrane becomes inflamed, resulting in

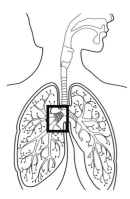

stepped-up mucus production. Over time, excess mucus can clog the bronchioles, cutting off air flow to the lungs. Coughing is the body's way of ridding the lungs of this mucus buildup.

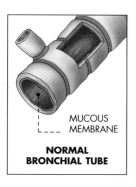

MUCOUS
MEMBRANE

**NORMAL
BRONCHIAL TUBE**

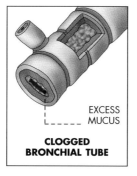

EXCESS
MUCUS

**CLOGGED
BRONCHIAL TUBE**

Herbal Therapies

A wide variety of herbs act as soothing expectorants. A sampling of therapies follows; for more, seek the advice of a professional herbalist.

For acute or chronic bronchitis, *coltsfoot (Tussilago farfara)* may relax bronchial tubes that are constricted or in spasm and help loosen phlegm. To prepare an infusion, add a cup of boiling water to 1 or 2 tsp coltsfoot; steep for 10 minutes. Drink it as hot as possible, three times daily. *Mullein (Verbascum thapsus),* believed to have an anti-inflammatory

Steaming toward Recovery

Humidity is helpful in treating both acute and chronic bronchitis, as moisture in the air can loosen phlegm and make it easier for you to expectorate. To be effective, however, humidifying devices must be used properly.

The warm steam distributed by vaporizers works well when used in a relatively small space, such as a bathroom; in an average room, most vaporizers aren't powerful enough to generate enough steam. Be sure to clean the vaporizer regularly to prevent the spread of germs.

Some devices can actually be hazardous to your health. Cool-mist humidifiers, often used in homes with dry air, must be cleaned daily with bleach; otherwise, they can spread germs and encourage mold or mildew, increasing your chances of developing lung infections.

effect on mucous membranes, can also be prepared as an infusion according to the same directions. Expectorants appropriate for chronic bronchitis include aniseed *(Pimpinella anisum),* elecampane *(Inula helenium),* and *garlic (Allium sativum).*

Homeopathy

For acute and chronic bronchitis, take the following three times a day, for up to four days: To treat fever, cough, and tightness in the chest with anxiety, use *Aconite* (12x). For loose white phlegm, cough, and irritability, use *Kali bichromicum* (12x). For loss of voice, cough, thirst, sore throat, and exhaustion, use *Phosphorus* (12x). Consult a homeopath for the remedy that's best for you.

Nutrition and Diet

To strengthen the immune system, nutritionists often recommend *vitamins A, B complex, C,* and *E,* along with the minerals *selenium* and *zinc.* Some suggest you also avoid mucus-producing foods, found mainly in the dairy group (although goat's milk generally causes less mucus production than cow's milk) as well as in refined starches (white-flour–based products) and processed foods. ■

B

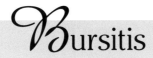

Bursitis

Symptoms

■ Pain, inflammation, and swelling in the shoulders, elbows, hips, knees, or joints of the hands or feet, particularly during stretching or extension when exercising, lifting, or otherwise pushing the joint beyond its normal limits.

■ Restricted range of motion in a joint, with or without immediate pain.

Call Your Doctor If

■ pain in a joint persists more than a few days; a prescribed anti-inflammatory medication may be the best treatment. You may also need a doctor's diagnosis to determine whether you are experiencing tendinitis, a strained ligament or tendon, or the onset of arthritis.

■ swelling persists after you take a painkiller or anti-inflammatory agent as prescribed; you may need to have a physician drain fluid from the affected joint or you may need to undergo corticosteroid treatment.

W herever your bones, tendons, and ligaments move against each other, particularly near joints, the points of contact are cushioned by small fluid-filled sacs called bursae. When a joint is overused, or when it stays under pressure or tension for extended periods of time, a nearby bursa can become inflamed. The sac fills with excess fluid, causing pressure on surrounding tissue and on the bursa sac itself. The immediate signal is pain, often accompanied by inflammation, swelling, and tenderness in the area.

One of the most common sites for bursitis to strike is the shoulder, which has the greatest range of motion of all the body's major joints. The pain is generally felt along the outside top of the shoulder. The discomfort of bursitis tends to be most severe after a night's sleep and will typically subside somewhat with normal activity. Other places that are prone to bursitis are the elbows, hips, and knees.

Treatment Options

Bursitis tends to heal itself with rest, but in the meantime the pain and inflammation can be relieved through a variety of remedies—including aspirin or an over-the-counter nonsteroidal anti-inflammatory drug (NSAID).

One particularly valuable alternative technique is diathermy, or deep-heat therapy, which should be performed under the direction of a sports physician, licensed physical therapist, or trainer. It not only can relieve the discomfort and inflammation of bursitis but also can soothe tense muscles, nerves, and tendons.

■ Acupuncture
Treatment by a trained acupuncturist can bring quick relief of bursitis pain.

■ Bodywork
An injured or stressed joint needs rest for natural healing to occur. In the short term, massage around the affected area stimulates circulation and relaxes surrounding muscles; it may also reduce tension in the joint area. Be careful, however, not to massage the affected area directly, because direct pressure on the bursa may irritate it further.

Poor body alignment and too much tension in

Bursitis

the muscles when performing a sport or a repetitive task can lead to bursitis. By teaching an improved use of the body, the Alexander technique may help eliminate these harmful habits.

Chiropractic

Following your chosen method of pain relief, a chiropractor can use mobilization techniques and other forms of physical therapy to restore a joint's active range of motion.

Flower Remedies

Bursitis is sometimes treated with rose-essence flower remedies. One particularly effective treatment to reduce inflammation is to apply *Rescue Remedy* in cream form to the painful joint three or four times a day. Rescue Remedy is a combination of five other flower remedies: *Cherry Plum, Clematis, Impatiens, Rock Rose,* and *Star-of-Bethlehem.*

Herbal Therapies

To increase blood circulation, reduce inflammation, and alleviate muscle tension, an herbalist might recommend a 5-ml tincture of the following herbs, taken orally three times a day: 2 parts each willow (*Salix* spp.) bark, cramp bark (*Viburnum opulus),* and celery (*Apium graveolens)* seed, along with 1 part prickly ash (*Zanthoxylum americanum).*

Mix equal parts *lobelia* (*Lobelia inflata)* and cramp bark to make a tincture that you can rub into your muscles as needed to ease the tension associated with bursitis pain.

Homeopathy

After evaluating the nature of the bursitis pain, a homeopath may prescribe regimens of *Belladonna, Bryonia,* or *Rhus toxicodendron.*

Hydrotherapy

For acute pain, use an ice pack (a bag of frozen vegetables works well) on the affected area. Leave it in place for five minutes, then remove it for one minute; repeat this procedure three times. For chronic symptoms, try alternating hot and cold compresses.

Hydrotherapists also recommend a warm castor-oil pack applied directly to the area. To make a castor-oil pack, soak a piece of white cotton or wool flannel in castor oil and squeeze out the excess. Heat the soaked cloth in a microwave oven for one to one and a half minutes. Place the pack over the affected area, cover it with plastic, and wrap with an old towel to prevent the castor oil from staining your clothes or any surfaces.

You can reuse the pack several times; store it in a plastic bag in the refrigerator. Discard the pack when the cloth begins to change color.

Nutrition and Diet

Vitamin C, vitamin A, and *zinc* are recommended for making tissue-building collagen and for repairing injured tendons and bursa tissue. Good dietary sources of vitamin C are citrus fruits and potatoes; cod-liver oil is a good source of vitamin A. In addition, *vitamin E* is considered effective in promoting the healing of damaged tissue. Follow the recommendations of a trained dietitian for amounts and duration when taking vitamin supplements. Another approach reported to be helpful in recurring cases of bursitis involves *vitamin B_{12}* injections, which should be administered by a licensed health-care practitioner.

Yoga

After initial therapy to relieve pain and reduce inflammation, and after you have given the affected joint time to rest, yoga exercises are a practical long-term way of loosening and strengthening your muscles and joints.

Home Remedy

In the early stages of bursitis, the best approach is to apply an ice pack to the joint and to keep the joint rested if possible. Both of these steps work well to reduce inflammation.

Prevention

Warming up before strenuous exercise and cooling down afterward is the most effective way to avoid bursitis and other strains affecting the bones, muscles, and ligaments. ∎

C

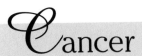 Cancer

Symptoms

In its early stages cancer usually has no symptoms, but eventually a malignant tumor will grow large enough to be detected. As it continues to grow, it may press on nerves and produce pain, penetrate blood vessels and cause bleeding, or interfere with the function of a body organ or system. The following symptoms may signal the presence of some form of cancer:

- A change in the size, color, shape, or thickness of a wart, mole, or mouth sore.
- A sore that resists healing.
- Persistent cough, hoarseness, or sore throat.
- Thickening or lumps in the breasts, testicles, or elsewhere.
- A change in bowel or bladder habits.
- Any unusual bleeding or discharge.
- Chronic indigestion or difficulty swallowing.
- Persistent headaches.
- Unexplained loss of weight or appetite.
- Chronic pain in bones.
- Persistent fatigue, nausea, or vomiting.
- Persistent low-grade fever, which may be constant or intermittent.
- Repeated instances of infection.

Call Your Doctor If

- you develop symptoms that may signal cancer, are not clearly linked to another cause, and persist for more than two weeks. You should schedule a medical examination without delay. If the cause of your symptoms is cancer, early diagnosis and treatment will offer a better chance of cure.

Throughout our lives, healthy cells in our bodies divide and replace themselves in a controlled fashion. Cancer starts when a cell is somehow altered so that it multiplies out of control. A tumor is a cluster of abnormal cells. Most cancers form tumors, but not all tumors are cancerous. Benign, or noncancerous, tumors—such as freckles and moles—stop growing, do not spread to other parts of the body, and do not create new tumors. Malignant, or cancerous, tumors crowd out healthy cells, interfere with body functions, and draw nutrients from body tissues. Cancers continue to grow and spread in a process called metastasis—eventually forming new tumors in other parts of the body.

The term "cancer" encompasses more than 100 diseases affecting nearly every part of the body, and all are potentially life threatening. The four major types are carcinoma, sarcoma, lymphoma, and leukemia. Carcinomas—the most commonly diagnosed cancers—originate in the skin, lungs, breasts, pancreas, and other organs and glands. Lymphomas are cancers of the lymphatic system. Leukemias are cancers of the blood and do not form solid tumors. Sarcomas arise in bone, muscle, or cartilage, and are relatively rare.

What Causes Cancer?

The fundamental cause of all cancer is a change, or mutation, in the nucleus of a cell. For a healthy cell to turn malignant, its genetic code must be reprogrammed for constant, uncontrolled cell division. Substances that either start or promote the process are called carcinogens, and there are many types. Scientists theorize that about 10 million of the 300 trillion cells in a human body die and are replaced every second. With such a high rate of cell activity, the potential for occasional malignant cell mutation is high. In a healthy person, special cells from the body's immune system somehow recognize mutant cells and destroy them before they multiply. Nevertheless, some mutant cells may occasionally evade such detection and survive, causing cancer.

Risk Factors for Cancer

Any habit, trait, or use of a substance that increases the odds of getting cancer is called a risk factor, and the risk for nearly all cancers increases with age. In-

Cancer

Yoga

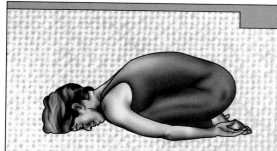

Child • *This position can help relieve stress and strengthen your immune system. Sit on your heels, knees together. With your arms at your sides, palms up, bend from the hips and extend your upper body over your knees, bringing your forehead toward the floor; hold for 20 seconds. Then slowly sit up.*

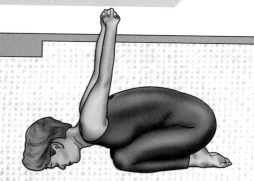

Yoga Mudra • *This position may help bolster your immune system. Sit on your heels, knees together. Bring your arms behind you, fingers clasped. Move your forehead to the floor and stretch your arms overhead; hold for 15 seconds, breathing deeply. Bring your arms back down; slowly raise your torso.*

herited, or familial, predisposition is a risk factor, although its influence varies from case to case. Researchers continue to identify genes that, when flawed, strongly predispose a person to a particular type of cancer. Such genetic predisposition is considered an influential risk factor but by no means guarantees that the person will develop the cancer.

Environmental risk factors relate to where and how we live. Most common cancers are linked to one of three environmental risk factors: smoking, sunlight, and diet. Smoking is linked to cancer of the lung, head-and-neck area, bladder, kidney, stomach, cervix, and pancreas, as well as to some leukemias. Overexposure to sunlight is linked to skin cancer. Diet is associated with some cancers of the gastrointestinal tract and may be linked to others, such as cancer of the breast, prostate, and uterus. Eating habits suspected of promoting cancer include overconsumption of alcohol, fat, and foods that have been smoked, cured, pickled, or charred. Lack of dietary fiber or antioxidant vitamins and minerals is also believed to be a risk factor.

Many substances in the environment have been identified as carcinogens, but in most cases a very high level of exposure is needed to cause cancer. Environmental carcinogens include various chemicals, gases, and other substances found in air, water, foods, pesticides, tobacco smoke, cleaning products, paints, and many industrial settings; excessive ionizing radiation—the type in x-rays, nuclear radiation, and radioactive waste; and certain viruses, such as HIV and the hepatitis B, papilloma, and Epstein-Barr viruses.

All these factors may contribute to cancer, yet cancer is not caused by any single factor. Cancer results from a "multifactor hit" of age, inherited predisposition, general health, and carcinogenic exposure. For example, some people exposed to particular carcinogens will develop cancer, while others, exposed just as intensely to the same carcinogens, will not. And as far as we know, most people who get a particular form of cancer are not strongly predisposed to it genetically. Thus, everyone's cancer risk profile is complex and unique.

Treatment Options

A comprehensive cancer program combines both curative and supportive treatment. Curative treatment attempts to terminate or slow the disease with some combination of surgery, radiation therapy, chemotherapy, and possibly, hormone therapy or immunotherapy. When cancer is no longer detected, a patient is said to be in remission. Generally, patients who remain cancer free for five or more years are considered cured. Some cancers cannot

CONTINUED

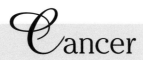

Cancer

be cured, but all can be treated, and in most cases the patient will improve.

Supportive treatment by nurses and other professionals accompanies cancer treatment. The goal is to relieve pain and other symptoms; maintain general health; and provide emotional, psychological, and logistical support to patients and their families. Similar supportive treatment is available to rehabilitate patients after curative treatment. Supportive therapy such as hospice care for cancer patients nearing the end of their lives provides relief from pain and other irreversible symptoms. Most mainstream care is geared toward providing supportive treatment through the resources of a cancer treatment center. The best complementary cancer therapies, which are generally provided outside a hospital, also provide excellent supportive care.

Alternative and unconventional treatments for cancer are numerous and varied. While some legitimate therapies offer real support, many questionable therapies offer no benefits, may be dangerous, and may harm patients by delaying appropriate care. It is important to keep in mind that even the most promising unconventional therapies rarely cure cancer and should replace standard treatment only after consultation with your doctor. Instead, supportive therapies should complement conventional care.

Appropriate complementary therapies improve quality of life, help alleviate symptoms such as pain and nausea, and may relieve physical and emotional stress. The act of seeking complementary therapy is beneficial in its own right by giving patients a sense of control over their illness. Before trying any complementary cancer therapy, research it thoroughly to make sure it is potentially beneficial and absolutely safe. Then check with your doctor to be sure it will not compromise standard treatment.

Acupuncture

Acupuncture has proved to relieve pain associated with many major illnesses. Although scientific study has not fully documented its effectiveness in treating cancer pain and side effects such as nausea and vomiting, it is a safe therapy that many cancer patients find beneficial. Acupuncture may also help patients feel stronger and thus better able to cope with their cancer. Consult a practitioner of Chinese medicine.

Bodywork

By promoting relaxation, bodywork therapies such as massage, qigong, and reflexology ease muscle tension and may alleviate other symptoms such as nausea and chronic pain. Because many bodywork therapies provide comforting physical contact, they can lessen the anxiety, depression, and isolation that cancer patients often feel.

Exercise

Physical activity can help control fatigue, muscle tension, and anxiety. The best exercises are those that calm the mind as well as strengthen the body, such as walking or swimming.

Herbal Therapies

Thousands of herbs are used by folk healers worldwide to treat cancer. But no herbal remedy cures cancer, despite claims to the contrary. Because some herbs contain toxic ingredients, check with your doctor before taking any herb to relieve symptoms. Herbs may alleviate side effects resulting from conventional treatment: **Horsetail** (*Equisetum arvense*) may help prevent hair loss after chemotherapy, and **ginger** (*Zingiber officinale*) may lessen nausea associated with chemotherapy or radiation. Consult your herbalist for other possibilities.

Some cancer sufferers report relief from pain, nausea, and vomiting using traditional Chinese medicine. Most practitioners recommend herbal remedies not to cure cancer but to relieve the side effects of conventional treatment. Researchers are studying plants used in traditional Chinese medicine to identify constituents that may combat cancer cells directly or stimulate the immune system to do so. These plants include **astragalus** (*Astragalus membranaceus*), **dong quai** (*Angelica sinensis*), and **Asian ginseng** (*Panax ginseng*).

Homeopathy

Homeopathic remedies do not treat cancer directly, but some can alleviate the side effects of radiation and chemotherapy. **Nux vomica** (12x) and **Phos-**

Cancer

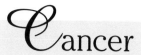

phorus (12x) may be particularly helpful in alleviating nausea. Consult a professional homeopath for the remedies appropriate for you.

Mind/Body Medicine

Some mind/body therapies work to improve quality of life through behavior modification; others encourage expression of emotions. Behavior therapies such as guided imagery, progressive muscle relaxation, hypnotherapy, and biofeedback are used to alleviate pain, nausea, vomiting, and the anxiety that may occur in anticipation of or after cancer treatment; they may also be used to bolster the immune system in its fight against cancer cells. Individual or group counseling, as well as art or music therapy, lets patients confront problems and emotions caused by cancer and receive support from fellow patients. Patients who pursue these types of therapies tend to feel less lonely, less anxious about death, and more optimistic about recovery.

Nutrition and Diet

Scientific evidence suggests that nutrition can play a role in cancer prevention. But no diet has been shown to slow or cure cancer. Vitamins, minerals, and other nutrients may inhibit cancer by neutralizing carcinogens, ensuring proper immune function, or preventing tissue and cell damage. Researchers are particularly interested in antioxidants—*vitamins A* (particularly beta carotene), *C,* and *E,* and *selenium*—but are also studying *folic acid, vitamin B_6, magnesium, zinc,* and coenzyme Q10, among others.

Because an excess of some vitamins can be harmful, many experts are cautious about dietary supplements. Instead, they advise a varied diet that includes lots of fresh fruits, vegetables, and whole grains; avoids processed, smoked, cured, fried, or barbecued foods; emphasizes lean cuts of meat and low-fat seafood; and minimizes sugar, fats, and alcohol. Many customized diets for cancer emphasize vegetarianism; indeed, patients who follow a nutritionally sound vegetarian diet do tend to feel better. Unfortunately, many anticancer diets also promote fasting, purging, and taking supplemental "immune-boosting" vitamins, minerals, and other concoctions that do not treat cancer and

may be both harmful and expensive. As a rule, patients should avoid any diet that claims to cure cancer, advocates abandoning standard treatment, causes severe weight loss or weakness, requires severe food restriction, or costs a lot of money.

Home Care

Relieving pain:
- In addition to taking prescribed medication, try relaxation techniques such as yoga, meditation, or massage given by a friend or spouse.

Other tips:
- Join a cancer support group.
- Get plenty of rest.
- Rather than feeling compelled to maintain a "positive attitude," express your emotions honestly. Don't worry if you sometimes feel depressed or afraid: These are normal reactions that will not make your cancer worse.
- Fill your days with activities you enjoy. Reading a good book, listening to music, and talking with friends are simple pleasures—but surprisingly therapeutic.
- Contact the American Cancer Society and the National Cancer Institute for free information about cancer prevention, diagnosis, treatment, and tips for managing cancer symptoms.

Prevention

- Do not smoke or use chewing tobacco.
- Stay out of the sun. Outdoors, use sunscreen to protect your skin from ultraviolet rays.
- Drink alcohol only in moderation.
- Exercise regularly to keep your body active.
- Get regular screening for cancer as part of your annual physical checkup.
- If your work exposes you to known carcinogens, be sure to follow all safety guidelines.
- To limit exposure to carcinogenic chemicals at home, avoid aerosol cleaning products; clean up spills and wash hands after using cleaning products; wear rubber gloves when using pesticides; and open doors and windows to allow fumes to escape when using chemicals, stains, or paints indoors. ∎

Carpal Tunnel Syndrome

Symptoms

- A tingling or numb feeling in the hand, usually just in the thumb and the first three fingers.

- Shooting pains in the wrist, forearm, and sometimes extending to the shoulder, neck, and chest.

- Difficulty clenching the fist or grasping small objects.

- Sometimes, dry skin and fingernail deterioration.

Call Your Doctor If

- the pain and numbness persist and you have not been able to find relief; your doctor can perform tests to confirm the diagnosis. Your arm and hand may have to be immobilized in a cast for several weeks, or in the worst case you may need surgery.

- you feel pain in your wrist, hand, or fingers after a fall or other accident; you may have a broken bone.

- your hands or fingers feel painful and stiff, especially if the joints become swollen; you may be suffering from a form of arthritis.

- pain in the hands and fingers is more intense at night; this may signal late-onset diabetes.

C *arpal tunnel syndrome (CTS) is one of several names for painful and disabling injuries to the thumb, fingers, and wrists, and sometimes to the elbows and other joints. As a group, these conditions are called repetitive stress injuries (RSI). The warning signs are tingling and numbness in the affected joints—typically the fingers—especially after the regular workday, or when you're ready to go to sleep, or on awakening.*

Many people think CTS came in with the computer keyboard. In fact, injuries to the carpal tunnel and other major nerve passages have been around a long time; but with so many fingers tapping away at computer keyboards, the problem is more widespread than ever. The same symptoms can develop from any repetitive manual activity, from playing sports or musical instruments to using power tools or waiting on tables. Some authorities believe that a pyridoxine (vitamin B_6) deficiency can also induce the symptoms.

Treatment Options

The following treatments complement the need to reduce inflammation, rest the damaged wrist, and take the necessary steps to correct the habits or activities that caused the problem in the first place.

Acupuncture
Acupuncture may provide relief by stimulating circulation, calming nerves, and releasing the body's own painkilling agents. In addition to inserting needles around the sore wrist, an experienced practitioner may treat the back, shoulders, and neck.

Chiropractic
A chiropractor will probably employ spinal adjustment of the neck and upper back to restore normal nerve activity. He or she may also manipulate the wrist, forearm, and shoulder, as well as applying a splint or brace.

Herbal Therapy
Make a soothing compress by simmering 1 to 2 oz of fresh grated ***ginger*** *(Zingiber officinale)* in 4 oz of boiling water. Dip a soft, folded cloth into the decoction and apply the hot compress to the affected area, covering it with a dry cloth to retain the heat.

Carpal Tunnel Syndrome

Discontinue this treatment if the ginger irritates your skin or if it doesn't improve your condition.

Homeopathy

Try the following: **Arnica** (6x to 30c) for swelling and bruising caused by overuse or misuse of the joints; **Ruta** (6x to 12x) for tendon inflammation; and **Rhus toxicodendron** (6x) for pain. Or see a licensed homeopath for a more specific analysis.

Massage

Massage therapy may help in cases where pressure from soft tissues, lack of blood flow, and stress are thought to be the cause. Because CTS can involve other areas besides the wrist, massage may be used on hand, wrist, arm, shoulder, or neck areas.

Nutrition and Diet

Supplemental **vitamin E** in amounts up to 800 IU daily is reported to help reduce tissue inflammation. **Vitamin C** supplements up to 1,000 mg may be beneficial in tissue restoration. **Vitamin B$_6$,** or pyridoxine, is reported to help nerve inflammation and enhance blood circulation. Because high-protein diets inhibit the absorption of B$_6$, reduce your protein intake. Start with 50 mg a day, or try a **vitamin B complex** supplement; symptoms should ease within the month.

Osteopathy

Osteopathic physicians may recommend manipulation of the joint and surrounding soft tissue to improve circulation and nerve function.

Yoga

Yoga positions that relax the neck and back may help, but avoid hand and neck stands, as well as positions that include arm twists, any of which could harm already sensitive nerves.

Home Remedies

A few simple exercises and a cold pack may be the best treatment for reducing the discomfort of an RSI. One effective exercise is opening and closing your fist 12 or more times. Or try the following:

- With palms facing each other, press your fingertips together 20 times, rest, then repeat.
- Holding your hands over your head, rotate them at the wrists clockwise for 20 seconds, then do the same exercise counterclockwise.
- Strengthen hand and forearm muscles with a spring-style or foam-rubber grip exerciser.

Prevention

The natural position of the hand in most normal activities is straight or slightly bent at the wrist, with the thumb more or less in line with the forearm. Bending the hand forward or backward at the wrist for extended periods stresses the carpal nerves, so learn to keep your wrist and hand as straight as possible when you work. Take breaks and exercise your hands and wrists every hour. If you work at a keyboard, use a wrist support to help prevent unnatural bending and make sure your desk and chair height are correct for your stature. ∎

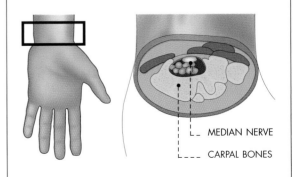

The Wrist

The wrist is a complicated, vulnerable joint. The median nerve—which runs from the forearm to the fingertips and controls movement of the fingers and thumb—passes through a tunnel formed by carpal bones and a tough layer of ligaments. If the median nerve is stressed or pinched, your fingers feel numb or tingly and you may lose feeling in your hand.

MEDIAN NERVE

CARPAL BONES

Cholesterol Problems

Symptoms

A high level of cholesterol in the blood does not have obvious symptoms but can be a risk factor for other conditions that do have recognizable symptoms, including angina, atherosclerosis, heart disease, high blood pressure, stroke, and other circulatory ailments.

- Soft, yellowish skin growths or lesions called xanthomas may indicate a genetic predisposition to an inability to process cholesterol and triglycerides in a normal fashion.

- Obesity and diabetes may be associated with high cholesterol levels.

- In men, impotence may be due to arteries affected by excessive blood cholesterol.

Call Your Doctor If

- you detect soft, yellowish skin growths on yourself or on your children. You should ask about being tested for a predisposition to high cholesterol.

- you develop symptoms of atherosclerosis, angina, or heart disease, such as pain in the lower legs, dizziness, unsteady gait, or thick speech. Any of these conditions may be associated with high blood cholesterol, and each requires medical intervention.

Don't wait for symptoms before having your cholesterol checked. Some doctors recommend a yearly test for total blood cholesterol and for LDL- and HDL-cholesterol levels.

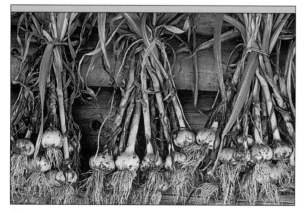

Garlic • *Members of the onion family, including garlic, may help lower your cholesterol levels, thus decreasing your risk of heart attack and stroke.*

Cholesterol is a type of fat, or lipid, found in every cell of your body and is especially concentrated in your brain, liver, and blood. Cholesterol supports such vital functions as cell building, nerve insulation, hormone production, and digestion. Your body produces all the cholesterol you need. The problem is that it's easy to get too much cholesterol into your bloodstream through a fatty, high-cholesterol diet.

Every day, the average American consumes 400 to 500 mg of cholesterol in food. High cholesterol wreaks havoc on the body, increasing the risk for atherosclerosis, heart disease, and stroke.

Types of Cholesterol

In the bloodstream, cholesterol binds with protein molecules to form various types of so-called lipoproteins. Lipoproteins are classified on the basis of their protein content as high-density (more protein) or low-density (less protein). High-density lipoprotein (HDL), known as good cholesterol, is a dense, compact microparticle that transports excess cholesterol to the liver, where it is altered and expelled in the bile. Low-density lipoprotein (LDL) is a larger, less dense particle that tends to remain in the body. LDLs can deposit too much cholesterol in artery walls, impeding normal blood flow and initiating the formation of blood clots. They are an important factor in the risk for coronary heart disease—and are hence known as bad cholesterol.

Everyone has both HDLs and LDLs, but in different proportions. A higher level of HDL relative to LDL is associated with decreased risk for cholesterol problems.

Treatment Options

Alternative therapists offer a range of natural ways to control your cholesterol levels. All can be pursued independently, and many can be combined with drug therapy if your therapist considers that necessary. The following list of treatments will let you customize your own program. To be safe, advise your doctor if you are using any alternative therapeutic substances or methods before mixing them with prescription drugs.

Cholesterol Problems

Ayurvedic Medicine

An Ayurvedic physician might recommend the combined formulas *Abana* and *Geriforte,* or the powder of the root *punarnava* combined with Indian bdellium. Indian bdellium's ability to control cholesterol levels has been compared with that of some synthetic drugs, with claims that it lowers LDL- and raises HDL-cholesterol levels without side effects. Indian bdellium is known as gugulipid *(Commiphora mukul)* in some Western herbal and health food stores.

Chinese Medicine

Traditional Chinese healers treat various forms of chronic heart disease, along with factors like high cholesterol, with acupuncture and an herbal therapy that employs **polygonum** *(Polygonum multiflorum)*. Because Chinese herbs almost always work in combinations rather than individually, you should consult a trained herbalist for an appropriate prescription.

Exercise

Evidence suggests that even though exercise alone cannot lower total cholesterol, moderate exercise several times a week can help raise HDL levels in many people. Vigorous exercise may raise HDL levels even higher, although at some point athletes apparently reach an "HDL plateau."

Herbal Therapies

Herbs reputed to have cholesterol-lowering properties include alfalfa *(Medicago sativa),* **turmeric** *(Curcuma longa),* **Asian ginseng** *(Panax ginseng),* and fenugreek *(Trigonella foenum-graecum).* You might also consult a nutritionally oriented doctor about the benefits of phytosterol tablets. Phytosterols are plant compounds structurally comparable to cholesterol that effectively block uptake of cholesterol in the liver.

Nutrition and Diet

The basic dietary rules for lowering cholesterol are simple: Avoid saturated fats and dietary cholesterol. Experts recommend a high-fiber diet with not more than 30 percent of your daily calories obtained from fat; some say 20 percent. Saturated fats derived from animal products and tropical oils should be kept to a minimum, so avoid eating deep-fried foods and pay attention to nutrition labels on packaged foods. For cooking, replace saturated fats that are solid at room temperature, such as butter and shortening, with liquid monounsaturated fats such as olive, canola, or flaxseed oil. There is evidence that consuming moderate amounts of monounsaturated fat—found in such foods as nuts, seeds, and avocados—may actually lower LDL cholesterol. Eat more vegetables, fruits, and grains, which are cholesterol free and rich in fiber.

Garlic and onion are believed to lower cholesterol, but reports vary on how much you should eat in order to benefit. It's safe to say that the more you eat, preferably raw, the better the effect. Eating grapes may help reduce blood cholesterol, thanks to flavonoid compounds in their skins. Look for grape-seed oil—squeezed from grape seeds after wine pressing—for cooking and for salad dressings. Vitamins, minerals, and nutrients thought to reduce cholesterol include **vitamins E, C,** and **A** (beta carotene), L-carnitine, pantethine, **chromium, calcium, copper,** and **zinc.** To keep your menus lively, try incorporating rice bran, artichokes, shiitake mushrooms, and chili peppers—all believed to help lower cholesterol.

Select foods that contain water-soluble fiber, which offers an excellent defense against high blood cholesterol. Foods on the high-fiber list are grapefruit, apples, beans and other legumes, psyllium seed, barley, carrots, cabbage, and oatmeal.

Prevention

- Keep your weight in check.
- Eat wisely every day—no more than 300 mg of cholesterol and at the very most 30 percent of your total calories from fat.
- Exercise several times a week—vigorously if you can, but moderate exercise is better than none at all.
- Track your progress. Have your blood cholesterol level tested periodically. At-home test kits are generally unreliable.
- If you smoke, quit. ■

Chronic Fatigue Syndrome

Symptoms

- Recent onset of debilitating fatigue.

- Fatigue that is not a result of exertion and that is unrelieved by rest.

- Persistent low-grade fever.

- Muscle soreness and weakness.

- Sleep disorders (insomnia or oversleeping).

- Swollen, tender lymph nodes.

- Migrating joint pain without swelling or redness.

- Forgetfulness, confusion, inability to concentrate.

- Recurrent sore throat.

- Headaches.

- Long-lasting malaise following physical exertion.

- Symptoms that persist for six months and result in a substantial reduction of activities.

Call Your Doctor If

- you have overwhelming fatigue and no identifiable, obvious reason for it, such as stress. Your doctor will need to rule out other illnesses that share symptoms with chronic fatigue syndrome, such as depression, thyroid problems, mononucleosis, arthritis, lupus, and cancer.

C hronic fatigue syndrome, or CFS—also known as chronic fatigue and immune dysfunction syndrome (CFIDS), chronic Epstein-Barr virus (CEBV), and myalgic encephalomyelitis (ME)—first came to public attention in the mid-1980s. It primarily strikes young urban professionals, with Caucasian women under age 45 accounting for 80 percent of cases; however, anyone, even a child, is susceptible. The cause is not known, but stress may affect the immune system, leaving it susceptible to an autoimmune disorder.

Treatment Options

A number of alternative therapies can help control the various symptoms of CFS. But be sure to check with your doctor for an accurate diagnosis before embarking on a course of treatment.

Acupressure

Applying gentle pressure to the gallbladder points may help relieve fatigue and depression while aiding your immune system. See the Gallery of Acupressure Techniques *(pages 18-31)* for help in finding the Gall Bladder 20 and 21 points on your shoulders and neck. This sequence can be done once or more a day or whenever symptoms appear. Pregnant women should press Gall Bladder 21 lightly.

Acupuncture

An acupuncturist may undertake a series of treatments to attempt to normalize and balance the immune system. In Chinese medicine, enhancing vital energy, nourishing the blood, and strengthening the spirit can be part of the therapeutic strategy.

Herbal Therapies

Goldenseal *(Hydrastis canadensis)* has been shown to increase white blood cell activity in some tests. **Echinacea** *(Echinacea* spp.*)* and shiitake *(Lentinus edodes)* mushrooms contain oligosaccharides, known to be extremely potent immune stimulators; take in moderate doses only, as advised by a qualified herbalist. **Gotu kola** *(Centella asiatica)* or **ginkgo** *(Ginkgo biloba)* may help you to be more alert; take 10 to 15 drops of the herb, in tincture form, twice a day. There are many other herbs that may be helpful; consult with a qualified herbalist.

Chronic Fatigue Syndrome

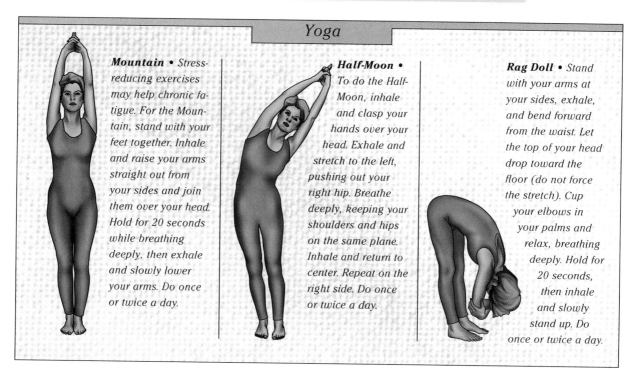

Yoga

Mountain • *Stress-reducing exercises may help chronic fatigue. For the Mountain, stand with your feet together. Inhale and raise your arms straight out from your sides and join them over your head. Hold for 20 seconds while breathing deeply, then exhale and slowly lower your arms. Do once or twice a day.*

Half-Moon • *To do the Half-Moon, inhale and clasp your hands over your head. Exhale and stretch to the left, pushing out your right hip. Breathe deeply, keeping your shoulders and hips on the same plane. Inhale and return to center. Repeat on the right side. Do once or twice a day.*

Rag Doll • *Stand with your arms at your sides, exhale, and bend forward from the waist. Let the top of your head drop toward the floor (do not force the stretch). Cup your elbows in your palms and relax, breathing deeply. Hold for 20 seconds, then inhale and slowly stand up. Do once or twice a day.*

The Chinese herbal formula *Bu Zhong Yi Qi Wan* (Tonify the Middle and Augment the Chi Pills) is used to treat CFS; it may help boost your energy levels. Another mixture, *Xiao Chai Hu Wan* (Minor Bupleurum Pills), is especially helpful if CFS first began with flulike symptoms. A Chinese medicine practitioner may recommend a commercially prepared mixture called Astragalus Ten Formula, which combines **Asian ginseng** (*Panax ginseng*), licorice (*Glycyrrhiza uralensis*), **astragalus** (*Astragalus membranaceus*), and other herbs. Some patients report improvement after taking this formula regularly.

Mind/Body Medicine

Meditation, progressive relaxation, guided imagery, qigong, and yoga *(above)* may help ease CFS symptoms without being tiring. In fact, they may provide an energy boost because they reduce stress.

Nutrition and Diet

One theory holds that a nutritional deficiency may be a contributing factor causing CFS, so it's important to maintain a healthful diet. Avoid caffeine; alcohol; refined sugar; white flour; salt; and fried, preserved, high-fat foods in favor of whole grains; beans; rice; fish; and fresh fruits and vegetables. Add edible seaweeds, shiitake (*Lentinus edodes*) mushrooms, and **licorice** (*Glycyrrhiza glabra*) to your diet. Eating two cloves of **garlic** (*Allium sativum*) a day may help boost your immune system's antiviral and antibacterial activity.

Coenzyme Q and **vitamin B_{12}** are nutritional supplements that may lessen symptoms. Some evidence suggests that a combination of malic acid and **magnesium** may help relieve fatigue and muscle pain. Egg lecithin taken with meals may enhance immunity and promote energy. Other immune-system-enhancing vitamins are **vitamin C** and mixed carotenoids—including beta carotene (**Vitamin A**). **Vitamins B_5** and **B_6, zinc, selenium, manganese,** and **chromium** all play a role in strengthening the immune system as well.

Home Remedies

Make sure you don't attempt more activity than you can handle. Get plenty of rest, pay attention to your diet, and exercise lightly on a regular basis. ∎

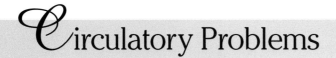Circulatory Problems

Symptoms

■ Cramplike pain, muscle fatigue, and aching in the legs; the blood vessels in your calves, thighs, feet, or hips may be blocked, possibly due to hardening of the arteries *(see Atherosclerosis).*

■ Bulging, bluish vessels in an aching leg; you may have varicose veins.

■ A painful vein; you may have phlebitis.

■ A finger, toe, or other body part that feels numb after exposure to cold weather, then becomes red and painful once it is warmed; you could be suffering from frostbite.

Call Your Doctor If

■ you experience sudden and severe localized pain, and the affected area turns pale and cold; you may have a fully blocked blood vessel, which can lead to tissue death.

■ you develop skin ulcers, localized skin discoloration, or nonhealing sores; these may be signs of obstructed blood flow.

■ you are experiencing pain in leg muscles while walking or resting; your blood flow may be dangerously restricted.

Most of us experience the discomfort of tired, stiff, aching legs every now and then. Many people, however, must cope with this sensation on a daily basis. This condition, called intermittent claudication, results from blocked arteries in the pelvis, thighs, or calves and most often is caused by atherosclerosis, commonly known as hardening of the arteries.

But interruptions in normal blood flow through arteries and veins can be brought on by a variety of conditions. Weakened arterial walls, for example, can balloon out and form pockets that trap blood. Veins can stretch, causing their internal valves to malfunction, and vascular disease can cause blood vessels to constrict. Most of the time the discomfort caused by circulatory irregularities is confined to the buttocks and legs, but it can also affect other parts of the body.

Treatment Options

Many nonconventional treatments for poor circulation are attempts to strengthen weak blood vessels or widen their openings, thus allowing greater blood flow to distant parts of the body. Some alternative therapies also help to ease the discomfort or reduce the inflammation and swelling associated with circulatory problems.

Bodywork
Yoga can promote blood flow and help alleviate the discomfort of poor circulation. See Yoga *(pages 182-183)* for more information about yoga's benefits.

Chelation Therapy
Many people seek relief through chelation therapy, which involves injecting the chemical EDTA into the bloodstream. This treatment, however, is controversial and far from universally accepted.

Chinese Medicine
A traditional healer may advise a combined program of acupuncture, herbal therapy, and massage. Chinese herbs are also used in specific combinations to treat circulatory problems.

Herbal Therapies
An extract of the small, thorny **hawthorn** *(Crataegus laevigata)* tree promotes circulation by dilating

Circulatory Problems

blood vessels, particularly coronary arteries. And **ginkgo** *(Ginkgo biloba)* has a well-documented record of medicinal success. Studies show that concentrated extracts from the leaves of the ginkgo tree may help improve circulation by dilating the arteries. If you have a blood-clotting disorder, consult a doctor before using ginkgo, since the plant contains a substance thought to suppress the blood's clotting ability. Ginkgo has also been shown to cause mild side effects, including excitability and digestive problems.

Taken orally, an Asian herb called **gotu kola** *(Centella asiatica)* appears to benefit circulation by strengthening blood vessel walls. **Cayenne** *(Capsicum annuum* var. *annuum)* and **ginger** *(Zingiber officinale)* may stimulate circulation by dilating arterioles and capillaries near the skin's surface. Butcher's-broom *(Ruscus aculeatus)* is believed to alleviate swelling and inflammation caused by many circulatory disorders. Both cayenne and butcher's-broom also work well topically, as an oil or a lotion.

Hydrotherapy

A long soak in a warm bath, followed by a brisk rub with a towel dipped in cold water, can ease general discomfort brought on as a result of poor circulation. Add a decoction of thyme leaves or larch needles (larch is a type of pine) to the bathwater for a stimulating effect. Soak cold feet in a warm footbath for 15 minutes. To promote circulation in the legs, alternate hot and cold footbaths (one to two minutes in hot water, 30 seconds in cold water) for 15 minutes. WARNING: Diabetics or others with reduced temperature sensitivity in their feet or legs must use extra caution to avoid burns.

Massage

Massage has been proved to increase blood flow and improve circulation, and can provide some of the benefits of exercise for those unable to exercise. Avoid massaging varicose veins directly; it will damage the vessel walls and make the veins worse. People with blood clots should not have massage.

Neural Therapy

Intended to restore electrical conductivity in the body through injections of anesthetics, neural ther-apy is popular in Germany for a range of conditions, including some circulatory problems. WARNING: Neural therapy should be used only as a complement to orthodox medical treatment, not as a substitute. This technique is not recommended for patients who have cancer, diabetes, or renal failure, or for people who are allergic to local anesthetics.

Nutrition and Diet

As a rule, your diet should be low in fat and high in fiber. Emphasize whole grains and fresh fruits and vegetables. Avoid caffeinated drinks, since caffeine causes blood vessels to constrict. If you suffer from cold hands and feet, don't fall for the "warming" properties of hot toddies. Alcohol can make you feel warmer, but it ultimately impairs your ability to stay warm. Alcohol makes it more difficult for you to maintain your body temperature in cold weather and may even promote hypothermia.

If you suffer from hardened arteries, eat more fish. Not only is fish low in fat and high in nutritional value, but it also boosts levels of high-density lipoprotein (HDL), the "good" cholesterol that purges blood vessels of fatty deposits. For dessert, try pineapple. Studies suggest that an enzyme in pineapple called bromelain enhances circulation while reducing inflammation. Bromelain is also available as a supplement and works best if taken on an empty stomach.

Reflexology

Stimulate all reflex areas on the feet; the reflex areas for the adrenal glands may be particularly helpful. In addition, working the reflex areas analogous to the localized problem areas may enhance circulation. *(See Reflexology, page 169, for more information on area locations.)*

Home Remedies

- Take regular walks or bike rides to enhance circulation in your legs. Do simple exercises, such as arm windmills, to get the blood flowing elsewhere.
- If you are taking birth-control pills, switch to another form of contraception.
- If you smoke, quit. ■

Common Cold

Symptoms

- Head and chest congestion, possibly with a runny nose and difficulty breathing.
- Sore throat.
- Sneezing.
- Dry cough that may occur only at night.
- Chills.
- Burning, watery eyes.
- Vague achiness all over your body.
- Headache.

Call Your Doctor If

- your newborn (two months or younger) has cold symptoms. For infants, the common cold can be a serious illness.
- congestion makes it hard for you to breathe, or your chest makes a whistling sound (a wheeze) when you breathe. You may have asthma.
- your throat hurts and your temperature is 101°F or higher; or your cold symptoms worsen after the third day. You may have a bacterial infection (such as strep throat), sinusitis, or bronchitis.
- your temperature is 103°F or higher. You may have pneumonia. Seek medical care immediately.
- your cold symptoms occur suddenly with exposure to certain triggers—such as pollen, cats, or perfume—and/or the symptoms continue for weeks. You probably have an allergy.

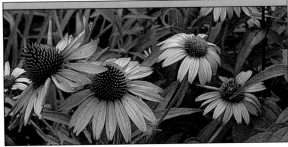

Echinacea • *A popular garden perennial, the herb echinacea contains ingredients that may help the body fight organisms such as those responsible for the common cold.*

*T*he aptly named common cold is the most frequent infection in all age groups in the United States. Cold symptoms are triggered when a virus attaches itself to the lining of your nasal passages or throat. Your immune system responds by attacking the germ with white blood cells called neutrophils. If your immune system cannot recognize the virus, the response is "nonspecific," meaning your body produces as many neutrophils as possible (usually more than are needed) and circulates them to the infected sites. This all-out attack kills many viruses, but it doesn't affect the 200 or so viruses that cause colds. Extra neutrophils clumping together at infection sites are what cause the achiness and inflammation of a cold, complete with vast amounts of mucus in the nose and throat.

Cold symptoms begin between one and four days after you are infected by a cold virus and typically last for about three days. During the time you have symptoms, you are contagious (meaning you can pass the cold to others). The illness usually goes away in a week or so without any special medicine.

Treatment Options

Begin to treat your cold as soon as you feel the first symptom. Especially with herbal remedies, an early response often results in a faster and easier recovery. (Pregnant or nursing mothers should check with their doctor before using herbal remedies.)

Aromatherapy

Herbal steam can reduce congestion, and if the vapor temperature is 110°F or higher, it will also kill cold germs on contact. Choose **eucalyptus globulus** (E. globulus), wintergreen (Gaultheria procumbens), or **peppermint** (Mentha piperita). Place fresh leaves in a bowl and pour in boiling water. Place a towel over your head, lean over the bowl to create a steam tent, and breathe the vapors.

Herbal Therapies

Taken at the first sign of symptoms, **echinacea** (Echinacea spp.) can reduce a cold's intensity and duration, often even preventing it from becoming a full-fledged infection. Echinacea apparently stimulates the immune response, enhancing resistance to all infection. It is most palatable in capsules and

Common Cold

tincture. **Goldenseal** *(Hydrastis canadensis)* helps clear mucus from the throat. It also contains the natural antibiotic berberine, which can help prevent bacterial infections that often follow colds. Take 10 to 15 drops of either herb in an alcohol-free form, known as glycerite tincture, two to three times a day for seven to 10 days.

For a good "cold tea," combine equal parts elder *(Sambucus nigra)*, **peppermint** *(Mentha piperita),* and **yarrow** *(Achillea millefolium)* and steep 1 to 2 tsp of the mixture in 1 cup hot water. This blend can help the body handle fever and reduce achiness, congestion, and inflammation.

Garlic *(Allium sativum)* appears to shorten a cold's duration and severity. Any form seems to work: capsules or tablets, oil rubbed on the skin, or whole garlic roasted or cooked in other foods. If you elect capsules, take three of them, three times daily, until the cold is over.

The Chinese herbal formula *Yin Qiao Pian* is said to be very effective for stopping a cold at the outset. *Sang Ju Yin Pian* (Mulberry Chrysanthemum Pills) is another cold remedy.

Homeopathy

Cold symptoms often respond well to homeopathic remedies. The dosage is 12c, taken every two hours for a maximum of four doses. **Gelsemium** may help if you have chills, aching arms and legs, and fatigue, or if your throat hurts. When your runny nose feels as though it burns, your eyes water constantly, and you sneeze often, try **Allium cepa.** If you feel irritable and have a runny nose that becomes congested at night, take **Nux vomica.** For a barking cough, a burning sore throat, and a bitter taste that lingers in your mouth, try **Aconite.** To prevent a cold, take one dose **Ferrum phosphoricum** (6x) every morning during cold season.

Lifestyle

Refrain from smoking, especially when you have a cold. Smoking assaults the mucous membranes and lungs, increasing your susceptibility to all sorts of respiratory infections, including colds. Once you have a cold, smoke irritates the already-inflamed tissues, making healing and recovery more difficult.

Nutrition and Diet

Good nutrition is essential for resisting and recovering from a cold. Eat a balanced diet. Take supplements as needed to ensure you are receiving the recommended dietary allowances for **vitamin A,** the **vitamin B complex (vitamins B_1, B_2, B_5, B_6, folic acid),** and **vitamin C,** as well as the minerals **zinc** and **copper.** If your diet is deficient in zinc, your body is low in neutrophils, and you're an easy mark for all types of infections, including colds. Zinc is available as a tablet or throat lozenge. While you have a cold, avoid dairy products, which tend to make mucus thicker. You also should avoid caffeinated and decaffeinated beverages and white sugar, which weaken the immune system.

"Jewish penicillin," also known as chicken soup, has been heralded as a cold therapy since the 12th century. Recent scientific evidence supports the notion that the soup reduces cold symptoms, especially congestion. Something (yet to be determined) in the chicken soup keeps neutrophils from clumping together and causing inflammation.

Any food spicy enough to make your eyes water will have the same effect on your nose, promoting drainage. If you feel like eating, a hot, spicy choice will help your body fight your cold.

Home Remedies

- Get plenty of rest. You may find you need 12 hours or more of sleep per night while you're fighting a cold.
- Keep your body hydrated by drinking up to eight glasses of fluid each day; this will replace the fluids lost through perspiration and your runny nose and minimize congestion.

Prevention

A strong immune system is the best defense against all infections. Boost your body's natural resistance by eating well, not smoking, and drinking plenty of fluids every day. Minimize contact with people who have colds, or at least don't share towels, silverware, or beverages with them. Cold viruses often survive for hours on doorknobs, money, and other surfaces, so wash your hands frequently. ∎

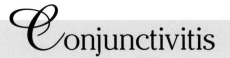 Conjunctivitis

Symptoms

- Burning, itchy eyes that discharge a heavy, sticky mucus may indicate bacterial conjunctivitis, commonly known as pinkeye.

- Copious tears, a swollen lymph node, and a light discharge of mucus from one eye are signs of viral conjunctivitis.

- Redness, intense itching, tears in the eyes, and sometimes an itchy, runny nose may indicate allergic conjunctivitis.

Call Your Doctor If

- you physically injure your eye. Eye injuries can become infected and lead to corneal ulcers, which can endanger your eyesight.

- your eyes become red when you wear contact lenses. Remove the lenses immediately and see your ophthalmologist; you may have a corneal infection.

- the redness in your eye affects your vision and is accompanied by severe pain or an excessive yellow or green discharge. You may have a staph infection or a streptococcal infection.

- your conjunctivitis frequently recurs or appears to be getting worse after a week of home treatment; you may have a bacterial or viral infection.

- your newborn baby's eyes are inflamed and are not producing tears; this may indicate a form of conjunctivitis known as ophthalmia neonatorum, which must be treated immediately by a physician to prevent permanent eye damage.

T *he conjunctiva—the transparent membrane that lines your eyeball and your eyelid—can become inflamed for various reasons. Conjunctivitis is caused by a bacterial or viral infection or by an allergic reaction to pollen, smoke, or other material that irritates your eyes. In most cases, the inflammation clears up in a few days. Although conjunctivitis can be highly contagious, it is rarely serious and will not damage your vision if detected and treated promptly.*

Bacterial conjunctivitis, commonly known as pinkeye, usually infects both eyes and produces a heavy discharge of mucus. Viral conjunctivitis is usually limited to one eye, causing copious tears and a light discharge. Allergic conjunctivitis produces tears, itching, and redness in the eyes, and sometimes an itchy, runny nose.

Ophthalmia neonatorum is an acute form of conjunctivitis in newborn babies. It must be treated immediately by a physician to prevent permanent eye damage or blindness.

Treatment Options

Alternative therapies rely on natural remedies in order to soothe irritated eyes and ease the itching and inflammation.

Aromatherapy
Myrtle hydrosol (myrtle water) will ease eye inflammation. Put it into a sterile spray bottle and carefully direct a light spray at the eyes.

Ayurvedic Medicine
An Ayurvedic physician may recommend an eyewash made from the root of barberry, the fruit rind of pomegranate, or the flower of jasmine.

Chinese Medicine
A qualified practitioner of Chinese medicine can prescribe a regimen of acupuncture or an herbal remedy such as *Niu Huang Shang Qing Wan* (Calculus Bovis Clear the Upper Pills).

Herbal Therapies
Using an eyecup, wash the eye several times a day with one of the following solutions. In each case, cool and strain the eyewash through a sterile cloth before using.

Conjunctivitis

- 1 tsp dried *eyebright* *(Euphrasia officinalis)* steeped in 1 pt boiling water.
- 2 to 3 tsp *chamomile* *(Matricaria recutita)* in 1 pt boiling water.

Homeopathy

Depending on your symptoms, take the following remedies four times daily for one or two days:
- for stinging eyes and red, puffy eyelids that are relieved by cold compresses, *Apis* 12x.
- for bloodshot eyes, sharp, splinterlike pains, and a gritty feeling, *Argentum nitricum* 12x.
- for itchy eyes with a sticky, yellow discharge, *Pulsatilla* 12x.

Hydrotherapy

Place an ice-cold compress on your eyes for 20 minutes, alternating eyes every two or three minutes. Stop for 30 minutes or an hour, then reapply for 20 minutes. If only one eye is infected, treat it two minutes on, two minutes off; don't use the same compress on the healthy eye because you might spread the infection. Or try placing a hot compress over each eye for one to five minutes, followed by a potato poultice—made of grated raw potato wrapped in a porous cotton or muslin cloth—covered with a cold washcloth.

For chronic conjunctivitis, alternate hot and cold compresses—three minutes hot, one minute cold—repeated four times. Finish with cold.

Home Remedies

You can cleanse and soothe irritated eyes with a prepared boric acid eyewash, or try the herbal eyewashes above. To relieve the discomfort of bacterial or viral conjunctivitis, apply a warm compress for five to 10 minutes, three to four times a day. For allergic conjunctivitis, place a cool compress or a cool, moist tea bag on your closed eye. If the condition does not improve in five days, consult an ophthalmologist.

Prevention

Bacterial and viral conjunctivitis are highly contagious. Unless you take preventive measures, the condition may spread to your other eye or to other people.
- Wash your hands often and well.
- Keep your hands away from the infected eye.
- Do not share washcloths, towels, pillowcases, or handkerchiefs with other family members.
- Change your washcloth, towel, and pillowcase after each use, and wash them thoroughly.
- Do not use other people's eye cosmetics, particularly eye pencils and mascara.

If your child gets pinkeye, you should keep him or her out of school for a few days. It is not uncommon for conjunctivitis to spread from one student to an entire class. ■

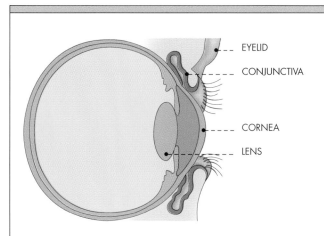

EYELID
CONJUNCTIVA
CORNEA
LENS

A Protective Layer

The conjunctiva is a thin, protective membrane that covers the exposed white of the eye and the inside of the eyelid. Bacterial conjunctivitis—sometimes called pinkeye—is the result of an infection that makes the conjunctiva red, teary, and itchy, with a thick greenish yellow discharge. When conjunctivitis is caused by an allergy, the discharge is clear and watery.

Constipation

Symptoms

- Hard, compacted stools that are difficult or painful to pass.

- No bowel movements in three days for adults, four days for children.

Call Your Doctor If

- your constipation is associated with fever and lower abdominal pain, and your stools are thin or loose; these symptoms may be an indication of diverticulitis.

- you have blood in your stools; this may be from a fissure or a hemorrhoid but could also be a sign of colorectal cancer; changes in your bowel movement pattern, such as passing pencil-thin stools, may also signal colorectal cancer.

- your constipation develops after you start a new prescription drug or take vitamin or mineral supplements; you may need to discontinue use or change the dosage.

- you or your child has been constipated for two weeks, with recurrent abdominal pain; this could be a sign of lead poisoning or another serious ailment.

- you are elderly or disabled and have been constipated for a week or more; you may have an impacted stool.

Yoga

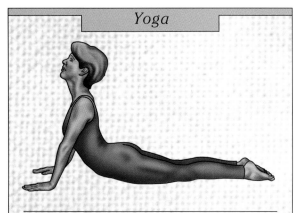

Cobra • *This position helps tone the abdominal organs. Place both forearms on the floor, elbows under your shoulders. Slowly straighten your arms and arch your back until your abdomen is off the ground. Relax and slowly uncurl, lowering your torso to the floor.*

Y our digestive system is remarkably efficient: In the space of a few hours it extracts nutrients from the foods you eat and drink, processes them into the bloodstream, and prepares leftover material for disposal. That material passes through 20 or more feet of intestine before being stored temporarily in the colon, where water is removed. The residue is excreted through the bowels, normally within a day or two.

Some people—including many alternative therapists—say we should move our bowels one to three times a day to remain healthy, but this remains controversial. Regularity very much depends on your diet, your age, and your daily activity. Nonetheless, the longer fecal material sits in the colon, the harder the stool becomes and the more difficult it is to pass. A normal stool should not be either unusually hard or soft, and you shouldn't have to strain unreasonably to pass it.

Our busy modern lifestyles may be responsible for most cases of constipation: not eating enough fiber or drinking enough water, not getting enough exercise, and not taking the time to respond to an unmistakable urge to defecate. Emotional and psychological problems can also lead to constipation.

Treatment Options

Most health professionals approach constipation as a lifestyle problem. Corrective measures include increasing fiber consumption, exercising regularly, and setting a routine time to move your bowels. You should seek the advice of a doctor if your problem is chronic or severe.

▪ Acupressure

Digestion may be improved by steady finger pressure on Stomach 36, four finger widths below the kneecap just outside the shinbone. Maintain pressure for one minute, then switch legs. To verify the location, flex your foot; you should feel a muscle bulge at the point site.

As an aid to relieving constipation, try applying pressure to Large Intestine 11, on the outer edge of the inside elbow crease. With the arm bent, press deeply into the point with your thumb for one minute, then repeat on the other arm. *(See the Gallery of Acupressure Techniques, pages 18-31, for exact point locations.)*

Constipation

Exercise

Walking for 20 to 30 minutes at a pace fast enough to get the heart pumping, or a good session at some other exercise, helps stimulate the bowels. Doctors say regular exercise, besides offering cardiac benefits, is an excellent way to correct chronic constipation. People should become accustomed to regular exercise when they are young so that it becomes a healthy, lifelong habit.

Herbal Therapies

Your health food store will have a selection of potentially useful herbal remedies. Try small amounts to test the effect they have on you or take them as recommended by a naturopath. Avoid herbal laxatives containing senna *(Cassia senna)* or buckthorn *(Rhamnus purshiana);* they can damage the lining and injure the nerves of the colon, and you can become dependent on them.

Homeopathy

For relief of mild constipation, you can find prepared remedies at a health food store. If your stools are soft but you have to strain to pass them, try remedies containing **Bryonia.**

Lifestyle

Simply recognizing the need to move the bowels solves many cases of constipation. Children respond to praise for sitting on the toilet and having regular bowel movements, and they can be trained at an early age.

For people who are convinced that regular bowel habits are important, the treatment is simple: Sit on the toilet every day at the same time for about 10 minutes, even if you don't have an urge to move your bowels. The best time is after a meal, because food in the stomach stimulates the colon to move. Be patient: It may take a couple of months before this new habit begins to work for you. Remember, however, to heed your body's own signals and to never resist the urge to move your bowels at other times.

Nutrition and Diet

Almost all Americans should eat more fiber. The American Dietetic Association recommends 30 grams of fiber a day, yet many people consume less than half that amount. Increasing your fiber intake is easy: Eat more raw fruits and vegetables—especially peas, beans, and broccoli—bran cereals, whole-wheat bread, and dried fruits such as raisins, figs, and prunes. A bonus is that most of these foods are rich in vitamins and minerals yet lower in calories than most processed foods.

It is never too early to start a healthy diet. Children as young as six months can be fed whole-grain cereals, which have more fiber and more nutrients than processed cereals. Even fast-food addicts can be tempted into snacking on fruit and raw vegetables. Otherwise, try a soluble or insoluble fiber supplement like **psyllium** *(Plantago psyllium),* which becomes gelatinous when combined with water and adds bulk to the stool. Drink 1 to 2 rounded tsp of powdered psyllium a day, stirred into a glass of cold water or juice, or include an equal amount of powdered flaxseed *(Linum usitatissimum),* available in many health food stores. Psyllium generally works within two days, but you can take it every day and not become dependent on it.

Insoluble fibers, including wheat bran, work as well as psyllium but may give you gas for a few weeks until your system adjusts to the change. You can mix bran with fruit juice, canned fruit, or cereal, or sprinkle it into sandwiches. Start by taking 1 tbsp a day, and gradually increase it to 3 or 4 spoonfuls.

An old folk remedy for stimulating the bowels is to drink a glass of warm water containing the juice of a whole lemon after waking in the morning and 15 minutes before each meal.

Prevention

The key to preventing constipation is simple: Drink adequate amounts of water—six to eight glasses a day is a good rule—and get sufficient fiber by eating fruits, vegetables, and grains. Fiber is critical because a large proportion of our stool is made up of bacteria, and fiber gives bacteria a good foundation to grow on. Ample bacterial action results in a larger volume of stool and better bowel function. ∎

Cough
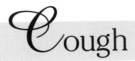

Symptoms

More important than the cough itself are aspects of it that provide clues to its cause:

- Frequency and duration of the cough.

- Length of the coughing spell.

- Type of material being coughed up (mucus or phlegm, blood).

- Color of the sputum (white, clear, green, yellow, pink, blood-specked).

- Consistency of the material coughed up (thick, thin, frothy).

- Presence or absence of accompanying pain.

Call Your Doctor If

- your cough lasts for more than seven to 10 days; it may be a sign of a serious disease.

- your cough is producing yellow, green, pink, or rust-colored sputum.

- your cough is exhausting, persistent, and accompanied by any of the following signs: hoarseness, sore throat, shortness of breath, wheezing, chest pains or tightness, fever of 101°F or higher, headache, back and leg aches, fatigue, rashes, or weight loss. A cough combined with one or more of these symptoms indicates an underlying ailment.

*A*lthough it is usually unwelcome and involuntary, a cough is not itself an illness but rather a protective reflex. Generally, the reflex kicks in when the membranes lining the respiratory tract secrete excessive mucus or phlegm. These secretions help to protect your airways from infections and irritants by trapping and flushing out viruses, bacteria, and foreign particles. Coughing is your body's way of getting rid of this accumulation. The sudden burst of air in a cough not only helps to keep the breathing passages open but also helps to clear the lungs and bronchial tubes. But be aware that severe coughing could indicate such serious infections as pneumonia or bronchitis.

Treatment Options

Most coughs are not dangerous. Therefore, if you have a nonproductive (dry) cough accompanied by a runny or stuffed-up nose, a sore throat, and sneezing, you have all the classic symptoms of a common cold, and you should just let it run its course.

The following therapies may ease the discomfort of an acute or chronic respiratory infection, but they will not treat the infection itself. It's best to use cough remedies for no longer than seven to 10 days and preferably only for temporary relief from nighttime coughing.

Acupressure

Sometimes a coughing fit can make the muscles in the upper back contract or go into spasm. To relieve the pain this causes, apply pressure to Lung 5 *(opposite)*.

Herbal Therapies

A wide variety of herbs act as stimulating or relaxing expectorants that help the body remove excess mucus from the airways. Stimulating expectorants increase the quantity of and then liquefy viscous sputum so it can be cleared out by coughing. Relaxing expectorants loosen the sputum and are soothing if you have a dry, irritating cough.

Since most herbal traditions have remedies for specific types of coughs, you might want to check the many possibilities with an herbalist. However, a basic herbal tea for cough that can be taken several times a day for three days consists of 2 parts **coltsfoot** (*Tussilago farfara*), 2 parts **marsh mallow** (*Althaea officinalis*), 2 parts **hyssop** (*Hyssopus officinalis*), 1 part aniseed (*Pimpinella anisum*), and 1 part **licorice** (*Glycyrrhiza glabra*). Add to 1 cup boiling water, steep for 20 minutes, and drink while hot.

There are many good Chinese herbal cough medicines available in Asian food stores. Among them are Fritillaria and Loquat Cough Mixture, King To's Natural Herb Loquat Flavored Syrup, and *San She Dan Chuan Bei Ye.*

■ Homeopathy

Homeopaths recommend different remedies and dosage schedules for the beginning and later stages of various types of coughs. For relief of early symptoms, take one dose four times a day; for relief of persistent symptoms, take one dose twice a day for four days. If a dry cough comes on suddenly with fever and restlessness, try **Aconite** (12c). If you are often thirsty and have painful bouts of dry coughs that intensify with the slightest movement, try **Bryonia** (12c). If your throat tickles and you get violent coughing fits whenever you lie down, try *Drosera* (12c). If the slightest draft of cool air initiates a tickling cough, take *Rumex crispus* (12c). If your cough is accompanied by hoarseness, difficulty in breathing, and considerable rattling in the chest, take *Antimonium tartaricum* (12c), which is particularly good for a well-established, productive cough.

■ Nutrition and Diet

The best thing to do for a cough is to drink plenty of liquids; usually this means four to six large glasses a day. A large intake of fluids will loosen the mucus and make coughing it up easier. Warm liquids, or just plain water, are best for this purpose. Try to avoid caffeinated or alcoholic beverages, which are diuretics that cause you to lose more liquid than you take in.

Most health professionals agree that you might speed recovery by drinking fresh fruit and vegetable juices. Some practitioners recommend **vitamin C** supplements; others consider a well-balanced diet just as effective.

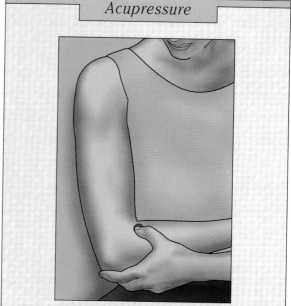

Acupressure

Lung 5 • *Pressing this point may help ease coughing spasms. Bend your right elbow and make a fist; place your left thumb on the outside crease of the elbow alongside the taut tendon. Press firmly for one minute, and repeat on the other arm. Do three times.*

Home Remedies

Besides drinking plenty of liquids, including herbal teas, rubbing your throat and chest with essential oil of **eucalyptus globulus** (*E. globulus*) or **myrrh** (*Commiphora molmol*) may give you relief. A simple rub might help you breathe more easily, cough less, and get a good night's sleep.

Another way to reduce persistent night coughing is to sleep with the head of your bed raised six to eight inches. This prevents the pooling of secretions and the return of the irritating acidic contents from your stomach to your esophagus, which you may be breathing in *(see Sore Throat).* Try to avoid caffeine and peppermint.

You can make an effective expectorant with organic honey and a large onion. Slice the onion into rings, place in a deep bowl, cover with honey, and let stand 10 to 12 hours. Strain and take a tablespoon of this mixture four or five times a day. ■

D

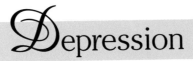
Depression

Symptoms

With major depression, you may experience four or more of the following:

- Persistent sadness, pessimism.
- Feelings of worthlessness, helplessness, hopelessness, or guilt.
- Loss of interest or pleasure in usual activities, including sex.
- Difficulty concentrating.
- Insomnia or oversleeping.
- Weight gain or loss.
- Fatigue, lack of energy.
- Anxiety, agitation, irritability.
- Thoughts of suicide or death.
- Slow speech; slow movements.

In children and adolescents:

- Insomnia, fatigue, headache, stomachache, dizziness.
- Apathy, social withdrawal, weight gain or loss.
- Drug or alcohol abuse, a drop in school performance, difficulty concentrating.
- Isolation from family and friends.

For dysthymia (minor but chronic depression), your symptoms will be less intense, fewer in number, but longer lasting.

Call Your Doctor If

- you or your child has suicidal thoughts, or has other signs of either major depression or dysthymia; professional help is available.

CAUTION

There is a distinct difference between feeling "depressed" and having a depressive illness. If you have low spirits for a while, don't be concerned. However, if you feel you can't lift yourself out of your misery, you should seek professional help.

Almost all of us feel low sometimes, usually because of a disturbing event in our lives. But ongoing depression—or suffering a period of what is known as major depression—is a serious condition that can lead to an inability to function or may even lead to suicide. Sufferers experience not only a depressed mood but also more harmful symptoms, including lack of interest in their usual activities, extreme fatigue, sleep problems, or feelings of guilt and helplessness. They are more likely to lose touch with reality, occasionally even having delusions or hallucinations.

Major depression often goes undiagnosed because it is confused with the normal low feelings that may arise because of a specific life situation. Also of concern is minor but chronic depression, also known as dysthymia, which can last two years or more. Although the exact causes are unknown, researchers currently believe that both forms are caused by a malfunction of the brain's neurotransmitters, chemicals (particularly norepinephrine and serotonin) that modulate moods.

Treatment Options

Treatment for depression varies according to the cause of the condition and its severity. Conventional methods include psychotherapy, antidepressant drugs, and electroconvulsive therapy. Alternative therapies are particularly effective for minor depression, but for more serious depressions they should be considered as complementary treatments, not replacements for conventional methods. Major or chronic depression should be treated by a psychiatrist.

In addition to the remedies mentioned below, you may want to consider acupressure or acupuncture, which may be helpful in relieving some symptoms; see a qualified, experienced practitioner. Massage, which is both soothing and energizing and enlivens the body, may also help. Try it once a week, if possible.

■ Aromatherapy

Aromatherapy may ease mental fatigue and help with sleep. The essential oils that may benefit depression are basil, **clary sage** (Salvia sclarea), jasmine, rose, and **German chamomile** (Matricaria recutita). The oil may be placed in a bowl of steaming

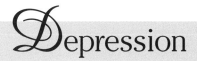Depression

water (2 or 3 drops), in a bath (5 or 6 drops), or on the edge of your pillow (1 or 2 drops).

Exercise

Physical activity should be a part of any therapy for depression; it improves blood flow to the brain, elevates mood, and relieves stress. Even if used alone, exercise can often bring startling results. Studies show that jogging for 30 minutes three times a week can be as effective as psychotherapy in treating depression. Pick an exercise you like and do it daily, if possible. Any exercise is fine; the more energetic and aerobic, the better.

Herbal Therapies

An experienced herbalist will recommend a particular combination of herbs tailored to your specific symptoms. For a general prescription for depression, one suggestion is 2 parts *St.-John's-wort (Hypericum perforatum),* 1 part oat *(Avena sativa)* straw, 1 part *lavender (Lavandula officinalis),* and 1 part *mugwort (Artemisia vulgaris) leaf.* Take 5 ml of the tincture three times a day for at least one month. St.-John's-wort, taken in any of its forms, is a traditional depression remedy in Europe. However, some herbalists report that its effects are unpredictable: Sometimes the herb gets remarkable results, other times it has no effect at all.

A combination of several Chinese and Western herbs known as Aspiration is believed to help lift depression. The formula addresses physical symptoms as well as psychological ones, including loss of appetite, chest constriction, and constipation. It is most effective when taken in conjunction with regular aerobic exercise, daily practice of a relaxation technique, and a good diet. Another Chinese herbal formula, Gather Vitality, may help with insomnia or oversleeping, aching limbs, and fatigue. Consult a practitioner of Chinese medicine.

Mind/Body Medicine

Many mind/body practices are helpful with depression. Music and dance can lift the spirits and energize the body. Meditation and relaxation techniques, such as progressive muscle relaxation, both stimulate and relax. Other choices include transcendental meditation and the exercise tech-

niques of yoga, t'ai chi, and qigong. Choose one or two that suit you and practice daily.

Anecdotal evidence suggests that EEG (brainwave) biofeedback is effective in reducing the intensity of all types of depression. The number of training sessions depends on the severity of the depression; dysthymia may average 20 sessions, and major depression may need 30 to 60.

Nutrition and Diet

Because depressive symptoms are exacerbated by nutritional deficiencies, good nutrition is important. Increase your intake of healthful foods such as whole-grain cereals, lean meats, fruits and vegetables, fish, and low-fat dairy products. It's very important to avoid alcohol, but also stay away from junk food, sugar, aspartame, and caffeine, which give you a sudden spurt of energy or a high feeling but then bring you down.

Recent clinical studies strongly suggest that *vitamin B complex* and *folic acid* (400 mcg daily) are useful in treating depression. The antioxidant *selenium* (100 mcg daily) was shown to have a mood-elevating effect when taken in regions where food is deficient in selenium. And many European studies show that the amino acid supplement L-tryptophan, known to increase the synthesis of serotonin, is of value in relieving depression. Although L-tryptophan, which is the amino acid tryptophan in its synthetic form, is no longer available in the U.S., tryptophan can be found in certain foods, such as milk, turkey, chicken, fish, cooked dried beans and peas, brewer's yeast, peanut butter, nuts, and soybeans. Eat plenty of these foods together with a carbohydrate (potatoes, pasta, rice), which will ease the brain's uptake of tryptophan.

Prevention

Some forms of depression may not be preventable, since current theory suggests that they may be triggered by neurochemical malfunctioning in the brain. However, there is good evidence that a low mood may often be alleviated or prevented by good health habits. Proper diet, exercise, vacations, no overwork, and making time to do things you enjoy all help keep the blues at bay.

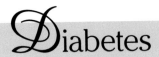iabetes

Symptoms

- Excessive thirst.

- Increased appetite.

- Increased urination (sometimes as often as every hour).

- Weight loss.

- Fatigue.

- Nausea, possibly vomiting.

- Blurred vision.

- In women, frequent vaginal infections and, possibly, the cessation of menstruation.

- In men, impotence.

- In men and women, yeast infections.

Call Your Doctor If

- you develop any of the above symptoms; diabetes requires medical intervention.

- you feel nauseated, weak, and excessively thirsty; are urinating very frequently; have abdominal pain; and are breathing more deeply and rapidly than normal—perhaps with sweet breath that smells like nail polish remover. You may need immediate medical attention for ketoacidosis.

- you feel weak or faint; are experiencing a rapid heartbeat, trembling, and excessive sweating; and feel irritable, hungry, or suddenly drowsy. You could be developing hypoglycemia and may need to eat or drink something quickly to avoid more serious complications.

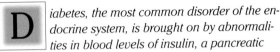

iabetes, the most common disorder of the endocrine system, is brought on by abnormalities in blood levels of insulin, a pancreatic hormone that helps your system convert blood glucose, or blood sugar, into energy. Type I diabetes—sometimes called insulin-dependent diabetes mellitus (IDDM) or juvenile, or juvenile-onset, diabetes—results from a shortage of insulin. Type II diabetes—also known as non-insulin-dependent diabetes mellitus (NIDDM) or adult-onset, or stable, diabetes—results from the body's inability to process the hormone effectively. About 90 percent of all diabetics have this form.

Diabetics need to keep an eye on their blood sugar levels every day to prevent an attack of hypoglycemia, in which available levels of blood sugar are too low to fulfill the body's energy needs. Hyperglycemia, or high blood sugar, can bring about a serious diabetic condition that is known as ketoacidosis, in which the blood becomes increasingly acidic from the accumulation of toxic by-products called ketones. These compounds are produced as the body breaks down fat for energy.

People with diabetes stand a higher-than-normal chance of developing heart disease and circulatory problems, and a number of them suffer from diabetic neuropathy, which causes a gradual deterioration of portions of the nervous system.

Treatment Options

Since diabetes that is incorrectly treated can be life threatening, you should never try to treat the disease without the help of a doctor. All diabetics should be under a physician's care and should always discuss any possible treatments thoroughly with the doctor.

■ Exercise

In laboratory tests, exercise has been shown to increase the tissue levels of **chromium,** which the body uses to regulate blood glucose and cholesterol levels. For Type I and Type II diabetics, exercise has also been found to increase the body's ability to use available insulin so that fewer insulin injections are needed. WARNING: If you have Type I diabetes, keep in mind that exercise lowers your blood glucose; you should have a carbohydrate snack before exercising, and eat or drink again if you experience the warning symptoms of a hypoglycemic attack.

Although diabetics can benefit from moderate exercise, you should check with your doctor before engaging in weightlifting or other forms of exertion that involve pushing or pulling very heavy objects; these activities raise blood pressure and may aggravate any eye problems that stem from diabetes.

■ Herbal Therapies

Check with a practitioner to make sure herbs are appropriate for your condition. Remember: If you need insulin to manage your diabetes, there is no herbal substitute for the hormone.

Diabetics in one study who ate crackers made from the powdered form of **burdock** (Arctium lappa) after a starchy meal had a lowered incidence of hyperglycemia. A topical cream made with **cayenne** (Capsicum annuum) may relieve the pain associated with peripheral neuropathy, which is a type of diabetic neuropathy.

Supplementing the diet with fenugreek (Trigonella foenum-graecum) seeds has been shown in clinical and experimental studies to reduce blood glucose and insulin levels while lowering blood cholesterol levels. **Garlic** (Allium sativum) may lower blood pressure as well as levels of cholesterol.

Ginkgo (Ginkgo biloba) extracts can increase blood flow to small capillaries and the small blood vessels that supply the brain. For diabetics, ginkgo may prove helpful by increasing circulation in the legs; such circulation problems are a major difficulty for diabetics and lead to many amputations.

Onion (Allium cepa) may free up insulin to help metabolize glucose in the blood, thus lowering blood glucose levels. Both raw and boiled onion extracts have been found to have this effect. Onion is also considered beneficial in maintaining a healthy cardiovascular system.

Chinese herbal medicines, including **Asian ginseng** (Panax ginseng), are frequently used to alleviate some symptoms of diabetes. Ginseng is often used in combination with other Chinese herbs; consult a practitioner for a comprehensive treatment plan.

■ Mind/Body Medicine

Any sort of practice that will lower your stress level, such as biofeedback, meditation, hypnotherapy, or other relaxation techniques, may help control your blood sugar.

■ Nutrition and Diet

The high-carbohydrate, high-plant-fiber (HCF) diet, an alternative to the diet plan usually recommended by doctors, calls for people with diabetes to follow these daily guidelines in planning their meals: Eat 70 to 75 percent complex carbohydrates, 15 to 20 percent proteins, and only 5 to 10 percent fats. The HCF diet is said to boost insulin's ability to promote blood glucose as an energy source, improve cholesterol levels, reduce the incidence of hyperglycemia and hypoglycemia, and help with weight loss for Type II diabetics. A modified version of the HCF diet further restricts what foods may be eaten but increases the allowable amount of complex carbohydrates.

Okra and peas can help stabilize blood sugar levels and provide fiber in a diet high in complex carbohydrates. Research suggests that cinnamon can lower insulin requirements in Type II diabetics; seasoning your food with as much as ¼ tsp at every meal may help regulate blood sugar levels.

Diabetics should avoid sugar, as it can worsen all of the effects of diabetes. Nutritionists also emphasize the importance of certain vitamins and minerals, including the following: **vitamins B₆, B₁₂,** and **C,** and **manganese, zinc, potassium,** and **copper.** Consult your practitioner to determine proper dosages.

Prevention

Because of the apparent link between obesity and Type II diabetes, you can reduce your chances of developing the disease by slimming down if you are overweight. This is especially true if diabetes runs in your family.

A good exercise program and a nutritionally balanced diet can greatly limit the effects of both Type I and Type II diabetes. If you smoke, quit; smoking can significantly increase the risk of heart disease, particularly for diabetics. ■

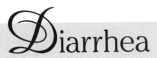Diarrhea

Symptoms

- Frequent or watery stools, possibly with abdominal cramping, may be a result of overeating fiber-rich foods or drinking too much coffee.

- Recurrent stools with mucus, possibly accompanied by lower abdominal pain that worsens with eating or stress; you may have irritable bowel syndrome.

- A sudden attack of frequent, watery stools that may be bloody, possibly accompanied by nausea, fever, and abdominal cramping. You may have a case of gastroenteritis.

Call Your Doctor If

- you have recurrent, foul-smelling stools that are pale or yellowish; stomach cramps; weakness. These are signs of malabsorption.

- you have watery bowel movements accompanied by nervousness, insomnia, or excessive sweating. You may have diabetes or a thyroid problem.

- you have loose stools, possibly with visible blood; these are signs of various disorders, including colorectal cancer.

- you have episodes of frequent, watery stools accompanied by coughing, wheezing, and a flushed face; these symptoms may be an indication of a carcinoid tumor (a growth in the intestine that could be benign or malignant).

- you have watery stools that may be black; abdominal pain; and possibly, bright red bleeding; you could have diverticulitis. Call your doctor today to obtain a proper diagnosis.

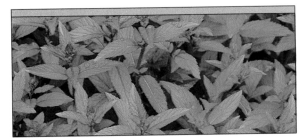

Peppermint • *Peppermint's medicinal value comes from its primary chemical constituent, menthol, a natural antispasmodic. A cup of peppermint tea helps to relax the muscles lining the digestive tract, thereby relieving the spasms that may accompany diarrhea.*

D iarrhea, a general term used to describe the frequent passage of loose, watery stools, is the body's way of cleaning out the digestive system—a process that usually occurs with unpleasant efficiency and some abdominal pain. Not many people make it through life without suffering at least one or two bouts of diarrhea.

Technically speaking, diarrhea is not a disease itself but rather a symptom of some other problem. The culprit can be as simple as a spicy meal or as serious as colorectal cancer. One of the most common forms is traveler's diarrhea, a variety of gastroenteritis brought on by the ingestion of food or water that has been contaminated by microorganisms as a result of improper handling. Many North Americans who have visited Latin America, the Middle East, Africa, or Asia are all too familiar with this condition, which is marked by four or five watery stools per day, abdominal cramps, nausea, and fever.

Stress or depression can lead to a type known as emotion-induced diarrhea. Diarrhea can also be caused by malabsorption—a digestive disorder in which fats and nutrients are not properly absorbed by the intestines—or by any number of other conditions, including diverticulitis, Crohn's disease, colitis, and diabetes.

In most cases of diarrhea, symptoms clear up within a few days. However, if your pain is severe or prolonged; if your stool contains blood, pus, or mucus; or if you show signs of dehydration (constant thirst, sunken eyeballs, dry lips), you should see a doctor immediately.

Treatment Options

Ayurvedic Medicine

An Ayurvedic physician may recommend a combined formula such as *Diarex* or *Bonnisan,* depending on the nature of the problem. Acute diarrhea may respond to a blending of equal parts yogurt and water with $\frac{1}{8}$ tsp of fresh ginger. Chronic cases may respond to a powder of the fruit of beleric myrobalan.

Chinese Medicine

Many people find relief from diarrhea through acupuncture and specific combinations of Chinese herbs. Consult a qualified practitioner for treatment tailored to your specific needs.

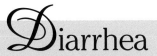

Diarrhea

Exercise

Stress can bring on a case of diarrhea or contribute to its intensity. Regular physical activity helps reduce stress.

Herbal Therapies

Taken three times daily, **peppermint** *(Mentha piperita)* or **chamomile** *(Matricaria recutita)* tea may ease intestinal spasms and cramps. You can also buy aloe vera juice: Sip half a cup slowly, twice a day.

Homeopathy

Several homeopathic remedies are used to treat diarrhea; you can choose a remedy by the accompanying symptoms:

- For burning pain when passing stools, **Arsenicum album** (12x).
- For abdominal pain, *Colocynthis* (12x).
- For watery, painless stools, **Phosphorus** (12x).

Hydrotherapy

Practitioners rely on a variety of hydrotherapy techniques for treating diarrhea. These include a heating compress to the abdomen and a 15-minute hot fomentation twice daily. Charcoal capsules are also used: Take two capsules with eight ounces of water after each bout of diarrhea.

Another common remedy is a hot half bath: After a bath in very warm water followed by a cold friction rub or shower, you are put in bed, wrapped in blankets, and allowed to sweat for 30 minutes to an hour. During the procedure, the practitioner monitors your temperature and makes sure you have plenty of water to drink.

Massage

Administered by a skilled practitioner, gentle massage to the midsection of the body can help improve intestinal activity and soothe the discomfort of diarrhea. A petrissage technique that is safe to use on the abdomen is the hand-on-hand stroke. See the Gallery of Massage Techniques, pages 124-129.

Nutrition and Diet

The best advice for diarrhea sufferers is to drink plenty of clear liquids, even if you're not thirsty.

Slightly salty or sweet drinks—broths, sweetened tea, ginger ale, and soda, for example—are particularly helpful. Stay away from citrus drinks and milk or milk products. Also avoid foods that are high in fiber, such as grains and most fruits. When your condition starts to improve, ease your way back into a normal diet by concentrating on foods that are easily digestible, such as bland cereal, gelatin, soft-boiled eggs, white rice, applesauce, and cooked carrots.

To help replace vital stores of potassium lost to diarrhea, many nutritionists recommend ripe bananas. You can make your own nourishing potassium broth at home. In a big pot of water, simmer 2 cups chopped carrots and 2 cups chopped potatoes for 45 minutes. Drink 2 to 3 cups of the liquid each day. This broth rehydrates the body, replaces lost minerals, and will help you feel better faster.

Sound Therapy

Music and relaxation, a music therapy program in which clients practice stress-reduction techniques to music until the sound itself triggers the relaxation response, can help relieve diarrhea linked to stress or tension.

Sound-healing approaches include projecting sound into the body and toning; the sound vibrations created during these treatments are said to positively affect the body's internal energy balance.

Prevention

When traveling to developing countries, be careful about what you eat and drink. Don't eat foods that are raw or unpeeled, and don't drink water from a tap, well, or stream unless you know it's been sterilized. Better to play it safe and drink only bottled beverages—served without ice. Remember that harmful bacteria trapped in ice will be released into your glass when the ice melts. Keep the following homeopathic remedies in your travel bag in case you do get a case of Montezuma's revenge:

- **Arsenicum album** (12x) for burning diarrhea.
- **Nux vomica** (12x) for painful, cramping diarrhea from bad food or water.
- **Phosphorus** (12x) for painless diarrhea that is exhausting. ■

*E*arache
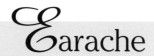

Symptoms

- Pain in the ear that is either sharp and sudden or dull and throbbing, accompanied by fever, nasal congestion, and muffled hearing, may indicate otitis media (middle ear infection). A child with otitis media may tug at the ear and cry when lying down at night.

- Itching in the ear, later with sharp or dull pain that worsens when you pull on the earlobe, may indicate swimmer's ear. There may also be a yellowish discharge, and possibly fever and temporary hearing loss.

- Sudden ear pain, usually after an injury or infection, may indicate a ruptured eardrum. There may also be bleeding or pus discharge from the ear, dizziness, ringing in the ear, or partial hearing loss.

Call Your Doctor If

- body temperature rises above 101°F or 102°F; a fever signals the possibility of a more serious infection requiring medical attention.

- you or your child frequently develops otitis media; repeated bouts with the disorder can lead to hearing loss or more serious infections.

- you suspect that you or your child has hearing problems; an infection may be affecting the ability to hear.

- you suspect that your young child has otitis media.

- you suspect you have a ruptured eardrum; you may need antibiotics or in some cases surgery.

P *ain in the ear can indicate any of a number of conditions, from excessive earwax to TMJ syndrome (pages 358-359). But it is most often the result of otitis media, or infection of the middle ear. Earache is also often caused by swimmer's ear—inflammation and possibly infection of the outer ear canal.*

Treatment Options

Most treatments try to rid the ear of infection or provide relief while the infection clears up on its own. Controversy surrounds the use of antibiotics. For example, research indicates that 80 percent of otitis media cases are viral in origin and therefore will not respond to antibiotics. But many doctors, particularly in the U.S., are concerned that without antibiotics, bacteria lurking inside the middle ear can grow out of control, possibly causing a serious complication such as hearing loss or mastoiditis. To be on the safe side, many American physicians treat all otitis media cases as if bacteria were present.

Aromatherapy
Lavender (*Lavandula angustifolia*) oil may help reduce inflammation and pain. For swimmer's ear, gently rub the area around the outer ear with 3 to 5 drops of lavender oil diluted in 1 tsp vegetable oil.

Ayurvedic Medicine
To open and drain the Eustachian tubes, Ayurvedic physicians massage the lymph nodes outside the ears. The massage is complemented with a drink made with the herb amala, a source of vitamin C.

Herbal Therapy
Mullein (*Verbascum thapsus*) oil, which has anti-inflammatory properties, may help soothe and heal an inflamed ear canal. Put 1 to 3 drops in the infected ear every three hours. Because ear-drop solutions cannot penetrate the middle ear, they should be reserved for outer ear infections. CAUTION: Do not use ear drops if there's a chance that the eardrum is ruptured.

Homeopathy
In the early stages of an ear infection with sudden onset and feverish restlessness, use **Aconite** (30c).

$\mathscr{E}$arache

For children with otitis media who are very irritable and in great pain, try **Chamomilla** (30c). When a child is weepy, clingy, feels better in the open air, and has a yellowish green discharge from the nose, use **Pulsatilla** (30c) every four to six hours. If the pain is severe, take 30c every half-hour until the pain abates, then take it every four to six hours.

■ Nutrition and Diet

The following supplements will help fight a viral infection:

- **Vitamin C.** Daily dosage: Your child's age times 500 mg. (WARNING: High doses of vitamin C can cause diarrhea; spread the dose out evenly during the day. Many people cannot tolerate more than 1,000 mg every two hours.)
- **Zinc.** Daily dosage: Your age times 2.5 mg. Do not take more than 50 mg per day without consulting a nutritionist.
- Bioflavonoids. Daily dosage: Your child's age times 50 mg, with 250 mg as the maximum.

■ Osteopathy

Consult an osteopathic practitioner for therapies, such as craniosacral manipulative therapy, that may help drainage of the Eustachian tubes.

Home Remedies

- Warmth, perhaps provided by a hot compress, relieves the symptoms of ear infection. Hot footbaths and inhalations of steam may also help.
- Gargling with salt water helps soothe an irritated throat and clear the Eustachian tubes.
- For swimmer's ear, make sure you keep the infected ear canal dry during the healing process, even while showering. Use earplugs or a shower cap.
- Some people find relief with over-the-counter nasal sprays, which act as decongestants. Used for more than three days, however, sprays can become habit forming and lead to rebound congestion, or a worsening of your condition.

Prevention

Because bottle-fed babies are more likely to get otitis media, it is better to breast-feed your infant, if possible, to prevent ear infections. (If you must bottle-feed, never lay your baby down and prop the bottle up.) Also, because allergies can cause otitis media, remove as many environmental pollutants from your home as you can, including dust, cleaning fluid and solvents, and tobacco smoke.

Food allergies may play a role in otitis media, so if you or your child is susceptible to the disease, try cutting back on milk, wheat products, corn products, and food additives, as these tend to be more allergenic than other foods. ■

Middle Ear Infection

Excess fluid in the middle ear normally drains harmlessly into the throat via the Eustachian tube. But if this tiny conduit becomes infected—perhaps by the same organisms that bring on a cold or the flu—it can swell shut, trapping fluid in the middle ear and promoting further infection. This fluid buildup causes painful pressure that, without proper treatment, can eventually burst the eardrum.

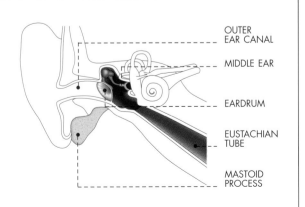

OUTER EAR CANAL

MIDDLE EAR

EARDRUM

EUSTACHIAN TUBE

MASTOID PROCESS

*E*ndometriosis

Symptoms

- Sharp abdominal pains before, during, or just after menstrual periods.

- Sharp abdominal pain during intercourse.

- Menstrual periods that are abnormally heavy, especially if they produce large clots and last more than seven days.

- Infertility.

Call Your Doctor If

- you suspect you are suffering from endometriosis. It is essential that you see a doctor for a proper diagnosis, which can be made only by laparoscopy—visual examination with a slim, lighted instrument that is inserted into the abdominal cavity through a small incision.

N ormally, the endometrium, the tissue lining a woman's uterus, is found only in the uterus. However, in a woman with endometriosis, microscopic bits of this tissue migrate outside the uterus, become implanted on other organs and tissues, and grow there. These lesions, or areas of abnormal tissue, usually develop within the abdominal cavity, but in rare cases they can affect organs such as the lungs.

Like the endometrium itself, the transplanted tissue responds to the hormones estrogen and progesterone by thickening and then bleeding every month. But because the transplanted tissue is embedded in other tissue, the blood it produces cannot escape and ends up irritating the surrounding tissue, causing the formation of cysts, scars, and adhesions.

Treatment Options

Endometriosis can be managed, but symptoms often return when treatment is stopped. Menopause usually ends the symptoms, but in women who take estrogen during and after menopause, symptoms may continue.

Most alternative remedies aim at relieving symptoms. But since they tend not to affect lesions directly, they are sometimes less effective than

Yoga

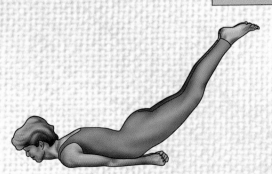

Locust • To tone the muscles in the pelvic area, lie on your stomach with your arms under your body. Squeeze your buttocks as you press down with your arms. While inhaling, raise your legs, keeping them straight as you press outward through the toes and heels. Hold for 15 seconds, exhale and release. Do once or twice a day.

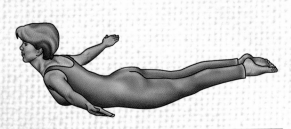

Boat • This exercise strengthens the spine and conditions the pelvic area. Lying on your stomach, inhale and lift your head, chest, arms, and legs off the floor. Stretch your arms behind you and hold the position for 15 to 20 seconds, then exhale and relax back onto the floor. Do once or twice a day.

Endometriosis

Endometrial Tissue

Special tissue called endometrium is flushed out of the uterus as part of the natural menstrual process. If fragments of endometrial tissue become implanted on other organs in the pelvic cavity, they can cause pain and abnormal bleeding. Left untreated, the tissue growths and the blood they produce can eventually form cysts that disrupt the function of the reproductive organs.

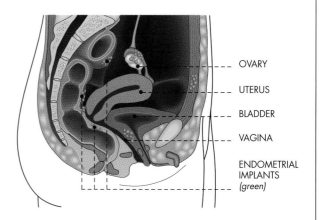

- - - OVARY
- - - UTERUS
- - - BLADDER
- - - VAGINA
ENDOMETRIAL IMPLANTS *(green)*

conventional treatment, which may involve hormone therapy or, in severe cases, surgery.

▓ Acupressure

You may be able to alleviate cramping by applying pressure to Spleen 6, located on the inside of the leg two inches above the ankle. Do not use this point if you are pregnant.

▓ Herbal Therapies

Some herbal formulas may relieve pain. **Skullcap** *(Scutellaria lateriflora)*, **black cohosh** *(Cimicifuga racemosa)*, and **wild yam** *(Dioscorea villosa)* may address underlying hormonal problems. **Valerian** *(Valeriana officinalis)* may help you relax, but do not take it for longer than a month unless directed by your practitioner. Life root *(Senecio aureus)* and black cohosh enhance the health of pelvic organs. Black haw *(Viburnum prunifolium)* and cramp bark *(Viburnum opulus)* are useful for cramping. Consult a medical herbalist for specific formulas.

▓ Nutrition and Diet

The body contains hormonelike substances called prostaglandins that, among other things, play a role in muscle contractions and thus contribute to menstrual cramping. Eating foods rich in natural antiprostaglandins—including mackerel, sardines, salmon, and cod—may therefore help reduce symptoms. You may choose to take these nutrients

in the form of fish-oil supplements and cod-liver oil.

A daily multivitamin-multimineral supplement containing **vitamin B complex** (50 to 100 mg), **vitamin E** (400 to 600 IU), **calcium** (1,000 mg), and **magnesium** (400 to 600 mg) may help balance estrogen and prostaglandin levels and reduce menstrual cramps. To relieve cramping, avoid caffeinated and decaffeinated beverages and white sugar.

Home Remedies

- Apply a heating pad or moist heat, and drink warm beverages to help relax cramping muscles. Exercise moderately to boost production of endorphins, your body's natural painkillers.
- To ease tension, drink herbal teas made with herbs such as **chamomile** *(Matricaria recutita)* and **passionflower** *(Passiflora incarnata)*.

Prevention

- Avoid exposure to dioxin, which recent evidence has shown may play a role in causing some instances of endometriosis.
- If you use tampons, change them frequently, especially when your flow is heavy, and consider discontinuing tampons or alternating them with sanitary napkins; these measures may help prevent menstrual flow from backing up—one theory for the cause of endometriosis. ■

Fever and Chills

Symptoms

■ A higher-than-normal body temperature (usually above 98.6°F), with or without other symptoms; possibly chills, especially while the fever is climbing.

■ Fever (102°F to 106°F) that comes on abruptly, possibly accompanied by chills, headache, malaise, diarrhea, runny nose, dry cough, sore throat, or aches in muscles or joints. You may have the flu or some other viral infection.

■ Fever after several hours in the heat; you could have heat exhaustion.

Call Your Doctor If

■ you have fever with a severe headache and a stiff neck, possibly accompanied by nausea, vomiting, sensitivity to light, drowsiness, or confusion. These are signs of meningitis.

■ a baby or child has fever with convulsions, shaking, and/or a blue color to the face. Call 911 or your emergency number immediately.

■ a child under age 12 has fever along with earache, rash, swollen jaw, noisy breathing, runny nose, red eyes, or dry cough. The problem could be an ear infection, croup, measles, German measles, chickenpox, or mumps.

■ you have fever accompanied by throbbing face pain, especially when a tooth is touched. You probably have a tooth abscess; call your dentist now for emergency treatment. *(See Toothache, pages 362-363.)*

I t may be difficult to appreciate the benefits when your body feels like it's on fire, but fever is a remarkable and extremely valuable defense mechanism. Fever itself is not an illness; it's a symptom of one. An elevated temperature is one of the first indications that foreign invaders have entered your body and that your immune system is responding to the threat. Perhaps more important is the direct role fever plays in battling these intruders. By turning up the heat, the body actually slows the growth of disease-causing bacteria and viruses, rendering them more vulnerable to defender cells of the immune system.

A fever is often preceded by chills or a sensation of overwhelming coldness. Although the two would seem to have contrasting effects, fever and chills are actually part of the same process. When the body comes under attack, blood vessels constrict and retreat inward to prevent heat loss. The skin begins to feel colder, prompting the body to fire up its heat-generating mechanism—shivering. This rapid, involuntary muscle movement quickly warms you up.

Although fever is usually the result of an infection, it can also be brought on by a number of other conditions. Fever is often a symptom of dehydration or anxiety, for example, and it can accompany such serious disorders as nerve disease and cancer. But just because you have a fever doesn't always mean there's something wrong with you. In healthy people, vigorous exercise can raise the body temperature well above normal.

Treatment Options

■ Acupressure

Applying pressure to a number of points is often recommended for fever, chills, and other symptoms that may accompany the flu; Spleen 6 and Stomach 36 are recommended for stimulating natural resistance to colds and flu *(see the Gallery of Acupressure Techniques, pages 18-31, for the locations of these points).* Large Intestine 11 *(opposite)* may help fight fever and strengthen your immune system.

■ Ayurvedic Medicine

An Ayurvedic physician may recommend one of the following remedies, depending on the exact nature of your constitution: for general fever and

ℱever and Chills

chills, a powder or milk decoction of the root of *shatavari* or an infusion or powder of Indian basil; for fever and colds without chills, an infusion or powder of mint; for general fever, solidified starch from a decoction of *guduchi*.

Flower Remedy

The Bach **Rescue Remedy** is often recommended for fever. Consult a naturopath or other practitioner familiar with flower remedies.

Herbal Therapies

For an herbal approach to stimulating your immune system, try taking ½ tsp each of tincture of **goldenseal** (*Hydrastis canadensis*) and **echinacea** (*Echinacea* spp.) twice a day. An infusion of **boneset** (*Eupatorium perfoliatum*) may relieve aches and fever: Simmer 1 cup boiling water with 2 tsp of the herb for 10 to 15 minutes; drink a cupful every hour, as hot as you can stand it. To combat chills, try taking 30 drops of **yarrow** (*Achillea millefolium*) or elder (*Sambucus nigra*) flower tincture every four hours until your chills are gone.

Homeopathy

Homeopathic remedies are particularly good for fevers; homeopathic physicians find them more effective than conventional medications such as aspirin, acetaminophen, or ibuprofen. A practitioner might recommend the following: for a mild or moderate fever, **Ferrum phosphoricum;** for acute fever, **Aconite** or **Belladonna;** for fever with extreme chills, **Bryonia.**

Hydrotherapy

Most hydrotherapists would not try to reduce a slight fever (between 99°F and 102°F) and in some cases might even attempt to encourage or increase the fever to enhance its germ-fighting abilities. Consult a healthcare practitioner familiar with hydrotherapy techniques.

To lower a fever, a hydrotherapist might recommend a wet sheet pack: Place two blankets on a bed, leaving a substantial portion of each blanket hanging over the sides. Spread a wet, wrung-out cotton sheet on the bed and have the patient lie on it. Wrap the sheet first around the trunk and legs,

then the arms; fold the sheet under at the feet to cover them completely. Next, cover the patient with a blanket, using a towel at the neck and shoulders to prevent draft. The sheet pack should remain in place for 12 to 20 minutes. Repeat the application once if necessary.

Nutrition and Diet

Fever can leave you exhausted, so it's important to rebuild your body's defenses through a nutritious diet once the storm has passed. When your temperature returns to normal, be sure to eat plenty of vegetables, fruits, proteins, and whole-grain cereals.

Home Remedies

- Avoid dehydration by drinking plenty of fluids, including water, tea, fruit juice, and broth.
- Suck on cubes of ice or frozen fruit juice.
- Take a warm bath; water that is too cool can make you shiver, possibly raising your body temperature even more. Sponging off with water can also help, but be careful not to get chilled.
- Eat if you feel hungry, but don't force it. The old myth about starving a fever is just that—a myth.

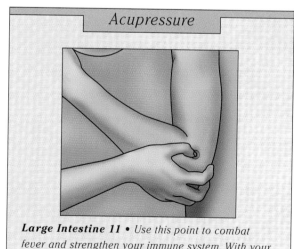

Acupressure

Large Intestine 11 • *Use this point to combat fever and strengthen your immune system. With your arm bent, use your thumb to press deeply on the outer edge of the elbow crease. Repeat on the other arm.*

F

*F*lu

Symptoms

- Fever—usually between 101°F and 102°F, but occasionally as high as 106°F—sometimes alternating with chills.

- Sore throat.

- Dry, hacking cough.

- Aching muscles.

- General fatigue and weakness.

- Nasal congestion, sneezing.

- Headache.

Call Your Doctor If

- you experience any of these symptoms and your immune system is already weakened by cancer, diabetes, AIDS, or other conditions; or if you have a serious illness like chronic heart or kidney disease, impaired breathing, cystic fibrosis, or chronic anemia. You may be at risk for developing serious secondary complications and need to be carefully monitored as long as symptoms last.

- your fever lasts more than three or four days, you become short of breath while resting, or you have chest pain. You may have developed pneumonia.

I nfluenza—commonly shortened to "flu"—is an extremely contagious viral disease that appears most frequently in winter and early spring. The infection spreads through your upper respiratory tract and sometimes goes into your lungs. The virus typically sweeps through large groups of people who share indoor space, such as schools, offices, and nursing homes.

Although both colds and influenza stem from viruses that infect the upper respiratory tract, the symptoms of influenza are more pronounced and its complications more severe. Influenza occurs most commonly in school-age children, but its most severe effects are felt by infants, the elderly, and people with chronic ailments. Specific strains of the disease can be prevented by injections of antibodies in a flu vaccine, but after influenza—or any other viral infection—has started, there is no cure except to let it run its course.

Treatment Options

Alternative therapies may help strengthen your body's ability to fight the virus and can help ease temporary flu symptoms.

Aromatherapy

In flu season, when those around you are coming down with the virus, protect yourself by gargling daily with 1 drop each of the essential oils of **tea tree** (Melaleuca alternifolia) and lemon in a glass of

---

Acupressure

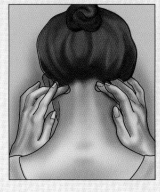

Gall Bladder 20
To help relieve flu symptoms, including headaches and eyestrain, place the tips of your middle fingers in the hollows at the base of your skull, about two inches apart on either side of the spine. Press firmly.

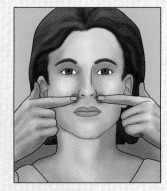

Large Intestine 20
This point can help relieve nasal congestion associated with the flu. Using your index or middle fingers, press hard on the outer edge of the nostrils at the base of the nose.

Flu

warm water; stir well before each mouthful. Do not swallow. If you come down with the flu despite your best preventive efforts, 10 to 20 drops of tea tree in a hot bath may help your immune system fight the viral infection and ease your symptoms. Be sure to use a pure, unadulterated form of tea tree oil; adulterated forms can be irritating to the skin.

If you have a congested nose or chest, add a few drops of essential oils of **eucalyptus globulus** (*E. globulus*) or **peppermint** (*Mentha piperita*) to a steam vaporizer. If you are asthmatic, be cautious the first time you try this; if you have not been exposed to essential oils before, inhaling the vapor may actually precipitate an attack.

■ Herbal Therapies

For an herbal approach to stimulating your immune system, try taking ½ tsp each of tincture of **goldenseal** (*Hydrastis canadensis*) and **echinacea** (*Echinacea* spp.) twice a day. If flu symptoms appear, chew a clove of raw **garlic** (*Allium sativum*) for its antiviral properties, but do not eat raw garlic on an empty stomach.

An infusion of **boneset** (*Eupatorium perfoliatum*) may relieve aches and fever and clear congestion: Simmer 1 cup boiling water with 2 tsp of the herb for 10 to 15 minutes; drink a cupful every hour, as hot as you can stand it. To combat chills, try taking 30 drops of **yarrow** (*Achillea millefolium*) or elder (*Sambucus nigra*) flower tincture every four hours until your chills are gone.

■ Homeopathy

For homeopathic self-care, try one of the following remedies in 6c or 30c dosages every six to eight hours for a day or two. If you don't notice an improvement in your condition after 24 hours, try another homeopathic remedy.

- If you feel tired, weak, and chilled, with a dull headache and stuffy nose, try **Gelsemium.**
- If you feel general achiness with irritability and have a headache that is worse when you move around, and if you are thirsty for cold fluids and have a dry hacking cough, try **Bryonia.**
- If you are restless, chilled, and thirsty, with a dry mouth, hoarse voice, and aching joints, try **Rhus toxicodendron.**

■ Nutrition and Diet

Eat **vitamin C**-rich fresh fruits and vegetables like citrus fruits, Brussels sprouts, and strawberries, or take 1,000 mg of vitamin C every two to three hours when awake. Increase **zinc** intake with lean meats, fish, and whole-grain breads and cereals.

■ Reflexology

To support your respiratory system, press your thumb into the solar plexus/diaphragm area on your foot for a few seconds, or massage the area with your thumb. (*See Reflexology, page 169, for more information on area locations.*)

Home Remedies

- If you have a sore or scratchy throat, try a salt-water gargle. Dissolve 1 tsp salt in 1 pt warm water. Gargle whenever your throat is uncomfortable, but don't swallow the mixture.
- Use a heating pad on body aches.
- When you feel like eating, try bland, starchy foods like dry toast, bananas, applesauce, cottage cheese, boiled rice, rice pudding, cooked cereal, and baked potatoes. These foods provide a gentle transition for your digestive system when you have not been eating regularly.
- Don't drink alcoholic beverages; they leave you dehydrated and can lower your body's ability to fight illness and secondary infection.

Prevention

The most effective preventive measure against influenza is to be inoculated every fall against strains that have developed since the previous outbreak. If you are vaccinated against one or more type A and B strains, you may still come down with flu, but your symptoms are likely to be milder than they would have been had you not had a vaccination.

- Give up smoking and alcohol; both lower your resistance to infection.
- Avoid sleeping in a room with someone who has the flu; the virus is easily spread in the air.
- Wash your hands often to kill viruses you may have picked up by touching contaminated objects like doorknobs or phone receivers. ■

$\mathcal{F}$ood Poisoning

Symptoms

Generally, food poisoning causes some combination of nausea, vomiting, and diarrhea that may or may not be bloody, sometimes with other symptoms.

- Abdominal cramps, diarrhea, and vomiting, starting from one hour to four days after eating tainted food and lasting up to four days, usually indicate bacterial food poisoning.

- Vomiting, diarrhea, abdominal cramps, headaches, and fever and chills, beginning from 12 to 48 hours after eating contaminated food—particularly seafood—usually indicate viral food poisoning.

- Vomiting, diarrhea, sweating, dizziness, tearing in the eyes, excessive salivation, mental confusion, and stomach pain, beginning about 30 minutes after eating contaminated food, are typical indications of chemical food poisoning.

- Partial loss of speech or vision, muscle paralysis from the head down through the body, and vomiting may indicate botulism, a severe but very rare type of bacterial food poisoning.

Call Your Doctor If

- you recognize symptoms of botulism. You need immediate medical treatment for a life-threatening illness.

- you recognize symptoms of chemical food poisoning. You need immediate medical treatment to avoid potential damage to one or more of your vital organs.

- the vomiting or diarrhea is severe and lasts for more than two days. You are at risk of becoming dehydrated, which can be dangerous.

Y ou can get food poisoning after eating food contaminated by viral, bacterial, or chemical agents. Food poisoning causes mild to acute discomfort and may leave you temporarily dehydrated. Mild cases last only a few hours or at worst a day or two, but some types—such as botulism or certain forms of chemical poisoning—are severe and possibly life threatening unless you get medical treatment.

Types of Food Poisoning

Many bacteria can cause food poisoning. People who have a staph infection or are infected with staph bacteria can transmit them to food they are preparing. People who eat or drink contaminated food or water can get traveler's diarrhea, usually caused by the bacterium *E. coli*. Bacteria can contaminate poultry, eggs, and meat, causing salmonella poisoning; though potentially fatal, most cases cause only mild discomfort. Harmful bacteria grow in cooked and raw meat and fish, dairy products, and prepared foods left at room temperature too long; dishes made with mayonnaise are notorious culprits.

Canned goods—especially home-canned produce—can harbor an anaerobic bacterium that is not destroyed by cooking. This bacterium causes botulism, a rare but potentially fatal food poisoning. Infants may develop botulism from eating honey because their immature digestive systems cannot neutralize its naturally occurring bacteria.

Raw seafood—especially contaminated shellfish—may bring on viral food poisoning. Certain mushrooms, berries, and other plants are naturally poisonous to humans and should never be eaten; potato sprouts and eyes also contain natural toxins. Toxic mold can form on improperly stored fruit, vegetables, grains, and nuts. Chemical food poisoning can be caused by pesticides or by keeping food in unsanitary containers.

Treatment Options

Vomiting and diarrhea are the body's way of flushing poison out of your system, so don't take any antiemetic or antidiarrheal medicine for 24 hours after your symptoms develop. Once you can keep fluid in your stomach, drink clear liquids for about

$\mathcal{F}$ood Poisoning

12 hours. Then eat bland foods like white rice, cooked cereals, and clear soups for a full day.

Because repeated vomiting or diarrhea can remove large amounts of water from your system, dehydration is a potentially dangerous complication, especially in children and older adults. You must see that lost fluids are replaced promptly and completely. If you cannot keep liquids down, intravenous fluid replacement may be necessary.

■ Acupressure

See the illustration below, right, for an effective acupressure technique to relieve the nausea associated with food poisoning.

■ Chinese Medicine

Among practitioners of Chinese medicine, *Po Chai* and Pill Curing are well-known herbal formulas for treating food poisoning.

■ Flower Remedy

The remedy **Crab Apple** is often recommended for food poisoning. Consult a naturopath or other practitioner familiar with flower remedies.

■ Herbal Therapies

For nausea, try **ginger** *(Zingiber officinale):* Take two capsules or a cup of ginger tea every two hours as needed. An infusion of meadowsweet *(Filipendula ulmaria),* **catnip** *(Nepeta cataria),* or **slippery elm** *(Ulmus fulva)* may help soothe the stomach: Steep 2 tsp of the herb in a cup of boiling water for 15 minutes; drink three times daily.

■ Homeopathy

Try any of the following over-the-counter remedies in 12c potency every three to four hours until symptoms improve: **Arsenicum album,** *Veratrum album,* **Nux vomica,** or *Podophyllum.*

■ Hydrotherapy

For symptom relief, alternate hot and cold compresses on your abdomen, with five minutes of hot followed by 10 minutes of cold. Hydrotherapists also recommend taking medicinal charcoal internally. Take two to three capsules after each bout of diarrhea; dissolve the tablets in water and drink.

■ Nutrition and Diet

After symptoms subside, restore strength by eating foods like white rice, bland vegetables, mashed potatoes, and bananas. To restore essential bacteria to your digestive tract, eat plain yogurt with active *Lactobacillus acidophilus* cultures, or take *Lactobacillus acidophilus* capsules. Avoid unfermented milk products, which may be difficult to digest.

Prevention

- Always wash your hands before preparing any food; wash utensils with hot soapy water after using them to prepare any meat or fish.
- Don't thaw frozen meat at room temperature. Thaw it gradually in a refrigerator, or thaw it quickly in a microwave oven and cook at once.
- Avoid uncooked marinated food and raw meat, fish, or eggs; cook all such food thoroughly.
- Don't eat any food that looks or smells spoiled, or any food from bulging cans or cracked jars.
- Set your refrigerator at 37°F; never eat cooked meat or dairy products that have been out of a refrigerator more than two hours.
- To relieve general nausea, try pressing Pericardium 6—on your inner forearm, two finger widths from the wrist *(below).* ■

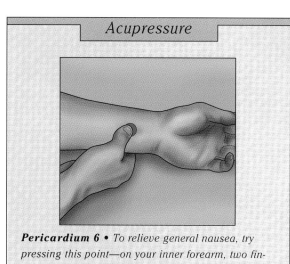

Acupressure

Pericardium 6 • *To relieve general nausea, try pressing this point—on your inner forearm, two finger widths from the wrist crease—for one minute. Repeat on the other arm.*

G

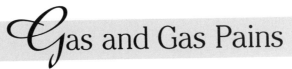

Gas and Gas Pains

Symptoms

- Abdominal bloating and pain.
- Belching.
- Flatulence (passing rectal gas).

Call Your Doctor If

- you have persistent, unexplained bloating for more than three days; you may have a more severe abdominal disorder.
- you have severe abdominal pain; you may have appendicitis.
- you have pain in your upper right abdomen; you might have gallstones or a stomach ulcer.
- you are flatulent, are losing weight, and have pale, foul-smelling bowel movements; you might have a malabsorption disorder, in which your intestines are not able to digest fat.

*G*as and gas pains are a normal part of your digestive process. People may typically pass gas more than 10 times a day, but you can greatly exceed that average and still be perfectly healthy. You can usually prevent and treat gas and gas pains without professional care, but if you have other symptoms, you should consult a doctor to find out if you have a more serious health problem.

Treatment Options

Changes in diet—avoiding or limiting milk products, alcohol, carbonated beverages, and high-fiber foods like beans—can go a long way toward solving problems with excessive gas. Many people rely on over-the-counter medications containing the active ingredient simethicone, which can help break up gas bubbles in the large intestine. Alternative medicine offers a wide variety of natural treatments as well.

Acupressure

Pressing the following points may help to alleviate gas pains: Conception Vessel 6, Large Intestine 4, Spleen 6, and Stomach 36. *(See the illustration opposite and the Gallery of Acupressure Techniques, pages 18-31, for information on point locations.)*

Acupuncture

A practitioner can provide treatment for gas using the same points used in acupressure as well as Conception Vessel 8, where heat might be applied instead.

Exercise

Moderate exercise after meals can help move gas through your system more quickly. In addition, following a regular program of exercise stimulates digestion and promotes the reabsorption and expulsion of gas.

Herbal Therapies

Anise water, made by steeping 1 tsp aniseeds in 1 cup water for 10 minutes, may be helpful. Teas made with **peppermint** *(Mentha piperita),* **chamomile** *(Matricaria recutita),* or fennel *(Foeniculum vulgare)* may also relieve gas pains.

Gas and Gas Pains

Homeopathy

Carbo vegetabilis is the most commonly used homeopathic remedy, but **Lycopodium** is used as well. **Nux vomica** is used for gas associated with constipation, and **Chamomilla** is preferred for gas in infants. Talk to a homeopath about which is most suitable for you.

Hydrotherapy

To relieve gas pains, apply a hot compress (a washcloth soaked in hot water and then wrung out) to the abdomen for several minutes, then follow with a cold friction rub: Soak a washcloth in ice water, wring it out, and rub it briskly over the abdomen for about half a minute.

Nutrition and Diet

Increase your fiber intake slowly and try avoiding beans, peas, and fermented foods such as cheese, soy sauce, and alcohol. Asafetida powder dispels intestinal gas and may be used as a spice with beans. Drink fewer carbonated drinks. Avoid mixing proteins and carbohydrates at the same meal. Do not overeat, and eat fewer different food items at one sitting. For people who are lactose intolerant, replacing cow's milk with soybean milk or using lactose-reduced dairy products may help.

Reflexology

Stimulate stomach areas to encourage stomach digestion, liver area to trigger bile secretion, gallbladder area to trigger release of stored bile, intestine areas to stimulate regular contractions in both intestines, and pancreas area to encourage the secretion of digestive enzymes. *(See page 169 for area locations.)*

Yoga

Any of the yoga postures that compress and stretch the abdomen help stimulate digestion and thus reduce gas and bloating. Try the Boat, Bow, Cobra, or Pigeon *(see the Gallery of Yoga Positions, pages 184-193).*

Home Remedies

Dissolve a teaspoon or two of superfine white, green, or yellow French clay (available at health food stores) in water and drink at least once daily (but not with meals). The clay absorbs impurities and intestinal gas; check with your doctor to make sure it won't absorb medications you may be taking as well.

Prevention

One of the main methods of preventing gas and gas pains is also the primary treatment: Avoid foods that generate gas in your system. Try to become more aware of the air that you swallow. You can avoid some gas, for instance, by not gulping your food; chew your food slowly and thoroughly. ■

Acupressure

Conception Vessel 6 • *Pressing on Conception Vessel 6 may help relieve gas pains. Measure three finger widths below the navel, then press inward on this point as far as you can, using your index finger. Inhale slowly and deeply, relaxing as you exhale.*

---

*G*laucoma

Symptoms

- Teary, aching eyes, blurred vision, occasional headaches, and progressive loss of peripheral vision are signs of chronic glaucoma.

- A sudden onset of severe throbbing pain, headaches, blurred vision, rainbow halos around lights, redness in the eye, dilated pupils, and sometimes nausea and vomiting are signs of acute glaucoma.

- Blurred vision, headaches, and halos around lights following an eye injury are signs of secondary glaucoma.

- In infants, teary or cloudy eyes, unusual sensitivity to light, and enlarged corneas are signs of congenital glaucoma.

Call Your Doctor If

- you have symptoms of acute glaucoma. You need immediate medical attention to prevent potentially permanent eye damage or blindness. You should also be monitored by a physician during treatment so that reduction in eye pressure can be verified.

More than two million adult Americans suffer from glaucoma, making it one of the leading causes of blindness. Chronic glaucoma, which accounts for 90 percent of cases in the United States, usually appears in middle age and seems to have a genetic component: 1 out of 5 sufferers has a close relative with the condition.

Other forms of glaucoma are less common but are no less serious. Acute, or narrow-angle, glaucoma accounts for less than 10 percent of reported cases, but it comes on quickly and requires urgent medical attention. If left untreated, it can irreversibly damage the optic nerve, which carries images from the eye to the brain, causing blindness—sometimes in a matter of days.

Secondary glaucoma is usually associated with another eye disease or disorder, such as an enlarged cataract, uveitis (an inner-eye inflammation), an eye tumor, or an eye injury. People suffering from diabetes are also susceptible to neovascular glaucoma, a particularly severe form of the disease. Congenital glaucoma is an extremely rare inborn condition affecting babies.

Treatment Options

Alternative approaches to treating glaucoma emphasize prevention and maintenance of eye health. Natural remedies may help keep glaucoma at bay or—if you are already under a doctor's care—may complement conventional treatment.

Acupuncture

Performed in conjunction with herbal therapy and a nutritious diet, acupuncture may help relieve tension and reduce pressure in the eye. The acupuncturist will concentrate on points along the bladder, gallbladder, liver, and kidney meridians.

Herbal Therapies

A variety of herbs have properties that address the factors contributing to glaucoma.

- Bilberry *(Vaccinium myrtillus)*—or its American equivalent, huckleberry—helps maintain collagen balance and prevents the breakdown of ***vitamin C.*** Eat 2 to 4 oz three times a day whenever the fresh berries are available.
- *Cannabis sativa,* also known as marijuana, contains the chemical compound tetrahydro-

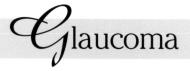 Glaucoma

cannabinol (THC). Clinical studies have demonstrated that it reduces the inner-eye pressure that causes glaucoma. Though a controlled substance, cannabis can be prescribed by a licensed professional to treat glaucoma.

■ Hydrotherapy

Hydrotherapy may be used to stimulate circulation in the eye. Soak a cloth in hot water, wring it out, and place it on your eyes for up to three minutes. Then do the same with a cold compress. Alternate each compress three times.

■ Mind/Body Medicine

Eye exercises may relieve the stress and eyestrain caused by overworked eyes and many other eye problems, including glaucoma.

■ Nutrition and Diet

Studies suggest that *vitamin C* lowers inner-eye pressure and restores collagen balance, making it especially useful if you are unresponsive to oral medications or eye drops. Foods high in vitamin C include cauliflower, broccoli, turnip greens, strawberries, grapefruits, and oranges. Alternatively, take up to 3,000 mg of a vitamin C supplement daily. *Chromium* and *zinc* may also deter glaucoma, as most people with the disease exhibit defi-

ciencies of these minerals, as well as of thiamine *(vitamin B₁).*

When used with traditional drug therapies, rutin is said to reduce inner-eye pressure and restore collagen balance. It can be found in supplement form at health food stores. See the product label or ask your doctor for appropriate dosages.

■ Reflexology

According to reflexology therapists, the nerve endings where your toes meet the rest of your foot influence the nerves in your visual system. Try working the base of the second and third toes, and up the shaft and both sides of the big toe; this may also help improve the blood supply to the eyes.

Prevention

Early detection is crucial. Only an ophthalmologist can diagnose the condition, but you must be aware of the warning signs. So if you sense that your vision is deteriorating—especially if you are over 40—a complete eye examination is a must.

If you are already near- or farsighted, a balanced diet and eye exercises may help prevent glaucoma. If you have diabetes or high blood pressure, stick diligently to your prescribed treatment to reduce the risk of developing glaucoma. ■

Fluid Buildup

Fluid normally drains from the eye through the drainage angle—located between the cornea and the iris—and out through the tiny Schlemm's canal. Chronic, or open-angle, glaucoma (inset, right) occurs when fluid is produced faster than it can drain out. Acute, or narrow-angle, glaucoma (inset, far right) occurs when the iris blocks the drainage angle.

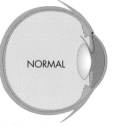

NORMAL

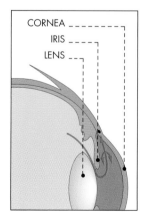

CHRONIC (open-angle)

CORNEA
IRIS
LENS

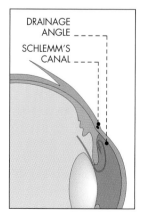

ACUTE (narrow-angle)

DRAINAGE ANGLE
SCHLEMM'S CANAL

*G*out

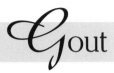

Symptoms

- Sudden, intense pain in a joint, typically the big toe or ankle, sometimes the knee.

- Swelling, inflammation, and a feeling that the joint is very hot.

- In extreme cases, alternating chills and fever.

- Usually strikes unexpectedly and may recur, but the symptoms typically do not last more than a week.

Call Your Doctor If

- severe pain in a joint recurs or lasts more than a few days, especially if the pain is accompanied by chills or fever; you may be experiencing the early signs of rheumatoid arthritis.

Without warning and, for some reason, in the middle of the night, it strikes—an intense pain in a joint, most often the big toe. With prompt treatment, the pain and inflammation of gout disappear after a few days, but they may recur at any time. Nine out of 10 sufferers are middle-aged men, and about half of them have a hereditary predisposition to the ailment.

Gout is uncommon in women and very rare in children. Men who are overweight or are suffering from high blood pressure are particularly prone to gout, which is actually a form of arthritis brought on by an excessively high level of uric acid in the blood. Specifically, it is the body's reaction to irritating crystalline deposits in the space between the bones in a joint.

Treatment Options

Nonconventional approaches to treating gout begin with reducing the immediate pain and inflammation, then continue with controlling excessive uric acid production. If you suspect that you have gout, you should consult a physician; left untreated, uric acid deposits can eventually cause irreversible damage to the kidneys and other tissues.

Acupuncture
Because acupuncture can be administered to areas other than the swollen joint, this procedure may be better tolerated than direct treatments, such as massage, by patients in the initial stages of gout. See a professional for treatment, which will focus on providing relief from the symptoms of acute pain and inflammation.

Herbal Therapies
Drink an infusion of 2 tsp celery *(Apium graveolens)* seed or gravelroot *(Eupatorium purpureum)* in a cup of water, three times a day, to stimulate elimination of uric acid. Do not take herbal teas if colchicine has been prescribed.

Homeopathy
A homeopathic physician may consider predisposition to gout in an overall constitutional treatment. *Colchicum,* or autumn crocus, from which colchicine is extracted, can be effective in relieving the pain of an attack. ***Bryonia*** may help when there is

Acupressure

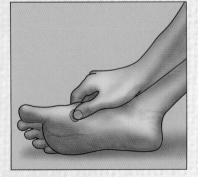

Spleen 3 • *To relieve the pain of a gouty toe, locate the indentation on the inside of the affected foot, just behind the bulge made by the large joint of the big toe. Maintain pressure on the point site with your thumb for 60 seconds. Repeat on the other foot.*

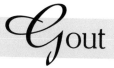 Gout

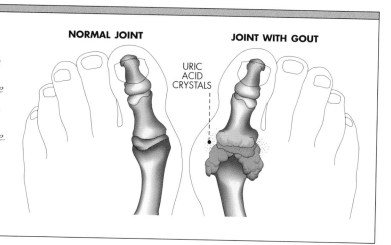

Joint Problems

Gout occurs when the body is unable to rid the blood of excess uric acid. Crystals of the chemical accumulate between the bones of certain joints, most commonly in the big toe. The result can be sudden and severe pain, inflammation, and in severe cases, joint deformity.

NORMAL JOINT

JOINT WITH GOUT

URIC ACID CRYSTALS

severe pain from slight movement of the affected joint. Other mixed homeopathic remedies may include dilute doses of **Arnica, Ledum,** *Urtica urens, Benzoicum acidum,* **Lycopodium,** and **Pulsatilla.**

■ Nutrition and Diet

In general, gout seems more common in people with diets that include meat and animal fats and is unusual in those following vegetarian diets. Dietary regimens for preventing attacks of gout in people showing a hereditary predisposition to the disease usually eliminate red meat and meat extracts such as bouillon and gravies; yeast and other enzyme-producing products; organ meats such as liver, sweetbreads, and kidneys; shellfish and certain kinds of preserved fish, including sardines, herring, and anchovies.

Vitamin C (1,000 mg three times a day) may help with the excretion of uric acid; consult a physician or healthcare practitioner familiar with nutritional therapies when taking large doses of vitamin C, which can cause some side effects. Some naturopathic practitioners also recommend supplementing the diet with 1 to 2 tbsp of flaxseed oil a day.

Several authorities report favorable results in treating the pain of chronic gout by having patients eat fresh or canned cherries—up to 8 oz a day—or drink cherry juice. Similar effects are claimed for strawberries, blueberries, and other red-blue berries.

Drinking plenty of clear, nonalcoholic fluids—fruit juices, herbal teas, or water—helps to dilute the urine and promote excretion of uric acid through continued flushing of the kidneys.

■ Reflexology

To help restore balance to the kidneys, the organs responsible for uric acid production, a reflexology practitioner will work the appropriate areas related to the kidneys; this should be done on both feet. In addition to affecting the kidneys, this technique may also serve to break up deposits of uric acid crystals that have become concentrated in the feet.

Home Remedies

The first concern in an attack of gout is to reduce pain and inflammation. If you can stand it, apply a plastic bag containing a few ice cubes or a bag of frozen vegetables to the joint; this will help relieve painful swelling. Wrap the cold bag in a soft cloth or towel and hold it against the painful area for up to five minutes at a time, then repeat as needed.

Prevention

If gouty arthritis runs in the family, men in particular should moderate their intake of alcohol, fats, and foods high in purines (chemicals essential to the production of uric acid), and they should keep their weight within recommended ranges. ■

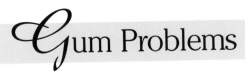 Gum Problems

Symptoms

- Swollen, red gums that may bleed easily.

- Localized pain, loose teeth, and bad breath, which suggest periodontitis, an inflammation of the periodontal ligament; x-rays may reveal some bone loss in the jaw area.

- Extremely painful, inflamed gums coated with a grayish white mucus; sometimes accompanied by a mild fever, malaise, bad breath, excess saliva, and painful swallowing. These are signs of Vincent's angina, also known as trench mouth.

- Sudden and unexplained severe bone loss around molars and incisors, especially in young African American girls; this is indicative of juvenile periodontitis.

- Extremely sore, swollen gums that bleed easily; perhaps accompanied by earaches, a sinuslike infection, nosebleeds, fever, weight loss, and malaise. You may have Wegener's granulomatosis, a rare but potentially fatal disease.

Call Your Dentist If

- you have any of the groups of symptoms listed above; timely treatment can help prevent the spread of infection and potentially save teeth.

Periodontal disease (gum disease)—an infection of the gums and other tissues that support the teeth—is one of the most prevalent of all chronic diseases. A diet rich in refined sugars is largely to blame, but modern dentistry and good toothbrushes and toothpastes have helped offset some of the pernicious effects of our eating habits; as a result, only 8 percent of adults ever develop severe gum problems. That rate would be even lower if people made an effort to cut back on highly processed foods, notorious for their refined-sugar content, and took dental hygiene more seriously.

Treatment Options

The best treatment for periodontal disease is prevention. If you do develop gum problems, seek professional treatment and advice. Many alternative therapies exist for gum problems, including rinses and pastes that will reduce plaque, fight infection and inflammation, and slow bleeding. But these remedies are no better than conventional commercial products at reaching below the gum line to areas where periodontitis blossoms. You still need to see a dentist regularly to ward off the risk of severe gum disease and tooth loss.

Acupuncture
A licensed acupuncture practitioner may choose areas that would stimulate the immune system to help fight off infections in the gums and reduce inflammation and pain.

Herbal Therapies
Massage gums with an infusion of **goldenseal** (Hydrastis canadensis) or **myrrh** (Commiphora molmol) to fight infection. Gargle with bayberry (Myrica spp.) or prickly ash (Zanthoxylum americanum) to stimulate circulation. A combination of **sage** (Salvia officinalis) and **chamomile** (Matricaria recutita) in an infusion makes an excellent mouthwash. You might also try gargling with **echinacea** (Echinacea spp.) tea made with 1 ml echinacea tincture in a small glass of water. Make a tea by boiling 1 to 2 tsp of the root in 1 cup of water; simmer for 10 minutes. Or drink Roman chamomile (Anthemis nobilis) or myrrh tea to fight inflammation in the gums. CAUTION: Do not use myrrh if you are pregnant.

Gum Problems

Homeopathy

For tender, bleeding gums and excessive salivation try **Mercurius vivus;** take orally twice a day for three days. If you continue to have problems, see a professional homeopath.

Massage

Massaging the gums can improve circulation and speed healing. Use the rounded part of your fingertips and move along your gum line inside your mouth, or from the outside press on the gums through your cheek. A stimulator brush, which has only two rows of bristles and is used without toothpaste, can also be therapeutic.

Nutrition and Diet

Crucial for healthy gums is a diet low in refined sugars and high in fiber. Other important nutritional elements include **vitamins A** (especially beta carotene), **C,** and **E,** as well as **zinc,** flavonoids (present in onions), and **folic acid** (particularly for pregnant women and women on oral contraceptives). Gingivitis, the earliest stage of periodontal disease, is common in scurvy patients, a reflection of vitamin C's vital role in maintaining a healthy mouth.

Home Remedies

You can make a wide assortment of mouthwashes and toothpastes at home. Some of the most effective ingredients include:

- a combination of baking soda and hydrogen peroxide, for brushing your teeth or as a mouth rinse.
- a mixture of bayberry and prickly ash as a gargle.
- cashew oil, **vitamin E** oil, or poultices of **goldenseal** or **myrrh** massaged into the gums, to speed healing and protect against infection.

Prevention

For proper dental care you need to floss daily, brush longer, rinse with a mouthwash, and massage your gum line. Always floss first, to loosen food particles and plaque, then brush your teeth gently but thoroughly with a soft brush using a circular motion. Rigorous horizontal brushing with hard bristles can cause your gums to recede. Mouthwashes combat bacteria, but they should not be substituted for brushing, which you should do two or three times a day.

The American Dental Association (ADA) recommends that you visit your dentist once or twice a year to get rid of intractable plaque and calculus, but some dentists believe that excellent at-home dental hygiene keeps the plaque and calculus from ever forming. To achieve "excellence" you have to spend at least 15 minutes twice a day working on your teeth, and another 15 minutes a day massaging your gums. ∎

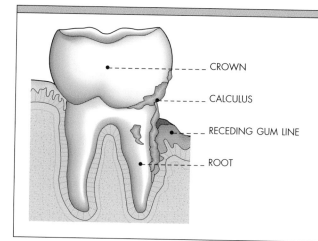

CROWN

CALCULUS

RECEDING GUM LINE

ROOT

Periodontal Disease

A bacterial film called plaque can accumulate along the gum line at the base of the teeth if not brushed away. Plaque hardens into calculus, which irritates the gums and causes them to recede. Pockets that form between the gums and teeth collect more plaque and calculus, causing destruction of the bone and ligament supporting the tooth, eventually resulting in tooth loss.

Common Ailments

$\mathcal{H}$ay Fever

Symptoms

Attacks, often seasonal, of:

- Prolonged, sometimes violent sneezing.
- Itchy, painful nose, throat, and roof of mouth.
- Nasal discharge.
- Stuffy, runny nose.
- Postnasal drip, resulting in coughing.
- Watery, itchy eyes.
- Head and nasal congestion.
- Ear pressure or fullness.
- Lethargy; sleep disturbance or insomnia.

Call Your Doctor If

- your condition becomes so severe that it interferes with your life and you're unable to control it with alternative therapies or over-the-counter medications. Your physician may administer prescription drugs, such as non-sedating antihistamines, to help.

- a secondary infection develops in congested sinus cavities; signs are fever, pain, a yellow or green discharge, postnasal drip, and sinus or tooth tenderness.

Acupressure

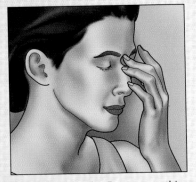

Governing Vessel 24.5 • *Pressure on this point may help relieve symptoms of hay fever. Place the tip of your middle finger at the top of the bridge of your nose, between your eyebrows. Press lightly for two minutes and breathe deeply. Do three to five times, at least twice a day.*

Hay fever is an immune disorder characterized by an allergic response to pollen grains and other substances. There are two types: seasonal, which occurs only during the time of year in which certain plants pollinate, and perennial, which occurs all year round. Typically, if you suffer from hay fever in the spring, you're probably allergic to tree pollens. Grass and weed pollens may be causing your allergic reaction during the summer. In autumn ragweed may plague you, and fungus spores cause problems from late March through November.

People with perennial hay fever are usually allergic to one or more of these outdoor agents. Perennial hay fever can also be brought on by other allergy-causing substances, or allergens. These include house-dust mites, feathers, and animal dander (the tiny skin flakes animals shed along with fur), all of which may be found in pillows, down clothing and bedding, shower curtains, heavy draperies, upholstery, and thick carpeting. Another common allergen, mold, is usually found in damp areas such as bathrooms and basements.

Treatment Options

Conventional medicine has several approaches for treating hay fever, from over-the-counter antihistamines to allergy shots. A number of alternative therapies can also help with symptom control and as preventive measures.

Aromatherapy

To ease sinus irritation, combine 5 ml **niaouli** (*Melaleuca viridiflora*), .5 ml **German chamomile** (*Matricaria recutita*), and 3 drops **peppermint** (*Mentha piperita*) essential oil; moisten your face and then spread a drop of this blend over your skin.

Herbal Therapies

For symptom relief, take two capsules of **nettle** (*Urtica dioica*) every 15 minutes during an attack, then four times a day as a maintenance dose. To help reduce inflammation, try inhaling the steam from **ginger** (*Zingiber officinale*) tea: Mix 2 tsp chopped or grated ginger in 2 cups boiling water and let simmer for 20 minutes. Breathe in the steam for five to seven minutes. You can use the same tea reheated to repeat this treatment several times a day.

*H*ay Fever

Regular doses of **parsley** *(Petroselinum crispum)* may help with hay fever; it is thought to work by reducing your body's production of histamine.

You may be able to slow down your body's production of mucus with goldenrod *(Solidago virgaurea),* **garlic** *(Allium sativum),* or **yarrow** *(Achillea millefolium).* Bathe irritated eyes with compresses soaked in either **eyebright** *(Euphrasia officinalis)* or **chamomile** *(Matricaria recutita);* make a tea from the leaves and dilute it by 50 percent with water or saline solution before using it to soak the compresses.

▨ Homeopathy

For watery, hot eyes, a burning nasal discharge with sneezing, and symptoms that feel worse late at night, try **Arsenicum album. Pulsatilla** can help if your symptoms—thick, yellow mucus accompanied by a loss of taste and smell—are made worse by warm rooms but are better outdoors. If you have watery, itchy eyes and a runny but not irritated nose, try *Euphrasia;* if, on the other hand, your nose is irritated and your eyes are watery but not itchy, try **Allium cepa.** Homeopathic practitioners recommend that you consult with a homeopath for the best treatment for conditions like hay fever because it often takes comparing as many as 15 different homeopathic remedies to find the right choice for a given individual and his or her symptoms.

▨ Nutrition and Diet

Nutritionists believe that refined sugar and casein, the protein in dairy products, are mucus-producing substances that are best avoided during hay fever season. Taking a commercial preparation of chelated **calcium** and **magnesium** may help regulate histamine production. A diet high in fruits and vegetables will supply large amounts of **vitamin C** and bioflavonoids, which help stabilize the body's cells that contain histamine. Supplements of quercetin, a bioflavonoid, may also control histamine; take 250 mg four times a day, before or between meals.

Some researchers believe that honey has a desensitizing and antiallergic effect that may relieve some hay fever symptoms. Two months before the season starts, begin eating 2 tsp daily of raw honey that comes from a nearby hive. Or chew (but don't

---

Homemade Decongestant

Make your own decongestant by simmering grapefruit, orange, or lemon peels, including the pith, in water mixed with honey until the peels are spongy, stirring occasionally. Be careful not to overcook—you don't want candied fruit. Eat one piece when symptoms start and one piece every evening at bedtime during hay fever season. Substances in the peel and white rind act as anti-inflammatory agents and will dry mucous membranes. Lemon is considered a stimulating expectorant that may help release mucus from your lungs.

---

swallow) a bite-size piece of honeycomb for five to 10 minutes twice a day. Check with your doctor first to avoid potential allergic reactions.

Many people with hay fever are also allergic to certain foods and may experience symptoms as a result of eating such foods as eggs, nuts, fish, shellfish, chocolate, dairy products, wheat, corn, citrus fruits, or food colorings or preservatives.

Prevention

The best way to combat the allergens that are assaulting you is to avoid them. Stay indoors between six and 10 o'clock in the morning and on days when the pollen count is high. The pollen count drops on rainy days and climbs when it's hot, sunny, and windy outside.

Keep windows—in your home and car— closed and the air conditioning turned on. Change ventilation system filters in your home once a month. Remove allergens from the air with ionizing air cleaners. Prevent mold in damp basements by using space heaters and dehumidifiers.

Try to keep your grass no more than an inch high in the spring and summer so that it won't pollinate. If you do yard work, wear a filtered mask and protective glasses. Wash your face, hands, and hair and rinse your eyes when coming in from outdoors to avoid leaving traces of pollen on your pillow. ■

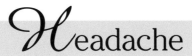 Headache

Symptoms

If your headache is:

- A dull, steady pain that feels like a band tightening around your head, you have a tension headache.

- Throbbing, and it begins on one side and causes nausea, you have a migraine. Visual disturbances, such as flickering points of light, may precede the headache.

- A throbbing pain around one red, watery eye, with nasal congestion on that side of your face, you have a cluster headache.

- A steady pain behind your face that gets worse if you bend forward and is accompanied by congestion, you have a sinus headache.

Call Your Doctor If

- a severe headache is accompanied by vomiting, limb weakness, double vision, slurred speech, or difficulty in swallowing; you may have a cerebral hemorrhage or an aneurysm—get medical help now.

- your headache is of a kind you've never had, occurs first thing in the morning, is persistent, brings on vomiting, and abates during the day; you may have high blood pressure or in very rare cases a brain tumor. See your doctor without delay.

- you have a high fever, light hurts your eyes, the pain is severe and is accompanied by nausea and a stiff neck; you may have meningitis—get medical help now.

- after a head injury, you are drowsy, with dizziness, vertigo, nausea, or vomiting; you may have a concussion. See your doctor without delay.

Although painful, most headaches are minor problems treatable with aspirin or another analgesic. But if they are severe, recur often, or are attended by other symptoms, you may need to take additional steps, including consultation with your doctor.

Major Types of Headaches

Tension headaches, which afflict almost everyone at some point, bring on a dull, persistent, non-throbbing pain that can make your head feel as if it's gripped in a vise. The muscles of your neck may seem knotted, and certain areas on your head and neck may be sensitive to touch. Tension headaches can be short lived and infrequent, or enduring and chronic. They are commonly triggered by stress; but eyestrain, poor posture, too much caffeine, or the grinding of teeth at night can also cause them.

Migraines are the most debilitating of headaches; they can be completely incapacitating. A migraine usually begins with an intense, throbbing pain on one side of the head. This pain may spread and is often accompanied by nausea and vomiting. A migraine can last from a few hours to three days and can cause oversensitivity to light, odors, and sound. The various symptoms of migraines seem linked to changes in the diameter of blood vessels in the head, possibly due to an imbalance in a brain chemical known as serotonin.

Cluster headaches are so named because they tend to come in bunches. Typically they begin several hours after a person falls asleep and are sometimes preceded by a mild aching sensation on one side of the head. The pain—severe, piercing, and usually located in and around one red, watery eye—is generally accompanied by nasal congestion and a flushed face. It lasts from 30 minutes to two hours, then diminishes or disappears, only to recur perhaps a day later. The root cause is unknown.

Sinus headaches are marked by pain in the forehead, nasal area, eyes, and possibly the top of the head; they also sometimes produce a feeling of pressure behind the face. Inflammation or infection of the membranes lining the sinus cavities can give rise to such headaches, as can suction on the sinus walls, which occurs when nasal congestion creates a partial vacuum in the sinuses. Sinus headaches

$\mathcal{H}$eadache

Cluster Headache

Although their exact cause is unknown, cluster headaches may arise from pressure on nerves around the eyes. Swollen sinus tissue may press against portions of these nerves, causing these electrical pathways to short-circuit and emit pain signals.

Tension Headache

Of the various types of tension headaches, one is thought to be linked to disorders in certain muscles in the head and the neck. Pain can be localized around any of these muscles or can spread to affect a broad portion of the scalp.

Sinus Headache

With a sinus headache, congestion within the sinus cavities leads to swelling that puts pressure on surrounding tissue and nerves, causing pain to radiate across the face.

NERVES ------
AREAS OF PAIN --

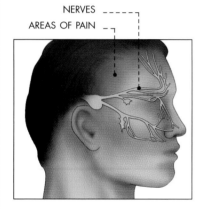

MUSCLES ------
AREAS OF PAIN --

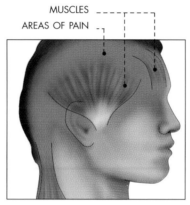

SINUS CAVITIES --
AREAS OF PAIN --

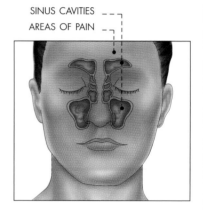

typically result from hay fever and other seasonal allergies, or from a cold or the flu.

Treatment Options

Alternative medicine, used alone or with conventional therapies, can be effective in dealing with headaches. Most of these remedies address the underlying causes. In particular, craniosacral therapists hope to relieve tension inside the head by manipulating the bones and membranes of the skull. Because tension so often figures in headaches, relaxation techniques are a staple of therapy.

■ Acupressure

Follow the illustrations at the top of page 273 to locate pressure points associated with headache relief. These techniques are often used in combination with one of the aromatherapy oils below.

■ Aromatherapy

The following oils may ease tension or migraine headaches. Moisten your fingertips with one or two drops of **lavender** *(Lavandula angustifolia)* essential oil blended with a so-called carrier oil such as sunflower oil, then massage your temples with a circular motion; repeat in the hollows at the sides of your eyes, behind your ears, and over your neck. For a sinus headache, try the same techniques using **Eucalyptus globulus** *(E. globulus)* or wintergreen *(Gaultheria procumbens)*. For any headache, inhale a blend of lavender, **rosemary** *(Rosmarinus officinalis),* and **peppermint** *(Mentha piperita).*

■ Chiropractic

Some tension headaches are caused by posture that puts unnecessary strain on muscles. A chiropractor may be able to remove the strain through spinal or cervical manipulation and realignment.

CONTINUED

*H*eadache

◼ Exercise

Regular physical activity can release endorphins, the body's natural painkilling agents. Exercise may also help dilate blood vessels; this increases blood flow and may counteract the constricting action that occurs at the onset of most migraines.

To nip a tension headache in the bud, try the following exercise while breathing deeply and thinking calm thoughts: While seated, inhale and gently tip your head back until you're looking up at the ceiling (be careful not to tip your head back too far, since this can compress the cervical spine); exhale and bring your head forward until your chin rests on your chest; repeat twice.

◼ Herbal Therapies

Perhaps the most widely recommended herbal remedy for treating and preventing migraines is **feverfew** *(Tanacetum parthenium),* which is

thought to work by blocking excessive secretion of serotonin, a neurotransmitter. When blood vessels constrict in the initial stage of a migraine, serotonin is released; feverfew may help counteract this by dilating those blood vessels. Chewing a leaf or two daily is one approach to prevention, but this can occasionally cause mouth ulcers; as a substitute for the leaves, you can use 125-mg capsules. To offset an acute attack, take three or four capsules right away, then continue this dosage every four hours; don't exceed 12 capsules in a day.

Migraines brought on by stress may benefit from a combination of equal parts **hawthorn** *(Crataegus laevigata),* linden *(Tilia* spp.), wood betony *(Pedicularis canadensis),* **skullcap** *(Scutellaria lateriflora),* and cramp bark *(Viburnum opulus),* taken three times a day as a tea or tincture. For migraines accompanied by nausea, try taking 500 mg of dried **ginger** *(Zingiber officinale)* with water at the onset of the warning stage, if your headache pattern includes an aura; repeat every two hours if needed. Three daily doses of **goldenseal** *(Hydrastis canadensis)* in tincture, tea, or powdered form may help reduce sinus headache pain.

Tension headaches may respond to three daily infusions of **valerian** *(Valeriana officinalis)* when combined with skullcap and **passionflower** *(Passiflora incarnata).* Cluster headaches may get quick relief from several daily applications inside the nostrils of an over-the-counter ointment made from **cayenne** *(Capsicum annuum* var. *annuum).* The same ointment applied to the skin is also said to be effective in preventing migraines. Because cayenne is hot and can cause painful skin burns, it's best used under a doctor's care.

◼ Homeopathy

A range of homeopathic medicines are available to treat specific types of headaches. For a throbbing headache that is worse on the right side when lying down, try **Belladonna.** For "splitting" headaches that feel worse with motion, noise, light, or touch, try **Bryonia.** For sinus pain with a thick nasal discharge, consider **Kali bichromicum.** For tension headaches accompanied by nausea or vomiting, try **Nux vomica.** For migraines or other chronic headaches, see a homeopathic practitioner.

OF SPECIAL INTEREST

A Headache Diary

Keeping a headache diary can help you pinpoint the factors causing your specific headache patterns. The diary should provide answers to these 10 questions:

1. *When did you first develop headaches?*
2. *How often do you have them?*
3. *Do you experience symptoms prior to the headaches?*
4. *Where is the pain exactly?*
5. *How long does it last?*
6. *At what time of day do the headaches occur?*
7. *Does the eating of certain types of food precede your headaches?*
8. *If you're female, at what time in your monthly cycle do they occur?*
9. *Are the headaches triggered by physical or environmental factors, such as odor, noise, or certain kinds of weather?*
10. *What words most accurately describe the pain of your headache: throbbing, stabbing, blinding, piercing . . . ?*

---

eadache

Headache

Acupressure

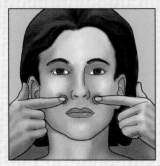

Stomach 3 • *Sinus headaches may be relieved by pressing this point. While looking in a mirror, place your index fingers at the bottom of your cheekbones, fingertips directly under the pupils of your eyes. Press firmly for one minute. Repeat three times.*

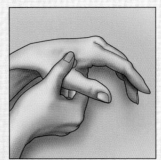

Large Intestine 4 • *Pressing this point may help relieve sinus headaches. Using the thumb and index finger of your right hand, squeeze the web of your left hand for one minute. Repeat this on the right hand. Do not use if pregnant.*

■ Massage

Massage therapy can relieve headache-producing tension in the muscles of your head, neck, shoulders, and face. Try giving yourself a 10-minute scalp massage: Place both middle fingers on your forehead at your hairline; using gentle pressure, gradually work them back to the crown of your head; tracing your hairline, repeat this motion in half-inch increments until you reach your temples; rotate your fingers on both sides for a few minutes; then bring both thumbs to the base of your skull along your hairline and massage both sides of your skull up to your crown to release any tightness.

■ Mind/Body Medicine

Meditation and progressive relaxation therapies are effective in reducing stress, which can cause tension headaches. Biofeedback training can also be helpful in controlling stress. Migraine headaches, too, can be treated through a biofeedback method called thermal biofeedback, in which you learn to increase the temperature of your hands and feet. Warming these extremities involves dilating the vessels that carry blood to them—a process that, in turn, may reduce abnormal blood vessel constriction in the skull and possibly result in diminished migraine frequency, intensity, and duration.

■ Nutrition and Diet

Among the foods sometimes associated with migraines are chocolate, aged cheeses, citrus fruits, processed meats containing sodium nitrates or the food additive MSG, and red wine. Keeping a food diary can help you identify foods to eliminate.

Magnesium relaxes constricted blood vessels; low levels of magnesium may contribute to migraine and cluster headaches. Supplemental doses of 200 mg three times a day may be preventive. Taking 50 to 200 mg of *niacin* (vitamin B_3) and niacinamide at the first hint of pain may help keep blood vessels dilated, possibly reducing the initial constriction phase of migraine headaches and thus avoiding an attack.

■ Osteopathy

Osteopaths believe headache pain stemming from pressure on nerves or blood vessels can be eased by neuromuscular manipulation and soft-tissue massage of your head, neck, and upper back.

Home Remedies

- Holding an ice pack or a bag of frozen vegetables against your forehead while soaking your feet in hot water may stop a migraine if done right away.
- At the first sign of a headache, drink three glasses of very cold water, then retire with a cold compress to a dark, quiet room to sleep (without a pillow).
- Inhaling pure oxygen from a tank kept near your bed may offset nighttime attacks of a cluster headache. But be sure to consult a doctor on how to use the oxygen. ■

Common Ailments

Hearing Problems

Symptoms

People often do not recognize a hearing problem until it is brought to their attention by a relative or a friend. Symptoms can include:

- An inability to hear or distinguish some or all sounds in one or both ears.

- Difficulty understanding conversation when many people are talking in the background.

- A need to turn up the volume on the television or radio louder than other people find comfortable.

Hearing problems are sometimes accompanied by dizziness, earache, discharge or bleeding from the ear, ringing or roaring noises in the ear, or in rare cases, weakness of facial muscles.

Call Your Doctor If

- you notice any hearing problems; it is important that you receive a timely medical evaluation, because early treatment may enable you to avoid permanent damage and regain full hearing.

- you experience a sudden and total hearing loss in one or both ears; this may indicate a severe reaction to medication, a tumor on the auditory nerve, or a neurological problem. Seek medical care as soon as possible.

- you have some hearing loss and your ear secretes pus or fluid; this may indicate an ear infection or a perforated eardrum.

- your hearing loss is accompanied by dizziness and nausea; these may be signs of otitis media, Ménière's disease, or another condition that needs medical attention.

S ome 28 million people in the United States have a hearing problem significant enough to interfere with their ability to understand conversations and communicate with others. Doctors divide hearing loss into two main categories. Conductive hearing loss occurs when something interferes with the transfer of sound waves from the outer to the inner ear. Sensorineural hearing loss results from damage to the inner ear or to the nerves that transmit sound impulses from the inner ear to the brain. Sounds may reach the inner ear, but they are not perceived because the necessary messages aren't sent correctly to the brain. Sometimes a person has a mixture of both types of hearing loss.

Treatment Options

In most cases of conductive hearing loss, once the underlying cause of the problem has been treated, hearing returns. With sensorineural hearing loss, however, the damage tends to be permanent. The following therapies primarily address the underlying problems that may be causing temporary loss of hearing.

Acupuncture

Acupuncture cannot restore hearing that has been lost as a result of permanent damage to the nerves or hearing mechanisms of the ear. However, in some such cases it may enable patients to discriminate better among the sounds they can hear. Acupuncture may also be used to help treat ear infections that may be causing temporary hearing problems. And it can sometimes be effective in alleviating tinnitus, or ringing in the ears. Consult a licensed acupuncture practitioner.

Herbal Therapies

Several herbs may help heal ear infections that might lead to hearing problems. **Garlic** *(Allium sativum),* which has been shown to act as a natural antibiotic, is considered very effective. Put 1 to 3 drops of garlic oil in your ear three times daily. You can buy the oil in a health food store or make your own: Slice several garlic cloves and put them in 1 oz of olive oil for up to seven days; strain and store in the refrigerator, being sure to warm the oil before using.

Hearing Problems

For ear drops, some naturopathic physicians use **mullein** *(Verbascum thapsus)* oil either alone or in combination with garlic oil. Herbalists also recommend **ginger** *(Zingiber officinale),* another natural antibiotic, both in tincture and in tea form. To make ginger tea, put 1 tbsp of the fresh root in 1 cup boiling water; let simmer for 10 minutes. Drink several times a day.

The anti-inflammatory properties of either **echinacea** *(Echinacea* spp.) or **goldenseal** *(Hydrastis canadensis)* may help heal an ear infection. Either herb can be taken in glycerin tincture form (10 to 15 drops in ear two or three times a day for seven to 10 days).

Ginkgo *(Ginkgo biloba),* which has been shown to improve circulation, is sometimes recommended for inner ear disturbances and partial deafness. It is available in herb stores in a variety of forms; the recommended dosage is 40 mg of the dried herb or 1 to 2 tsp of the liquid extract three times a day.

Yoga

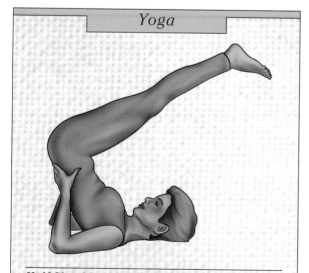

Half Shoulder Stand • *This position can improve blood circulation to the ears. Lie on your back and bring your knees toward your forehead, supporting your hips with your hands. Inhale and extend your legs, keeping them at a right angle to your back (above). Take a few deep breaths, then exhale and lower your legs.*

■ Homeopathy

For acute or chronic hearing problems, homeopaths recommend a variety of medications. Consult an experienced practitioner for specific remedies and dosages.

■ Nutrition and Diet

In some cases, hearing may be improved by reducing salt, which can cause fluids to be retained in the ear, where they can press against the hearing organs. If you are prone to repeated ear infections, avoid dairy products, which some alternative practitioners believe create excess mucus in the body, especially in children. Some evidence indicates that **vitamin A** supplements (5,000 to 10,000 IU a day) may help hearing loss, particularly if the condition is accompanied by tinnitus, a ringing or roaring sensation in the ears.

Prevention

- Wear earplugs if you are exposed to noise levels that may be harmful to your ears. Cotton balls are not sufficient, as they do not block enough sound. They can also become lodged deep in the ear canal.
- Do not listen to loud music with earphones.
- If you are at a concert and the music hurts your ears, put on earplugs or leave immediately. The overamplified sound may cause permanent damage.
- Educate your children about the danger of loud recreational noise.
- If you ride a subway, wear earplugs or cover your ears with your hands as the trains pass. The roar of the trains can damage your ears.
- Place pads under noisy countertop household appliances such as blenders.
- To lower the risk of infectious diseases that may lead to permanent hearing loss, make sure your children receive all of their immunizations on time.
- If your ears frequently tend to get severely blocked with wax, clean them periodically with hydrogen peroxide.
- Be sure to report any sudden hearing loss to your doctor immediately. ■

Heartburn

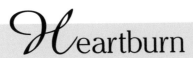

Symptoms

- A burning feeling in the chest just behind the breastbone that occurs after eating and lasts a few minutes to several hours.

- Chest pain, especially after bending over or lying down.

- Burning in the throat—or hot, sour, or salty-tasting fluid at the back of the throat.

- Belching.

Call Your Doctor If

- you experience heartburn along with any of the following: difficulty swallowing, shortness of breath, sweating, dizziness, vomiting, diarrhea, extreme abdominal pain, fever, or black or bloodstained bowel movements. You may have a serious medical problem, and it could be a heart attack; call for medical help now.

- you take an antacid to relieve heartburn and do not feel relief within 15 minutes. This may also be a sign of a heart attack; call for medical help now.

- your heartburn is aggravated by exercise and relieved by rest. This can be a sign of heart disease.

- you have chronic heartburn (daily or almost daily). Your esophagus is being repeatedly burned by stomach acid, which can lead to esophagitis, esophageal scarring, stomach ulcers, or cancer.

CAUTION

Antacids can mask or aggravate some ailments. Do not take antacids without consulting your doctor if you have high blood pressure, an irregular heartbeat, kidney disease, chronic constipation, diarrhea, colitis, any kind of intestinal bleeding, or any symptoms of appendicitis. Pregnant or nursing mothers should consult a physician before taking any medication, including antacids.

D*espite its name, heartburn has nothing to do with the heart. It is an irritation of the esophagus caused by stomach acid. With gravity's help, a muscular valve called the lower esophageal sphincter, or LES, keeps stomach acid in the stomach. The LES is located where the esophagus meets the stomach—below the rib cage and slightly left of center. Normally it opens to allow food into the stomach or to permit belching; then it closes again. But if the LES opens too often or too far, stomach acid can reflux, or seep, into the esophagus and cause a burning sensation.*

Occasional heartburn isn't dangerous, but chronic heartburn can indicate serious problems. Heartburn is a daily occurrence for 10 percent of Americans and 50 percent of pregnant women. It's an occasional nuisance for another 30 percent of the population.

Treatment Options

Most physicians advocate antacids for occasional heartburn. A variety of antacids available over the counter work by curtailing the production of stomach acid. Alternative practitioners rely primarily on herbal remedies to reduce acid and on relaxation therapies to lessen stress.

Acupressure

To relieve heartburn, use deep thumb pressure to massage these points for at least one minute: Stomach 36, Spleen 6, and Pericardium 6. See the illustrations opposite and the Gallery of Acupressure Techniques *(pages 18-31)* for point locations.

Chinese Medicine

Taken once or twice, a tea made from 10 grams orange peel, 4 slices fresh **ginger** *(Zingiber officinale)*, 10 grams poria *(Poria cocos)*, 10 grams agastache *(Agastache rugosa)*, and 3 grams **licorice** *(Glycyrrhiza glabra)* may alleviate heartburn. This mixture should not be taken daily.

Herbal Therapies

Ginger *(Zingiber officinale)* tea can diminish heartburn quickly, and **chamomile** *(Matricaria recutita)* tea's calming effects are especially helpful for stress-related heartburn. **Slippery elm** *(Ulmus fulva)* tea is also soothing and is reputed to have

*H*eartburn

strong anti-inflammatory qualities. Mix 1 part powdered bark in 8 parts water, simmer for 10 minutes, and drink ½ cup, three times daily.

Homeopathy

Specific heartburn symptoms often respond well to homeopathic remedies. The dosage is 12x, taken every 15 minutes; repeat up to three times, then repeat the series once if needed. After eating spicy foods, take **Nux vomica;** after rich foods, take *Carbo vegetabilis;* and for burning pain, take **Arsenicum album.**

Hydrotherapy

Placing an ice pack over your stomach for five to 10 minutes before eating may help prevent an attack of heartburn. To relieve heartburn, drink charcoal slurry: Stir 1 tbsp charcoal powder (available at health food stores) into a 10-oz glass of water; let the black powder settle to the bottom of the glass and drink the slurry water on top. Keep in mind that charcoal can interfere with the body's absorption of any medications you may be taking at the time.

Nutrition and Diet

Certain foods commonly relax the LES, including tomatoes, citrus fruits, garlic, onions, chocolate, coffee, alcohol, and peppermint. Try to avoid these foods, as well as dishes high in fats and oils (animal or vegetable), which often lead to heartburn. In general, try to refrain from eating large meals;

Acupressure

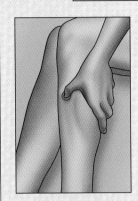

Stomach 36 • *To find this point, measure four finger widths below the kneecap just outside the shinbone. To verify the location, flex your foot; you should feel a muscle bulge at the point site. Apply steady pressure with a finger or thumb, then repeat on the other leg.*

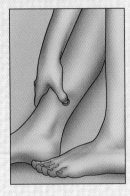

Spleen 6 • *Measure four finger widths up from the top of the right inside anklebone. With your thumb, press near the edge of the shinbone. Repeat on the other leg. (Do not use this point if you are pregnant.)*

---

instead, eat four or five small meals each day, and eat slowly. This, along with maintaining a weight in proportion to your height, will minimize abdominal pressure—and heartburn.

Prevention

Heartburn is often preventable. The keys are maintaining a reasonable weight, avoiding foods that cause stomach acid to reflux into your esophagus, getting adequate rest and exercise, and minimizing stress. Certain medications, especially some antibiotics and aspirin, can also lead to heartburn, so seek alternatives when possible.

Chew your food slowly and thoroughly, and avoid eating within two to three hours of bedtime. If you must lie down after eating, lie on your left side; your stomach is lower than your esophagus in this position. ■

> ## OF SPECIAL INTEREST
>
> ### The Milk Myth
>
> *Milk is not a remedy for heartburn. The soothing effect felt when drinking milk is deceiving; once in the stomach, milk's fat, calcium, and protein cause increased acid secretion and worsened heartburn. Mints are also often credited with alleviating heartburn, but they don't: Mint actually relaxes the lower esophageal sphincter, making heartburn more likely.*

Heart Problems

Symptoms

The symptoms listed below apply to several types of heart conditions. Bear in mind, however, that each type of heart disease has its own set of indicators; that most symptoms associated with heart disease could be caused by other conditions; and that some forms of heart disease may have no noticeable effects.

- Tight, suffocating chest pain, often associated with angina and heart attack.

- Sharp, piercing chest pain, which is a common sign of pericarditis.

- Sensations of fluttering, thumping, pounding, or racing of the heart, known as palpitations.

- Shortness of breath.

- Fluid retention in the legs, ankles, abdomen, lungs, or heart.

- Lightheadedness, weakness, dizziness, or fainting spells.

Call Your Doctor If

- you experience unusual chest pain, particularly if it persists or recurs. It may be heartburn, but it could also indicate a heart attack.

- you experience recurrent disturbances of your heartbeat (heart arrhythmias). If frequent or persistent, irregular heartbeats may signal a serious heart condition.

- you suddenly become dizzy, lightheaded, weak, or faint. Even if the cause is not heart disease, it could be serious.

T he human heart is built for amazing endurance—there are billions of beats in an average lifetime—but, like any other part of the body, it can break down. Heart problems vary widely in their nature and severity. They may be transient or chronic, slow developing or sudden, inconvenient or deadly. Some types of heart disease, closely linked to diet and lifestyle, are preventable; others are due to genetic inheritance, infections, or other uncontrollable factors. Two of every five Americans will die of heart disease; the daily toll is approximately 2,500 people. Fortunately, the death rate is declining steadily, thanks largely to improved medical care and widespread public education.

Types of Heart Problems

Arrhythmias

Arrhythmias are disturbances in the heart's normal beating pattern. The irregularities occur in many forms, each with its own potential causes and treatments. A heartbeat that is abnormally rapid is called tachycardia; a heartbeat that is too slow is known as bradycardia. Mild, isolated disturbances —such as the sensation of a skipped beat—are normally harmless. But recurrent problems should be checked by a physician. Serious arrhythmias can be a consequence of other heart diseases but may also occur independently.

Congenital Heart Disease

Should anything go awry in the formation of the heart during prenatal development, a baby will be born with one or more congenital heart defects. Such defects are quite common, occurring in about seven of every 1,000 babies. The exact causes of defects are generally hard to pin down; genes and environmental factors inside the mother's body may both contribute. Chromosome abnormalities, including the one that causes Down syndrome, have been linked to many congenital heart defects. Infections, such as German measles, contracted during pregnancy by the mother may also result in congenital heart disease for the child.

Congenital heart defects range widely in their effects. Some are apparent immediately, but others do not produce noticeable symptoms until adulthood. Minor conditions, such as some heart mur-

$\mathcal{H}$eart Problems

murs, often clear up on their own, but the most severe conditions cannot be corrected and are fatal.

Coronary Heart Disease

The most common of all heart problems, coronary heart disease is characterized by blockages in the coronary arteries. This blockage brings about a reduction in blood flow to the heart muscle, depriving it of vital oxygen. Usually, the disease stems from atherosclerosis.

Severe coronary heart disease can lead to congestive heart failure, a general weakness of the heart that results in ineffective pumping action. Coronary heart disease can also result in painful episodes of angina or a heart attack or, in the worst case, sudden cardiac death. For both men and women, the likelihood of heart disease increases significantly after the age of 65.

Heart Valve Disease

The heart has four valves, which open and close to permit blood flow between the heart's four chambers and connected blood vessels. A defective valve may fail either to open properly, obstructing blood flow, or to close properly, allowing blood leakage. Congenital heart disease and various inflammatory conditions are among the causes of valve disorders.

Pericardial Disease

Any disease of the pericardium, the membranous sac surrounding the heart, is classified as pericardial disease. One of the more common is an inflammatory condition called pericarditis. It is usually caused by a viral infection, a connective-tissue disease such as lupus or rheumatoid arthritis, or trauma to the pericardium. Pericarditis often follows open-heart surgery.

Excess fluid buildup within the pericardium is a frequent symptom of the disease. Listening with a stethoscope, a doctor may detect the disease upon hearing a characteristic scratching sound called a pericardial rub. Acute cases are marked by fever and sharp pain in the center of the chest.

Primary Myocardial Disease

Diseases of the heart muscle, or myocardium, are collectively referred to as primary myocardial disease, or cardiomyopathy. When diseased, the myocardium becomes abnormally stretched, thickened, or stiff. The many possible causes of the problem include connective-tissue diseases, genetic heart conditions, metabolic disorders, reactions to certain drugs or toxins such as alcohol, and viral infections. Often, the precise cause of cardiomyopathy is unknown. In any event, either the myocardium becomes too weak to pump efficiently, or

---

Pumping Blood

Oxygen-depleted blood enters the right atrium through the superior and the inferior venae cavae and flows through the tricuspid valve to the right ventricle, then through the pulmonary valve and artery into the lungs. Oxygenated blood from the lungs enters the left atrium through the pulmonary veins, enters the left ventricle through the mitral valve, and is pumped back to the body through the aortic valve and aorta.

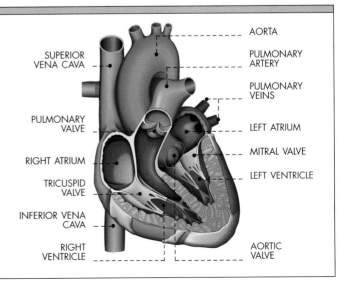

SUPERIOR VENA CAVA —
PULMONARY VALVE —
RIGHT ATRIUM —
TRICUSPID VALVE —
INFERIOR VENA CAVA —
RIGHT VENTRICLE —

AORTA
PULMONARY ARTERY
PULMONARY VEINS
LEFT ATRIUM
MITRAL VALVE
LEFT VENTRICLE
AORTIC VALVE

CONTINUED

*H*eart Problems

stiffening prevents filling of the heart with blood. Symptoms can include chest pain, shortness of breath, swelling of the feet and ankles, and light-headedness.

Treatment Options

Natural therapies that focus on diet, nutrition, herbalism, and purification of the body through exercise, stress reduction, and detoxification can significantly reduce the body's vulnerability to certain types of heart disease, although some cannot be prevented. Once heart disease begins to produce noticeable symptoms, you must seek medical attention. Conventional care aims to stabilize the condition immediately, to control symptoms over the long term, and to provide a cure when possible. A number of alternative therapies are beneficial complements to the conventional methods.

▪ Bodywork
Since all forms of bodywork help the body to relax, any of them might be useful in preventing and controlling heart disease. The reason is simple: Relaxation reduces stress, and stress has been identified as a likely risk factor for coronary heart disease. You can put yourself in the hands of a bodywork

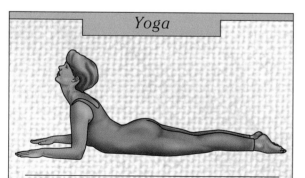

Yoga

Sphinx • *This position may help to reduce stress. Lie on the floor. Place both forearms on the floor with your palms down and your elbows directly under your shoulders. Inhale and push your chest away from the floor as far as comfortably possible without lifting your elbows. Hold for a few deep breaths, then relax and exhale.*

therapist, or you can study yoga or qigong. See also Mind/Body Medicine *(right)*.

▪ Chelation Therapy
Chelation therapy is sought annually by thousands of Americans who suffer from angina and atherosclerosis. Advocates claim that it is safer and cheaper than, and as effective as, many conventional drug or surgical treatments. Critics contend that while chelation therapy is useful in treating certain conditions, cardiovascular disease is not necessarily one of them.

▪ Chinese Medicine
Practitioners of traditional Chinese medicine generally view heart disease as arising from heart weakness or blocked energy flow. Depending on the symptoms, standard treatment would involve prescribed herbal remedies plus massage, acupuncture, and dietary recommendations.

▪ Chiropractic
While chiropractic medicine is inappropriate for acute care of heart conditions, it can help in long-term treatment. A chiropractic physician would recommend suitable diet and lifestyle changes, and would also perform skeletal manipulation when appropriate. Some studies indicate that regular chiropractic manipulation may reduce hypertension.

▪ Herbal Therapies
The plant world is full of herbs that can affect the heart. The therapeutic properties of some have been rigorously documented. The effects of others, such as motherwort *(Leonurus cardiaca)* and **yarrow** *(Achillea millefolium),* are not as well researched yet perhaps no less valid. Certain herbs, such as foxglove *(Digitalis purpurea)* and lily of the valley *(Convallaria majalis),* contain compounds called cardiac glycosides that make them particularly potent. Because of their potentially dangerous side effects, they should be administered only by a qualified medical herbalist. Many of the gentler "heart" herbs do not contain cardiac glycosides yet still improve cardiovascular function. The most noteworthy of these is **hawthorn** *(Crataegus laevigata).* Any herbal treatment of the heart should be

$\mathcal{H}$eart Problems

supervised by a medical herbalist and approved by your doctor. For further herbal recommendations, see Atherosclerosis, Cholesterol Problems, Circulatory Problems, and High Blood Pressure.

Lifestyle

If you smoke, quit. You should also get in the habit of exercising, since physical activity strengthens the heart and the blood vessels, reduces stress, and has been shown to reduce blood pressure while also boosting levels of HDL, or "good," cholesterol. A number of studies indicate that drinking alcohol in moderation may actually reduce the risk of heart disease. But more than one drink a day, and a few drinks per week, is not recommended.

Mind/Body Medicine

Learning to relax can help prevent and treat heart disease. While success varies from person to person, stress-reduction techniques have been shown to moderate high blood pressure, heart arrhythmias, and emotional responses such as anxiety, anger, and hostility that have been linked to coronary heart disease, angina, and heart attack. Some relaxation techniques that have proved beneficial are meditation, progressive relaxation, prayer, and biofeedback training.

Nutrition and Diet

Even modest changes in diet and lifestyle can significantly reduce the risk of heart disease. Most people know that eating foods low in cholesterol, saturated fat, and salt will help keep blood pressure low and decrease the formation of plaques, or calcified fatty deposits, in blood vessels. Less known to most people are the specific vitamins, minerals, and nutrients, such as **magnesium, potassium, niacin** (vitamin B_3), many other **B-complex vitamins, vitamin E,** coenzyme Q10, L-carnitine (an amino acid), and the fatty acids in fish oils, that may protect against heart and arterial disease.

Prevention

- To stabilize both blood pressure and cholesterol levels and to keep your weight in check, try to eat more fruits, vegetables, and grains,

---

OF SPECIAL INTEREST

The Risks for Women

A 50-year-old woman arrives in the emergency room complaining of severe chest pain and difficulty in breathing. The attending physician orders tests and eventually finds that the patient's coronary arteries are smooth and free of clots. In medical parlance, this patient is said to have Syndrome X—a condition that presents the classic symptoms of angina or heart attack without the classic cause, coronary artery blockage.

Until recently, cardiologists had done little to explain Syndrome X. (It is still under study, but one theory holds that it is caused by circulation problems in small vessels of the heart.) Lack of interest stemmed in part from lack of concern: Nearly two-thirds of Syndrome X patients are women, and traditionally women were thought to get heart disease only rarely. However, statistical evidence is challenging that notion—and changing attitudes about women and heart disease.

Among other things, the evidence indicates that heart disease is the number one killer of American women. Half of all women in the United States eventually die of heart disease, and six times as many die of heart attacks annually as succumb to breast cancer.

Women tend not to display the textbook symptoms of heart disease. Part of the reason could be that some traditional diagnostic and treatment tools (such as exercise stress tests) do not work as well for women as for men. Still, the death rate for women who have undergone coronary bypass surgery is twice as high as that for men, probably because women's blood vessels are smaller. However, the same risk factors (such as smoking and high blood pressure) apply to both sexes.

---

and fewer foods that are salty, high in fat, or fried. Avoid or decrease your intake of white sugar and stimulants, including caffeinated and decaffeinated beverages, to lessen vascular spasms and help lower blood pressure.
- Exercise regularly to tone your heart and blood vessels and to shed excess pounds.
- Don't smoke. ∎

ℋemorrhoids

Symptoms

- Bright red anal bleeding that may streak the bowel movement or the toilet tissue.

- Tenderness or pain during bowel movements.

- Painful swelling or a lump near the anus.

- Anal itching.

- A mucous anal discharge.

Call Your Doctor If

- you experience any anal bleeding for the first time, even if you believe you have hemorrhoids. Colon polyps, colitis, Crohn's disease, and colorectal cancer can also cause anal bleeding. An accurate diagnosis is essential.

- you have been diagnosed with hemorrhoids and you have anal bleeding that is chronic (daily or weekly) or more profuse than the streaking described above. Although rare, excessive hemorrhoidal bleeding can cause anemia.

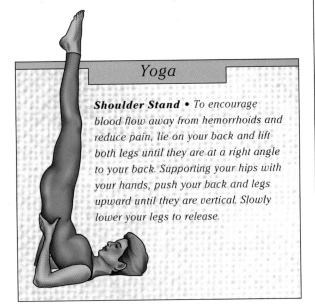

Yoga

Shoulder Stand • *To encourage blood flow away from hemorrhoids and reduce pain, lie on your back and lift both legs until they are at a right angle to your back. Supporting your hips with your hands, push your back and legs upward until they are vertical. Slowly lower your legs to release.*

Hemorrhoids are essentially varicose veins of the rectum. The hemorrhoidal veins are located in the lowest area of the rectum and the anus. Sometimes they swell, so that the vein walls become stretched, thin, and irritated by passing bowel movements. When these swollen veins bleed, itch, or hurt, they are known as hemorrhoids, or piles. Hemorrhoids are classified into two general categories:

Internal hemorrhoids lie far enough inside the rectum that you can't see or feel them, and usually don't hurt. Bleeding may be the only sign of their presence. External hemorrhoids lie within the anus and are often painful. If an external hemorrhoid prolapses, or enlarges and protrudes outside the anal sphincter (usually in the course of passing a stool), you can see and feel it.

Hemorrhoids are the most common cause of anal bleeding and are rarely dangerous, but you must see your physician for a definite diagnosis.

Treatment Options

Most hemorrhoid treatments aim to minimize pain and itching. The efficacy of over-the-counter remedies, the basic ingredient of which is some form of lubricant, such as lanolin, is debatable; plain petroleum jelly often works just as well. Some remedies also contain an anesthetic to relieve pain. Creams or ointments are best; suppositories usually go too far up into the anal canal to help. The following remedies can also help alleviate hemorrhoid discomfort. If symptoms persist, contact your doctor.

Acupuncture

The most responsive point for relieving hemorrhoid pain is Governing Vessel 20. Others that may augment this are Stomachs 25 and 36, Governing Vessel 14, and Large Intestine 11. A technique known as deep drainage can be extremely effective; see a licensed practitioner for this and other acupuncture treatments.

Herbal Therapies

Applied twice daily, pilewort *(Ranunculus ficaria)* ointment can reduce the pain of external hemorrhoids: Simmer 2 tbsp fresh or dried pilewort in 7 oz petroleum jelly for 10 minutes. Allow to cool before using; store leftover ointment in a closed

Hemorrhoids

container. Pilewort may also be taken as a tea. Witch hazel (*Hamamelis virginiana*) applied to external hemorrhoids can also help.

■ Homeopathy

More than a dozen remedies, each taken at 12x, can help hemorrhoid pain. Choosing the right one requires attention to your symptoms and, usually, a homeopath's help. For a sore, bruised, and perhaps bleeding anus, try *Hamamelis. Aesculus* can ease sharp, spiking rectal pain that is worsened with bowel movements, and **Sulphur** can reduce burning and itching aggravated by warmth.

■ Hydrotherapy

Warm (not hot) sitz baths are often recommended for hemorrhoid discomfort: Sit in about three inches of warm water for 15 minutes, several times a day, especially after a bowel movement.

■ Massage

This technique moves matter through the intestines, helping to prevent the constipation that contributes to hemorrhoids. Begin on your left side. Lie on your back, raise your knees, and using your fingers or your palm to make long, sweeping strokes, stroke from a point just below your ribs toward your feet; then stroke across your abdomen from the right to left just below your rib cage. Finally, point your fingertips toward your feet, and drag your hand up your right side from pelvis to ribs. Repeat each stroke three to six times.

■ Nutrition and Diet

Prevent constipation by following a high-fiber diet. Meals and snacks should consist primarily of vegetables, fruit, nuts, and whole grains, and as few refined foods and meats as possible. If this is a big change for you, introduce the new foods slowly, to avoid gas. If you aren't able to eat enough high-fiber food, supplement your diet with **psyllium** stool softeners or bulk-forming agents. (Avoid laxatives, which cause diarrhea that can further irritate the swollen veins.) Drink up to eight glasses of fluid each day; if your life is especially active or if you live in a hot climate, you will need more.

Monitor your sodium intake. Excess salt in the diet causes fluid retention, which means swelling in all veins, including hemorrhoids.

■ Yoga

Yoga can encourage blood flow away from hemorrhoids, reducing pain, inflammation, and bleeding. Try the Shoulder Stand *(opposite)*, Half Shoulder Stand, Plow, and Bridge, holding each posture for a few minutes each day. *(See the Gallery of Yoga Positions, pages 184-193, for more information.)* A good complement for these postures is lying on a slant board with your head down for 15 minutes daily.

Home Remedies

- Try not to sit for hours at a time, but if you must, take breaks: Once every hour, get up and move around for at least five minutes. A doughnut-shaped cushion can ease hemorrhoid pressure and pain.
- Insert petroleum jelly just inside the anus to make bowel movements less painful.
- Dab witch hazel (*Hamamelis virginiana*), a soothing anti-inflammatory agent, on irritated hemorrhoids to reduce pain and itching.
- Bathe regularly to keep the anal area clean, but be gentle: Excessive scrubbing, especially with soap, can intensify irritation.
- Don't sit on the toilet for more than five minutes at a time, and when wiping, be gentle. If toilet paper is irritating, try dampening it first, or use cotton balls or alcohol-free baby wipes.
- When performing any task that requires exertion, be sure to breathe evenly. It's common to hold your breath during exertion, but if you do, you're straining, and contributing to hemorrhoid pain and bleeding.

Prevention

A healthful diet and lifestyle are good insurance for preventing hemorrhoids, whether you already suffer hemorrhoid symptoms or are intent on never having them. Regular exercise is also important, especially if you work a sedentary job. Exercise helps in several ways: It keeps weight down, makes constipation less likely, and enhances muscle tone. ■

High Blood Pressure

Symptoms

In the vast majority of cases, there are no clear warning signs of hypertension (high blood pressure). If symptoms do occur, they may include:

- Headaches, chest pain or tightness, nosebleeds, and numbness and tingling; you may have severe hypertension.

- Excessive perspiration, muscle cramps, weakness, palpitations, and frequent urination; you may have secondary hypertension, possibly caused by kidney disease, a tumor, or an adrenal gland disorder.

Call Your Doctor If

- while taking antihypertensive drugs you experience worrisome side effects, such as drowsiness, constipation, dizziness, or loss of sexual function. Your doctor may need to prescribe a different drug.

- you are pregnant and develop hypertension; high blood pressure can affect not only your health but also that of your unborn child.

- you are experiencing severe headaches, blurred vision, nausea, and confusion or memory loss; you may have malignant hypertension, the name for hypertension that causes organ damage. Malignant hypertension can result in stroke or heart attack if left untreated.

- your diastolic pressure—the second number in a blood pressure reading—suddenly shoots above 130; you may have malignant hypertension.

Blood pressure—the force of blood pushing against artery walls as it courses through the body—naturally rises and falls with changes in activity or emotional state. It's also normal for blood pressure to vary from person to person, even from one area of your body to another. But when blood pressure remains consistently high, corrective steps should be taken.

Treatment Options

Many alternative therapies for high blood pressure focus on relaxation techniques. Others are attempts to get closer to the physiological roots of the problem, either by changing the patient's habits or lifestyle, or by influencing the operation of the heart and blood vessels.

Bodywork
Regular sessions of massage or shiatsu can help lower blood pressure by promoting relaxation. Both therapies employ touch and manipulation to reduce tension in the body.

Chinese Medicine
Traditional Chinese healers treat high blood pressure by coupling acupuncture with herbal and massage therapy. Acupuncture may benefit people with moderate hypertension, but it is not recommended for those with severe cases. Chrysanthemum flower *(Chrysanthemum indicum)*, peony *(Paeonia lactiflora)* root, eucommia *(Eucommia ulmoides)* bark, and prunella *(Prunella vulgaris)* are among the many Chinese herbs that might be prescribed in combination formulas for high blood pressure.

Herbal Therapies
Hawthorn *(Crataegus laevigata)*, used to treat many circulatory disorders, may help reduce high blood pressure. Over time, the herb may help dilate blood vessels while also moderating heart rate. Hawthorn tea can be prepared at home by steeping the dried flowers and berries in hot water for 10 to 15 minutes. Research indicates that ample consumption of **garlic** *(Allium sativum)* and onion *(Allium cepa)* can help reduce blood pressure. **Valerian** *(Valeriana officinalis)*, used only when need-

High Blood Pressure

ed, may work as a relaxant for people experiencing undue stress. *(See also Stress.)*

Mind/Body Medicine

A number of methods, including biofeedback, meditation, and hypnotherapy, call on the mind to relax the body and, practiced over time with guidance from trained professionals, may help lower blood pressure. Positive imagery—picturing yourself floating in calm water, for instance—can also work well for some people.

Nutrition and Diet

Adjusting the foods you eat will help keep your blood pressure in check. Your diet should be high in fiber and low in fat and salt. With these pointers in mind, emphasize fruits, vegetables, and whole grains. Enhance the flavor of your food with seasonings other than salt, and avoid processed foods, which tend to be high in sodium. You should also watch what you drink. Studies suggest that caffeine elevates blood pressure, at least temporarily, while moderate use of alcohol may lower it. But keep cocktails to a minimum; more than two ounces of alcohol per day can aggravate hypertension.

Of the vitamins and minerals that help lower blood pressure, *potassium* has one of the best track records. To get the 3,000 to 4,000 mg per day that researchers recommend, start eating more fresh vegetables and fruits, especially potatoes and bananas. According to several studies, daily doses of *calcium* (800 mg) or *magnesium* (300 mg) can help. Fish is a good source of fatty acids, which help relax arteries and thin the blood. Although it does contain sodium, celery is especially beneficial because it also contains ingredients believed to relax blood vessel walls.

Yoga

Mainly because of its relaxing effects, yoga is highly recommended for hypertension.

Home Remedies

- Adopt a healthful diet. Eat lots of fruit, vegetables, and whole grains. Give up salty foods and add seasonings other than salt to your meals. Go easy on alcohol and caffeine.
- Exercise regularly to shed extra pounds and get your blood flowing. Activities such as walking, jogging, cycling, and swimming lower blood pressure over the long term.
- If you smoke, quit.

Prevention

You can help keep your blood pressure at a healthful level and reduce your risk of heart disease by making a few changes in your lifestyle.

- Watch what you eat. Stay away from salt and fat, concentrating instead on foods that are high in fiber, *calcium,* and *magnesium.*
- Get plenty of exercise. Regular aerobic workouts condition the heart and keep blood vessels dilated and working properly, as do daily yoga and stretching exercises.
- If you are overweight, try to trim down. Even a small reduction can make a big difference.
- If you smoke, now is the time to stop. ∎

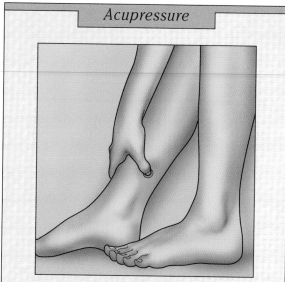

Acupressure

Spleen 6 • *Pressure on this point may help regulate blood pressure. The point is four finger widths up from the inner anklebone, near the edge of your shinbone. Press gently with your thumb for one minute, then switch legs. Do not use if you are pregnant.*

285

$\mathcal{I}$mmune Problems

Symptoms

In general, problems with your immune system manifest themselves as a tendency to catch colds, the flu, and various other infections more frequently than usual; to get easily tired; or to develop allergies. For specific symptoms of immune system disorders, see Allergies, Arthritis, Asthma, Chronic Fatigue Syndrome, Diabetes, Hay Fever, and Multiple Sclerosis.

Call Your Doctor If

■ you suspect you have an immune system disorder; you need to be properly diagnosed so that you can be properly treated.

T *he job of the immune system is to seek out, recognize, and destroy pathogens—disease-causing substances or organisms, such as bacteria and viruses. In fighting off these trespassers, your body produces such symptoms of illness as fever and malaise.*

An overactive immune system results in autoimmune disorders. In these cases, for reasons that aren't clear, the immune system mistakes healthy tissues for foreign invaders and attacks them. Another type of immune error occurs when the system overreacts to something harmless, as with allergies. The opposite occurs when the immune system fails to respond adequately, resulting in immunodeficiency diseases such as AIDS.

For people who are generally healthy, the immune system can become temporarily depressed. When this happens, your body becomes more susceptible to infections, which hit you harder and stay with you longer than they would otherwise. A number of things can temporarily weaken the immune system, including environmental toxins, stress, poor diet, lack of exercise and sleep, and abuse of alcohol and tobacco.

Treatment Options

A number of alternative therapies are available for various autoimmune disorders. Consult the entries on multiple sclerosis, arthritis, and diabetes for possible remedies. The alternative choices suggested in the sections on allergies and hay fever may be helpful for those problems. Always seek the advice of a healthcare practitioner before embarking on alternative treatments.

In addition to the remedies below, you might want to try acupuncture, massage, or homeopathy, which may help with your specific symptoms. For each method, consult a specialist in the field.

■ Herbal Therapies
Echinacea (*Echinacea* spp.), long thought to be a potent immunostimulant, may have antiviral and antibacterial properties as well. **Garlic** *(Allium sativum)* may have anti-infective and immune-enhancing qualities. Mushrooms such as shiitake *(Lentinus edodes)*, enokidake *(Flammulina velutipes)*, and reishi *(Ganoderma lucidum)* may promote production of antibodies.

*I*mmune Problems

Various Chinese preparations may also be helpful: Dried slices of the remedy known as polyporus, from the mushroom *Polyporus umbellatus,* can be made into a tea and drunk for a tonic effect on the immune system. **Astragalus** *(Astragalus membranaceus)* tea or tincture may help combat viral infections and enhance the functioning of immune cells. The traditional *Xiao Chai Hu Wan* (Minor Bupleurum Pills) may strengthen the immune system. **Asian Ginseng** *(Panax ginseng)* may improve immune functioning by protecting against the damage caused by free radicals.

■ Mind/Body Medicine

Research into the mind's effect on the immune system, called psychoneuroimmunology, has produced some findings on the relationship between happiness and health. One study has confirmed earlier reports that stress depresses immunity and that feeling good boosts it. Moreover, the data turned up an unexpected discovery: It seems that the impact of positive experiences such as expressions of love or feelings of accomplishment continues for two days, whereas the effects of negative events such as criticism or arguments last only one day. This suggests that the affirming consequences of happiness are more powerful and longer lasting than the negative effects of sadness—by 2 to 1.

Progressive relaxation techniques such as meditation, yoga, and qigong can promote a deep sense of relaxation and reduce stress. Regular exercise is considered to be another effective way to relieve stress.

■ Nutrition and Diet

Nutritionists may recommend a diet high in fresh vegetables and fruit, whole grains, brown rice, low-fat dairy products, fish, and poultry, and low in refined sugars, white flour, junk foods, red meats, and saturated fats. A daily antioxidant multivitamin containing the U.S. recommended daily allowance of **vitamins A, B complex, C,** and **E,** with **zinc, selenium,** and other trace minerals, can play a role in shoring up immunity. *(See Atherosclerosis for more information on antioxidants.)*

One theory holds that juice or water fasts may release a hormone that enhances the immune system. Fasts also cut down on the system's work load, because less energy is expended to process food allergens. Fasts are best attempted under the care of a doctor or nutritionist, who will advise you on how to safely begin and end one, as well as about some of the side effects to expect. Don't fast if you're pregnant or diabetic, or if you have a heart condition or an ulcer.

Prevention

- Avoid overeating and overindulging in alcohol, caffeine, and tobacco. Get plenty of rest, exercise regularly, and eat a balanced diet.
- Don't assault infections with antibiotics right away unless your physician deems it necessary. The immune system grows stronger with every battle won, so helping it fight with remedies less powerful than antibiotics—such as vitamins, homeopathic remedies, and herbal therapies—will allow the immune system to do its job.
- As much as possible, avoid radiation exposure, harmful chemicals, and prolonged use of immunosuppressive drugs such as corticosteroids, all of which can damage immunity. ■

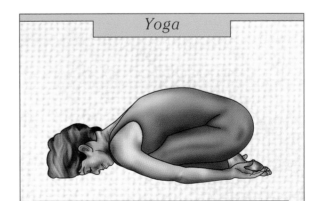

Yoga

Child • *The Child may help strengthen your immune system. Sit on your heels, thighs together. Exhale slowly while bending forward from your hips. Bring your forehead to the floor. Breathe deeply for 20 seconds, then inhale as you arise. Do this once, three or four times a day.*

I

*I*ncontinence

Symptoms

- Inability to control urination.
- Involuntary urination when coughing, laughing, sneezing, running, or performing other physical activity.

Call Your Doctor If

- you have become unable to control your urination after an illness such as a bladder infection or after taking a new medication. Sudden loss of urinary control may also indicate neurological damage.
- self-help remedies for controlling your urination are not working.

A lthough it is typically age related, incontinence—the involuntary loss of urine—is not, as is commonly believed, an inevitable consequence of aging. The condition often reflects an underlying disorder and is usually treatable, even in the elderly. With proper care, about 70 percent of cases can be improved or cured.

If left untreated, however, the condition will not improve and may actually worsen. Incontinence can lead to bladder or urinary tract infections. And the presence of leaked urine on the skin may cause uncomfortable rashes or other skin disorders. In those instances where treatment doesn't work, patients can avoid such complications by using special absorbent pads and other aids designed to help manage the problem.

Types of Incontinence

Medical professionals group incontinence into three major categories, although many people—women especially—experience symptoms of more than one. With stress incontinence, the muscles surrounding the urethra are so weakened that they can no longer resist a sudden increase in bladder pressure. Coughing, sneezing, laughing, exercising, or otherwise moving in a way that puts sudden pressure on the bladder can cause leakage—but usually only a few drops. With urge incontinence, the bladder, like that of an infant or toddler, simply contracts whenever it is full; the patient has no control over the sudden urge to void. Overflow incontinence occurs when a patient can no longer feel the sensation that signals when it is time to void. The bladder never empties normally and remains at least partially full; excess urine just spills out, usually in relatively small amounts.

Treatment Options

Most cases of incontinence can be cured or, at the very least, greatly improved with treatment. Many conventional practitioners routinely recommend two nonmedical approaches—Kegel exercises *(opposite)* and biofeedback—for patients suffering from stress incontinence. Bladder retraining is another useful technique. For seven days you keep a written record of how much you drink, how often

Incontinence

you urinate, and how much urine you produce. You then start urinating at scheduled intervals, usually every 30 or 60 minutes. Gradually, over a period of several weeks, you will increase the length of time between visits to the toilet.

If the condition persists or worsens, see a doctor for a full evaluation. Conventional approaches—including surgery—may be necessary.

■ Acupuncture

Acupuncturists believe that incontinence results from a deficiency of kidney and spleen chi. To restore the balance of chi in the affected parts, practitioners stimulate the specific points related to these organs and their channels. Consult a professional acupuncturist.

■ Biofeedback

Studies have shown that biofeedback techniques can lead to complete bladder control in up to 25 percent of incontinent patients and to substantial improvement in another 30 to 50 percent. Treatment sessions typically involve inserting a catheter through the urethra into the bladder and then slowly filling the bladder with fluid while the patient uses biofeedback techniques to control the urge to urinate.

■ Homeopathy

For stress incontinence, particularly in the elderly, try *Causticum,* which is said to restore vitality to aging tissue. For both stress and urge incontinence, particularly when a person is rising from a prone position, try **Pulsatilla,** thought to relieve irritation of the lining of the urinary tract system and restore it to proper functioning.

■ Nutrition and Diet

Try to keep your weight down. Excess weight puts pressure on bladder muscles, weakening them.

The straining that accompanies constipation can also weaken bladder muscles. Avoid constipation by increasing the fiber in your diet; eat more whole-grain foods and fruits and vegetables.

Avoid alcohol, caffeine, decaffeinated drinks, sugar and sugar substitutes, spicy foods, and acidic fruits and juices—all of which can irritate the bladder and trigger leaks. Foods to which you are sensitive can also cause bladder irritation.

Home Remedies

- Double void: After urinating, wait a few seconds, then try again. Pouring cool water over the urinary opening after voiding can help.
- If you are a woman with stress incontinence, try crossing your legs when sneezing or coughing. This simple practice can be very effective in stopping leakage.
- Try bouncing on a minitrampoline for exercise; after several days, the pelvic floor muscles become strengthened enough to help prevent stress incontinence. ■

Kegel Exercises

Women with stress incontinence can use Kegel exercises to strengthen the pelvic floor muscles that support the uterus and bladder and control contractions of the vagina and urethra. While urinating, slowly contract the pelvic floor muscles, halting the flow of urine. Hold for up to 10 seconds and repeat several times. You can also do the exercises at other times, while standing, sitting, or lying down.

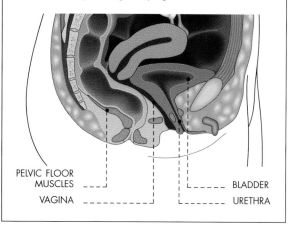

PELVIC FLOOR MUSCLES — — — —

VAGINA — — — — — — — — —

BLADDER

URETHRA

I

$\mathcal{I}$ndigestion

Symptoms

- Heartburn.
- Gas or belching.
- Abdominal pressure and/or pain, which can radiate toward the chest.
- Mild nausea.
- Vomiting.

Call Your Doctor If

- any abdominal pain continues for more than six hours; this may indicate appendicitis, stomach ulcers, gallstones, or another serious problem or disease. You may need emergency care.

- you experience indigestion with any of the following: prolonged vomiting, vomiting of blood, black or bloody bowel movements, severe upper abdominal pain, pain radiating into your neck and shoulder, shortness of breath, or feeling weak or faint. Your indigestion may be part of a larger problem, such as gallstones, gastritis, pancreatic trouble, stomach ulcers, or possibly cancer. Or you might be having a heart attack; get medical help immediately.

- you have repeated bouts of indigestion accompanied by abdominal pain, fever, or dark urine. Your discomfort may indicate gallstones, stomach ulcers, or liver disease.

- your indigestion consistently follows your eating dairy products. You may suffer from lactose intolerance.

I ndigestion is a catchall term for assorted stomach discomforts. Symptoms of indigestion are cues that normal digestion has been interrupted for one or more reasons. If stomach acid enters the esophagus, for example, you may feel heartburn. Swallowing too much air while eating or drinking can induce a distended stomach and cause excessive belching. Stomach infections or inflammation can bring on gastritis. Sufferers of irritable bowel syndrome may regularly experience abdominal pain, bloating, and diarrhea.

Indigestion may be occasional or chronic (daily or almost daily). Though uncomfortable, indigestion itself is not life threatening. It can accompany serious problems, however, and should not be ignored.

Common Causes

Everyone—all ages, men and women alike—feels occasional indigestion. The likelihood increases with age as the digestive system gradually becomes less efficient. Occasional or chronic indigestion may be brought on by overeating; overindulging in alcohol; frequent use of analgesics—such as aspirin—and other pain relievers; eating while under stress; or eating food that does not agree with your system.

Two common causes of chronic indigestion are obesity, which increases pressure in the abdomen, and smoking, which increases the production of stomach acid and relaxes the sphincter between the esophagus and stomach. Overeating—even if it doesn't lead to obesity—is also a major cause of indigestion and of a general weakening of the digestive system. In addition, about half of all chronic indigestion sufferers are infected with the bacterium *Helicobacter pylori*. This bacterium is known to cause stomach ulcers, and researchers are trying to determine if it causes other kinds of indigestion as well.

Treatment Options

Because indigestion sufferers may have several disorders at once, healers suggest diverse therapies. Fortunately, there are many choices for relief. With most alternative treatments, patience is essential. Quelling persistent indigestion may take weeks or

Indigestion

even months. Remember, however, that indigestion can result from a number of causes, so no single remedy will help everyone.

If it is determined that your indigestion is caused by *Helicobacter pylori,* you may need to see a doctor for a prescription of antibiotics to treat the infection.

Acupressure

To reduce symptoms of indigestion, massage the following for at least one minute: Large Intestine 4 and Stomach 25 and 36. If gas is also a problem, add Bladder 60 and Spleen 6. *(See the Gallery of Acupressure Techniques, pages 18-31, for information on point locations.)*

Aromatherapy

The essential oils of **tarragon** *(Artemisia dracunculus),* **rosemary** *(Rosmarinus officinalis),* and marjoram can reduce spasms of the digestive tract. Take 1 drop of one of these oils internally with either honey or a so-called carrier oil such as almond oil.

Ayurvedic Medicine

Shatavari may speed up digestion and alleviate many indigestion symptoms. Ayurveda bitters—including those from the trunk wood and bark of the common teak tree *(Tectona grandis)*—may also enhance digestion. Other remedies include infusions or powders made from mint, chamomile, and fennel seeds. Combined formulas include *Gasex* for adults (two to three tablets chewed after meals) and *Bonnisan* for children (consult a practitioner for dosages appropriate for the age of your child).

Herbal Therapies

Various teas may calm digestive distress. To reduce stomach acidity, drink meadowsweet *(Filipendula ulmaria)* tea once or twice daily, before meals (add 1 tsp to 1 cup boiling water, steep for 10 minutes, then filter). If you also feel stressed, add **lavender** *(Lavandula officinalis)* or **chamomile** *(Matricaria recutita).* If bloating or gas is a problem, try a tea of **peppermint** *(Mentha piperita),* chamomile, or lemon balm *(Melissa officinalis).*

Certain herbs are reputed to promote digestion and soothe and heal the esophagus, making them particularly appropriate for indigestion with heartburn. About 30 minutes before eating, drink ½ cup of tea made from **goldenseal** *(Hydrastis canadensis),* barberry *(Berberis vulgaris)* bark, gentian *(Gentiana lutea)* root, or Oregon grape *(Mahonia aquifolium)* root.

A number of Chinese herbal formulas, including *Po Chai* and Pill Curing, are effective against certain types of acute indigestion. A practitioner of Chinese medicine can prescribe a remedy that's appropriate for your condition.

Hydrotherapy

Place a hot-water bottle over the abdomen after meals. A hot compress or moist abdominal bandage can also help relieve indigestion.

Massage

Gentle massage properly applied to the abdomen can help speed digestion and alleviate the discomfort of indigestion. See the hand-on-hand petrissage technique in the Gallery of Massage Techniques, page 125.

Home Remedies

- Refrain from smoking, especially before eating.
- Try one or several of the herbal teas above to relieve your specific symptoms.
- Relax after eating. Exercise diverts blood from the stomach, making digestion less efficient.
- If you frequently chew gum, stop for a while to see if your symptoms dissipate. It's common to swallow air when chewing gum, which can cause indigestion.

Prevention

Indigestion is universal; it's almost impossible to avoid it forever. You can encounter it less often, however, if you chew your food well, watch your weight, avoid overeating (especially foods rich in fat) or overindulging in alcohol, avoid your "trigger" foods, and abstain from smoking. ■

Insomnia

Symptoms

■ Persistent trouble falling asleep.

■ Failure to sleep through the night.

■ Waking up earlier than usual.

Call Your Doctor If

■ you experience disturbed sleep for more than a month without apparent cause. You may need referral to a sleep-disorder specialist to monitor your sleep patterns and test for underlying physical ailments.

■ your insomnia is associated with a life-changing event, such as the loss of a job or a loved one. You may need sleep medication for a brief period.

■ you never seem to get enough sleep and fall asleep without warning during the day. You may be suffering from narcolepsy.

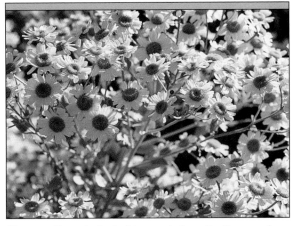

Chamomile • *An herbal tea made from the flowers of the German chamomile (Matricaria recutita) plant can be very calming and soothing. You can buy prepared bags of chamomile tea or make your own by steeping 2 tsp flowers in 8 oz piping hot water for 10 minutes.*

A fter infancy, humans function the way the world turns—on a natural cycle that repeats itself about every 24 hours. During this daily cycle—which is known as the circadian rhythm—most adults sleep between six and eight hours, usually at night and without interruption. Although a few nights of poor sleep do no harm, prolonged insomnia can have serious consequences.

Insomnia can be described in terms of both duration and severity. Transient insomnia is associated with a temporary disturbance of one's normal sleeping pattern and usually lasts no more than several nights. Short-term insomnia, lasting two or three weeks, can accompany worry or stress and typically disappears when the apparent cause is resolved. Chronic insomnia is a more complex disorder with potentially serious effects.

Narcolepsy is characterized by attacks of irresistible drowsiness during the day, disrupting the pattern of a person's normal activity. A narcoleptic may not sleep well at night but suffer sleep attacks during the day.

Treatment Options

Many poor sleepers simply need help relaxing. If you're a habitual insomniac and trying to get to sleep just makes you feel more awake, the following remedies may help reduce your worry about sleep while relaxing your body and mind. If the root cause of insomnia is stress, any treatment must address the underlying problem.

■ Aromatherapy

A relaxant effect may be provided by oils of Roman chamomile *(Anthemis nobilis),* **lavender** *(Lavandula angustifolia),* neroli, rose, or marjoram. Add a few drops to your bathwater or sprinkle a few drops on a handkerchief and inhale.

■ Exercise

Moderate exercise—a 20- to 30-minute routine three or four times a week—will help you sleep better and give you more energy. Tailor the routine to your physical condition and exercise in the morning or afternoon, not close to bedtime. Breathing exercises can promote relaxation; here's a routine you can do anywhere, anytime:

■ Exhale completely through your mouth.

Insomnia

- Inhale through your nose to a count of four.
- Hold your breath for a count of seven.
- Exhale through your mouth for a count of eight. Repeat the cycle three times.

Herbal Therapies

Half an hour before bedtime, drink a calming herbal tea made with **chamomile** *(Matricaria recutita),* lime blossom *(Tilia cordata),* **passionflower** *(Passiflora incarnata),* or hops *(Humulus lupulus);* for insomnia from nervous tension, use vervain *(Verbena officinalis)* or **skullcap** *(Scutellaria lateriflora).* **Valerian** *(Valeriana officinalis)* is effective and seldom causes morning sleepiness: Brew valerian tea or take about 20 drops of tincture in water at bedtime; experiment to find the dosage that suits you best. Note that valerian, like any sleeping aid, acts as a central nervous system depressant and should not be used every night.

Homeopathy

For insomnia, a homeopathic practitioner may prescribe **Nux vomica** if the cause is anxiety or restlessness, **Ignatia** if the insomnia is related to grief, *Coffea* if it is related to excitability, or *Muriaticum acidum* if it stems from emotional problems.

Massage

Massage can promote relaxation and better sleep. While this may not be possible on a daily basis, it is a good complement to full-body exercises that may have caused stiff, tight muscles. Sessions with a massage therapist, or a massage routine performed by a partner, can be especially helpful when the insomnia is due to stress and anxiety, as well as muscular stiffness or discomfort.

Mind/Body Medicine

Meditation, yoga, and biofeedback can reduce tension and promote better sleep. Visualization, or guided imagery, may help you relax: Hold a peaceful image in your mind before bedtime.

Nutrition and Diet

Melatonin, a hormone secreted naturally by the pineal gland, is said to induce sleep without producing negative side effects; try a capsule nightly at bedtime for two weeks. The dosage should range anywhere from .3 to 1 mg. You may want to start by trying the lowest dose, which has proved effective with some people. Because experience with this hormone is limited, you may also want to consult your healthcare practitioner.

Calcium and **magnesium** taken 45 minutes before bedtime have a tranquilizing effect. Use a 1:1 ratio, in tablet or capsule form.

High or low blood sugar can disrupt sleep patterns. To help stabilize blood sugar, avoid sweets and fruit juices. To actuate the brain's sedative neurotransmitters, eat starchy food—a plain baked potato, a slice of bread, or an apple—half an hour before bedtime.

Warm milk, a traditional sleep aid, may provide a benefit that is more psychological than physiological. It does contain tryptophan, a sleep-inducing amino acid, but it also contains many other amino acids that compete to enter the brain.

Home Remedies

Be sure your bedroom is quiet and dark. Earplugs and eye masks may help; some light comes in even through closed eyelids.

Both children and adults may have trouble sleeping if they are overstimulated by activity or by watching television just before bedtime. A quarter-hour of quiet conversation, light reading, or soft music may make all the difference.

If you wake up at night and can't go back to sleep, remain quiet and relaxed. Sleep is normally punctuated by periods of restlessness, or even waking. Be patient; sleep usually returns.

Prevention

Try not to be rigid about when and how much you sleep. Worrying about a sleep schedule can just make it harder to fall asleep. If you prefer taking a nap during the day and sleeping less at night, do so. The total amount of sleep you get in 24 hours is more important than your daily schedule. ■

Irritable Bowel Syndrome

Symptoms

- Constipation or diarrhea shortly after meals, over a period of several months, usually accompanied by abdominal cramps or bloating and increased intestinal gas.

- Bowel movements different in frequency or consistency from your normal pattern.

Call Your Doctor If

- you have pain in the lower left abdomen, fever, and a change in the frequency of bowel movements; you may have diverticulitis.

- you discover blood in your stools; you could have colon polyps or colorectal cancer.

- you have a fever, or you have been losing weight unexpectedly; such symptoms may signal disorders such as ulcerative colitis or Crohn's disease.

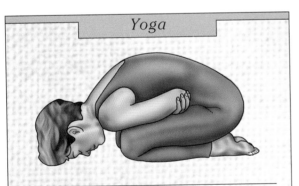

Yoga

Abdominal Massage • *To ease bowel spasms, sit on your heels, thighs together. Place your left fist on the right side of your abdomen, press your right elbow over it, and cup your left elbow in your right hand. Exhale, bend forward, and bring your forehead to the floor. Breathe deeply. Relax and gently massage the area with your fist 15 to 20 seconds. Rise and massage your abdomen with your fingers. Repeat on your left side. Do twice daily.*

*I*rritable bowel syndrome (IBS), which is sometimes referred to as spastic colon or spastic colitis, is the most common of all digestive disorders. The most frequently encountered symptom is abdominal pain with diarrhea or soft, frequent stools. In other cases, IBS comes with abdominal cramps and painful constipation, usually following meals. Whatever the specific symptoms, your digestion appears to be normal but your bowel movements become abnormal and stay that way for several weeks or longer. Irritable bowel syndrome affects 10 to 15 percent of adults at some time in their lives, often during periods of significant change or stress.

Treatment Options

Various herbal and dietary remedies may be effective in preventing or soothing the discomfort of diarrhea and constipation. Relaxation techniques may be particularly effective in coping with stress-related aspects of the problem.

Acupuncture

An acupuncturist will determine an appropriate approach by asking you questions about stresses in your life that may be at the root of the problem. Treatment for IBS typically involves 10 to 12 sessions in which needles are inserted along the liver, spleen, and kidney meridians. For symptomatic relief of diarrhea, the acupuncturist will probably insert the needles near the navel and left knee. To treat a bad bout of diarrhea, the practitioner may employ moxibustion, in which heat is applied near the points, for quick relief.

Exercise

Walking at an aerobic pace for 20 to 30 minutes gets the heart pumping, stimulates the digestive process, and relaxes the body. Vigorous noncompetitive exercise is also recognized as an effective way of combating and controlling stress. (Competitive sports, however, can add to stress for many individuals.) Yoga *(see the illustration at left)* not only conditions the muscles and connective tissue but also is thought to tone the internal organs, including the digestive tract, and release excess tension from the body.

Irritable Bowel Syndrome

Herbal Therapies

For diarrhea, make a carob *(Ceratonia siliqua)* tea: Pour 1 cup hot water over 1 tsp roasted carob powder. Drink three times a day.

To calm an overactive gastrointestinal tract, try a European favorite: Take one or two enteric-coated **peppermint** *(Mentha piperita)* oil capsules between meals, three times daily. Reduce the dose if you have a burning sensation when you move your bowels. Another option is peppermint tea: Steep 1 tbsp dried peppermint leaves in a cup of boiling water for 30 minutes; drink three to four cups a day. Infusions of **chamomile** *(Matricaria recutita),* **marsh mallow** *(Althaea officinalis)* root, bayberry *(Myrica* spp.), or **slippery elm** *(Ulmus fulva)* also are soothing to the intestinal tract and can be made the same way.

Homeopathy

A homeopathic practitioner will determine which remedy is appropriate to get at the root cause of the IBS. For relief of occasional diarrhea, try prepared remedies available in health food stores. **Ignatia** may be helpful if you are having spasms of pain and diarrhea after emotional upsets. If you are passing offensive-smelling gas and mucus in the stools, take **Mercurius vivus.** If sudden cramplike pains are relieved by bending over, take *Colocynthis.* If your stools are soft but you have to strain to pass them, try **Nux vomica.**

Mind/Body Medicine

A number of techniques have been found helpful for IBS, including training in muscle relaxation. After four to six weeks of daily practice, you will learn how to relax your previously tense muscles and relieve symptoms brought on by stress.

Biofeedback training is another technique that has become accepted by more and more conventional doctors and often is covered by insurance. In one form of biofeedback, painless electrodes are placed on the forehead to monitor muscle tension as an indicator of stress. Patients are taught to relax their muscles by actuating audio or visual signals that indicate the level of tension in the muscle.

Of all the relaxation techniques, the most familiar may be hypnotherapy. A practitioner uses the power of suggestion to teach a patient in a hypnotic state how to relax the smooth muscles of the intestines. Guided imagery, often taught by yoga instructors and massage therapists, can also teach you new ways to relax yourself.

Nutrition and Diet

Certain foods may contribute to IBS by irritating your gastrointestinal tract. Most things that people say taste good—from hamburgers and fries to ice cream and chocolate—are made with lots of fat. Whether it's vegetable oil or animal fat, or saturated or unsaturated, dietary fat overload is something many people simply can't handle. Other known irritants to some people's digestive tracts are eggs and dairy products, spicy foods, and stimulants, including caffeinated beverages and white sugar; decaffeinated beverages are also a problem, as are other forms of sugar such as molasses, corn syrup, and fructose.

If you are like most Americans, you are not eating enough fiber. To correct a dietary fiber imbalance:

- gradually increase the amount of fresh fruits and vegetables, whole grains, and bran in your diet, or
- take 1 tbsp bran stirred into a glass of fruit juice or water every day, or
- take soluble fiber, like **psyllium** *(Plantago psyllium)* seed. Stir 1 tbsp into a glass of cold water and drink once a day. When you are taking supplemental fiber, be sure to drink several extra glasses of plain water a day. You may experience a certain amount of intestinal gas at first, but it should subside as your body adjusts to the new regimen.

Prevention

Healthy outlets for stress are great preventives to many gastrointestinal problems, including IBS. Get regular exercise—anything from a brisk 20-minute walk to a round of golf or tennis or a half-hour's worth of swimming laps. And take 10 minutes twice a day to just relax and let go of tensions. ■

Kidney Disease

Symptoms

- Frequent thirst and urge to urinate.
- The passing of very small amounts of urine.
- Swelling, particularly of the hands and feet, and puffiness around the eyes.
- Unpleasant taste in the mouth and urinelike odor to the breath.
- Persistent fatigue or shortness of breath.
- Loss of appetite.
- Increasingly higher blood pressure.
- Pale skin.
- Excessively dry, persistently itchy skin.
- In children: increased fatigue and sleepiness, decrease in appetite, and eventually, poor growth.

Call Your Doctor If

- you are experiencing any of the symptoms listed above. Although any of them may indicate another disorder, each is one of the warning signs of kidney disease, which is a life-threatening illness. Consult your doctor without delay.

CAUTION

Because many drugs are excreted through the kidneys, if you have been diagnosed with kidney disease you need to consult with your doctor before taking any over-the-counter medications. You may be told to avoid ibuprofen and acetaminophen, for example, which have been implicated as possible contributors to kidney disease.

T he kidneys, two fist-sized organs located on either side of the spine just above the waist, perform a life-sustaining role. They cleanse the blood by removing waste and excess fluids, maintain a healthful balance of various body chemicals, and help regulate blood pressure.

When the kidneys become diseased or damaged, they can suddenly or gradually lose their ability to perform these vital functions. Waste products and excess fluid then build up inside the body, causing a variety of symptoms, particularly swelling of the hands and feet, shortness of breath, and a frequent urge to urinate. If left untreated, diseased kidneys may eventually stop functioning. Loss of kidney function is a very serious and potentially fatal condition.

Types of Kidney Disease

Kidney disease is classified as either acute (when loss of function occurs suddenly) or chronic (when deterioration takes place gradually, perhaps over many years). The chronic form can be particularly insidious: It may not show symptoms until considerable, often irreparable, damage has been done.

The causes of chronic kidney disease are often difficult to pinpoint. Most are the result of another disease or condition, such as diabetes, high blood pressure, or atherosclerosis—all of which impede the flow of blood inside the kidneys. Lupus and other diseases of the immune system that affect blood vessels may also trigger kidney disease by causing the kidneys to become inflamed.

Some chronic kidney diseases are inherited; others are congenital—the result of some sort of urinary tract obstruction or malformation that the person was born with and that predisposes the victim to kidney infections and diseases.

Chronic kidney disease may also result from long-term exposure to toxic chemicals or to drugs, including certain illegal drugs, such as heroin. Researchers also suspect that excessive amounts of vitamin D and protein, particularly in the diets of the elderly or the very ill, may harm the kidneys. But in many chronic cases, the precise cause remains unknown.

Acute kidney disease can occur within a matter of days following the onset of any medical con-

Kidney Disease

dition that suddenly and dramatically reduces the flow of blood to the kidneys. Examples are a heart attack, a traumatic injury such as one sustained in an automobile accident, a serious infection, or a toxic reaction to a drug.

Inhaling or swallowing certain toxins, including methyl, or wood, alcohol; carbon tetrachloride; antifreeze; and poisonous mushrooms, can also cause the kidneys to suddenly malfunction. Marathon runners and other endurance athletes who do not drink enough liquids while competing in long-distance athletic events may suffer acute kidney failure due to a sudden breakdown of muscle tissue, which releases a chemical called myoglobin that can damage the kidneys.

Treatment Options

Kidney disease is a life-threatening condition that requires medical care. Alternative treatments may be used to supplement that care, but before trying them you should discuss them thoroughly with your doctor.

Medications, especially those that control diabetes and high blood pressure, can sometimes help slow the progress of chronic kidney disease. Some medical practitioners have found that certain restrictive diets are useful, particularly if the condition is caught early (see Nutrition and Diet, right). But if these measures fail, and the kidneys deteriorate to the point where they no longer function, there are only two treatments: dialysis, in which artificial devices clean the blood of waste products, or a kidney transplant.

■ Chinese Medicine

Traditional Chinese health practitioners use several herbs in the treatment of kidney disorders. However, because many herbs can be harmful to the kidneys, you should always consult your physician before taking the advice of an herbalist or ingesting any herbal remedies.

■ Homeopathy

Homeopathic remedies are generally safe for the treatment of chronic kidney conditions. However, the remedies should be prescribed by a practitioner skilled in both conventional and alternative medicine, and they should never be used as a substitute for conventional medicine.

■ Nutrition and Diet

Although the approach remains controversial in conventional medical circles, a growing number of physicians now encourage dietary changes to help manage chronic kidney disease. Some studies have shown that rigid adherence to a diet that severely restricts protein can delay or even prevent continued kidney deterioration. This is especially true of people whose kidney disease is the result of diabetes. Studies have shown that diabetics who follow a diet that keeps their blood glucose levels within a tight range can help retard the progress of kidney disease.

Special restricted diets can decrease the work load on diseased kidneys, keep body fluids and chemicals in balance, and fend off a buildup of waste products in the body. Although such diets should be specifically tailored to each patient's individual needs, they all typically incorporate the following general restrictions:

- protein: no more than 1 gram per kilogram of body weight per day.
- *potassium:* no more than 2 grams per day.
- *phosphorus:* no more than 1 gram per day (usually accomplished by adhering to protein restrictions).
- *sodium:* in advanced cases of kidney disease, no more than 2 grams per day.

Calcium supplements (1,500 mg per day) are frequently recommended to counteract the bone weakening that often accompanies kidney disease.

■ Yoga

Postures that stretch the kidney area, such as the Cobra and the Locust, can be helpful.

Prevention

Kidney disease has been linked to certain chemicals found in common household products. Read labels carefully and avoid exposure to these chemicals: cadmium, carbon tetrachloride, chloroform, ethylene glycol, oxalic acid, and tetrachloroethylene. ■

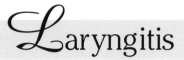 Laryngitis

Symptoms

- Hoarseness and loss of voice.
- Pain when speaking.
- Tickling and rawness in the throat.
- A constant need to clear the throat.
- Loss of voice that is accompanied by the flu, a cold, or pneumonia.
- Fever (occasionally).

Call Your Doctor If

- hoarseness and discomfort last more than a week; this could signal a bacterial infection or a more serious disorder.
- you develop laryngitis after being exposed to environmental toxins, such as poisonous fumes or noxious odors; such exposure might have caused more damage than just a simple inflammation of your vocal cords.
- laryngitis occurs along with or as a result of alcohol abuse or chronic bronchitis, both of which require a doctor's care.
- a child's hoarseness turns into a sharp, barking cough, which could indicate a severely restricted airway or, possibly, croup.

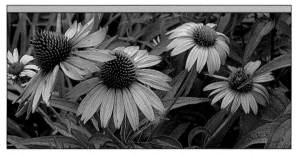

Echinacea • This attractive plant, known by gardeners as purple coneflower, is valued by herbalists for its roots. Echinacea root has antibacterial, antiviral, and immune-boosting properties that help wipe out the illness causing laryngitis.

I f you lose your voice, or if the sounds coming out of your mouth sound higher or lower than normal, you may have laryngitis. Specifically, this disorder is an inflammation of the mucous membrane of the larynx, or the part of your windpipe that contains the vocal cords. Your vocal cords open and close during the course of normal speech (right). If they become swollen, perhaps as a result of a viral or bacterial infection, overuse, or in some cases, an allergic reaction to a certain food, the sounds you make become distorted. You'll be hoarse, or you may lose your voice.

Treatment Options

Viral laryngitis usually goes away by itself in a few days, so a persistent case is a warning sign that something other than a virus may be causing your symptoms. To treat laryngitis, alternative practitioners often prescribe methods to soothe the raw throat or boost the immune system.

Acupuncture

A recent study found that many patients with laryngitis or tonsillitis benefited from acupuncture. Consult a licensed acupuncturist for treatment.

Aromatherapy

The essential oils of **thyme** *(Thymus vulgaris),* cypress, **rosemary** *(Rosmarinus officinalis),* and sage can help relieve the discomfort of laryngitis; place a few drops on a handkerchief and inhale.

Ayurvedic Medicine

An Ayurvedic physician may recommend one of the following remedies for laryngitis: an infusion or powder of cloves or of the fruit of beleric myrobalan, an infusion of ginger or mint, a milk decoction or powder of licorice root.

Chinese Medicine

For acute laryngitis, a practitioner of Chinese medicine may prescribe *Hou Yan Wan,* or Throat Inflammation Pills (also known as Laryngitis Pills).

Herbal Therapies

To help restore the voice, try gargling with a tea made from red sage *(Salvia officinalis* var. *rubia),*

ℒaryngitis

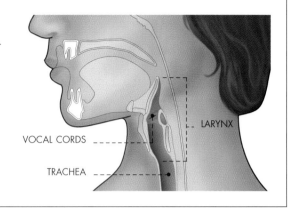

The Larynx and Voice Loss

The vocal cords are two taut bands that stretch across the larynx—a boxlike chamber at the upper part of the trachea, or windpipe. Air passing through these bands causes vibrations that produce sounds, which are shaped and modified by the tongue, teeth, and lips into speech. When the vocal cords are inflamed or infected because of laryngitis, the voice typically becomes hoarse or muted.

VOCAL CORDS

TRACHEA

LARYNX

bayberry (*Myrica* spp.), or white oak (*Quercus alba*) bark. A tincture of **echinacea** (*Echinacea* spp.) every hour for two days is thought to help boost the immune system. Mix 10 drops of the tincture in a glass of water and swallow.

■ Homeopathy

If laryngitis is a result of overuse or trauma to the vocal cords, use **Arnica** (6x or 12x) every hour; if you notice no improvement after four or five hours, try another preparation. For laryngitis that is accompanied by dryness of the throat and the feeling of a plug in the larynx, use *Spongia tosta* (12x) four times a day. For laryngitis accompanied by a dry, croupy cough that comes on suddenly after exposure to cold weather or with the first signs of a cold, use **Aconite** (6x or 12x) every two hours. If these remedies don't work, consult a practitioner.

■ Hydrotherapy

To soothe the discomfort of laryngitis, use a heating compress, which goes on cold but heats up as the body responds to the treatment.

Begin by placing a warm washcloth on your neck for two or three minutes. Soak a long, wide cotton cloth in cold water, then wring it out thoroughly and wrap it loosely around your neck. Next, wrap wool flannel (a wool scarf works nicely) around the cotton and secure it with a safety pin. Leave the compress in place for at least 30 minutes, preferably overnight. Follow the treatment with a quick cold sponge to the area. Change the

compress every eight hours and allow the skin to dry for at least an hour between treatments.

■ Nutrition and Diet

Drinking plenty of fluids, eating lots of raw fruits and vegetables, and reducing your intake of refined carbohydrates may help speed your recovery from laryngitis. To boost your immune system, supplement your daily diet with 1,000 to 3,000 mg **vitamin C,** 10,000 to 20,000 IU of beta carotene (**vitamin A**), and garlic.

Home Remedies

- Rest your body as well as your voice—completely. If you must speak, whisper; do not engage the vocal cords at all.
- Drink plenty of liquids, such as water or tea mixed with a little honey or lemon.
- Inhale steam from a pot of boiling water.
- Apply warm compresses to your throat.

Prevention

To prevent laryngitis, avoid straining your voice and give it proper rest after overuse. If you're prone to laryngitis, try to stay away from cigarette smoke or other environmental toxins. If you think your laryngitis stems from an allergy to a certain kind of food, experiment by removing suspected items from your diet, then reintroduce them one by one while monitoring the effect. *(See Allergies.)* ■

$\mathcal{M}$énière's Disease

Symptoms

- Intermittent dizziness (vertigo), sometimes accompanied by nausea and vomiting, pallor, and exhaustion.

- Hearing problems, including increasing hearing loss, tinnitus (a ringing, roaring, or buzzing sound in the ears), a sensitivity to loud noises, and the sensation of not hearing the same sounds in both ears.

- A feeling of fullness in the ears.

- Headache.

Call Your Doctor If

- you suspect you have Ménière's disease, which requires a medical evaluation.

- you have recurrent episodes of dizziness; difficulty in maintaining balance may point to problems in your inner ear that need medical attention.

- you find it more and more difficult to hear; a gradual loss of hearing over time may indicate a problem in any part of your ear (inner, middle, or outer) or in your brain.

- sounds are perceived differently by each ear; this may be a sign of other types of inner ear disorder in addition to Ménière's disease.

M énière's disease, first described more than a century ago by French physician Prosper Ménière, is characterized by numerous symptoms, all relating to problems in the inner ear. Attacks of the disease can be triggered by anxiety, tension, or excessive salt intake. Though the cause of the disorder is still in question, it is known that it involves an overabundance of endolymph, the fluid that fills the inner ear, home of the sensory organs for hearing and balance.

Treatment Options

Because scientists haven't yet found a cure for Ménière's disease, most treatment is directed at alleviating the symptoms and dealing with the psychological impact of the disorder. Conventional treatment often begins with medications to reduce pressure and fluid in the inner ear and to reduce feelings of dizziness. Surgery is reserved as a last resort for patients with extremely serious cases.

Acupuncture
For dizziness, consult an acupuncturist for stimulation at the following ear points: neurogate, sympathetic, kidney, occiput, adrenal, and heart. For chronic cases, an acupuncturist may treat body points on the kidney, triple warmer, and spleen meridians. *(See Acupuncture, pages 34-35, for more information on point locations.)*

Aromatherapy
To relieve stress, bathe with essential oils of ***lavender*** *(Lavandula angustifolia),* geranium, and sandalwood. Or try a massage with lavender essence and ***German chamomile*** *(Matricaria recutita)* oil.

Bodywork
For chronic cases, consult an osteopath or chiropractor for adjustments to the head, jaw, and neck relating to movement restriction that might affect the inner ear. For acute cases of dizziness, a reflexologist might suggest working the ear reflex; this and other areas that may prove beneficial to work are illustrated above, right. A craniosacral therapist may be able to alleviate your symptoms by gently moving the bones of your skull; this is believed to relieve pressure in the head.

*M*énière's Disease

Reflexology

To help relieve the symptoms of Ménière's disease, stimulate the ear area by walking your thumb along the base of the small toes and the shafts of the second and third toes. Walk your thumb up and down the upper portion of the spinal column area, and work the neck area on the big toe. Then stimulate the solar plexus area.

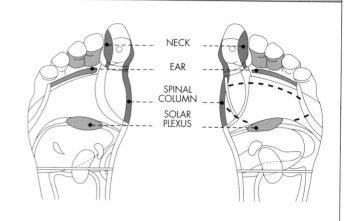

NECK
EAR
SPINAL COLUMN
SOLAR PLEXUS

Homeopathy

There are several homeopathic options, all of which call for a dosage of 12x every four to six hours. For dizziness in an acute attack that is made worse by a sensitivity to motion and is accompanied by a headache and a roaring or buzzing in the ears, try **Bryonia.** For dizziness and nausea in an acute attack, use *Cocculus.* For dizziness that is worse when lying down or turning over and is accompanied by sensitivity to light, try *Conium.* And for dizziness with nausea and vomiting that is aggravated by the least bit of motion or by closing the eyes and is accompanied by heightened noise sensitivity, try *Theridion.*

Mind/Body Medicine

In Ménière's disease, patients may undergo a vicious circle—attacks followed by anxiety and stress, which in turn provoke an attack. Various forms of massage therapy and yoga are excellent ways to reduce stress. And a number of communities across the country sponsor support groups.

Nutrition and Diet

Some nutritionists recommend a diet that increases calories, fat, and protein, but there is no evidence that such a regimen can cure the disease. Specialists also recommend a daily intake of the following: 2,000 mg of *vitamin C;* 50 mg each of *vitamins B₁, B₂,* and *B₆;* 20 mg of *zinc;* and other vitamins and minerals. If you have Ménière's disease, you may want to stay away from salt—which causes your body to retain fluid—and restrict your intake of liquids. Some experts speculate that lowering fluid levels in your body also helps relieve the buildup of pressure in your inner ear, but this has not been proved. A nutritionist or dietitian can help prescribe a diet for any specific problems you may have.

Home Remedies

- During an attack, lie still and try to relax.
- Try reducing your intake of liquids and salt; some people believe that lowering fluid levels in the body can help reduce the pressure of fluid buildup in the inner ear.
- Avoid caffeine, smoking, and alcohol, which may increase stress and interfere with a proper resting state.
- Try to get a good night's sleep.
- Avoid driving, swimming, climbing on ladders, and other activities in which an attack of dizziness might lead to a serious injury.

Prevention

The best way to prevent an attack of Ménière's disease is to reduce stress. Seek out enjoyment, perhaps through a hobby or a sport. Take time off to pursue things that give you pleasure: Listen to music, read a magazine, drink a relaxing tea— *chamomile (Matricaria recutita)* is a good choice— or simply take some time to sit and do nothing. ■

$\mathcal{M}$enopause

Symptoms

Not all women experience symptoms with the onset of menopause. If symptoms occur, they may include:

■ Hot flashes—sudden reddening or heating of the face, neck, and upper back, which may produce sweating. Flashes typically last only a few minutes.

■ Night sweats, which may disrupt sleep and lead to insomnia.

■ Pain during intercourse, caused by thinning of vaginal tissues and loss of lubrication.

■ Increased nervousness, anxiety, or irritability.

■ The need to urinate more often than before, especially during the night.

Call Your Doctor If

■ you experience bleeding after menopause; among other possibilities, it may be a sign of uterine cancer, so you should be checked by your doctor.

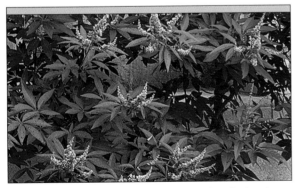

Chaste Tree • Used for centuries to manipulate the functioning of the female reproductive system, chaste tree can help relieve premenstrual syndrome and counter symptoms of menopause.

Menopause literally means the end of menstruation, but the term is also used to refer to the months and years before and after a woman's final period. Most women menstruate for the last time at about age 50, a few as early as 40, and a very small percentage as late as 60. Most women notice some physical changes—such as irregular periods and light menstrual flow—up to a few years before menstruation ceases.

As a woman ages, her ovaries slow and eventually cease their normal functions, including egg production. Even more significant, they decrease their production of estrogen and progesterone. As levels of these hormones—especially estrogen—decline, they cause changes throughout the body and particularly in the reproductive system, the most notable change being the end of menstruation. Decreased estrogen levels may also be responsible for the various symptoms associated with menopause, such as hot flashes and mood swings, which may or may not be present.

Some symptoms, including hot flashes and mood swings, are temporary and will pass as the body adjusts. But more serious problems can also result. Decreased levels of estrogen, for example, affect the way bones absorb calcium and can raise cholesterol levels in the blood; postmenopausal women thus face increased risk for developing both osteoporosis and cardiovascular diseases such as atherosclerosis.

Treatment Options

The most common approach to treating menopausal problems is to make up for the body's reduced production of estrogen. Known in conventional medicine as hormone replacement therapy, this technique is somewhat controversial because of certain side effects, so you should weigh the risks and benefits in consultation with your doctor.

■ Aromatherapy
Essential oils of ***clary sage*** *(Salvia sclarea),* sage, and geranium can help ease the symptoms of menopause. Put a few drops in the bath, or sprinkle the oil on a handkerchief and inhale.

■ Ayurvedic Medicine
Depending on your needs, an Ayurvedic physician may recommend the combined formula *Geriforte* or

Menopause

one of the following: the powder of *shatavari* root, boiled in milk to which clarified butter (ghee) has been added, taken three times daily; or the powder of Indian nut grass, steeped in a pint of water and taken with ginger and honey three times a day.

Bodywork

Many women find relief of menopausal symptoms through therapeutic touch, a method in which a healer holds his or her hands near the patient's body to sense and correct energy blockages. Consult a practitioner trained in this technique.

Herbal Therapies

A variety of herbs and foods may help relieve symptoms of menopause. Extracts and teas made from **black cohosh** (*Cimicifuga racemosa*) may supply beneficial amounts of phytoestrogen, or plant estrogen. Combinations of **chaste tree** (*Vitex agnus-castus*), motherwort (*Leonurus cardiaca*), **wild yam** (*Dioscorea villosa*), and other herbs may help reduce the frequency and discomfort of hot flashes, and may also relieve other symptoms. The herb **horsetail** (*Equisetum arvense*), thought to increase the absorption of calcium in the bones, may help prevent loss of bone density after menopause.

Some Chinese herbs—including **dong quai** (*Angelica sinensis*) and **Asian ginseng** (*Panax ginseng*)—may have estrogenic effects. Exact proportions are important, and some dosages are toxic; consult an herbalist. For hot flashes and night sweats, a Chinese medicine practitioner may recommend the formulas *Zhi Bai Ba Wei Wan* (Eight Flavor Pills) or *Liu Wei Di Huang Wan* (Six Flavor Pills).

Hydrotherapy

For relief from hot flashes, try a cold compress: Wet a cotton washcloth with ice water. Wring it out and apply it to the neck and chest. Hold the cloth in place for three minutes, rewetting it as needed to keep it cold. Dry the area after the treatment.

Mind/Body Medicine

Regardless of your religious affiliation or particular set of spiritual beliefs, prayer and meditation can be powerful tools to help you cope with the symptoms of menopause.

OF SPECIAL INTEREST

Menopausal Myths and Facts

Myth: *Menopause makes women emotionally unstable.*
Fact: *Most women experience no emotional problems; those that occur can be treated.*

Myth: *Menopause puts an end to sexual desire.*
Fact: *Vaginal dryness can make intercourse painful, reducing desire, but this is readily treated with vaginal lubricants or estrogen creams. Menopause itself can affect libido either positively or negatively; some women actually have increased libido with menopause.*

Myth: *Menopause disrupts a woman's life.*
Fact: *Most women experience few or no menopausal problems; 25 percent have moderate, treatable symptoms. In countries where age is respected, women report the fewest symptoms during menopause.*

Nutrition and Diet

Eating foods high in plant estrogens, such as soybeans and lima beans, may alleviate symptoms; additional sources include whole grains, other beans, nuts, and seeds.

Sound Therapy

A number of sound-healing and music-therapy techniques can be useful in treating the stress and other symptoms associated with menopause. Consult a music therapist or sound healer for a program that's right for you.

Home Remedies

- Raise your intake of **calcium** and **magnesium** and engage in weight-bearing exercises to avoid osteoporosis and maintain general good health.
- Take 400 to 800 IU of **vitamin E** daily to treat hot flashes and reduce the risk of cardiovascular disease. ■

$\mathcal{M}$enstrual Problems

Symptoms

- Menstruation does not occur. Called amenorrhea, this can come from pregnancy, overexercise, or anorexia nervosa.

- Menstruation is painful and produces clots. Called dysmenorrhea, this may be entirely normal, but it may also be caused by endometriosis; polyps, fibroids, or other lesions of the uterus; or an intrauterine device (IUD).

- Menstrual flow is heavy. Called menorrhagia, this can be a result of stress, endometriosis or other pelvic lesions, pelvic infection, or an IUD.

Call Your Doctor If

- you have heavy menstrual flow that fills a tampon or sanitary napkin within an hour; heavy flow can cause anemia.

- you have missed a period and think you may be pregnant; a late flow that is unusually heavy could indicate a miscarriage.

- you experience sharp abdominal pain before periods or during intercourse; you could have endometriosis.

- you get your period after menopause.

$\mathcal{M}$ *enstruation is a normal part of a woman's reproductive cycle. When an ovary releases an egg, it also releases the hormone estrogen, which stimulates the lining of the uterus to grow and engorge with blood. If the egg is not fertilized, the ovary releases progesterone, which makes the uterus shed its lining; the resulting menstrual flow typically consists of a few tablespoonfuls of blood and tissue fragments. This series of events repeats on a cycle of approximately 28 days until it is interrupted by pregnancy or ended by menopause.*

The degree of discomfort or pain a period causes, as well as the amount of menstrual flow, varies widely among individuals. Also, your own period may occasionally be heavier or more painful than usual. Such problems, while unpleasant, generally do not signal underlying disease. But you should be aware that the same complaints can sometimes indicate more serious conditions, such as endometriosis or an ovarian cyst.

The three main categories of menstrual irregularities are lack of period (amenorrhea), painful periods (dysmenorrhea), and heavy periods (menorrhagia). The following text explains these problems and what you can do about them.

LACK OF PERIOD

Although often no cause for concern, amenorrhea can be a sign of an underlying problem. It might indicate, for example, that you have low levels of estrogen in your system and are therefore at a greater risk of developing osteoporosis. Or it may signal a lack of progesterone and that you are at a greater risk for endometrial problems, including endometrial cancer. Also, of course, if you do not menstruate, you cannot become pregnant.

The lack of a period in a woman who has not yet begun to menstruate is known as primary amenorrhea; in a woman who has temporarily stopped menstruating, it is known as secondary amenorrhea. Primary amenorrhea has several causes, the most likely of which is that a girl has simply not yet reached puberty. (It is perfectly normal for puberty to occur as late as the age of 17.) But delayed puberty in a girl who is very thin or who exercises excessively is worrisome, because it could be an indication of anorexia nervosa; women who have very low body fat do not menstruate.

Primary amenorrhea can also point to other problems. In rare cases, for example, a girl might actually lack ovaries or a uterus and therefore not be able to menstruate. Or a tumor, an injury or trauma, or a structural defect might be interfering with some aspect of the menstrual cycle, from the production of hormones to the actions of the organs and tissues that the hormones affect.

Secondary amenorrhea can also be traced to injuries or structural abnormalities; one common cause is ovarian cysts. But factors such as stress can also disrupt the balance of hormones and thereby interrupt the normal cycle. Also, as in adolescence, extreme underweight can stop menstruation; if your period stops while you are dieting or in athletic training, you may be overdoing it. And, of course, amenorrhea could signal the onset of menopause or pregnancy.

PAINFUL PERIODS

Menstrual pain, or dysmenorrhea, is hardly unusual and in most cases is completely normal, even if troublesome. But there are situations in which painful periods may signal a condition that requires further evaluation by your doctor. And if your pain interferes with your normal activities, you should consider some of the treatments listed

---

OF SPECIAL INTEREST

Menstrual Myths and Facts

Myth: *A bath causes or worsens menstrual cramps.*
Fact: *Soaking in a warm bath can soothe and relax muscles, thereby reducing pain.*

Myth: *Menstruating women should restrict their activities, and even stay in bed and rest.*
Fact: *Women can carry on normal activities during their period. Exercise may actually help lessen pain by stimulating muscles to release endorphins.*

Acupressure

Conception Vessel 4 • *You may be able to correct irregular periods by working this point. Measure four finger widths down from your navel. Press your index finger firmly into your abdomen and hold for one to two minutes. Do this twice a day every day.*

here, which may help bring you relief.

If you have always had painful periods, they are probably the result of hormonal changes during your menstrual cycle. The factor most likely to be causing pain is that your body is producing an excess of prostaglandins—hormonelike substances that cause contractions of the uterus during menstruation and when a woman goes into labor. During menstruation, these contractions ensure that all the menstrual blood and tissue are expelled from the body, but excess prostaglandins can cause repeated contractions—and perhaps even spasms—which are experienced as cramping. It is common for these pains to persist throughout your reproductive years, but many women find that menstrual cramps become milder after they have had a baby.

Dysmenorrhea may, however, also be caused by an underlying condition, such as endometriosis, an infection, or growths in the uterus.

HEAVY PERIODS

A heavy period (menorrhagia) is a menstrual flow that lasts longer than eight days, saturates tampons or napkins within an hour, or includes large clots of blood. Heavy periods may be caused by various factors—a hormonal imbalance, endometriosis, a pelvic infection, uterine growths such as fibroids, or use of an IUD. Excessive bleeding may signal other irregularities in your cycle: lack of ovulation, low levels of progesterone, or an excess of prostaglandins. Heavy periods can cause iron deficiency anemia.

Treatment Options

Treatment for primary amenorrhea may involve no more than waiting to see if nature takes its course. For a girl who exercises strenuously or who is very thin, a healthcare professional may advise a lighter training regimen or an effort to gain weight. Treatment for anorexia nervosa might also be necessary. For secondary amenorrhea, if you think stress is to blame, take steps to reduce stress in your life; this alone may restore your cycle.

Most of the alternative therapies for menstrual cramps focus on promoting the relaxation of tense muscles or on reducing tension in general. Treatment for menorrhagia (heavy periods) may include **iron** and **folic acid** supplements to treat and prevent anemia.

In addition to the suggestions listed below, see the appropriate entries for treatment advice related to an underlying condition.

Acupressure
An acupressure technique that may prove effective in correcting irregular menstrual periods is illustrated on page 305. For relief of pain associated with menstrual cramps, use points known as Spleen 6 or Spleen 9. *(See the Gallery of Acupressure Techniques, pages 28-29.)*

Both acupressure and acupuncture use techniques that rely on spleen points to help control blood flow. See a practitioner for points and techniques to relieve excessive menstrual flow.

Aromatherapy
For painful periods, massage the lower abdomen, back, and legs with oil or lotion containing **German chamomile** (Matricaria recutita).

Practitioners of aromatherapy find that oils of geranium, juniper, and cypress, rubbed on the abdomen, may bring relief for sufferers of heavy menstrual flow.

Chiropractic
Chiropractic techniques can sometimes help relieve menstrual cramps; see a chiropractor for treatment.

Herbal Therapies
To help initiate menstrual flow, make a tincture of one part **chaste tree** (Vitex agnus-castus), two parts blue cohosh (Caulophyllum thalictroides), and two parts **mugwort** (Artemisia argyi) **leaf;** take 2 ml three times daily until menstrual flow begins.

To relieve cramps, drink a hot tea of 2 tsp cramp bark (Viburnum opulus) simmered for 15 minutes in 1 cup water; use this three times a day. Bilberry (Vaccinium myrtillus) and bromelain will also relax muscles. **Dong quai** (Angelica sinensis) and **feverfew** (Tanacetum parthenium) can relax uterine muscles; feverfew may work by inhibiting prostaglandin synthesis. **Valerian** (Valeriana officinalis) helps relax cramping muscles; however, it may be addictive and should be used only for a limited time. Consult an herbalist.

Evening primrose (Oenothera biennis) oil applied over painful areas can also bring relief, but don't use it if there's a chance you may get pregnant. In addition, a castor-oil pack placed over painful areas can be helpful.

Tension, anxiety, and painful spasms may be relieved with treatments of black haw (Viburnum prunifolium), **skullcap** (Scutellaria lateriflora), and **black cohosh** (Cimicifuga racemosa). Take equal parts of these herbs in 5-ml doses as needed.

Tea made from **yarrow** (Achillea millefolium) may help control bleeding associated with heavy periods. You may also benefit from taking a tincture made of equal parts life root (Senecio aureus), shepherd's purse (Capsella bursa-pastoris), and wild cranesbill (Geranium maculatum); take it twice daily in 5-ml doses.

A number of Chinese herbal formulas can help with menstrual problems. For a painful period, try the combination formula *Xiao Yao Wan* (Free and Easy Wanderer Pills); for excessive bleeding, *Yun*

ℳenstrual Problems

Yoga

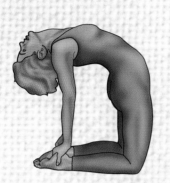

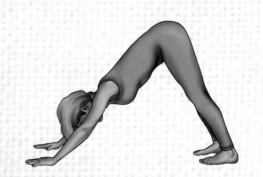

Camel • *Performing this position regularly may help relieve amenorrhea or painful periods. First, kneel down. Lean backward as you exhale, placing your palms on the soles of your feet and tilting your head back (above). Inhale as you squeeze your buttocks and press your pelvis forward. Breathe slowly and hold this position for 20 seconds.*

 To release, exhale as you sit back on your heels. Then inhale as you bring your body up, raising your head last. Breathe slowly and relax for 20 seconds. Do once or twice a day.

Downward Dog • *This pose helps release pelvic tension. From the Table position on your hands and knees, inhale and raise your pelvis to form an inverted V with your knees slightly bent.*

 Press your palms and heels into the floor as you breathe deeply, keeping your arms and shoulders open and your back and legs straight (above). Hold for 20 to 30 seconds. To release, exhale as you resume the Table position. Sit back on your heels, bring your head up, and relax before attempting to stand up again. Do this two or three times a day.

Nan Bai Yao may offer relief. See a practitioner of Chinese medicine for a diagnosis.

Nutrition and Diet

To address nutrient deficiencies that may be causing amenorrhea, take supplements of or eat foods rich in **zinc** (fish, poultry, lean meats) and **vitamin B complex** (brewer's yeast, wheat germ).

 Eating a balanced diet consisting of small meals throughout the day rather than three larger meals and avoiding sugar, salt, and caffeine may help relieve or prevent cramping. You may get relief from a multivitamin-multimineral supplement containing vitamin B complex, **calcium,** and **magnesium.** You can also take 50 mg of **vitamin B$_6$** twice a day. Because your goal is to keep your body relaxed, avoid caffeine and other stimulants.

Yoga

Poses for relaxation and the relief of cramps are described and illustrated in the box above.

Home Remedies

- Take extra calcium and magnesium to stop uterine muscle cramps and to lessen the flow.
- Take a warm, relaxing bath.
- Drink herbal teas containing yarrow to help control bleeding.
- Apply a castor-oil pack to the abdomen to relax the muscles and lessen the flow.

Prevention

Maintain normal weight for your build, which helps prevent excess fat and estrogens in the body. Overweight women tend to have abnormal menstrual periods, perhaps because of an increase in estrogen-secreting cells.

 Take a multivitamin-multimineral supplement including **vitamins A, B complex, C,** and **E,** as well as **calcium** and **iron.** ■

$\mathcal{M}$ononucleosis

Symptoms

The early symptoms of mononucleosis resemble those of the flu, including:

- Severe fatigue.
- Headache.
- Sore throat, sometimes very severe.
- Chills, followed by a fever.
- Muscle aches.

After a day or two, the following symptoms may appear:

- Swollen lymph nodes, especially in the neck, armpits, or groin.
- Jaundice (a yellow tinge to the skin and eyes).
- Bruiselike areas inside the mouth.
- Soreness in the upper left abdomen (from an enlarged spleen).

Call Your Doctor If

- you have these symptoms, particularly for longer than 10 days, or if you have a severe sore throat for more than a day or two; you need to be examined by a doctor to rule out other illnesses.
- you develop swollen lymph nodes all over your body, which may be a sign of tuberculosis, cancer, or human immunodeficiency virus.
- you develop abdominal pain, which may indicate a ruptured spleen. Seek emergency medical treatment immediately.

CAUTION

If you have mononucleosis, avoid the risk of rupturing your spleen by forgoing any strenuous exercise until you have fully recovered.

Mononucleosis, often referred to as mono, is a very common viral illness. About 90 percent of people over age 35 have antibodies to mono in their blood, which means that they have been infected with the disease, probably during early childhood. When mono strikes young children, the illness is usually so mild that it passes for a common cold or the flu. When it occurs during adolescence or adulthood, however, the disease can be much more serious. Most people who come down with mono feel much better within two or three weeks. But sometimes the disease lingers for a year or so, causing recurrent, but successively milder, attacks.

Treatment Options

Most people recover on their own without any treatment within two weeks. Practitioners of alternative medicine recommend rest and various treatments to help relieve the symptoms of the disease. They also offer remedies to help strengthen the body's immune system.

Aromatherapy

Lavender (*Lavandula angustifolia*), bergamot, and **eucalyptus globulus** (*E. globulus*) are sometimes recommended to relieve fatigue and other symptoms of mono. Add a few drops of the essential oils of one or more of these herbs to a warm bath.

Chinese Medicine

The Chinese herbal formula *Xiao Chai Hu Wan* (Minor Bupleurum Pills) is often prescribed for the treatment of mononucleosis; it helps the liver clear infections from the body. Acupuncture may also be beneficial; consult a practitioner of Chinese medicine for dosages and treatment.

Herbal Therapies

To help fight the infection, try **echinacea** (*Echinacea* spp.) in glycerin tincture form; use 15 drops two times a day. To reduce the fever associated with mono, try drinking a tea made from elder (*Sambucus nigra*) flowers or **yarrow** (*Achillea millefolium*). Drink either tea three times a day. Or if you prefer, take 2 to 4 ml of the tincture of either herb three times a day.

To help cleanse the lymphatic system, try a

$\mathcal{M}$ononucleosis

tea made from cleavers (*Galium* spp.) or wild indigo *(Baptisia tinctoria)*; drink three times a day. Alternatively, take 2 to 4 ml of tincture of cleavers or 1 ml of tincture of wild indigo three times daily.

To help with the anxiety and depression that sometimes accompany long-term bouts with mono, try **St.-John's-wort** *(Hypericum perforatum)* or vervain *(Verbena officinalis)*. Both herbs, when taken internally, appear to act as mild sedatives. Vervain is also recommended for jaundice, one of the symptoms of mono. Make a tea out of either herb and drink three times daily. Or take in tincture form: 1 to 4 ml of St.-John's-wort or 2 to 4 ml of vervain three times a day.

■ Homeopathy

Mononucleosis calls for a constitutional treatment—a set of remedies prescribed specifically for you, based on your symptoms and your medical history. Consult an experienced homeopath for such a treatment.

■ Mind/Body Medicine

Various relaxation techniques, such as meditation, biofeedback, and guided imagery, can be helpful in reducing stress, which can exacerbate the fatigue associated with mononucleosis.

■ Nutrition and Diet

To strengthen your immune system and help speed your recovery, eat plenty of whole (not processed) foods, especially fresh fruits and vegetables. Avoid foods that are high in saturated fats, animal proteins, and sugars, as they are difficult to digest and put stress on your body. Also avoid both caffeinated and decaffeinated beverages, which may weaken the immune system.

To maintain a better balance of blood sugar, and thus a more even energy level, eat four to six small meals throughout the day rather than three larger ones; try not to overeat at any one meal. Some people also find that eating a small portion of low-fat protein immediately on awakening in the morning and again in the evening before going to bed can help raise energy levels. Good choices of protein for this purpose include low-fat cheese as well as tofu, lentils, and other legumes.

Vitamin supplements may also enhance your immune system. Take **vitamin A** (2,500 to 10,000 IU daily), **vitamin C** (500 to 2,000 mg daily), and **vitamin B complex** (50 mg a day). You may also wish to try daily **magnesium** (200 to 500 mg), **calcium** (200 to 500 mg), and **potassium** aspartate (50 to 200 mg) supplements. Research has shown that these supplements can dramatically improve energy levels after six weeks of constant use.

■ Yoga

Yoga can help reduce fatigue. The exercises are gentle enough to be done even by someone with the illness. One recommended pose is the Cobra *(see the Gallery of Yoga Positions, page 186).*

Home Remedies

■ Rest your body. Do not plan to return to your normal activity level for at least a month.

■ Drink plenty of liquids to prevent dehydration.

■ For sore throat, use a saline gargle—½ tsp salt in a glass of warm water.

■ To help ease fatigue, massage your kidneys daily. With loose fists, rub your lower back for three to five minutes. A good occasion to do this is in the shower with warm water running down your back. ■

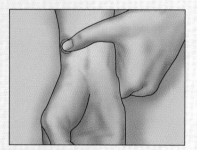

Acupressure

Lung 7 • *Pressing this point may bolster immunity and lung function. The point is located on the thumb side of the inner forearm, two finger widths above the crease in the wrist. Apply steady, firm pressure for one minute, then repeat on the other arm.*

Common Ailments

Motion Sickness

Symptoms

■ Sweating, dizziness, pallor, and nausea—sometimes leading to vomiting—while traveling by car, bus, train, ship, or airplane.

Call Your Doctor If

■ you are planning a trip and are concerned that you will be bothered by motion sickness that does not respond to alternative remedies; your doctor may prescribe antinausea drugs.

T he nausea and dizziness that afflict some people when they are traveling in a vehicle certainly cause discomfort, but they are not serious. The symptoms of motion sickness usually subside either once your body adjusts to your mode of travel or shortly after the trip ends. Motion sickness may occur because your brain is receiving conflicting information from your sensory organs.

Treatment Options

If you are prone to motion sickness, preparations for any trip should include measures to prevent the disorder or mechanisms to cope with it.

Acupressure

Much scientific research exists to substantiate the use of wrist point Pericardium 6 in relieving nausea. You might want to purchase acupressure wristbands to place over this point when you travel. When worn as directed, the nodules on the bands put pressure on points acupressure proponents say reduce nausea. The bands are often recommended by conventional physicians and alternative practitioners alike, and are sold in many pharmacies and travel-goods stores.

See the illustrations opposite for information on the location of Pericardium 6 and another point that may be helpful.

Aromatherapy

For relief of nausea, take 1 drop of the essential oil of **peppermint** *(Mentha piperita)* internally by mixing it with honey or a so-called carrier oil such as almond oil.

Ayurvedic Medicine

For adults, an Ayurvedic physician may prescribe the combined formula *Gasex* (two to three tablets chewed after meals); for children, *Bonnisan* (consult a practitioner for the proper dosage for your child's age). Another good remedy is an infusion or powder made from the bark and leaves of the neem tree.

Flower Remedies

The flower remedy **Crab Apple** is often recommended for motion sickness and other ailments

Motion Sickness

that cause nausea. Consult a naturopath or other practitioner familiar with flower remedies.

■ Herbal Therapy

Ginger (*Zingiber officinale*) is a favorite motion sickness remedy of naturopaths. The herb causes none of the side effects of antinausea drugs and can be drunk as a tea, eaten candied, or taken in capsule form (two capsules every four hours the day before and as needed during travel); it should be taken on an empty stomach.

■ Homeopathy

Homeopathic remedies sometimes come in kits that contain motion sickness remedies, which can be taken before and during travel as directed. One of the most effective is *Tabacum*.

■ Hydrotherapy

Placing an ice bag at the base of the skull and on the solar plexus for about 15 minutes can help relieve motion sickness. You might also try a hot compress on the abdomen, or bathing your feet in a pail of cold water (between 45°F and 55°F) for five to 10 minutes.

■ Massage

Properly administered, gentle massage to the chest and abdomen can help control motion sickness. First, however, you should make sure that your

queasy stomach is not a symptom of a more serious problem, and you should discontinue the massage if your nausea increases.

Prevention

There are many strategies you can use to lower your vulnerability to motion sickness. In addition to the suggestions above, the following may help:

- Get plenty of fresh air. Open a car window, get on the ship's top deck, or open the overhead air vent in a plane.
- Keep your head as still as possible, close your eyes or focus on the horizon or another stationary object, and sit where motion is felt the least—in the front seat of the car, amidships or in a forward cabin of the ship, or over the wings of the plane. Avoid sitting facing backward on a bus, train, or plane. Don't read while in motion.
- Eat light meals of low-fat, starchy foods and avoid strong-smelling or -tasting foods.
- Don't drink alcohol or smoke.
- If nausea does set in, try eating olives or sucking on a lemon; these foods make your mouth dry and help diminish nausea. Soda crackers may help absorb excess saliva and acid in your stomach. If you feel too sick to eat, try drinking ginger ale (made from real ginger) or any carbonated beverage. ■

Acupressure

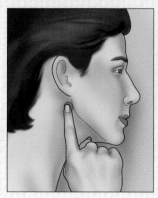

Small Intestine 17 • *To aid the ear's balancing mechanism, place your index fingers just below your earlobes in the indentations at the back of the jawbone. Apply light pressure while breathing deeply for one minute. Repeat one or two times.*

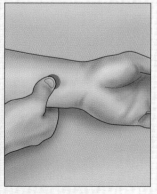

Pericardium 6 • *To help calm nerves and reduce nausea, place your thumb in the center of your inner wrist between the two forearm bones, two finger widths from the wrist crease. Press firmly for one minute, three to five times; then repeat on the other arm.*

Multiple Sclerosis

Symptoms

The first attack is generally mild, lasts only a few days, and is followed by a long period of remission—perhaps years—before the next episode. Symptoms vary considerably. They include:

- Weakness, stiffness (spasticity), or numbness in one or more limbs.

- Sensations of tingling, pins and needles, heaviness, a bandlike tightness around one or more limbs or the trunk of the body.

- Tremors, instability, or a lack of balance or muscular coordination.

- Blurred or double vision, or rapid, involuntary eye movement.

- Bladder or bowel incontinence.

- Fatigue: either a feeling of general tiredness or extreme exhaustion.

Call Your Doctor If

- you or someone you know has symptoms associated with multiple sclerosis. Because other diseases share some of the same symptoms, proper diagnosis and, if appropriate, treatment by a physician are essential.

- you are suffering from an acute attack. A number of conventional medications may help you cope with some of the symptoms: Steroid injections can help relieve pain; interferon beta cuts the frequency and severity of relapses; baclofen and dantrolene act to suppress spasticity; muscle relaxants relieve stiffness and pain; and amantadine, an antiviral drug, may promote stamina.

Multiple sclerosis, or MS, is a disease of the central nervous system, with effects that can range from relatively minor physical annoyances to major disabilities. The exact cause is unknown, but the root problem is electrical. Normally, most nerves in the body are insulated by a fatty substance known as myelin, which permits the efficient transmission of electrical impulses—the nerve signals. Multiple sclerosis occurs when this protective sheath becomes inflamed and ultimately destroyed in places, short-circuiting the electrical flow. Among the possible consequences are loss of muscular coordination, impaired vision, and incontinence. Repeated inflammation of the nerves produces scarring (sclerosis), which happens too rapidly for healing to take place; the effects of the lesions become permanent.

Treatment Options

If you have MS, it is imperative that you seek evaluation and treatment by a conventional medical doctor. Although the disease cannot be cured, its symptoms can be alleviated by certain medications. A number of alternative remedies can also help you cope with the discomfort associated with MS. You'll need professional guidance for some of the therapies described below, but you can learn to do many of them yourself at home.

Acupuncture

With MS patients, the goal of acupuncture is to reduce fatigue and limb stiffness and relax muscles.

Apitherapy

Many people with MS have found relief with apitherapy, also known as bee venom therapy (BVT). The recommended treatment involves two sessions per week of painful stings from a live honeybee for four to six months. When an already inflamed area is stung and becomes swollen, the body's natural anti-inflammatory agents act to shrink swelling, in the process reducing the original inflammation.

BVT causes temporary stinging, itching, swelling, and reddening, and it has been known to cause fatal shock in some people and severe allergic reactions in others. Be sure to check with your doctor before embarking on a series of treatments.

Multiple Sclerosis

Bodywork

Regularly working your muscles will help keep them from atrophying. The Feldenkrais method is a series of lessons to retrain your neuromuscular system and expand your range of motion. Massage can also relieve discomfort and maintain circulation.

Exercise

Physical activity is highly recommended for MS patients—although exercise should not be performed during an attack or too strenuously at other times, as overexertion can bring on an attack. Swimming, stretching, and low-impact aerobics are all within the range of many people with MS, and even patients in wheelchairs can exercise to some degree.

Gentle stretching is particularly helpful for the spasticity, stiff gait, and foot dragging that can accompany MS. Performing gentle stretches in cool water can also help relax spastic limbs. Studies show that regular yoga exercises increase secretions of the adrenal medulla, a nervous system stimulator, which can help to slow degeneration.

Nutrition and Diet

Certain foods can bring on attacks in some MS sufferers. Among problem foods are milk and dairy products, caffeine, yeast, and gluten (found in wheat, barley, oats, and rye). Ketchup, vinegar, wine, and corn can also prove problematic.

A number of special diets attempt to correct the fatty imbalance in MS sufferers. Two approaches (sometimes used together) appear to be the most effective: One is to increase the intake of fatty acids; the other, to decrease the intake of saturated fats. The latter tactic is the more common, though in many recommended diets, saturated fats are not the only targets for reduction or elimination.

The best-known diet for MS sufferers is the Swank Diet, devised by Dr. Roy Swank of the Oregon Health Sciences University. In many cases it has apparently slowed the course of the disease and reduced attacks. Very low in saturated fats, the diet calls for specific amounts of polyunsaturated oils—sunflower, safflower, and sesame oils, for example, as well as oils in beans, leafy green vegetables, and most fish. It also includes proteins, supplements of cod-liver oil, and high doses of vitamins. Butter, margarine, shortening, and hydrogenated oils (such as coconut and palm oil) are strictly forbidden. In the first year, you are advised to avoid red meat and other foods high in saturated fats.

Supplements figure in many diets recommended for MS sufferers. Linoleic acid, found in sunflower oil and known for its role in regulating the immune system, is said to reduce the severity of MS attacks and to produce longer remissions.

Nerve sheaths may be strengthened with 5 daily grams of lecithin (kept refrigerated). Coenzyme Q, or CoQ10, in 30-mg doses two or three times a day, may help cells utilize more oxygen. ■

Myelin Loss

Myelin, a fatty substance that sheathes and protects the fiberlike axons of cells in the central nervous system, also speeds electrical signals as they travel along nerve pathways to carry out movement and other vital processes. Multiple sclerosis causes myelin to disintegrate, thereby obstructing signal flow and potentially leading to progressive loss of motor coordination and other functions.

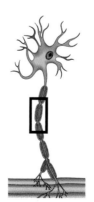

NERVE CELL

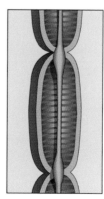

MYELIN SHEATH

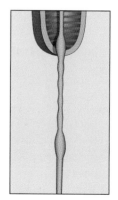

ABSENCE OF MYELIN

*M*uscle Cramps

Symptoms

Once you've experienced a muscle cramp, you'll probably recognize any future ones by the nature of the pain they cause. Common symptoms include:

- Sudden, painful spasm or tightening of a muscle, especially in the legs.

- Hardening of the affected muscle.

- In some cases, visible distortion or twitching of the muscle beneath the skin.

- In other cases, extremely severe cramps in the arms and legs, beginning without warning, and sometimes affecting the abdominal muscles as well. These symptoms are typical of heat cramps.

- Persistent cramping pains in lower abdominal muscles, which may occur along with back problems or during menstruation.

Call Your Doctor If

- you have frequent muscle cramps.

- your cramp lasts more than an hour and has not responded to your own treatment.

CAUTION

Cramping pain in your chest and arm muscles may indicate a heart problem. Call your doctor or get medical help immediately. If you suffer from circulatory problems, diabetes, heart disease, or deep varicose veins, or if you have had a stroke or been warned that you might be susceptible to one, avoid massage until you talk to your doctor.

F *rom a stitch that grabs your side while you're running to a spasm in your calf awakening you in the dead of night, muscle cramps can be an all too common source of discomfort. Normally, a muscle at work contracts, then releases and lengthens when the movement is finished or when another muscle exerts force in the opposite direction. But sometimes a muscle contracts with great intensity and stays contracted, refusing to stretch out again; this is a muscle cramp.*

Muscles contract or lengthen in response to electrical signals from nerves; minerals such as sodium, calcium, and magnesium, which surround and permeate muscle cells, play a key role in the transmission of these signals. Imbalances in these minerals—as well as in certain hormones, body fluids, and chemicals—or malfunctions in the nervous system itself can foul up the flow of electrical signals and cause a muscle to cramp.

Physical overexertion depletes fluids and minerals and can lead to cramping, particularly in people who work or exercise in conditions that overheat their bodies. If you are not careful to drink plenty of fluids, activities like working in the garden on a hot summer day can cause heat cramps. And if you do not take steps to alleviate them, heat cramps can progress to much more serious heatstroke and heat exhaustion.

Treatment Options

There are simple techniques for easing common, occasional muscle cramps *(see Home Remedies, opposite)*, but if you suffer from frequent or severe cramps, see your doctor. Frequent cramps might indicate a more serious illness. And severe cramps in your chest, shoulders, or arms can be symptoms of a heart attack; call immediately for medical help.

Acupressure
If the cramp is in your calf, try applying pressure for two to three minutes at the lower end of the calf muscle bulge.

Aromatherapy
The essential oils of Roman chamomile, ***bay laurel** (Laurus nobilis)*, and ***peppermint** (Mentha piperita)* may help relax tight muscles and soothe the pain of a muscle cramp; add a drop or two to a base oil and massage the muscle.

*M*uscle Cramps

Ayurvedic Medicine

An Ayurvedic physician may recommend massaging the affected area with oil of *shatavari* or applying a paste of ginger and turmeric.

Chinese Medicine

Chinese medicine offers a number of treatments for muscle cramps, including acupuncture and herbal medicine. Consult a practitioner.

Herbal Therapies

An infusion of **ginkgo** *(Ginkgo biloba)* may help improve circulation and relieve leg spasms. Pour a cup of boiling water onto 2 tsp of the dried herb and steep for 15 to 20 minutes; drink three times a day. An herbalist might prescribe Japanese quince *(Chaenomeles speciosa)* as an antispasmodic for cramps in the calves.

Homeopathy

Over-the-counter homeopathic preparations (in tablet form) of *Cuprum metallicum* (6c), sucked slowly, may relieve the spasm and ache.

Hydrotherapy

Use alternating hot and cold compresses: Soak one washcloth in hot water and another in ice water. Wring out the warm cloth, then place it over the affected area for three minutes. Wring out the second cloth and place it over the same area for 30 seconds. Repeat this alternating technique two more times. For severe cramping, do the procedure morning and evening; once a day for minor problems.

Or try a hot vinegar pack: Heat a pan of equal parts vinegar and water, then soak a towel in the mixture. Wring out the towel and apply it to the affected body area for five minutes. Remove the towel and apply a cold towel for five minutes. Cover with wool. Repeat these hot-cold applications three times, making sure to finish with cold.

Massage

A skilled practitioner can relieve cramping by applying massage directly to the affected area and using other cramp-releasing techniques. Massage is also useful for soothing the area and reducing tension once a cramp has released.

Nutrition and Diet

Nutritionists recommend taking **vitamin E** supplements (200 IU daily) to prevent night cramps. You may also find relief by increasing your intake of **calcium.** Good sources include milk, cheese, yogurt, dark green leafy vegetables, and canned fish. A 400-mg supplement taken before bed may help prevent night cramps.

Home Remedies

To relieve a typical cramp, you need to make the muscle stop contracting—by either stretching it or massaging it, or both. You can stretch a calf muscle simply by standing on your toes on the edge of a stair and slowly lowering your heels until you feel a good stretch without pain. For a greater stretch, stand facing a wall, put your hands or forearms against the wall, and—keeping your feet flat on the floor—slide backward until you are leaning against the wall from several feet away. For even more stretch, keep edging your feet backward.

Try this technique for massaging away a cramp: From a sitting position, stretch your heel down, pointing your toes up—toward your head. To give resistance, put your other foot against the top of the foot on the cramping side; then after the cramp releases, firmly squeeze your calf with your hand. Begin at the edges of the cramp and move in toward the center with gentle pressure. For an obstinate cramp, immerse the muscle in a hot bath, perhaps while stretching and massaging it. To treat heat cramps, drink plenty of cool water. This is also the best way to prevent heat cramps: Drink a cup of cool water before and after exercise, and every 15 minutes during exercise. If you use a sports beverage instead, drink one that is low in sugar (which can bring on stomach cramps). Dilute juices with 3 parts water.

Prevention

Practicing yoga regularly will greatly decrease the occurrence of leg cramps by stretching the muscles and increasing circulation. See the Gallery of Yoga Positions *(pages 184-193)* for recommended routines to follow. ■

Common Ailments

$\mathcal{N}$ausea

Symptoms

Symptoms of gastroenteritis, also called stomach flu or intestinal flu, include:

- Nausea and vomiting.
- Diarrhea.
- Abdominal cramps and pain.
- Fever.
- Weakness.

Any of a variety of mild to severe stomach symptoms may indicate gastritis. The most common are:

- Upper abdominal discomfort or pain.
- Nausea.
- Diarrhea.
- Loss of appetite.

Call Your Doctor If

- you have nausea with shortness of breath, chest pain, and sweating; these are signs of a heart attack.

- you experience nausea and severe headache, possibly with vomiting (these symptoms may worsen with exposure to bright light); you could have a migraine or meningitis.

- you have nausea accompanied by increased thirst and urination, dehydration, and possibly a fruity odor on your breath; you could have diabetes.

- you have severe nausea with pain starting in the upper abdomen and moving to the right shoulder blade; you may have gallstones.

- you have nausea that lasts one to two weeks, headache, malaise, and fatigue, perhaps accompanied by a sore throat, fever, and rash; possible disorders include mononucleosis, strep throat, and scarlet fever.

Everyone has experienced the sick-to-your-stomach feeling of nausea at some point in life. Characterized by an urge to vomit, nausea is not itself an illness but rather a sign that things are not quite right in the digestive system or elsewhere in the body. The cause can be a relatively minor, temporary condition like motion sickness or anxiety, or as serious and life threatening as a heart attack or cancer of the stomach.

In many cases, nausea is brought on by a case of gastroenteritis, a general term that applies to many types of irritation and infection of the digestive tract. The most common cause of gastroenteritis is a virus that can spread quickly through an office, school, or day-care center. Food poisoning, bacteria, and parasites may also be the culprit, and sometimes drinking excessive amounts of alcohol can irritate your digestive tract enough to cause gastroenteritis.

Inflammation of the stomach lining, a condition known as gastritis, also commonly leads to nausea along with other symptoms such as vomiting, diarrhea, and general discomfort. Gastritis typically affects the elderly but can strike anyone at any age. It can be caused by certain medications, including aspirin, as well as by viral or bacterial infections.

Treatment Options

A number of alternative therapies can be extremely useful in treating nausea.

Acupressure
See the illustration opposite for an acupressure point that is particularly effective for relieving acute nausea and vomiting.

Aromatherapy
Essential oil of **peppermint** (*Mentha piperita*) can help calm the stomach and relieve a case of nausea. Take one drop internally by mixing it with honey or a so-called carrier oil such as almond oil.

Ayurvedic Medicine
A practitioner may recommend the combined formula *Gasex* for adults (two to three tablets chewed after meals) and *Bonnisan* for children (consult a practitioner for the dosage appropriate for your

Nausea

child's age). Other appropriate remedies include a hot or cold infusion of the leaves of the neem tree, and a tea made from coriander seeds.

Chinese Medicine

After a thorough evaluation of your overall constitution, a practitioner of Chinese medicine can prescribe a course of treatment, which may include herbal therapy or possibly acupuncture, to harmonize the digestive organs.

Flower Remedy

The flower remedy **Crab Apple** is often recommended for ailments causing nausea. Consult a naturopath or other practitioner familiar with flower remedies.

Herbal Therapies

Meadowsweet *(Filipendula ulmaria)* can reduce nausea and stomach acidity: Pour 1 cup boiling water on 2 tsp dried meadowsweet and steep for 15 minutes; drink three times daily. **Slippery elm** *(Ulmus fulva)* may also help calm your digestive tract when the worst symptoms have passed: Mix 1 part powdered slippery elm with 8 parts water and bring to a boil; simmer for 15 minutes. Drink half a cup three times a day.

    Chamomile *(Matricaria recutita)* tea can soothe the stomach: Steep 1 tsp of the herb in 1 cup of boiling water for 10 minutes. **Licorice** *(Glycyrrhiza glabra)* extract in capsule or liquid form may also help. Lemon balm *(Melissa officinalis)* is particularly good for digestive problems linked to anxiety. **Ginger** *(Zingiber officinale)* tea can help relieve nausea due to morning sickness, but check with your doctor before taking any herbal remedy.

Homeopathy

If symptoms are severe, take 12x dosages of one of the following homeopathic preparations every two hours until symptoms improve. If you do not feel any better after two or three doses, try another preparation:

- **Ipecac** for extreme nausea and vomiting.
- **Nux vomica** for symptoms caused by exhaustion, overeating, or drinking too much alcohol or coffee.

- **Bryonia** for nausea, a tender stomach, a dry mouth, and a sensation like a stone in your stomach.

Hydrotherapy

A cold footbath or ice bags at the base of the skull and on the solar plexus can help ease nausea. Another technique hydrotherapists often advise is placing a hot compress on the abdomen while applying a cold compress to the base of the skull.

Massage

Gentle massage of the chest and abdomen can provide relief from nausea. However, you must first make sure that your upset stomach is not a symptom of a more serious disorder. Massage is especially good for nausea related to anxiety and stress.

Nutrition and Diet

Limit or eliminate alcohol, caffeine, and carbonated drinks from your diet. When the worst symptoms have passed, eat more noncitrus fruit, cooked vegetables, and bland foods, and eat fewer refined carbohydrates such as white bread and white rice. Supplements of **zinc** and **vitamin A** may help heal the stomach lining after a bout with gastritis. ■

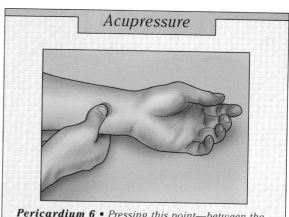

Acupressure

Pericardium 6 • *Pressing this point—between the two bones of the forearm, two finger widths from the center of the inner wrist crease—may help relieve nausea and stomach disorders. Press firmly for one minute, three to five times; then repeat on the other arm.*

$\mathcal{N}$euralgia

Symptoms

Neuralgia, or nerve pain, comes in many different forms: It may be sudden, shooting, sharp, burning, or stabbing, and it is sometimes accompanied by a background sensation of burning, itching, or aching, or by hypersensitivity to touch. It occurs in one part of your body, typically on one side. The pain may be intermittent or continuous; it can last for a few seconds or a few minutes, and it may recur, on and off, for days or weeks.

Call Your Doctor If

■ you suspect that the pain is caused by a spinal problem, a herniated disk, or a pinched nerve.

■ the symptoms include impaired bladder or bowel control or a dragging foot—signs of nerve damage; call your doctor immediately.

■ facial neuralgia spreads to an eye after a herpes attack; this could lead to blindness if untreated.

■ the pain becomes too great to bear; nerve damage could result.

N euralgia, as the name suggests, is nerve pain, occurring when a nerve is irritated or inflamed. The pain, spreading along neural pathways, may be fleeting or chronic and can range from mild to outright unbearable.

Types of Neuralgia

Only a few types of neuralgia are common. One, characterized by flashes of facial pain, is called trigeminal neuralgia, after the multibranched cranial nerve that is affected; the condition occurs mostly in people over age 50 and afflicts three times as many women as men. Nerves of the buttocks and legs are also vulnerable; irritation of the large sciatic nerve, for example, produces the neuralgia called sciatica. Another relatively common type is postherpetic neuralgia, which strikes after an attack of the type of herpes infection known as shingles and typically manifests itself as a continuous burning sensation.

Generally, the likeliest source of neuralgia is irritation or inflammation of a nerve or pressure on a nerve from bones or connective tissue. Such pressure may be due to a muscle or spinal injury, a prolapsed disk, or years of poor posture. Trigeminal neuralgia may stem from the pressure of a blood vessel on a nerve. In postherpetic neuralgia, the nerve inflammation is caused by a viral infection. In many cases of neuralgia, however, the reason for the nerve's irritated state is unknown.

Treatment Options

In addition to the therapies listed below, consider seeing a chiropractor or an osteopath; manipulations of the spine and of soft tissue can help relieve several types of neuralgia, including sciatica.

■ Acupuncture
Acupuncture has been shown to be extremely effective in treating neuralgia. If the pain is severe, five to 10 acupuncture sessions may be required.

■ Bodywork
In a series of lessons, an instructor trained in the Alexander technique can teach you to adjust your

$\mathcal{N}$euralgia

body posture and movements to prevent future attacks. Other bodywork techniques that may prove helpful include the Feldenkrais method and Aston-Patterning. See a trained therapist for therapeutic techniques specific to your problem.

■ Herbal Therapies

A cup of boiling water poured over 2 tsp **St. John's-wort** *(Hypericum perforatum)* and allowed to steep for 10 minutes has painkilling properties when drunk three times a day. Recent experiments on extracts from **black cohosh** *(Cimicifuga racemosa)* suggest that this herb may have anti-inflammatory qualities.

■ Homeopathy

For sharp, shooting pain with tingling and burning, try **Hypericum** (6x) once an hour for three to four doses. Consult a homeopath for other remedies specific to your symptoms.

■ Massage

Deep-tissue massage reduces pain by probing into successively deeper layers of muscle and connective tissue. This type of massage releases chronic tension and contraction in muscles and connective tissues that may be exerting pressure on a nerve. Consult a massage therapist experienced in treating pain conditions.

Massage will also help to reduce muscle tension that may be a result of the body trying to protect the painful, vulnerable area.

■ Nutrition and Diet

When an attack begins, a maximum dose of 50 mg **vitamin B$_6$** three times a day and **vitamin B complex** once a day may help; continue for one week only. For postherpetic neuralgia, add 400 IU **vitamin E** twice a day.

Making oats a regular part of your diet can improve the overall condition of nerves. A drink made from minced oat straw or oat grass steeped for two minutes in warm water and strained is thought to be a valuable tonic; use 1 to 4 grams daily. To soothe itching skin, bathe in water that has been run over oatmeal placed in a muslin bag and hung under the bathtub tap.

Areas of Pain

Neuralgia, or pain that results from a nerve that has been irritated or damaged, occurs in various forms

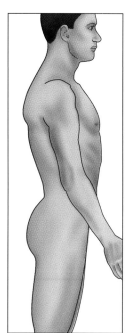

in different parts of the body. Trigeminal neuralgia, for example, affects the face. Intercostal neuralgia causes pain between the ribs, and sciatica strikes the lower back and legs. These locations are not exclusive, however; neuralgia can develop in any part of the body where a nerve has been damaged.

Home Remedies

■ A man suffering from trigeminal neuralgia can grow a beard to shield his face from the cold, exposure to which sometimes leads to an attack.

■ An old folk remedy calls for cutting a baked potato in half and applying the cooled halves to an afflicted area to draw out the pain.

Prevention

Learning how to sit, stand, and lift for proper back support is the best way to forestall some types of neuralgia. Several different bodywork therapies, as well as chiropractic and osteopathy, can teach you how to move properly to avoid attacks. Consult a licensed practitioner or a trained therapist. ■

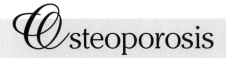

Osteoporosis

Symptoms

Osteoporosis is usually asymptomatic until a fracture occurs.

■ Backache.

■ A gradual loss of height and an accompanying stooped posture.

■ Fractures of the spine, wrists, or hips.

■ Loss of bone in the jaw.

Call Your Doctor If

■ you develop a backache or a sudden severe back pain, which can indicate a spinal compression fracture caused by osteoporosis.

■ dental x-rays reveal a loss of bone in the jaw, which can be an early sign of osteoporosis.

O *steoporosis, which means "porous bones," causes bones to gradually thin and weaken, leaving them susceptible to fractures. Although all bones are affected by the disease, those of the spine, hip, and wrist are most likely to break. In elderly people, hip fractures can be particularly dangerous, because the prolonged immobility required during healing often leads to blood clots or pneumonia. Women are more susceptible to osteoporosis, perhaps because their bones tend to be lighter and thinner, and because their bodies experience hormonal changes after menopause that appear to accelerate the loss of bone mass.*

Treatment Options

Because osteoporosis is difficult to reverse, prevention is the key to treatment. To prevent the disease or slow its progression, many doctors suggest hormone replacement therapy to postmenopausal women. Many doctors recommend the treatment only for women at high risk of osteoporosis, because hormone replacement therapy has been associated with an increased risk of serious health problems, most notably uterine and breast cancers. Alternative medicine offers effective preventive measures that focus on building and retaining strong bones.

■ Exercise

Studies have shown that weight-bearing exercises—those that put stress on bones, such as running, walking, tennis, ballet, stair climbing, aerobics, and weightlifting—reduce bone loss and help prevent osteoporosis. To benefit from the exercise, you must do it at least three times per week for 30 to 45 minutes. Swimming and bicycle riding, although good cardiovascular exercises, do not appear to prevent osteoporosis because they do not put enough stress on bones.

■ Herbal Therapies

Herbs traditionally used to prevent osteoporosis include **horsetail** *(Equisetum arvense)*, alfalfa *(Medicago sativa)*, **licorice** *(Glycyrrhiza glabra)*, **marsh mallow** *(Althaea officinalis)*, and sourdock *(Rumex crispus)*. Take daily in tea or tincture form.

Chinese medicine herbalists may recommend

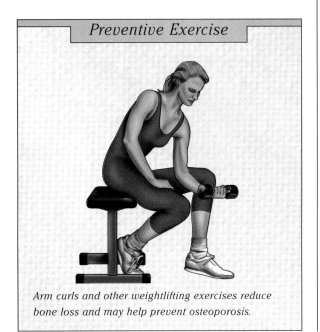

Preventive Exercise

Arm curls and other weightlifting exercises reduce bone loss and may help prevent osteoporosis.

Osteoporosis

a general herbal formula used for graceful aging, *Liu Wei Di Huang Wan* (Six Flavor Pills); it is said to help nourish and strengthen the bones. Consult a practitioner for appropriate dosages.

■ Homeopathy

In addition to a *calcium*-rich diet and exercise, homeopaths recommend treatments they believe help the body absorb calcium. Remedies are likely to include **Calcarea carbonica,** *Calcarea phosphorica, Calcarea fluorica,* or **Silica.** Consult a homeopath for remedies and dosages.

■ Nutrition and Diet

To ensure that women get enough calcium to build and maintain strong bones, health experts recommend eating plenty of foods rich in **calcium,** such as nonfat milk, low-fat yogurt, broccoli, cauliflower, salmon, tofu, and leafy green vegetables. According to a panel convened by the National Institutes of Health, women who are still menstruating or who are postmenopausal but taking hormone replacement therapy should consume 1,000 mg of calcium each day. Postmenopausal women who are not being treated with estrogen should get 1,500 mg daily. (One glass of nonfat milk provides only 300 mg of calcium.)

Because most women take in through their diet only half or a third as much calcium as they need, some practitioners recommend calcium supplements to make up the difference. Calcium supplements are available in many forms, but chelated forms, such as calcium citrate and calcium gluconate, appear to be more effective at reducing bone loss. Avoid using dolomite or bone meal as calcium supplements or calcium carbonate supplements labeled "oyster shell," as they may contain lead and other toxic metals.

To help the body absorb calcium, some practitioners suggest taking **vitamin D** supplements (400 to 800 IU). **Magnesium** supplements (250 to 350 mg) or trace minerals are sometimes prescribed as well. CAUTION: Calcium supplements can inhibit the absorption of salicylates, tetracycline, and other medications. Check with your practitioner before beginning a supplementation program.

In addition to eating calcium-rich foods, you should also avoid **phosphorus**-rich ones, which can promote bone loss. High-phosphorus foods include red meats, soft drinks, and those with phosphate food additives. Indeed, several studies have indicated that vegetarians tend to have denser bones later in life than meat eaters (other studies have shown no such difference).

To help keep estrogen levels from dropping precipitously after menopause and thus help prevent osteoporosis, some alternative practitioners advise postmenopausal women to consume more food containing plant estrogens, especially tofu, soybean milk, and other soy products.

Home Remedies

Here are two easy ways of increasing the amount of calcium in your diet:
- Add nonfat dry milk to everyday foods and beverages, including soups, stews, and casseroles. Each teaspoon of dry milk adds about 20 mg of calcium to your diet.
- Add a little vinegar to the water you use to make soup stock from bones. The vinegar will dissolve some of the calcium out of the bones, for a calcium-fortified soup. A pint can contain as much as 1,000 mg of calcium.

Prevention

- Eat foods rich in calcium, such as nonfat milk, low-fat yogurt, broccoli, salmon, tofu, sesame seeds, almonds, and leafy green vegetables.
- Eat foods that contain plant estrogens, especially tofu and other soy products.
- Avoid foods that can interfere with your body's absorption of calcium, such as red meats, soft drinks, and excessive amounts of alcohol and caffeine.
- Do weight-bearing exercises for 30 to 45 minutes at least three times a week.
- Do not smoke. Some studies have shown that women who smoke increase their risk of developing osteoporosis by 50 percent.
- Avoid antacids containing aluminum, as they can prevent calcium absorption by binding with phosphorus in the intestines. ■

Pain, Chronic

Symptoms

Any pain that, despite treatment, lasts longer than six months is medically defined as chronic. The condition may include weakness, numbness, tingling, or other sensations along with sleeping difficulties, a lack of energy, and depression. Some common forms of chronic pain are:

■ Continuing muscle pain, accompanied by cramping, soreness, swelling, and muscle spasms or stiffness.

■ Lingering back pain, which may be sharp or aching, constant or intermittent, localized, radiating, or diffuse.

■ Enduring joint pain, with tenderness and a sensation of heat in the affected area as well as radiating pain and a restricted range of motion.

Call Your Doctor If

■ your pain continues for several weeks and doesn't respond to over-the-counter analgesics and rest; early care may keep acute pain from becoming chronic.

■ your pain is unrelenting and unresponsive to prescription medications; your doctor may administer tests to rule out cancer or other possible causes.

■ the symptoms of your chronic pain change abruptly. You may be at risk of complications, or you may have developed a different, unrelated problem.

T ens of millions of Americans suffer from chronic pain. It can be mild or excruciating, episodic or continuous, merely inconvenient or totally incapacitating. The emotional toll of chronic pain can become part of a vicious circle: Stress and anxiety may actually decrease the body's production of its natural painkillers. Because of the mind/body links associated with chronic pain, effective treatment may require addressing psychological as well as physical aspects of the condition.

Treatment Options

Many people suffering from chronic pain are able to gain some control over it on their own. But others may need professional help. For them, pain clinics—special care centers devoted exclusively to dealing with intractable pain—are often the answer.

Acupuncture

Acupuncture may be used to reduce swelling and inflammation associated with chronic pain. The treatment may include placing needles along the large intestine meridian, considered the most effective of pain-relieving channels. One theory holds that acupuncture works by stimulating the release of endorphins, the body's natural painkillers. Because this therapy is thought to have a cumulative effect, it is most beneficial if done on a regular basis. For the best results, consult an acupuncturist who has experience treating a wide range of types of chronic pain.

Aromatherapy

Mix together the following essential oils with a carrier oil such as sweet almond oil and massage the blend into your skin at the site of the pain: *lavender (Lavandula angustifolia),* to reduce inflammation and relax muscles; *eucalyptus globulus (E. globulus),* to bring down swelling and accelerate healing; ginger *(Zingiber officinale),* to relieve pain and stiffness associated with arthritis and other types of degenerative joint disease.

Bodywork

The Alexander technique reeducates you in the way you move to avoid adding unnecessary ten-

Pain, Chronic

sion to skeleton-supporting muscles, thus preventing neck and back problems. This therapy has been shown to be especially helpful for correcting poor posture that can cause backaches.

Exercise
Research has shown that regular exercise can diminish pain in the long run by improving muscle tone, strength, and flexibility. Exercise may also release endorphins. Some exercises are easier for certain chronic pain sufferers to perform than others; try swimming, biking, walking, or rowing.

Herbal Therapies
To help decrease inflammation and pain, herbalists recommend applying **ginger** *(Zingiber officinale)* packs, prepared by soaking a clean cloth in ginger tea, for 10 minutes, three to four times a day. Topically applied dilutions of wintergreen *(Gaultheria procumbens)* oil—which contains methyl salicylate, an ingredient similar to that found in aspirin—may have an analgesic effect. Geranium *(Pelargonium odoratissimum)* and **white willow** *(Salix alba)* bark are natural painkillers. **Chamomile** *(Matricaria recutita)* is an antispasmodic and anti-inflammatory agent. Consult an herbalist to determine the best treatment for your specific condition.

Homeopathy
Try **Rhus toxicodendron** for joint, back, and arthritic problems that feel worse when first rising in the morning and become better with warmth. Persistent, acute pain may be relieved by **Kali bichromicum;** however, a constitutional remedy is often needed to help relieve pain in the long run. Consult your homeopath for the correct constitutional remedy for you.

Massage
Massage therapy may provide temporary relief of muscle stiffness and spasms by reducing muscle tension, which can produce sudden, involuntary contractions that lead to more pain, which in turn leads to more spasms. Massage with ice packs may interrupt pain messages sent along nerve pathways, replacing those messages with signals about temperature and, in this way, providing relief.

Mind/Body Medicine
Visualization, or guided imagery, may be a worthwhile pain-controlling technique. Try the following exercise: Close your eyes and try to call up a visual image of the pain, giving it shape, color, size, and motion. Now try slowly altering this image, replacing it with a more harmonious, pleasing—and smaller—image. Don't expect this imaging technique to work right away; it takes practice.

Another approach is to keep a diary of your pain episodes and the causative and corrective factors surrounding them. Review your diary regularly to explore avenues of possible change. Strive to view pain as part of life, not all of it.

Electromyographic (EMG) biofeedback may alert you to the ways in which muscle tension is contributing to your pain and help you learn to control it.

Hypnotherapy and self-hypnosis may help you block or transform pain through refocusing techniques. One self-hypnosis strategy, known as glove anesthesia, involves putting yourself in a trance, placing a hand over the painful area, imagining that the hand is relaxed, heavy, and numb, and envisioning these sensations as replacing other, painful feelings in the affected area.

Relaxation techniques such as meditation have been shown to reduce stress-related pain when they are practiced regularly. Regular, gentle yoga practice can be helpful in relaxing muscles, thus decreasing pain and tension.

If you can't get your mind off the problems that may be producing stress, visualize two lists; in one column, list the problems in order of priority, and in the other, visualize potential solutions to them. Place an imaginary check mark by each one after you've found a solution for it, then put both lists out of your mind and try the relaxation exercise again.

Nutrition and Diet
For chronic back pain, a beneficial regimen may be 500 mg of **vitamin C** three times a day with meals, 800 mg daily of **calcium** taken with 400 mg of **magnesium,** and 400 IU daily of **vitamin E.** CAUTION: Be sure to check with your doctor or a nutritionist before taking large doses of vitamin supplements. ∎

Common Ailments

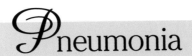Pneumonia

Symptoms

- A combination of low fever and chills, muscle aches, fatigue, enlarged lymph nodes in the neck, chest pain, sore throat, and coughing are typical symptoms of viral pneumonia.

- High fever, cough with thick yellow-green sputum that may contain blood, shortness of breath, rapid breathing, sharp chest pain that is worse when you breathe deeply, abdominal pain, and severe fatigue are symptoms of bacterial pneumonia.

- Loss of appetite and weight, fever, coughing with sputum, perhaps following a period of unconsciousness, may indicate aspiration pneumonia.

- In children, labored and rapid breathing, sudden onset of fever, cough, wheezing, and bluish skin are general signs of pneumonia.

Call Your Doctor If

- your symptoms indicate you have any form of pneumonia. You need immediate medical treatment to recover and avoid complications.

- your sharp chest pain does not respond to prescribed treatment; you have increased shortness of breath; or your fingernails, toenails, or skin becomes dark or develops a bluish tinge after diagnosis. Your lungs are not getting enough oxygen and you need medical assistance.

- you cough up blood; you may need additional treatment for a worsening infection.

Pneumonia is the relatively common inflammation caused by various viral, bacterial, and fungal infections or by exposure of the lungs to certain chemicals. In response, the lungs become congested with fluids and cells that leak from the affected tissue. If the inflammation is limited to one lobe of one lung, it is classified as lobar pneumonia; inflammation spreading from the bronchi to other parts of one or both lungs is bronchopneumonia. If both lungs are inflamed, the condition is called double pneumonia.

Treatment Options

If you are diagnosed as having pneumonia, various alternative therapies may help ease your symptoms and hasten your recovery.

Acupuncture
Acupuncture on the lung meridian may help your recovery from pneumonia by reducing cough and congestion, making you more comfortable, and improving your energy level. Consult a licensed practitioner for a complete evaluation so that the acupuncture treatments can be tailored to your specific condition.

Aromatherapy
Recovery from pneumonia may be helped if you add the essential oils of **eucalyptus globulus** (E. globulus), **lavender** (Lavandula angustifolia), **tea tree** (Melaleuca alternifolia), or pine to a warm bath or a vaporizer for steam inhalation.

Herbal Therapies
Since clearing the lungs of phlegm is an important part of the healing process, using traditional herbal expectorants to promote coughing can aid recovery. To make your own expectorant, combine 2 oz **licorice** (Glycyrrhiza glabra), 1 oz wild black cherry (Prunus serotina) bark, 1 oz **coltsfoot** (Tussilago farfara), ¾ tsp **lobelia** (Lobelia inflata), and 1 oz horehound (Marrubium vulgare). Simmer 1 tbsp of the mixture in 1 cup of water for five minutes; let the mixture steep for 10 minutes and strain it into a clean container. Adults should drink one cupful every two hours. Lobelia can be poisonous, so never use more than the recommended amount. Stop

Pneumonia
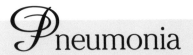

Evidence of Infection

Healthy lungs exchange carbon dioxide in the blood for oxygen through tiny air sacs called alveoli (inset, top). A pneumonic infection— whether it is caused by bacterial, viral, or chemical agents—makes tissue in the alveoli swell and fill with fluid (inset, bottom). Shallow, labored breathing brought on by an insufficient oxygen supply is often a symptom of pneumonia.

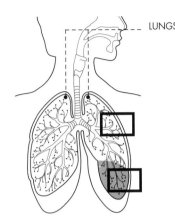

LUNGS

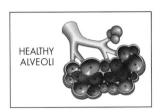

HEALTHY ALVEOLI

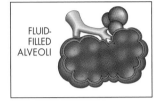

FLUID-FILLED ALVEOLI

using this mixture if you become nauseated, and never give it to children or pregnant women.

Homeopathy

Some recommended over-the-counter homeopathic remedies are **Aconite, Ferrum phosphoricum, Bryonia, Phosphorus,** and **Arsenicum album;** follow label directions. For lingering chest weakness after pneumonia, a homeopathic physician might prescribe *Stannum metallicum* or *Antimonium tartaricum.*

Massage

After the fever is gone, massage the chest and the upper back muscles to ease chest congestion. Adding a few drops of essential oil of **eucalyptus globulus** to the massage lotion may help to loosen and release phlegm.

Percussion massage techniques may help relieve congestion by dislodging phlegm so it can be coughed out. Use the cupping technique *(see the Gallery of Massage Techniques, page 128)* on the back and sides of the body over the area of the lungs. Allow the receiver to cough up phlegm as much as needed.

Nutrition and Diet

- Up to 1,000 mg of **vitamin C** an hour may offer substantial benefits in fighting pneumonia if started within two days of onset. Reduce the dosage if you develop diarrhea.
- From 25,000 to 50,000 IU of **vitamin A** daily, for not more than two weeks, may help support your respiratory and immune systems.
- **Zinc** supplements, up to 60 mg daily, may also help your immune system fight infection.
- 600 IU of **vitamin E** daily may help support damaged lung tissue.

Home Remedies

- A heating pad or hot-water bottle on the chest or back for 10 minutes several times a day can help relieve chest pain. Wrap the pad or bottle in a towel to prevent burning the skin.
- Try a traditional mustard poultice to loosen phlegm. Mix dry mustard with enough warm water to make a thick paste. Spread the paste on thin cotton or cheesecloth, fold, and place on your chest for several minutes, but don't overdo it: Mustard may cause blistering if it is left on bare skin too long.

Prevention

- Avoid smoking and exposure to tobacco smoke, which significantly damage the hairlike cilia that filter irritants from the lungs. Smoking weakens your ability to fight viral and bacterial agents that cause pneumonia. ■

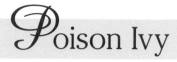Poison Ivy

Symptoms

- Patches of red, itchy skin, usually followed by small blisters, which fill with a clear fluid and eventually break open.

- Severe cases can develop into swollen, extremely painful areas filled with fluid.

- The rash rarely appears on the soles of the feet or palms of the hands.

Call Your Doctor If

- your rash stays red and itchy for more than two weeks; you may have another type of contact dermatitis, eczema, or lupus.

- the rash is near your eyes or covers a large part of your body. You may need medical intervention.

- you have severe allergic complications, such as generalized swelling, headache, fever, or a secondary infection.

- you have been exposed to or inhale the smoke from burning poison ivy, poison oak, or poison sumac. The toxin is not killed by fire and can cause severe allergic reactions internally as well as externally.

P oison ivy, poison oak, and poison sumac cause a short-lived but extremely irritating allergic form of contact dermatitis. The rash generally develops within two days, peaks after five days, and starts to decline after a week or 10 days. While some people survive exposure without ill effects, complete immunity is unlikely; people who seem immune at one time and place may find themselves vulnerable in other situations.

The leaves, stems, and roots of these plants contain the resin urushiol, which even in minute amounts can trigger an inflammatory allergic reaction on exposed skin. Urushiol can be transferred by fingers or animal fur and can remain on clothing, shoes, and tools for several months. Scratching the rash does not spread the poison to other parts of the body, but it can prolong the discomfort and cause a secondary infection.

Treatment Options

You can treat a mild case yourself using conventional or alternative remedies. Conventional over-the-counter topical remedies contain antihistamines, benzocaine, or hydrocortisone, which relieve the symptoms of poison ivy. Various alternative therapies help relieve itching and swelling. In addition to topical remedies, **vitamin C** injections are also said to provide relief. If you have complications from a severe case, you may need to see a doctor. If your case is so severe that general illness develops, your doctor may recommend injections of prednisone or another corticosteroid drug.

Herbal Therapies

The leaves of jewelweed (*Impatiens pallida*), which often grows near poison ivy, may neutralize urushiol if wiped over the skin immediately after contact. For relief from itching, try the following topical remedies:

- The leaves of the common plantain *(Plantago major)*. Make a poultice by mashing the leaves with a mortar and pestle. Apply the mashed leaves directly to the skin, then hold in place by covering with clean cotton or gauze strips.
- 1 tbsp salt in ½ cup water with enough cosmetic clay to make a paste; add 1 or 2 drops of oil of **peppermint** (*Mentha piperita*).

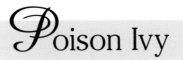 Poison Ivy

- Equal parts **goldenseal** *(Hydrastis canadensis)* root powder and green clay, available in health food stores.
- Osha *(Ligusticum porterii)* root tincture taken internally has an antihistamine effect that will reduce swelling. Take 20 drops of the tincture three times a day.

Homeopathy

Of all the over-the-counter homeopathic remedies available, **Rhus toxicodendron**—derived from the poison ivy plant itself—may be the most effective. Follow directions on the label.

Home Remedies

- Wash exposed skin with soap and water within 15 minutes of contact. If soap and water aren't at hand, but you're near a creek, wash with mud and water before waiting to wash again at home.
- Cover open blisters with sterile gauze to prevent infection.
- Make a paste with water and cornstarch, oatmeal, baking soda, or Epsom salt, and apply it to the rash. You can also use a paste made with baking soda and a few drops of witch hazel.
- Run hot water over the rash—as hot as you can stand it. The itching will intensify briefly, then abate, giving you several itch-free hours.

Prevention

The best way to deal with this poisonous threesome is to learn to recognize the plants, then steer clear of them. If you suspect contact with a poison plant, wash immediately and thoroughly with soap and water anything—your skin, clothes, shoes, tools—that might have picked up the plant's toxic resin. If you're going into poison-plant country, try one of the barrier lotions available from outdoor suppliers. The old folk tale about eating poison ivy leaves to make yourself immune is just that—a myth: Never eat the leaves or berries of wild plants. Many of them can cause dangerous reactions in humans. ∎

Identifying Poison Plants

Poison ivy—with its shiny green, sometimes reddish, yellow, or orange leaves—shares with poison oak a characteristic three-leaf pattern. Poison sumac has paired, pointed leaves, sometimes with greenish white berries. The maps below show the distribution (in green) of each type.

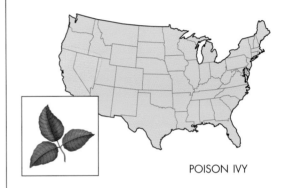

POISON IVY

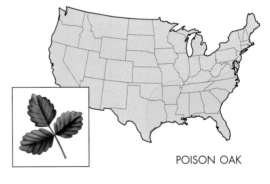

POISON OAK

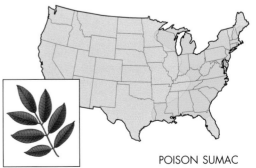

POISON SUMAC

Common Ailments

Premenstrual Syndrome

Symptoms

The symptoms of premenstrual syndrome recur during the same phase of the menstrual cycle, usually anywhere from seven to 10 days before your period begins. They may include any of the following:

- Bloating and fluid retention.
- Breast swelling and pain.
- Acne, cold sores, or susceptibility to herpes outbreaks.
- Weight gain of as much as five pounds (from retention of fluids).
- Headaches, backaches, and joint or muscle aches.
- Moodiness, anxiety, depression, or irritability.
- Food cravings, especially for sugary or salty foods.
- Insomnia.
- Drowsiness and fatigue, or conversely, extra energy.
- Hot flashes or nausea.
- Constipation, diarrhea, or urinary disorders.

A very small number of women with premenstrual syndrome may experience more intense symptoms:

- Fits of crying.
- Panic attacks.
- Suicidal thoughts.
- Aggressive or violent behavior.

Call Your Doctor If

- your symptoms are severe enough to interfere with your normal functions; your doctor may be able to offer treatments that will alleviate your symptoms.

P *remenstrual syndrome—commonly known as PMS—is a physical condition characterized by a variety of symptoms that typically recur during a particular phase of the menstrual cycle. Practically every woman experiences at least one PMS symptom sometime in her life. Specific symptoms vary from woman to woman. Although some adolescents suffer from PMS, most women first develop the symptoms during their twenties.*

Women most often affected by premenstrual syndrome are those who have experienced a major hormonal change, as may happen after childbirth, miscarriage, abortion, or tubal ligation. Women who stop birth-control pills may also notice an increase in PMS symptoms until their hormone balance returns.

Treatment Options

Remedies for PMS fall into two categories: hormonal treatments, prescribed by some conventional doctors, and nutritional and lifestyle changes, prescribed by both conventional and alternative practitioners. Hormones (usually estrogen or progesterone) are given in a variety of forms, including injection and vaginal or rectal suppositories. But because of the health risks associated with hormonal treatments, many women prefer to try alternative methods first. You may have to try several treatments, or a combination of them, before you find the right approach.

Aromatherapy

To relieve anxiety and irritability, add a few drops of **lavender** *(Lavandula angustifolia)* or **German chamomile** *(Matricaria recutita)* oil to a warm bath; juniper oil may also help. For breast tenderness, try adding 6 to 8 drops of geranium oil to a warm bath.

Herbal Therapies

Herbalists recommend a wide variety of herbs to help alleviate the many symptoms of PMS. **Chaste tree** *(Vitex agnus-castus),* for example, is sometimes prescribed because it is believed to help balance the body's hormones and relieve the anxiety and depression associated with PMS. **Dandelion** *(Taraxacum officinale),* whose leaves are thought to act as a powerful diuretic, is sometimes used to

$\mathscr{P}$remenstrual Syndrome

reduce the bloating and breast swelling caused by premenstrual fluid retention.

For relief from PMS symptoms, Chinese herbalists sometimes recommend *Xiao Yao Wan* (Free and Easy Wanderer Pills). Consult a practitioner for the appropriate dosage.

■ Lifestyle

Studies have shown that regular exercise lessens PMS symptoms, perhaps by stimulating the release of endorphins and other brain chemicals that help relieve stress and lighten mood. Getting enough sleep is also important for the successful treatment of PMS. Lack of sleep can exacerbate fatigue, irritability, and other emotional symptoms. Experts recommend that people who have trouble getting enough rest stick to a regular sleep schedule.

■ Mind/Body Medicine

Various relaxation techniques, such as yoga and meditation, can be helpful in reducing the anxiety, irritability, and other emotional symptoms that sometimes occur premenstrually. The Cobra, Bow *(below, right),* and Boat yoga positions are particularly recommended for PMS.

■ Nutrition and Diet

Dietary changes have been shown to effectively reduce PMS symptoms in some women. Try reducing your intake of caffeine, sugar, salt, dairy products, and white flour, which studies have shown can aggravate your symptoms. Many women also find that eating six or more small meals throughout the day rather than three large ones reduces their symptoms, perhaps by keeping insulin levels more constant.

Some PMS symptoms, such as mood swings, fluid retention, bloatedness, breast tenderness, food cravings, and fatigue, have been linked to a deficiency of *vitamin B6* or *magnesium.* Nutritionists recommend supplements of these nutrients: 50 to 100 mg of vitamin B6 daily, and 400 to 600 mg of magnesium daily, with a gradual increase if necessary. Supplements of *calcium, zinc, copper,* and *vitamins A* and *E,* as well as various amino acids and enzymes, are also sometimes prescribed. Consult an experienced nutritionist.

Some research has indicated that a dietary deficiency in fatty acids may contribute to PMS. Many women report that taking evening primrose *(Oenothera biennis)* oil, a substance that contains essential fatty acids, is effective. Your healthcare practitioner may recommend that you take one or two capsules (500 mg) up to three times a day throughout the month. Other dosage regimens are also recommended. Consult your healthcare practitioner.

Home Remedies

- Try to reduce stress and increase sleep during the week before your period.
- Exercise regularly.
- Try to manage your food cravings—particularly for chocolate; giving in to them may actually make your symptoms worse. Reach for fruit instead of sugary treats.
- As your period approaches, take long, warm baths to ease tension and stress.
- Use a hot-water bottle, a heating pad, or castor-oil packs to ease backaches and muscle aches associated with PMS.
- Abstain from alcohol before your period. It can aggravate PMS depression, headaches, and fatigue, and can trigger food cravings. ■

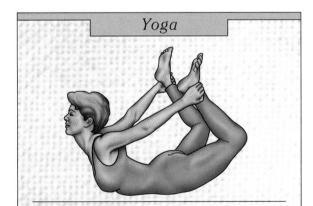

Yoga

Bow • *Try this position to relieve some of the symptoms of PMS. Lie on your stomach and grasp both ankles. While inhaling, squeeze your buttocks and slowly raise your head, chest, and thighs off the floor, pressing your ankles outward. Exhale and breathe slowly, then release.*

Prostate Problems

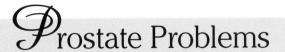

Symptoms

For an enlarged prostate:

- Difficulties in urination, including a weak or intermittent stream, unusual frequency (especially at night), straining, dribbling, or inability to empty the bladder.

For acute prostatitis:

- Frequent, difficult urination.

- A burning sensation when urinating.

- Sudden fever, chills.

- Pain in the lower back and in the area just behind the scrotum.

- Blood in the urine.

For chronic prostatitis:

- Frequent, difficult urination.

- Pain in the pelvis and genital area.

- Pain upon ejaculation, blood in the semen, or sexual dysfunction.

For prostate cancer:

- A frequent need to urinate, especially at night; starting or stopping the urine stream may be difficult.

- A painful or burning sensation during urination or during ejaculation.

- Blood in urine or semen.

Call Your Doctor If

- your symptoms lead you to suspect an enlarged or infected prostate. If allowed to progress, prostate problems can lead to bladder stones, generalized infection, or kidney failure.

- your symptoms lead you to suspect you may have prostate cancer. However, in the early stages prostate cancer rarely causes symptoms. The American Cancer Society recommends that all men over the age of 50 have an annual PSA (prostate-specific antigen) test in order to detect early cancer.

T he prostate is a walnut-sized gland that surrounds the male urethra—the tube that transports urine from the bladder through the penis. Its primary function is to produce an essential portion of the seminal fluid that carries sperm; the prostate also controls the outward flow of urine from the bladder. Because of this dual role, signs of prostate trouble can include both urinary and sexual difficulties.

Prostate problems occur in two principal forms: enlargement of the prostate, or BPH (for benign prostatic hyperplasia), which appears to stem from age-related changes in hormonal balance; and prostatitis, a bacterial infection, which may be either sudden and severe (acute prostatitis) or milder but persistent or recurrent (chronic prostatitis). Prostatitis is often the result of a urinary tract or bladder infection that has spread into the prostate gland. A chronic infection may follow an acute one. An enlarged prostate can be a sign of prostate cancer.

Treatment Options

Various alternative remedies aim to relieve symptoms or shrink an enlarged prostate gland. If your symptoms are severe, you should see a physician.

Ayurvedic Medicine

A practitioner may prescribe herbal remedies and exercises to increase circulation and relieve congestion in the prostate.

Chinese Medicine

Prostatitis and urethritis are considered conditions of damp heat and would be treated accordingly by a practitioner.

Herbal Therapies

An extract of the berries of the **saw palmetto** *(Serenoa repens)*, a scrubby tree of the American Southeast, is said to shrink an enlarged prostate and relieve symptoms. Other remedies include **Asian ginseng** *(Panax ginseng)*, flower pollen, **horsetail** *(Equisetum arvense)*, **nettle** *(Urtica dioica)*, true unicorn root *(Aletris farinosa)*, and the powdered bark of pygeum *(Pygeum africanus)*, an evergreen tree.

For prostatitis, pipsissewa *(Chimaphila umbellata)* and horsetail are used to treat chronic infec-

$\mathcal{P}$rostate Problems

An Enlarged Prostate

The prostate, a walnut-sized gland in a man's lower abdomen, lies at the base of the bladder and surrounds a section of the urethra, a tube that carries urine and semen out of the body. As indicated below, enlargement of the prostate can put increasing pressure on the urethra, making urination progressively painful and difficult.

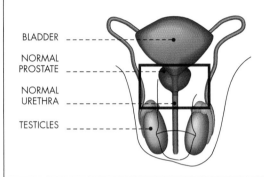

BLADDER
NORMAL PROSTATE
NORMAL URETHRA
TESTICLES

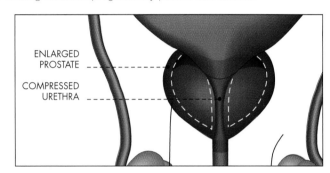

ENLARGED PROSTATE
COMPRESSED URETHRA

tion. Thuja *(Thuja occidentalis)* and pasqueflower *(Anemone pulsatilla)* are also suggested for inflammation of the prostate.

Homeopathy

Homeopathic practitioners may use various remedies to treat prostatic enlargement and prostatitis, among them *Berberis vulgaris* and *Staphysagria.*

Nutrition and Diet

Prostate enlargement may respond to nutritional therapies. **Zinc,** which is involved in many aspects of hormonal metabolism, is thought to promote prostate health and reduce inflammation; rich sources of zinc are oysters, wheat bran, whole oatmeal, pumpkinseeds, and sunflower seeds. **Vitamins C** and **E** may promote prostate health. The amino acids glycine, alanine, and glutamic acid are said to alleviate symptoms. The prostate may also benefit from large amounts of essential fatty acids, as found in flaxseed oil, walnut oil, sunflower oil, soybean oil, and evening primrose oil.

A recent study indicated that two to three servings a week of tomatoes—provided by food cooked in a tomato sauce, for example—may reduce the risk of prostate cancer, because of substances in the tomatoes called lycopenes.

Prevention

To prevent a recurrence of chronic prostatitis and promote prostate health:
- Take warm sitz baths.
- Drink water; dehydration stresses the gland.
- Avoid prolonged bicycle or horseback riding, or other exercises that irritate the area.
- Take supplements of **zinc** and **vitamin C.** ■

Yoga

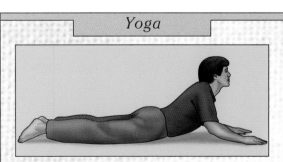

Cobra • *For an enlarged prostate, place both forearms on the floor, elbows directly under your shoulders. Inhale and push your chest up while pressing your pelvis against the ground. Hold for 15 seconds, breathing deeply, then slowly relax.*

Rashes and Skin Problems

Symptoms

The general warning signs of skin cancer include:

- Any change in size, color, shape, or texture of a mole or other skin growth.

- An open or inflamed skin wound that won't heal.

Symptoms of other skin problems are varied:

- Dry, reddish, itchy skin indicates some type of dermatitis, or skin inflammation, of which there are many types.

- Deep pink, itchy, raised patches of skin with white scales, typically on the scalp, knees, elbows, and upper body, could be signs of psoriasis.

Call Your Doctor If

- an existing mole changes size, shape, color, or texture; you develop a very noticeable new mole as an adult; or a new skin growth or open sore does not heal or disappear in a few weeks. You may have skin cancer.

- a child's rash progresses rapidly from a simple red flush to small bumps, then becomes a crusted, pimplelike inflammation that's extremely itchy; the child probably has chickenpox.

- a child has a red rash that spreads from the face downward and is preceded by fever, cough, and inflamed nasal passages; these are symptoms of measles.

- you have painless ulcers on the genitals and perhaps in the mouth, followed by red, circular, non-itching lesions on the skin, especially the palms and soles; you may have syphilis.

T he skin, largest of all human organs, is susceptible to a wide variety of disorders, ranging from short-lived and annoying rashes to painful, life-threatening skin cancer.

Common Skin Problems

Among the most common skin problems is a broad range of ailments known as dermatitis, a term that means skin inflammation. One familiar type, contact dermatitis, typically causes the skin to develop a pink or red rash, which may or may not itch. Pinpointing the exact cause of contact dermatitis can be very difficult. The culprit can be a poisonous plant, such as poison ivy or poison oak, or one among any number of other possible irritants, including certain flowers, fruits, vegetables, herbs, detergents, soaps, antiperspirants, and cosmetics.

Atopic dermatitis—also known as eczema—causes the skin to itch, scale, swell, and sometimes blister. Eczema usually runs in families and is often associated with allergies, asthma, and stress. Seborrheic dermatitis is a condition that causes greasy, yellowish scaling on the scalp and other hairy areas, as well as on the face and genitals. In infants, the disorder is called cradle cap.

Another familiar malady of the skin is psoriasis. Unpredictable, intractable, and unsightly, this is one of the most baffling and persistent of all skin disorders. Psoriasis is characterized by skin cells that multiply up to 10 times faster than normal, typically on the knees, elbows, and scalp. As underlying cells reach the skin's surface and die, their sheer volume causes raised, white-scaled patches. A variety of factors, ranging from stress to a bacterial infection, can precipitate an episode of psoriasis. Many doctors believe external stress, such as that associated with a new job or the death of a loved one, triggers an inherited defect in skin-cell production. Psoriasis is not contagious, and most outbreaks are relatively benign. With treatment, symptoms generally subside within weeks.

Types of Skin Cancer

Skin cancers fall into two basic categories: melanoma and nonmelanoma. Melanoma is cancer of me-

Rashes and Skin Problems

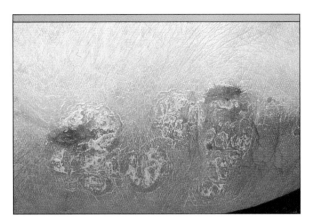

Psoriasis • *Usually occurring around the knees, elbows, and scalp, psoriasis is characterized by thick, silvery scales. There may be some itching but probably only a vague feeling of discomfort. Emotional stress and poor health can contribute to psoriasis; heredity is also a factor.*

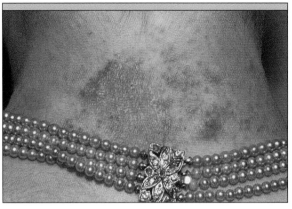

Contact Dermatitis • *This rash results from contact with various substances, including certain plants, cosmetics, jewelry, medications, and detergents. Symptoms include small bumps or blisters that develop—over a period of weeks or months—into a rash that is usually very itchy.*

lanocytes, cells in the epidermis that produce a protective pigment called melanin; the disease affects about 1 in 10 skin cancer patients. It can start in heavily pigmented tissue, such as a mole or birthmark, as well as in normally pigmented skin. Melanoma usually appears first on the torso, although it can arise on the palm of the hand; on the sole of the foot; under a fingernail or toenail; in the mucous linings of the mouth, vagina, or anus; and even in the eye. Melanoma, which is associated with infrequent but excessive sunbathing that causes scorching sunburn, is an extremely virulent, life-threatening cancer. It is readily detectable and always curable if treated early, but it progresses faster than other types of skin cancer and tends to spread beyond the skin. Once this occurs, melanoma becomes very difficult to treat and cure.

The two most common skin cancers—basal cell carcinoma (BCC) and squamous cell carcinoma (SCC)—are nonmelanomas, which are rarely life threatening. They progress slowly, seldom spread beyond the skin, are detected easily, and are usually curable. BCC, which accounts for nearly 3 out of 4 skin cancers, is the slowest growing; SCC is somewhat more aggressive and more inclined to spread.

Every malignant skin tumor in time becomes visible on the skin's surface, making skin cancer the only type of cancer that is almost always detectable in its early, curable stages. Prompt treatment of skin cancer is equivalent to cure.

Treatment Options

Alternative therapies can be very useful in the treatment of many common skin problems. They can also help combat the pain, nausea, fatigue, and headaches that frequently accompany conventional treatment of advanced skin cancer. However, the only acceptable treatment for cancer is conventional medical care. If you think you have skin cancer, see a doctor without delay.

■ Aromatherapy
Essential oils of **lavender** (*Lavandula angustifolia*), **thyme** (*Thymus vulgaris*), jasmine, and **German chamomile** (*Matricaria recutita*) may help soothe allergy-related eczema when they are used to scent a room. Add a few drops of one of these oils to a bowl of hot water. (Do not apply the oils directly to the skin.)

■ Flower Remedy
Rescue Remedy is a cream that can be applied to a rash or other irritation as often as two or three

CONTINUED

*R*ashes and Skin Problems

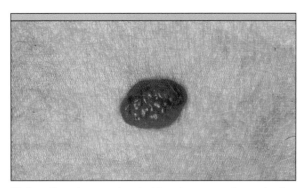

Mole • *Sometimes confused with melanoma, moles are benign growths that come in many shapes and sizes. They can develop at any age and on any part of the body. Most are dark and circular, and either smooth and flat or raised and wrinkled. If the color or size changes or if a mole starts to bleed, call your doctor.*

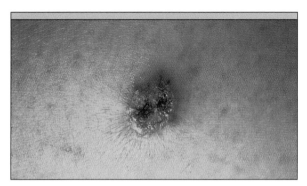

Basal Cell Carcinoma • *The most common type of skin cancer, basal cell carcinoma is a malignancy that grows slowly and rarely spreads to other organs. A small bump—typically in areas routinely exposed to the sun—develops a central crater that eventually erodes, crusts, and bleeds.*

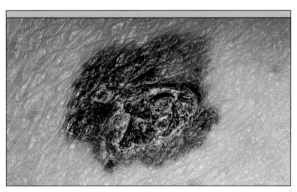

Melanoma • *The most serious form of skin cancer, melanoma may develop from an existing mole with an irregular border or in an area where there was no previous mole. The dark spot can become inflamed and change shape, color, size, and elevation. Call a doctor right away.*

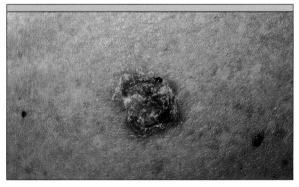

Squamous Cell Carcinoma • *Continual overexposure to the sun is the most frequent cause of this cancer. The tumor typically appears as a hard lump with a scaly, crusted surface. Growths usually develop on the lips, ears, hands, neck, and arms. This cancer can spread to internal organs.*

times a day. It can help reduce inflammation and speed the healing process.

▧ Herbal Therapies

Over the years, countless herbs have been used to treat skin ailments. Picking out what's right for your condition can be difficult, so seek help from a trained practitioner. The following are some substances herbalists consistently recommend.

Evidence suggests that evening primrose *(Oenothera biennis)* oil may effectively soothe itching associated with dermatitis and psoriasis. Some doctors believe it's as effective as corticosteroid drugs with fewer side effects, although people with liver disease or high cholesterol should use it only under medical supervision; pregnant women should avoid evening primrose oil because it can affect hormone levels.

Burdock *(Arctium lappa)* root, which boosts the immune system and helps reduce inflammation, and **dandelion** *(Taraxacum officinale)* root may also help reduce symptoms of dermatitis and psoriasis. Simmer 1 tbsp of either of these dried herbs in a cup of boiling water for 10 minutes; strain and drink hot, up to 3 cups a day. You may also take up to 1½ tsp fluidextract of burdock or dandelion root daily.

Homeopathy

For benign, short-term skin problems, an over-the-counter *Calendula* cream may soothe the inflammation. Taking **Rhus toxicodendron** (12x) three or four times a day may relieve the itching associated with a number of skin disorders, including contact dermatitis and chickenpox.

Don't try to choose homeopathic remedies on your own to treat a chronic, systemic condition such as psoriasis. Consult a qualified practitioner, who may recommend **Sulphur,** *Graphites,* **Lycopodium,** or **Arsenicum album.**

Light Therapy

Psoriasis and certain chronic types of dermatitis often respond to light therapy (also called phototherapy), in which patients receive timed exposure to ultraviolet rays from an artificial light source. In nearly all cases, the skin clears considerably in a matter of weeks.

Despite its apparent effectiveness, light therapy has its drawbacks. At four to eight sittings a month, treatment can be time consuming and relatively expensive. Light therapy may cause premature aging of the skin and increase a person's risk of developing skin cancer. In some instances, the skin condition can recur within a year.

Some people try to avoid the doctor's office or the hospital by using a tanning salon as their source of UV radiation. They won't find the healing rays they seek, however. Because of concerns about the risks of skin cancer, tanning salons must filter out the type of UV rays used in light therapy. Even patients who own a sunlamp should seek help from a healthcare professional. Only a qualified practitioner can tell you how much UV radiation you can tolerate without risking long-term damage to the skin.

Some light therapists recommend the use of indigo light to treat allergic hives and insect bites.

Nutrition and Diet

Fish oil high in EPA (eicosapentaenoic acid), from such fish as mackerel, herring, and salmon, may help reduce inflammation and itching. Because you would have to eat up to two pounds of fish a day to get enough EPA, try a 1,000-mg fish-oil capsule containing EPA four times a day; or try 1 tbsp cod-liver oil, also high in **vitamin A,** once a day; vitamin A plays a vital role in skin growth and maintenance.

Supplements of vitamin A (25,000 IU a day) and **zinc** (50 to 100 mg a day) may aid in skin healing, while **vitamin E** ointment or capsules (200 to 400 IU a day) can help relieve itching and dryness. **Vitamin B complex** containing **vitamin B_5** and **vitamin B_1** may also promote healthy skin: To help fight a case of psoriasis or dermatitis, the suggested dosage is 50 mg two or three times a day.

Home Remedies

- For dermatitis and mild forms of psoriasis, try mixing over-the-counter oatmeal or cornstarch preparations into a warm bath. Follow with application of a topical ointment (such as petroleum jelly or vegetable shortening) that helps the skin retain water and soothes inflammation. Take care not to stay in the bath too long: Lengthy immersion can strip the skin of essential oils.
- For scalp psoriasis, wash your hair with a coal-tar shampoo or with a mixture of cedarwood and juniper or lemon oils.

Prevention

If you are susceptible to skin cancer, take the following precautions whenever possible:

- Avoid intense sun exposure by staying out of it from late morning through early afternoon.
- Outside, wear a hat, long sleeves, trousers, and sunglasses that block UV radiation.
- Use a sunscreen with a sun protection factor of 15 or higher whenever you are outside.
- Consider taking a **B-complex** vitamin; B vitamins contain a compound called PABA, the active ingredient in many sunscreens. ■

*S*easonal Affective Disorder

Symptoms

Some or all of these symptoms are present during the fall and winter. Occasionally, seasonal affective disorder (SAD) occurs in summer, but with diminished rather than increased eating or sleeping symptoms.

- Depression, difficulty enjoying life, pessimism about the future.
- Loss of energy, inertia, apathy.
- Increased sleep, difficulty getting up in the morning.
- Impaired functioning: difficulty getting to work on time; tasks that are normally easy seem impossible.
- Increased appetite, weight gain.
- Carbohydrate cravings.
- Desire to avoid people.
- Irritability, crying spells.
- Decreased sex drive.
- Suicidal thoughts or feelings.

For children and adolescents:

- Feeling tired and irritable.
- Temper tantrums.
- Difficulty concentrating.
- Vague physical complaints.
- Marked cravings for junk food.

Call Your Doctor If

- you or your child suffers some of these symptoms with the onset of fall and winter and they seem to diminish or dissipate as spring and summer approach; your healthcare practitioner can help guide you to the most effective treatments for this condition.

*S*easonal affective disorder (SAD) is an extreme form of the "winter blues," bringing lethargy and curtailing normal functioning. It was only recently recognized as a specific disorder, but since 1982 much has been learned about it and how to treat it. People suffering from SAD undergo extreme seasonal differences in mood, as if they were split between a "summer person" and a "winter person."

Although a different kind of SAD can occur in the summer, its most common form begins gradually in late August or early September and continues until March or early April, when the symptoms begin to dissipate. Sufferers have been known to increase their sleep by as much as four hours a night and gain more than 20 pounds as they attempt to "hibernate" the winter away. Research suggests that SAD may affect 11 million people in the United States each year, and that an additional 25 million suffer a milder form that is indeed called the winter blues. Four times as many women suffer from SAD as men, and it tends to run in families.

The condition is thought to be caused by fluctuations in the brain chemical serotonin, which are triggered by inadequate amounts of outdoor light. Geographical location plays the largest role in determining a person's susceptibility to SAD; the nearer one lives to one of the poles, the greater the incidence.

Treatment Options

The most effective treatment for SAD is light therapy, sometimes combined with psychotherapy. However, a number of other alternative remedies have also proved helpful. For example, some healers believe that certain electrical emissions in the atmosphere—negative ions—improve a person's mood and health. In the last 30 years, scientists have developed small devices that emit negative ions into the atmosphere of a room. The negative ionizer seems particularly helpful for people with SAD (one study showed a 58 percent reduction of depression) and may be a good supplement to light therapy and medications.

Bodywork

A number of people with seasonal affective disorder have found relief of their symptoms through Therapeutic Touch. See Bodywork *(page 56)* for

Seasonal Affective Disorder

more information on this technique and on finding a qualified practitioner.

Chinese Medicine
SAD has been known to Chinese medicine for centuries and can be treated by acupuncture and Chinese herbs used in special combinations. Consult a practitioner for a course of treatment that is appropriate for your condition.

Energy Medicine
Polarity therapy, administered by a trained practitioner, can often be helpful in cases of SAD. See Energy Medicine *(pages 64-65)* for more information on this form of therapy.

Flower Remedies
The Bach flower remedy *Rescue Remedy* is often recommended for patients with seasonal affective disorder and may be particularly beneficial when used in combination with other flower remedies. Consult a naturopath or other practitioner familiar with flower remedies.

Hydrotherapy
To help promote relaxation and ease depression, soak in a hot bath containing a few drops of *lavender (Lavandula angustifolia)* or *German chamomile (Matricaria recutita)* essential oil. Consult a naturopathic physician familiar with hydrotherapy for other appropriate remedies.

Light Therapy
Light therapy can be used in different ways and may employ different types of light boxes, light visors, and lamps. All are designed to bring extra light to the eyes. Check to be sure a light box filters out harmful ultraviolet light.

Light boxes that generate strong full-spectrum light are the most beneficial (strong fluorescent light may cause problems such as dizziness, headaches, and even depression). Place the box on a table or desk where you can do paperwork, read, or make phone calls, and sit before it for periods varying from 15 minutes to 1½ hours a day.

Other light sources include larger boxes that stand on the floor, visors with lights attached, and dawn simulators—lights programmed to turn on by your bed on winter mornings before dawn.

Light boxes can be bought for several hundred dollars at special stores. Experts warn against constructing your own light box because of possible damage from ultraviolet light.

Massage
Administered by a trained professional, massage may be a useful adjunct to other therapies. Try three or four massage sessions to see if it works; one session is not enough to judge.

Mind/Body Medicine
Tapping the power of the mind and spirit can be of immense value in overcoming SAD. Various forms of meditation help relax the body and focus concentration, and for many people the power of prayer can be formidable therapy. Others find relief through guided imagery, in which patients are trained to use their imagination as a way to influence certain physiological conditions. Exercise can also be very helpful; in particular, engaging in a regular program of yoga is said to be a powerful way to rebalance the endocrine system and thereby decrease the symptoms of SAD.

Nutrition and Diet
People with SAD are apt to overeat in the winter, with cravings for sweets and starches. One SAD expert urges patients to avoid snacking on foods rich in carbohydrates and, instead, balance carbohydrates with protein or restrict carbohydrate-rich food to a single balanced meal a day.

Home Remedies

- Take a walk at lunchtime when the sun is high. Be outdoors as often as you can.
- Exercise as much as you are able.
- Take winter vacations in places with long days.
- Increase the natural light in your home by trimming low-lying branches near the house and hedges around windows.
- Paint your walls with lighter colors.
- Keep warm and enjoy the fun aspects of winter—such as wood fires, books, music. ■

$\mathcal{S}$exually Transmitted Diseases

Symptoms

Especially if you are a woman, you may experience no symptoms until you have developed serious complications, or you may notice:

- A vaginal, anal, or urethral discharge; the color may be white, yellow, green, or gray, or the discharge may be blood streaked, and it may have a strong odor.

- Genital and/or anal itching or irritation.

- A rash, blisters, sores, lumps, bumps, or warts on or around the genitals.

- Burning during urination.

- Swollen lymph glands in the groin.

- Pain in the groin or lower abdomen.

- Vaginal bleeding.

- Testicular swelling.

- Flulike symptoms.

- Painful intercourse.

Call Your Doctor If

- you have any of the above symptoms. Sexually transmitted diseases are contagious and may result in serious complications or death if left untreated.

Sexually transmitted diseases (STDs), once called venereal diseases, are among the most common of contagious diseases. As the name of this group implies, these infections can be contracted by means of vaginal, anal, or oral sex. You are at high risk if you have more than one sex partner and/or you don't use a condom when having sex. You are also at high risk for some of these diseases—notably AIDS and hepatitis B—if you share needles when injecting intravenous drugs.

Except for AIDS and hepatitis B, sexually transmitted diseases can be cured or managed if they are treated early. But because they may produce no early symptoms, you may not realize you have an STD until it has damaged your reproductive system, vision, heart, or other organs; hence the importance of prevention. Also, having an STD weakens the immune system and leaves you more vulnerable to other infections. Bacterial STDs include chlamydia, gonorrhea, and syphilis. Viral STDs include AIDS, genital herpes, genital warts, and hepatitis B. The microbes that cause STDs are found in semen, blood, vaginal secretions, and sometimes saliva. Most of the organisms are spread by vaginal, anal, or oral sex, but some, such as those that cause genital herpes and genital warts, may be spread through skin contact. You can get hepatitis B by sharing personal items, such as razors, with someone who has it.

Treatment Options

Don't try to treat an STD yourself. These diseases are contagious and serious. You must see a doctor. Bacterial STDs can be cured with antibiotics if treatment begins early enough. Although the alternative remedies listed here cannot cure STDs, they can reduce symptoms, speed healing, and strengthen your body's immune system.

Acupressure

To cleanse your system and build up energy, try massaging acupressure points Liver 3, on top of the foot between the big and second toes, and Liver 8, on the inside of the leg above the knee. Also try kneading Kidney 3, on the inside of the leg between the anklebone and the Achilles tendon. (See the Gallery of Acupressure Techniques, pages 18-31, for more information.)

Sexually Transmitted Diseases

Herbal Therapies

To treat syphilis, some herbalists advocate the following formula: Add 2 tbsp each of sarsaparilla (*Smilax* spp.) and sourdock (*Rumex crispus*) root to 1 qt boiling water. Simmer for five minutes and add 3½ tsp thyme. Steep covered for one hour. Drink 1 to 3 cups per day.

Calendula (*Calendula officinalis*), **myrrh** (*Commiphora molmol*), and thuja (*Thuja occidentalis*) may reduce the inflammation and discharge that accompany gonorrhea; use these herbs as a tea or douche. Apply calendula ointment to herpes sores to help them heal faster. Pipsissewa (*Chimaphila umbellata*), a woodland wildflower once used to flavor soft drinks, may also help, as could **uva ursi** (*Arctostaphylos uva-ursi*), **goldenseal** (*Hydrastis canadensis*), and **burdock** (*Arctium lappa*).

Saw palmetto (*Serenoa repens*), which contains berberine and stimulates the immune system, is useful in treating chlamydia and other genital infections, especially in men. You may drink it as a tea or take capsules. **Garlic** (*Allium sativum*) has been used by AIDS patients for its antibacterial and antiviral properties, and some studies have indicated that **hyssop** (*Hyssopus officinalis*) may be useful in treating Kaposi's sarcoma, a rare form of skin cancer that often strikes people with AIDS.

To cleanse your system, a doctor of Chinese medicine may prescribe an herbal formula tailored to your body's needs. This might include **gentiana** (*Gentiana scabra*), **Chinese foxglove root** (*Rehmannia glutinosa*), **dong quai** (*Angelica sinensis*), **bupleurum** (*Bupleurum chinense*), and licorice (*Glycyrrhiza uralensis*). Herbs such as coptis (*Coptis chinensis*) are considered helpful in strengthening the urinary and reproductive systems, especially when pelvic inflammatory disease is a complication.

Homeopathy

To treat gonorrhea, a homeopathic physician may want to attack the bacteria with antibiotics and then prescribe a remedy to strengthen your immune system and prevent recurrences. In addition to prescribing antibiotics to treat syphilis, he or she will ask you if any of your ancestors had this or any other sexually transmitted disease, on the theory that you could have inherited the tendency to contract syphilis. If so, a homeopath might prescribe a remedy such as *Syphilinum*, to help stimulate your immune system's response to the disease.

Nutrition and Diet

With your doctor's approval, try fasting for one to three days to clean out your system. Drink the juices of pomegranate and cranberry to flush out toxins from the urinary tract. Because antibiotics destroy beneficial intestinal bacteria as well as pathogenic kinds, eat yogurt containing live cultures or take acidophilus supplements.

Avoid high-fat, salty, processed foods, which may make your system too sluggish to fight off disease. To increase your body's resistance to infection, supplement your daily diet with **vitamin E** (200 IU) and **zinc** (15 mg).

Home Remedies

- Take hot baths to help reduce pain and inflammation associated with gonorrhea.
- Supplement antibiotic therapy with the herbs listed above.
- Use ice packs to reduce abdominal pain.
- Apply moist heat to infected joints to ease the pain of gonococcal arthritis.
- Douche with vinegar, yogurt, or lemon-juice solutions to relieve vaginal distress.
- Take zinc and **vitamins A, C,** and E to boost your immune system and to help treat some skin infections, such as herpes.
- Practice relaxation techniques to ease stress and speed healing.

Prevention

Always avoid sex with anyone who has genital sores, a rash, a discharge, or other disease symptoms. If you are in a high-risk group you should:
- Use latex condoms and water-based lubricants. Remember that condoms are not 100 percent effective at preventing disease.
- Avoid sharing towels or clothing.
- Wash before and after intercourse.
- Get a vaccination for hepatitis B.

$\mathcal{S}$hingles

Symptoms

- Slight fever, malaise, chills, upset stomach.

- Bruised feeling, usually on one side of your face or body.

- Pain (often in the chest) that is followed several days later by tingling, itching, or prickling skin and an inflamed, red skin rash.

- A group or long strip of small, fluid-filled blisters.

- Deep burning, searing, aching, or stabbing pain, which may be continuous or intermittent.

Call Your Doctor If

- you suspect an outbreak is beginning; antiviral drugs taken in the early stages may shorten the course of the infection.

- shingles on your face spreads near your eye; get treatment to avoid possible cornea damage.

- the affected area becomes secondarily infected with bacteria (indicated by spreading redness, swelling, a high fever, and pus); antibiotics may be necessary to help halt the spread.

- your rash lasts longer than 10 days without improvement; get treatment to avoid potential nerve damage.

- the pain becomes too great to bear; your doctor may prescribe a strong analgesic or a nerve block.

S *hingles is a reactivation of the herpes zoster virus—the same virus that causes chicken-pox—in which painful skin blisters erupt on one side of your face or body. Typically, this occurs along your chest, abdomen, back, or face, but it may also affect your neck, limbs, or lower back. The area can be excruciatingly painful, itchy, and tender. After one to two weeks the blisters heal and form scabs, although the pain continues.*

The deep pain that follows after the infection has run its course, known as postherpetic neuralgia, can continue for months or even years, especially in older people. Shingles usually occurs only once, although it has been known to recur in some people.

Treatment Options

No treatment has yet been discovered to prevent or halt shingles, and although steps can be taken to shorten its duration, frequently the virus must simply run its course. Because the pain following shingles is difficult to manage and can last so long—months or, in rare cases, years—the best approach is early and immediate treatment for the symptoms. Also, early medical attention may prevent or reduce the scarring that shingles can cause.

Your doctor may suggest medications to reduce inflammation and help you cope with the pain; antiviral drugs may help stop progression of the rash. The alternative treatments below are primarily intended for symptom relief and to help reduce inflammation.

Ayurvedic Medicine

A practitioner of Ayurvedic medicine might recommend a paste made from powdered turmeric; apply the paste to affected areas of your skin for pain relief and to speed healing.

Chinese Medicine

Acupuncture and Chinese herbal remedies may help both in the early stages of shingles and if there are chronic problems later. Consult a practitioner of Chinese medicine for specific treatment. One herbal formula that may be effective early on in the course of the disease is *Long Dan Xie Gan Wan* (Gentiana Drain the Liver Pills).

$\mathcal{S}$hingles

Flower Remedy

A Bach flower remedy known as **Rescue Remedy** cream may provide pain relief when applied to affected areas of the skin. Consult a practitioner such as a naturopathic physician who is familiar with flower remedies.

Herbal Therapies

Dabbing or sponging lesions with a solution of lemon balm *(Melissa officinalis)* may reduce inflammation. Make a 50-50 mixture of tincture and boiled, then cooled, water. Apply **calendula** *(Calendula officinalis)* lotion or ointment to lesions four or five times a day. Calendula helps the body fight the virus and desensitizes nerve endings. You can also try three daily applications of a commercially prepared gel made from an extract of **licorice** *(Glycyrrhiza glabra),* which appears to interfere with virus growth. An over-the-counter cream made from **cayenne** *(Capsicum annum* var. *annum)* might decrease the pain of shingles, but it is extremely hot and should be applied only after blisters have healed and never on broken skin.

Homeopathy

There are many effective homeopathic remedies for the symptoms of shingles, including **Rhus toxicodendron** (12x) for itchy, raised lesions and **Arsenicum album** (12x) for red, burning lesions. Consult a homeopathic physician for the best remedy for your particular case.

Hydrotherapy

For the first three or four days, try ice for 10 minutes on, five minutes off, every few hours. Later, apply cool, wet compresses soaked in aluminum acetate, available over the counter in the form of astringent solution, powder packets, or effervescent tablets.

Nutrition and Diet

For relief of postherpetic pain, take 1,200 to 1,600 IU of **vitamin E** daily, but for no more than two weeks, only under a physician's care, and only if you don't have high blood pressure. To alleviate symptoms once the disease has begun, take 500 mg one to three times a day of the amino acid L-lysine,

but only for one week. Studies have shown that this works best if you avoid foods containing the amino acid arginine, such as chocolate, cereal grains, nuts, and seeds. Taking 1,000 to 3,000 mg of **vitamin C** daily with meals may help your body fight the virus.

Home Remedies

- Keep the affected area clean, dry, and exposed to air (without clothes covering it) as much as possible. Don't scratch or burst the blisters. If the pain keeps you from sleeping, snugly bind the area with an elastic sports bandage.
- To desensitize nerve endings, crush two aspirin, mix them with 2 tbsp rubbing alcohol, and apply the paste to lesions three times a day. To cut down on itching, ask your pharmacist to make the following mixture: 78 percent calamine lotion with 20 percent rubbing alcohol, 1 percent phenol, and 1 percent menthol. You can apply this mixture continuously until your blisters scab over. Other remedies for itching include frequent applications of **vitamin E** oil, gel from the aloe vera plant, or fresh leeks that have been chopped in a food processor. Dusting colloidal oatmeal powder where clothes rub against your skin can also reduce pain. ■

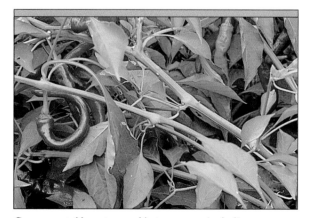

Cayenne • *Many types of hot peppers, including cayenne, contain a natural stimulant called capsaicin that can provide pain relief when applied to the skin in ointment form.*

Sinusitis

Symptoms

- Feeling of fullness in the face.
- Pressure behind the eyes.
- Nasal obstruction, difficulty breathing through the nose.
- Postnasal drip.
- Foul smell in the nose.
- Fever (possibly).
- Toothache (possibly).

Call Your Doctor If

- sinusitis develops into an inflammation around the eye (orbital cellulitis), which could cause damage to the eye and facial nerves.
- the condition does not improve within seven days; you may need a prescription for antibiotics.
- sinusitis recurs more than three times in a year, and periods between bouts grow shorter; you may have a chronic infection that could become serious.

Sinusitis is an infection or inflammation of the sinuses, the air-filled pockets in the bones of the face. One of the most common healthcare complaints in the U.S., sinusitis occurs when the mucus-producing linings of the sinuses become inflamed. By far the most frequent cause is blockage of the tiny drainage openings called ostia, perhaps as a result of an upper respiratory tract viral infection. Once these openings are clogged, foreign material can't get out, and invading bacteria cause the sinus walls to swell and fill with pus.

Treatment Options

Many alternative therapies attempt to relieve the pain of sinusitis and open the sinuses for drainage. Others aim to fight infection by boosting the immune system. If the sinuses are infected with bacteria, you may need antibiotics to kill the disease organisms before they cause further damage or spread to other sinuses.

Acupuncture

Acupuncture has been shown to be effective in the treatment of sinusitis. An acupuncturist may apply medium stimulation to various ear points— adrenal, forehead, internal nose, lung, and near the sinuses—to help drain the sinuses. Points on the stomach, bladder, and large intestine meridians can also help; consult a licensed practitioner.

Aromatherapy

Inhalants of **eucalyptus globulus** (E. globulus), pine, or **thyme** (Thymus vulgaris) may help break up your clogged sinuses. You may also alleviate the symptoms by holding menthol or eucalyptus packs over your sinuses.

Herbal Therapies

Bromelain tablets have been shown in controlled studies to reduce inflammation, nasal discharge, headache, and breathing difficulties. You can boost your immune system with **echinacea** (Echinacea spp.), **goldenseal** (Hydrastis canadensis), or **garlic** (Allium sativum), preferably raw. Breathing the steam of clove (Syzygium aromaticum) tea or **ginger** (Zingiber officinale) tea also provides some relief. To combat excessive mucus production, herbalists

Sinusitis

suggest elder *(Sambucus nigra)* flower, **eyebright** *(Euphrasia officinalis)*, **marsh mallow** *(Althaea officinalis)*, or goldenrod *(Solidago virgaurea)*.

The exact makeup of a prescribed Chinese herbal mixture depends on whether the sinusitis is "hot" (acute or infectious) or "cold" (chronic or allergic). Either way, the preparation may include the Chinese herb **ephedra** *(Ephedra sinica)*, a decongestant. (WARNING: Do not use ephedra if you have hypertension or heart disease.) A number of other Chinese herbs, among them honeysuckle *(Lonicera japonica)*, fritillary bulb *(Fritillaria cirrhosa)*, **tangerine peel** *(Citrus reticulata)*, xanthium fruit *(Xanthium sibiricum)*, and **magnolia flower** *(Magnolia liliflora)*, can also help relieve sinusitis symptoms.

■ Homeopathy

For acute sinusitis with thick, stringy mucus and pain in the cheeks or the bridge of the nose, use **Kali bichromicum** (30c) once or twice a day. For sinusitis with intense facial pain, alternating chills and sweat, and yellow-green discharge from the nose and mouth, use **Mercurius vivus** (30c) twice a day. For acute sinusitis with a clear, thin discharge, sneezing, headache, and a stopped-up nose at night, use **Nux vomica** (30c) twice a day. For sinusitis with light yellow or green nasal discharge accompanied by low spirits and lack of thirst, use **Pulsatilla** (30c) twice a day. If symptoms linger for more than two days, seek the advice of a professional homeopath.

■ Nutrition and Diet

A good, healthful diet including fruits and raw green leafy vegetables can help stimulate secretions and break up sinusitis. Nutritionists also suggest the following supplements to the diet: **vitamin C,** 500 mg every two hours; bioflavonoids, 1 gram per day; beta carotene **(vitamin A),** 25,000 IU per day; and **zinc** lozenges (consult a nutritionist for dosages). Stay away from foods that you suspect may trigger an allergic reaction.

Home Remedies

- Inhale steam from a vaporizer, a humidifier, a mixture of hot water and vinegar, or even a cup of tea or coffee. Steam is one of the best remedies for unclogging sinuses.
- Use warm compresses on your nose to help open your sinuses.
- Drink plenty of liquids.

Prevention

It's difficult to prevent sinusitis, but you can reduce your chances of having your sinuses become infected. First, avoid allergenic substances, which for some people include the dust in their beds and certain foods, such as dairy products and wheat. Whenever possible, avoid cigarette smoke. Note: People with diabetes, cystic fibrosis, and certain other diseases may be prone to sinusitis. ■

Acupressure

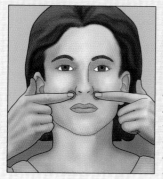

Large Intestine 20 •
This point may help relieve the pain, congestion, and swelling of sinusitis. Gently press the points on either side of your nose; apply pressure upward, underneath your cheekbones. Breathe deeply and hold for one minute.

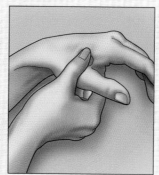

Large Intestine 4 •
To ease headache pain and congestion, press your right thumb into the webbing between the thumb and index finger of your left hand. Hold for one minute, then repeat on the other hand. (Do not use if you are pregnant.)

Common Ailments

$\mathcal{S}$ore Throat

Symptoms

The classic symptoms of a sore throat include a burning sensation or "scratchiness" in the back of the throat; pain, especially when swallowing; and, perhaps, tenderness along the neck. These symptoms may be accompanied by:

- Sneezing and coughing.
- Hoarseness.
- Runny nose.
- Mild fever.
- General fatigue.

Call Your Doctor If

- you also have a fever higher than 101°F without other cold symptoms; this may indicate a case of strep throat, which needs treatment.

- you also have flulike symptoms that don't get better after a few days; this may indicate infectious mononucleosis.

- any hoarseness lasts longer than two weeks; this could be a sign of throat cancer or oral cancer.

- your sore throat is accompanied by drooling, or you experience difficulty swallowing or breathing; this may indicate an inflamed epiglottis, the structure that overhangs the opening to the larynx, or an abscess in the back of the throat; these two uncommon conditions require medical attention.

Sore throat is one of the most common health complaints, particularly during the colder months, when respiratory diseases are at their peak. Typically the raw, scratchy, burning feeling at the back of your throat is the first sign that a cold or the flu is on the way. But a sore throat can also presage more serious conditions, so you should watch how it develops and call a doctor if it seems to be out of the ordinary.

Treatment Options

Most alternative therapies for sore throat are geared toward symptom relief, although some address the cause. A sore throat usually goes away on its own. However, if the pain persists or worsens after a few days, you should see your doctor.

Aromatherapy

To increase blood circulation and improve fluid drainage in sore areas, massage your throat and chest with a lotion made with 2 drops each of *eucalyptus globulus* (E. globulus) and cypress in 2 tsp of a carrier oil such as vegetable or almond oil.

Herbal Therapies

At the first sign of soreness, take three raw cloves of *garlic (Allium sativum)* a day. (Garlic is a natural antibiotic and antiseptic.) If garlic smell becomes a problem, try four garlic oil capsules instead. Teas made from either *goldenseal (Hydrastis canadensis)* or *echinacea (Echinacea* spp.) may also be effective. One of the best herbal treatments uses *ginger (Zingiber officinale),* which is noted for its anti-inflammatory properties. Simmer 2 tsp chopped fresh ginger in water for 20 minutes; breathe in the steam from this tea for five minutes and repeat two or three times a day.

A traditional Native American treatment is drinking a tea made from the inner bark of the *slippery elm (Ulmus fulva).* Put 2 tsp powdered bark in 1 cup water. Bring to a boil and simmer for 10 to 15 minutes.

Homeopathy

Homeopaths prescribe several remedies for sore throats. Consult a homeopathic practitioner or try those listed here:

Sore Throat

- If the pain comes on suddenly and is accompanied by great thirst and hoarseness, try **Aconite** (6c) three times a day.
- If the pain comes on suddenly and is accompanied by fever, headache, and restlessness, use **Belladonna** (6c) three times a day.
- If your sore throat has come on gradually and is accompanied by fatigue, try **Ferrum phosphoricum** (6c) three times a day.
- If the back of your throat is red and swollen and the pain is relieved by cold water or ice, try **Apis** (6c) three times a day.
- If your sore throat is accompanied by flulike symptoms, extreme sluggishness, and weakness, use **Gelsemium** (6c) three times a day.

▨ N u t r i t i o n   a n d   D i e t

At the first sign of soreness, take 500 to 6,000 mg of **vitamin C** daily to help fight the cold or other viral infection causing it. CAUTION: Unless your body is accustomed to megadoses of vitamin C, it cannot absorb more than about 1,000 mg every two hours; the excess will be passed off in your urine or, in some cases, result in diarrhea.

Home Remedies

- Get plenty of rest and drink a lot of fluids.
- Suck on a **zinc** lozenge (consult a nutritionist for dosages). Zinc can relieve sore throats and other cold symptoms but may cause nausea if taken on an empty stomach.
- To help relieve the pain, apply a warm heating pad or compress to your throat. You can also try a warm chamomile poultice: Mix 1 tbsp dried **chamomile** *(Matricaria recutita)* into 1 or 2 cups boiling water; steep for five minutes, then strain. Soak a clean cloth or towel in the tea, wring it out, then apply to your throat. Remove the cloth when it becomes cold. Repeat as often as necessary.
- Try steam inhalations to ease the pain. Run very hot water in a sink. With a towel draped over your head to trap the steam, lean over the sink while the water is running. Breathe deeply through your mouth and nose for five to 10 minutes. Repeat several times a day. ■

Acupressure

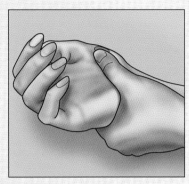

Lung 10 • *To help relieve the discomfort of a sore and swollen throat, try pressing on this point. Using your left thumb, apply pressure to the center of the pad at the base of your right thumb. Hold for one minute and repeat on the other hand.*

OF SPECIAL INTEREST

Homemade Gargles

To wash away mucus and irritants and bring relief from the pain of a sore throat, try any of the following gargles:

- *Salt water: Mix ½ tsp salt in 8 oz warm water.*
- *Sage: Put 1 to 2 tsp dried leaves in 1 cup boiling water; steep for 10 minutes, then strain and cool until lukewarm.*
- *Lemon: Mix the juice of one lemon in 8 oz warm water.*
- *Horseradish: Mix 1 tbsp pure horseradish, 1 tsp honey, and 1 tsp ground cloves in 8 oz warm water.*
- *Raspberry: Put 1 to 2 tsp raspberry leaf in 1 cup boiling water; steep for 10 minutes, then strain and cool until lukewarm.*
- *Cayenne pepper: Mix the juice of half a lemon, 1 tbsp salt, and ¼ tsp cayenne pepper (or more if you can tolerate it) in ½ cup warm water. The cayenne pepper temporarily reduces the amount of pain-causing chemicals produced by nerve endings in the throat.*

Stomach Ulcers

Symptoms

- Burning upper abdominal pain, particularly between meals, early in the morning, or after drinking orange juice, coffee, or alcohol, or taking aspirin; discomfort is usually relieved after taking antacids or eating a meal.

- Tarry, black, or bloody stools.

Call Your Doctor If

- you have been diagnosed with a stomach ulcer and begin experiencing symptoms of anemia, such as fatigue and a pallid complexion. Your ulcer may be bleeding.

- you have symptoms of a stomach ulcer and develop severe back pain. Your ulcer may be perforating the stomach wall. Call your doctor now.

- you have symptoms of a stomach ulcer and vomit blood or material that looks like coffee grounds, or you pass dark red, bloody, or black stools, or stools that resemble currant jelly. These symptoms indicate internal bleeding; call 911 or your emergency number now.

- you have an ulcer and become cold and clammy, and feel faint or actually do faint. These are symptoms of shock, usually resulting from massive blood loss; get emergency medical treatment.

 bout 1 out of 10 Americans will suffer from the burning, gnawing abdominal pain of an ulcer sometime in life. Stomach, or peptic, ulcers are holes or breaks in the protective lining of the stomach, the esophagus, or the duodenum, which is the upper part of the small intestine. The most common type are duodenal ulcers; the second most common are gastric ulcers, which develop in the stomach, followed by the comparatively rare esophageal ulcers, which are typically a result of alcohol abuse.

Although stress and diet have long been thought to cause ulcers, research conducted since the mid-1980s has persuasively demonstrated that the primary culprit in most ulcers is a bacterial infection; the bacterium Helicobacter pylori is present in 92 percent of duodenal ulcer cases and 73 percent of gastric ulcers.

Treatment Options

An ulcer should always be monitored by your doctor. When a bacterial infection has been diagnosed as the cause, the best treatment is with antibiotics, which can permanently cure the ulcer. Many people also use over-the-counter antacids for symptom relief. There are, however, a variety of alternative treatments that can aid in relieving pain and in healing ulcers.

Acupuncture
Acupuncture targeting the points associated with stress, anxiety, and stomach/gastrointestinal disorders may help with the treatment of peptic ulcers. Consult a licensed acupuncturist.

Herbal Therapy
Licorice (*Glycyrrhiza glabra*), which stimulates mucus secretion by the stomach, is frequently used in herbal treatments of ulcers. Herbalists and naturopathic physicians typically employ a special preparation of licorice rather than the tincture or tea form; consult an herbal practitioner.

Mind/Body Medicine
Biofeedback, meditation, and other relaxation techniques can help you learn how to deal effectively with stress, which increases stomach acid production and irritates ulcers.

$\mathcal{S}$tomach Ulcers

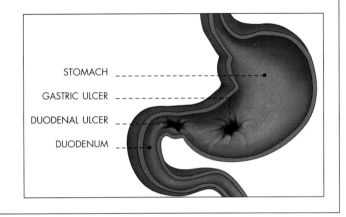

A Hole in the Stomach

A peptic ulcer is a break in the protective lining of the esophagus, the stomach, or the duodenum. Duodenal and gastric ulcers (inset) are the two commonest forms. Their typical symptoms are recurring pain in the upper abdomen and a bloated feeling after eating.

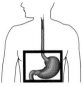

STOMACH

GASTRIC ULCER

DUODENAL ULCER

DUODENUM

▉ Nutrition and Diet

Some nutritionists recommend supplementing your intake of **vitamins A** and **E** as well as **zinc,** which increase the production of mucin, a substance your body secretes to protect the stomach lining. Another suggestion may include drinking about a quart of cabbage juice daily; its high content of glutamine is thought to expedite the growth of mucin-producing cells.

Home Remedies

- Cut down on milk. Although it may feel as though milk's coating properties are soothing your ulcer, milk actually stimulates stomach acid secretion, irritating the ulcer.
- Pick appropriate antacids. Like milk, calcium-containing antacids can stimulate stomach acid secretion. Experiments suggest that bismuth, an ingredient in some over-the-counter stomach medications, may help destroy the bacterium that causes some peptic ulcers.
- Be cautious when choosing over-the-counter pain relievers. Aspirin and nonsteroidal anti-inflammatory drugs (NSAIDs), such as ibuprofen, can cause ulcers and prevent an existing ulcer from healing. Your best choice may be acetaminophen, which does not cause or promote stomach ulcers.
- Learn how to deal with stress. While there is no evidence that stress causes ulcers, it can

exacerbate existing ones. Practicing relaxation techniques can help alleviate stress.

Prevention

- Avoid foods and beverages such as caffeinated drinks that irritate your stomach. Use common sense: If it upsets your stomach, avoid it. Spicy and fatty foods are common irritants.
- Eat foods with high fiber content. Fiber is thought to enhance mucin secretion. ▉

OF SPECIAL INTEREST

Can You Catch an Ulcer?

In 1982, two Australian doctors determined that the bacterium Helicobacter pylori played a significant role in the development of peptic ulcers, and further studies have shown antibiotics to be effective in treating ulcers caused by the bacterium. Does this mean that ulcers are contagious? The answer is murky. Not everyone infected with the bacterium develops an ulcer, and certainly other factors—such as heredity and excessive use of aspirin, tobacco, and alcohol—increase the chances of getting one. Still, research has shown that infected children are more likely to transmit the bacterium than adults are.

Stress

Stress is the reaction of our bodies and minds to something that upsets their normal balance. The human response to stressful events is an ancient one, dating back to a time when life was a constant struggle for survival. A good example of stress in action is the way you react when you are frightened or threatened. But not all stressful events are so sudden or so obvious as the threat of bodily harm. Stress occurs when there is an imbalance between the demands of life and our ability to cope with them. Any challenge that overwhelms us—a serious illness, the death of a family member, the loss of a job or a lover—can be stressful to the point of physical and psychological dysfunction.

Symptoms

■ Physical symptoms may include headache, fatigue, insomnia, digestive changes, neck pain or backache, loss of appetite, or overeating.

■ Psychological symptoms may include tension or anxiety, anger, reclusiveness, pessimism, resentment, increased irritability, feelings of cynicism, and inability to concentrate or perform at usual levels.

Call Your Doctor If

■ you have prolonged or acute symptoms. Excessive stress puts you at risk of other serious disorders, including immune problems, digestive disorders, diabetes, asthma, high blood pressure, migraine headaches, and possibly cancer.

■ you have symptoms of stress and any of the following: unusual patterns of sleep, appetite, and moods; physical movement that is unusually agitated or abnormally slow. You may have clinical depression.

Treatment Options

Some treatments once considered alternative are now widely used in the medical community—particularly those designed to promote physical and mental relaxation.

■ Aromatherapy
Essential oil of **lavender** *(Lavandula angustifolia)* can help reduce stress: Try 5 or 6 drops in a bath, or put 2 or 3 drops on a handkerchief and inhale from time to time. Other oils to try include Roman chamomile *(Anthemis nobilis)*, marjoram *(Origanum majorana)*, **lemon-scented eucalyptus** *(Eucalyptus citriodora)*, and lemon balm *(Melissa officinalis)*.

■ Ayurvedic Medicine
Two combined formulas, *Geriforte* and *Mentat,* may help reduce stress. The following remedies may also be useful: a milk decoction or powder of the root of winter cherry; a decoction or powder of the fruit of emblic myrobalan; or an infusion, powder, or pill of gotu kola.

■ Bodywork
The Alexander technique focuses on ways to eliminate stress-causing muscle tension and promote a restful breathing pattern.

■ Exercise
Vigorous aerobic exercise can reduce the level of pulse-quickening hormones released during stress and stimulate a sense of well-being. Even a walk

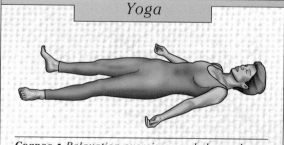

Yoga

Corpse • *Relaxation exercises can help you keep stress under control. For the Corpse, lie on your back, with your feet approximately 18 inches apart and turned out slightly. With palms up, place your hands about six inches from your hips. Close your eyes and breathe deeply for eight to 10 minutes.*

$\mathcal{S}$tress

around the block can help reduce anxiety. Try to schedule the exercise of your choice for 30 minutes at least three times a week.

Stretching exercises can relax tense upper-body muscles that accompany stress and affect breathing. Rotate your shoulders up, back, and then down. Inhale as the shoulders go back; exhale as they go down. Do the exercise four or five times, inhale deeply, and exhale. Repeat the cycle.

Flower Remedy

The Bach flower **Rescue Remedy** may help reduce stress. Consult a naturopath or other practitioner familiar with flower remedies.

Herbal Therapies

A traditional response to stress is to drink a cup of hot tea. Some herbalists suggest **chamomile** (*Matricaria recutita*), **passionflower** (*Passiflora incarnata*), **valerian** (*Valeriana officinalis*), or **American ginseng** (*Panax quinquefolius*) tea.

Hydrotherapy

Try a warm bath containing 1 drop of the essential oils of **lavender** (*Lavandula angustifolia*), jasmine, or **German chamomile** (*Matricaria recutita*).

Massage

By relaxing tense muscles and helping circulation, massage helps the mind relax. Between treatments, massage your temples, neck, shoulders, and face.

Mind/Body Medicine

Meditation brings relaxation and increased awareness. When you feel stressed, think affirmations such as "I can face this calmly. I control my own life." Or try visualization, or guided imagery, exercises. Visualizing a pleasant situation can bring physical as well as emotional benefits; combine a visualization session with soothing music. Many excellent teachers, books, and tapes are available to help you learn the technique.

Nutrition and Diet

How well you handle stress can be affected by your diet. Because it is easy to neglect nutrition when you are under stress, make an extra effort to eat a balanced diet—plenty of vegetables and fruit, as well as foods high in complex carbohydrates, moderate in protein, and low in fat. Avoid or reduce caffeine consumption: Excessive caffeine has been shown to increase anxiety.

Sound Therapy

A number of sound-therapy techniques can help reduce stress. See Sound Therapy (*pages 170-171*) for more information.

Home Remedies

There are many simple, inexpensive ways to manage stress on your own. For many people, a good way to start is by cutting out artificial stress relievers such as alcohol, which can mask symptoms and may become addictive. Try exercise instead. Take walks. Breathe deeply.

In times of stress, social support is crucial. People with close personal relationships are the most likely to recover from serious illness or injury, and stress is no different. The ability to form relationships with people—or pets, for that matter—can be a key to good health.

Prevention

While we can't—and perhaps shouldn't try to—change our personality or avoid stressful situations, we can learn to cope with them. Try the following:

- Cultivate outside interests and plan occasional diversions to break routine habits.
- Set up a regular sleeping schedule and get plenty of rest—without sleeping pills.
- Avoid the learned behaviors of hurry and worry, which can upset your sleeping, eating, and other schedules. Take time to enjoy your life.
- Make a list of things that trouble you. Ask yourself: What's the worst that can happen? Have I done what I can to prepare myself? Is this problem really worth worrying about?
- When you're facing a stressful situation, remember a bit of folk wisdom: Count to 10 and take a deep breath before saying or doing anything. A deliberate pause can be an instant tranquilizer. ■

Sty

Symptoms

- Sty: a red, hot, tender, uncomfortable, and sometimes painful swelling near the edge of the eyelid. *(See the photograph opposite, below.)*

- Chalazion: a relatively painless, smooth, round bump within a fat gland of the eyelid.

Call Your Doctor If

- either type of swelling does not subside within a few weeks.

- the swelling interferes with your vision.

- you have pain in the eye.

- you have recurrent sties. A sty can be a symptom of other ailments such as diabetes and chronic skin problems.

CAUTION

Although some alternative treatments may be helpful in relieving and preventing eyelid infections, never put any preparations in the eye itself unless specifically directed to do so by a physician. The surface of the eye is easily damaged by some antiseptics and medications. When applying any lotions or compresses to the eyelid, keep your eye closed.

A sty is a pimple or abscess on the upper or lower edge of the eyelid that signals an infected eyelid gland. Although sties are usually on the outside of the lid, they can also occur on the underside.

An external sty starts as a pimple next to an eyelash. It turns into a red, painful swelling that usually lasts several days before it bursts and then heals. Most external sties are short lived.

An internal sty (on the underside of the lid) also causes a red, painful swelling, but its location prevents the pus from appearing on the eyelid. The sty may disappear completely once the infection is past, or it may leave a small fluid-filled cyst or nodule that can persist and may have to be cut open.

A chalazion is also a sign of an infected eyelid gland, but unlike a sty, it is a firm, round, smooth, painless bump located usually some distance from the edge of the lid.

Sties and chalazions are usually harmless and rarely affect your eye or sight. They can occur at any age and tend to recur elsewhere on the lid.

Treatment Options

While painful and unsightly, most sties heal within a few days on their own or with simple treatment. Chalazions, too, often disappear on their own, but it might take a month or more.

If sties recur, your doctor may prescribe an antibiotic ointment or solution. Apply it to the eyelid (with your eye closed) as directed.

Although a chalazion will often disappear on its own, applying warm compresses to the lid and perhaps a corticosteroid ointment will help speed the process.

In some especially problematic cases that do not respond to home treatment, you may need to have an internal sty or a chalazion removed surgically. An ophthalmologist can perform this minor procedure in the office using a local anesthetic. The eyelid usually heals quickly.

Acupuncture

In traditional Chinese medicine it is believed that all types of boils, including sties, are caused by heat invasion. To diffuse the heat, an acupuncturist may insert needles into Spleen 10 and Large Intestine 11 *(see Acupuncture, pages 34-35, for point locations).*

Ayurvedic Medicine

An infusion made with Indian basil can be soaked in a piece of clean cloth or cotton ball and applied to the sty to provide relief. Be sure to read the caution at left about applying treatments to the eye. Consult a qualified practitioner of Ayurvedic medicine for further specific advice.

Flower Remedy

Bach **Rescue Remedy** cream, applied directly to the sty, may help the eyelid heal faster. Be careful when you apply the cream—avoid getting it in your eye.

Herbal Therapies

To help reduce the pain and inflammation of sties, herbalists recommend professionally prepared eye drops made from **eyebright** *(Euphrasia officinalis).* They may also prescribe an oral preparation of **burdock** *(Arctium lappa).*

Hydrotherapy

Hydrotherapy treatment for a sty consists of applying hot compresses to the affected eye for 10 to 15 minutes four times daily for several days. This not only relieves pain and inflammation but also helps the sty ripen faster. To make a hot compress, use a cotton cloth or washcloth. Soak it in hot water,

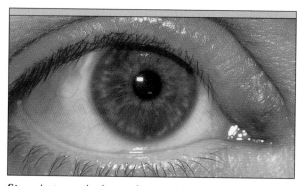

Sty • *A sty results from a bacterial infection at the root of an eyelash, typically at the inner corner of the eye. It causes the follicle of the eyelash to become inflamed (above); a pus-filled bump will form and then rupture. A sty can be painful, but it typically clears up on its own within a week.*

then wring it out; the cloth should be dry enough not to drip but wet enough to maintain a hot temperature for several minutes. Replace or remoisten the cloth as needed to keep it hot. Be sure to close your eye while you apply the compress. When the sty comes to a head, continue applying hot compresses to relieve pressure and promote rupture. Do not squeeze the sty; let it burst on its own.

Nutrition and Diet

If you have recurrent sties and chalazions, a nutritionist may recommend that you take supplements of **vitamins A** and **C,** which seem to promote healthy skin. You might also want to try a system-cleansing diet, consuming only raw fruits and vegetables, yogurt, herbal teas, fruit juices, and mineral water for up to a week. Naturopathic physicians believe that this diet, repeated at regular intervals, may keep sties from developing.

Home Remedies

The simplest—and often the most effective—treatment for sties and chalazions is to apply hot compresses, as described under Hydrotherapy, above. When the sty has come to a head, it will spontaneously rupture. You can also make a compress by wetting a tea bag with warm water and placing it on your eyelid, with your eye closed, for five minutes three to four times a day.

Prevention

If sties tend to recur, you need to cleanse the outside of your eyelids daily. Put a few drops of very mild baby shampoo into a teacup of warm water and stir. Using a clean cotton swab, gently brush the mixture over your eyelid once a day, keeping your lids closed. It is very important that you avoid contact of the eyelid with cosmetics, dirty towels, or contaminated hands.

Frequent application of hot compresses at the first sign of an infection will prevent further blockage of the lid glands. To keep the infection from spreading to other members of your household, be sure to use a clean, disposable cloth for compresses and do not share washcloths or towels. ■

Sunburn

Symptoms

- Mildly reddish to severely red or purplish skin discoloration; skin feels hot and tender. Sunburn appears one to six hours after exposure to sunlight and peaks within 24 hours, later fading to tan or brown.

- Small, fluid-filled blisters that may itch and eventually break; flaking or peeling skin that reveals the tender, reddened underlayer.

- Red, blistered skin accompanied by chills, fever, nausea, or dehydration. This severe stage of sunburn is considered a first-degree burn.

- Pain and irritation of the eye associated with overexposure to ultraviolet rays from sunlight or other sources.

Call Your Doctor If

- your sunburn blisters and is accompanied by chills, fever, or nausea. Severe sunburn requires professional care in order to limit the risk of infection and to prevent dehydration.

- your eyes are extremely painful and feel gritty. You should have your eyes examined by an ophthalmologist to determine whether the corneas are damaged.

Even though light-skinned people have the highest risk of getting sunburned, skin of any color can be damaged by the sun's rays. A sunburn is like any other kind of burn, except that it comes on more slowly. Skin that is reddened and feels hot to the touch can be self-treated and will heal in a matter of days. Sunburned skin that swells or blisters, causing localized pain and overall discomfort, is considered a first-degree burn. A sunburn that results in swelling and extensive blisters may be accompanied by fever, nausea, and dehydration.

Getting a severe sunburn early in life increases the risk of developing malignant melanoma, a type of skin cancer, years later. (See Rashes and Skin Problems, pages 332-335.)

The Sun's Dangerous Rays

Of the sun's ultraviolet (UV) radiation that penetrates Earth's atmosphere, UVA radiation generally only tans but may also take part in premature aging and wrinkling. UVB rays cause sunburn and the potential for skin cancer. Reflected sunlight from sand, water, or snow is as strong as direct sunlight; shade, clouds, clothes, sunglasses, and sunscreens do not provide complete protection. In addition, certain drugs can intensify the harmful effects of UV radiation; if you are concerned about the potential danger, ask your healthcare practitioner about the risk of photosensitivity.

Treatment Options

Few cases of sunburn require medical care. If the burn is very painful or widespread, a doctor may prescribe oral corticosteroids to relieve the discomfort. Treatment for extremely severe cases of sunburn—those involving extensive blistering, dehydration, or fever—usually requires bed rest and possibly hospitalization.

Ayurvedic Medicine

Fresh gel of aloe or a paste made from the herb Indian country mallow can provide relief when they are applied to the skin. A paste or the oil of sandalwood applied to the forehead may help cool the body. Consult a practitioner of Ayurvedic

$\mathscr{S}$unburn

medicine to find out about these and other traditional Indian remedies.

▪ Chinese Medicine

A traditional Chinese remedy for burns of any kind is *Ching Wan Hung* (Beijing Absolute Red); consult a practitioner of Chinese medicine for treatment.

▪ Flower Remedy

The flower remedy known as **Rescue Remedy** cream can be applied to sunburned skin to provide relief. Consult a practitioner such as a naturopathic physician who is familiar with flower remedies.

▪ Herbal Therapies

Over-the-counter preparations containing **aloe** (*Aloe barbadensis*) are excellent for relieving the dryness and irritation that accompany sunburn. Lotions, poultices, and compresses containing **calendula** (*Calendula officinalis*) will reduce inflammation and pain. **Echinacea** (*Echinacea* spp.) may be used on exposed new skin after peeling or blistering, to help prevent infection.

▪ Homeopathy

Cantharis (12x) taken orally every three to four hours for up to two days is recommended for relieving pain and helping to heal blisters.

▪ Hydrotherapy

A cool bath laced with several tablespoonfuls of baking soda or cider vinegar can relieve the pain, itching, and inflammation of a moderate sunburn.

Home Remedies

Apply cold compresses or calamine lotion to ease itchiness, take aspirin to relieve pain, and have a cool bath or shower for overall relief. Drink plenty of water, but avoid alcohol, which dehydrates the skin. Do not break any blisters; doing so will slow the healing process and increase the risk of infection. When your skin peels or the blisters break, gently remove dried fragments and apply an antiseptic ointment or hydrocortisone cream to the skin beneath. If you feel feverish or nauseated, drink lots of fluids and see a doctor immediately.

Prevention

The most effective way to prevent sunburn is to limit your exposure to direct sunlight, especially between 10:00 a.m. and 3:00 p.m. Take a look at your shadow: If it's shorter than your height, stay under cover.

- If you have to be outside in the midday sun, wear loose-fitting clothes, a broad-brimmed hat, and socks and shoes to protect your feet and ankles.
- Note that radiation exposure is greater at higher altitudes and southern latitudes.
- Any water surface reflects the sun's rays and can double the radiation dose. Protect your skin with a water-resistant sunscreen.
- Protect babies' sensitive skin from strong sunlight, and alert older children to the hazards of overexposure.
- Wear sunglasses that are rated for UV protection. In general, gray, brown, and green lenses—in order from most to least effective—can block out damaging UV rays. ▪

OF SPECIAL INTEREST

Screening the Sun

Two types of sunscreens are on the market. Physical sunblocks, such as zinc ointment, protect by creating a barrier between your skin and the sun. They're good for small areas, such as the nose and lips, but not for your whole body. Products containing para-aminobenzoic acid (PABA) block virtually all UVB rays—the kind most likely to cause sunburn—but offer only minimal protection against UVA rays.

Sunscreens carry a sun protection factor (SPF); a rating of SPF 15 is recommended for most people, but fair-skinned people who are in the sun all day need more. Apply sunscreen 30 minutes before you go out, and reapply it after a swim. Even if you don't swim, a waterproof sunscreen has more staying power. If PABA gives you a rash, try sunscreens containing cinnamates for UVB protection and avobenzone for UVA protection.

Common Ailments

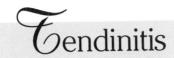Tendinitis

Symptoms

- Painful tenderness at or near a joint, especially around a shoulder, wrist, or heel (where it is known as Achilles tendinitis), or on the outside of an elbow (where it is called tennis elbow).

- In some cases, numbness or tingling.

- Stiffness that, along with the pain, restricts the movement of the joint involved.

- Occasionally, mild swelling at the joint.

- Persistence of the soreness, which may last or recur long after the tendon has had time to recover from the original injury.

Call Your Doctor If

- your pain doesn't ease up in seven to 10 days. You want to avoid letting chronic tendinitis set in; moreover, you may have another problem such as bursitis, carpal tunnel syndrome, phlebitis, or tenosynovitis.

- your pain is extremely severe and is accompanied by swelling and loss of function. You may have a ruptured tendon, which requires immediate medical attention.

CAUTION

If you have suffered a stroke or have diabetes, circulatory problems, or heart disease, avoid massage and applications of heat or cold until you consult your doctor.

T endinitis is an inflammation in or around a tendon, which is a cable of fibrous tissue that connects a muscle to a bone and transmits the force the muscle exerts. Tendons are designed to withstand bending, stretching, and twisting, but they can become inflamed because of overuse, disease, or injuries that leave them with torn fibers or other damage. The pain can be significant, and it will worsen if the damage progresses because of continued use of the joint. Most tendinitis heals in about two weeks, but chronic tendinitis can take more than six weeks to improve, often because the sufferer doesn't give the tendon time to heal.

Treatment Options

The goal of treatment is to restore movement to the joint without pain and to maintain strength in surrounding muscles while giving the tissues time to heal. Adequate rest is crucial. Returning too soon to the activity that caused the injury can lead to chronic tendinitis or torn tendons.

Ayurvedic Medicine
A paste of Indian bdellium applied directly to the affected area can help soothe the pain of tendinitis.

Bodywork
The Alexander technique—which teaches patients how to maintain good body alignment and reduce muscle tension—can have a healing effect on chronic tendinitis. The Feldenkrais method, Rolfing, and Aston-Patterning are other bodywork techniques that may also help heal chronic tendinitis.

Chinese Medicine
Acupuncture, if performed by a qualified practitioner, can be useful in treating tendinitis. A number of Chinese herbal liniments can also soothe tendinitis pain, including *Po Sum On* Medicated Oil, *Tieh Ta Yao Gin* (Traumatic Injury Medicine), and *Zheng Gu Shui*. Chinese herbalists might prepare a poultice of gardenia (*Gardenia jasminoides),* flour, and wine, which, together with *tui na*—a type of massage that uses the ball of the thumb to manipulate the area—may help to reduce swelling and to increase circulation.

Tendinitis

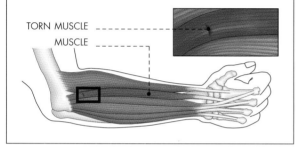

TORN MUSCLE

MUSCLE

■ Herbal Therapies

For pain, a naturopathic practitioner might suggest **white willow** *(Salix alba),* the natural form of aspirin, taken orally. Try comfrey *(Symphytum officinale)* salve, applied two or three times a day, to help relieve inflammation and to strengthen the tendon. Bromelain, an enzyme found in pineapples, is sometimes taken orally with the aim of reducing inflammation in soft tissues; bromelain should not be taken with meals, so take it at least 30 minutes before, or two hours after, eating.

■ Hydrotherapy

Use alternating hot and cold compresses: Soak one washcloth in hot water and another in cold. Wring out the warm cloth and place it over the affected area for three minutes; follow with the cold cloth for 30 seconds. Alternate them two more times, finishing with a cold cloth. Do this once or twice a day, as needed.

Or try a hot vinegar pack: Heat equal parts vinegar and water, then soak a towel in the mixture. Wring it out and apply it to the affected area for five minutes. Remove it, then apply a cold one for five minutes. Cover with wool. Repeat these hot-cold applications three times, finishing with cold.

■ Massage

If performed by a skilled practitioner, massage can help relieve tendinitis and promote the proper healing of the affected tissues; the friction technique is particularly effective for chronic tendinitis.

■ Nutrition and Diet

Research suggests that vitamin supplements may help heal tendinitis. Ask your doctor about taking daily supplements of **vitamin C** (1,000 mg), beta carotene (**vitamin A,** 10,000 IU), **zinc** (22.5 mg), **vitamin E** (400 IU), and **selenium** (50 mcg).

Home Remedies

Try the RICE treatment: rest, ice, compression, and elevation. Rest mainly means not using the joint, especially not for the same action that injured it. For ice, a bag of frozen vegetables will do if no ice pack is handy. Compression is best provided by an elastic sports bandage wrapping the area snugly, but not painfully tight. For elevation—to reduce fluid pressure in the injured area—put your ankle on a footstool or lift your elbow onto a chairside table.

Prevention

Include warmups, cooldowns, and stretches in your exercise routine. Vary your exercises, and gradually increase their level of difficulty. ■

OF SPECIAL INTEREST

Tendinitis on the Job

If your tendinitis is caused by tasks you perform at work and you cannot rest your injuries while keeping up with your duties, ask your supervisor for help in modifying your work habits. You may want to request a work-site inspection by an ergonomics specialist, who can analyze the situation and suggest changes. Try some stretches before and after work, and plan to take a five- to 10-minute period each hour to rest the injured area by undertaking tasks that do not involve its use.

Thyroid Problems

Symptoms

Hyperthyroidism:

- Weight loss despite increased appetite.

- Increased heart rate, higher blood pressure, and increased nervousness, with excessive perspiration.

- More frequent bowel movements, sometimes accompanied by diarrhea.

- Muscle weakness, trembling hands.

- Development of a goiter.

Hypothyroidism:

- Lethargy, slower mental processes.

- Reduced heart rate.

- Increased sensitivity to cold.

- Tingling or numbness in the hands.

- Development of a goiter.

Subacute thyroiditis:

- Mild to severe pain in the thyroid gland.

- The thyroid feels tender to the touch.

- Pain when swallowing or turning your head.

- Appearance of these symptoms shortly after a viral infection, such as the flu, mumps, or measles.

Call Your Doctor If

- you are feverish, agitated, or delirious, and have a rapid pulse; you could be having a thyrotoxic crisis, which is a sudden and dangerous complication of hyperthyroidism.

- you feel intensely cold, drowsy, and lethargic; you could be experiencing a myxedema coma, a sudden and dangerous complication of hypothyroidism that can cause unconsciousness and possibly death.

T hrough the hormones it produces, the thyroid gland influences almost all of the metabolic processes in your body. Thyroid disorders can range from a small, harmless goiter that needs no treatment to life-threatening cancer. The most common thyroid problems involve irregular production of thyroid hormones. Too much of these vital body chemicals causes a condition known as hyperthyroidism, possibly resulting in a goiter or Graves' disease. Insufficient hormone production, on the other hand, leads to hypothyroidism. Untreated for long periods of time, hypothyroidism can bring on a myxedema coma, a rare but potentially fatal condition that requires immediate hormone injections. Generally, though, most thyroid problems are not serious if properly diagnosed and treated.

Treatment Options

Alternative treatments will not completely suppress or replace thyroid hormones. Rather, they attempt to relieve some of the discomfort associated with thyroid conditions, or to improve the function of the thyroid gland through a variety of approaches ranging from diet supplements and herbal remedies to lifestyle changes and special exercises. You should always receive a professional evaluation for any thyroid disorder; most of these conditions require a course of treatment beyond the scope of home care alone.

Ayurvedic Medicine

For an enlarged thyroid, an Ayurvedic physician might prescribe an appropriate course of *panchakarma* therapy, make dietary recommendations, and suggest taking *Trikatu* pills (capsules containing dry ginger, black pepper, and Indian long pepper) and an infusion of Irish moss.

Chinese Medicine

Many thyroid problems can be treated through acupuncture or specific combinations of Chinese herbs. For hyperthyroidism, baked licorice *(Glycyrrhiza uralensis)* combination, **bupleurum** *(Bupleurum chinense)* and dragon bone combination, or bupleurum and peony combination may be helpful. Consult a qualified practitioner for dosages or techniques that are appropriate for your condition.

Thyroid Problems

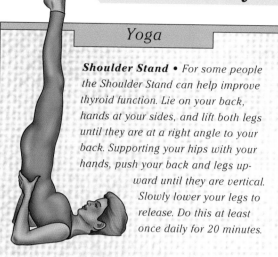

Yoga

Shoulder Stand • *For some people the Shoulder Stand can help improve thyroid function. Lie on your back, hands at your sides, and lift both legs until they are at a right angle to your back. Supporting your hips with your hands, push your back and legs upward until they are vertical. Slowly lower your legs to release. Do this at least once daily for 20 minutes.*

▪ Exercise

Aerobic exercise 15 to 20 minutes a day helps maintain good thyroid function. Regular physical activity is especially important if you are hypothyroid. (Ask your doctor before starting an exercise program.)

▪ Herbal Therapies

For relief from the symptoms of hyperthyroidism, try 4 parts bugleweed *(Lycopus* spp.), 2 parts motherwort *(Leonurus cardiaca),* 2 parts **skullcap** *(Scutellaria lateriflora),* and 1 part **hawthorn** *(Crataegus laevigata)* in a tincture three times a day. For insomnia due to hyperthyroidism, combine equal parts **valerian** *(Valeriana officinalis)* and **passionflower** *(Passiflora incarnata)* in a tincture and take half an hour before bedtime.

In the case of hypothyroidism, try a tea made from bladder wrack *(Fucus vesiculosus).* Three times daily, pour 1 cup boiling water on 2 tsp bladder wrack; steep for 10 minutes. Bladder wrack can also be taken in capsule form three times daily.

▪ Homeopathy

Thyroid (12x) is believed to help support the thyroid gland in cases of hypothyroidism; talk to your homeopathic practitioner to see if this remedy is appropriate for you.

▪ Hydrotherapy

For hypothyroidism, try alternating hot and cold compresses: Soak one facecloth in hot water, an-

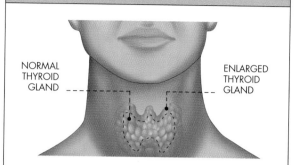

The Thyroid Gland

The thyroid gland, located at the base of the neck in front of the windpipe, needs iodide to produce necessary quantities of a vital bodily hormone. If the diet does not contain enough iodide, the gland simply begins to grow in an effort to meet its production quota. In some cases the enlarged thyroid, known as a goiter, becomes uncomfortable or overproductive and must be surgically removed.

other in cold. Wring out the hot cloth and hold it over the front of your neck for three minutes. Wring out the cold cloth and place it on the same spot for 30 seconds. Repeat this technique two more times— once a day for mild hypothyroidism, morning and evening for severe cases. Other therapies include a neutral bath (for hyperthyroidism), and a 30-second dip in a cold bath or a 30-second cold rinse at the end of a hot shower (for hypothyroidism).

▪ Nutrition and Diet

For hypothyroidism, avoid cabbage, peaches, rutabagas, soybeans, spinach, peanuts, and radishes, as these foods can interfere with the manufacture of thyroid hormones. Supplements of **vitamin C, vitamin E,** riboflavin **(vitamin B₂), zinc, niacin** (vitamin B₃), pyridoxine **(vitamin B₆),** and tyrosine might help boost thyroid production. However, if you have hyperthyroidism, eating the foods listed above might help lower your body's production of thyroid hormones. ▪

357

TMJ Syndrome

Symptoms

- Pain in front of the ears, especially upon awakening.

- Persistent pain in the facial muscles on one or both sides.

- A clicking or popping sensation when opening the mouth or working the jaw.

- Difficulty opening the mouth because it feels locked or painful.

- Recurring headaches.

Call Your Doctor If

- you have difficulty opening your mouth following an injury or a blow to the face. You may have dislocated or damaged one or both of your temporomandibular joints.

- you have persistent discomfort in your jaw that does not respond to painkillers, heat, massage, or rest. You may need a specialist's diagnosis and advice about more aggressive treatment to relieve both the symptoms and the cause.

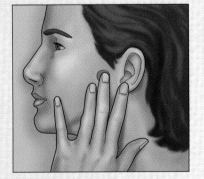

Acupressure

Stomach 7 • *Pressing this point may ease tension in the jaw. With your middle fingers, feel on either side of your jaw about one thumb width in front of your ears. Find a slight indentation along the upper jaw line, then press steadily for one minute.*

T he twin joints that connect the lower jaw, or mandible, to the temporal bones of the skull are relatively simple hinges with small disks of cartilage to protect the bony surfaces that rub against each other. The jawbreaking term for pain or discomfort in this area is temporomandibular joint (TMJ) syndrome, or myofascial pain dysfunction. Most people exhibit temporary symptoms of TMJ at some point in their lives, but some experience chronic pain that radiates through the face and around the neck and shoulders. Most cases of TMJ are due to excessive strain on the jaw muscle, a displaced disk, or degenerative joint disease.

Treatment Options

Acupuncture
Acupuncture relieves the symptoms of TMJ, including muscle tension in the jaw, headache, ringing in the ears, and referred neck pain. Acupuncture works by relaxing the muscles, which makes it effective for TMJ symptoms caused by stress.

Chiropractic
Chiropractic therapy is recommended for TMJ caused by muscle overuse and strain rather than by joint damage. A chiropractor not only treats the patient's back and body alignment but may also use physical therapy, interferential current, ultrasound, or diathermy on the affected joint, any of which can help relax the area and allow the chiropractor to stretch the muscles and manipulate the jaw.

Hydrotherapy
A few drops of the essential oils of **lavender** (*Lavandula angustifolia*) or St.-John's-wort (*Hypericum perforatum*) in warm bathwater may help you relax. To reduce inflammation of the TM joints, apply hot and cold compresses. Start with a hot towel for three minutes, then switch to a cold towel for half a minute; repeat two or three times a day for chronic conditions, or more frequently if acute.

Massage
When muscle tension is believed to play a role in TMJ, massage therapy may provide relief. Two areas can be massaged: One, the temporalis muscle, runs from just above and slightly forward of the top

TMJ Syndrome

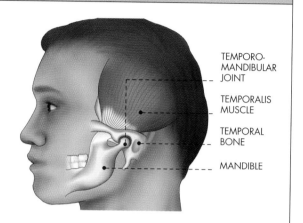

The Temporomandibular Joint

The temporomandibular joint is a hinge that joins the mandible, or jawbone, to the temporal bone of the skull. The large temporalis muscle and other ligaments and muscles keep the joint operating smoothly. If any component is forced out of alignment by such things as muscle tension, arthritis, a head injury, or an uncorrected bite, the joint may not move smoothly and can cause pain.

TEMPORO-MANDIBULAR JOINT

TEMPORALIS MUSCLE

TEMPORAL BONE

MANDIBLE

of your ear over to your temple; the other is on your jaw about an inch in front of your earlobes. Place a finger on either of these areas and then open and close your jaw, pressing your teeth together slightly when the jaw is closed. You will feel a muscle pop in and out as it contracts and relaxes. Place your thumb or your index and middle fingers on these areas, and massage lightly in little circles. Doing this for a minute or two at each spot can help relax muscles that cause tension around the joint.

Mind/Body Medicine

While relaxation techniques, hypnotherapy, and guided imagery can all alleviate the symptoms of TMJ, biofeedback is the most effective mind/body treatment. Biofeedback is a drug-free, noninvasive approach to eliminating tension and controlling stress-related pain, and can be self-administered after training by a professional therapist. Using electrical readings from the muscle that moves the jaw, practitioners can train a patient to control the tension in the overall area. Studies have shown that biofeedback works especially well for chronic TMJ sufferers and may help reduce pain and minimize clicking for a longer time than other treatments.

Nutrition and Diet

It is important for TMJ sufferers to reduce strain on jaw muscles and joints. Avoid hard foods like raw carrots and apples, and chewy foods like steak and bagels. If the pain in your jaw becomes really un-

bearable, try fasting or putting yourself on a liquid diet for a day or two; this is especially effective if you also speak only when it's absolutely necessary.

Osteopathy

For TMJ that is caused by a bad bite, osteopathy complements dental work. Before your dental work, an osteopathic physician will balance the appropriate muscles so that your dentist is not balancing your bite to an abnormal muscular pattern.

Home Remedy

Mouth guards for football and hockey players might help mild cases of TMJ due to bruxism (grinding of teeth during sleep). You'll find the guards in sporting goods stores.

Prevention

- To prevent TMJ caused by unconscious muscle strain or uneven pressure on the jaw, don't sleep with your head tilted or with the entire weight of your head concentrated on your chin—a common practice among people who sleep on their stomachs. Try sleeping on your side, or on your back without a pillow.
- If you feel tension in your jaw every morning, you may be unwittingly clenching or grinding your teeth. Ask a dentist or orthodontist about being fitted with a bite guard. ■

Tonsillitis
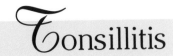

Symptoms

For tonsillitis:

- A very sore throat with red, swollen tonsils; there may be a white discharge or spots on the tonsils.

- Swollen and tender lymph nodes in the neck under the jaw.

- A low-grade fever and headache accompanying the other symptoms.

For tonsillar abscess:

- In addition to inflamed tonsils, severe pain and tenderness around the area of the soft palate, at the roof of the mouth, and difficulty swallowing.

- Distinctively muffled speech, as if the child is speaking with a mouthful of mashed potatoes, caused by swelling from the abscess.

Call Your Doctor If

- your child has symptoms of tonsillitis.

- your child has tonsillitis and starts drooling or having difficulty breathing, which may indicate a tonsillar abscess or epiglottitis, inflammation of the epiglottis. Call 911 or your emergency number now.

- your child has trouble breathing at night or experiences noisy breathing or episodes of sleep apnea, in which the child stops breathing for brief periods while asleep; these symptoms may indicate adenoid problems or overgrown tonsils.

- your child has recurrent bouts of tonsillitis; surgery may be indicated.

T he tonsils are masses of lymphatic tissue located at the back of the throat. They produce antibodies designed to help your child fight respiratory infections. When these tissues themselves become infected, the resulting condition is called tonsillitis. Most tonsil infections and tonsillar abscesses in elementary school age children are caused by the streptococcal bacterium, the same organism that causes strep throat.

Tonsillitis most commonly affects children between the ages of three and seven, when tonsils may play their most active infection-fighting role. But as the child gets older, the tonsils shrink, and infections become less common. Tonsillitis is usually not serious unless a tonsillar abscess develops. When this happens, the swelling can be severe enough to block your child's breathing. Secondary ear infections (otitis media) and adenoid problems are other possible complications.

Treatment Options

Some alternative therapies are effective in relieving the symptoms of tonsillitis. But be sure to first get a throat culture to rule out strep throat, which must be treated with antibiotics. Severe cases may warrant a tonsillectomy. A tonsillar abscess should be treated by a medical doctor before you start any alternative method.

Aromatherapy

A practitioner may recommend oregano and general treatment with a variety of essential oils.

Ayurvedic Medicine

The combined formula *Septilin* may be useful in treating tonsillitis. Other appropriate remedies include an infusion of mint; a powder of the fruit of beleric myrobalan mixed with honey; and a powder or pill of Indian bdellium.

Chinese Medicine

A practitioner of Chinese medicine may advise acupressure to relieve a sore throat, or acupuncture to combat chronic tonsillitis. Often-used herbal remedies include Honeysuckle and Forsythia Powder, thought to help soothe a sore throat in the early stages of tonsillitis; Superior Sore Throat Powder; and *Liu Shen Wan* (Six Spirit Pills).

Tonsillitis

Herbal Therapies

To reduce inflammation, herbalists suggest drinking a tea made from cleavers (*Galium* spp.): Add 1 tsp dried herb to 1 cup boiling water. A gargle made from **sage** *(Salvia officinalis)* is thought to help fight infection: Add 2 tsp to boiling water and steep for 10 minutes. Let your child gargle with the tea (as warm as she can tolerate it) for five minutes several times a day; make sure she does not swallow the tea. The steam from **ginger** *(Zingiber officinale)* tea may help shrink inflamed tonsils: Breathe in the steam for five minutes, three to four times a day.

Homeopathy

After determining if your child is suffering from acute or chronic tonsillitis, a homeopath may recommend one of the following remedies: for inflamed tonsils, **Belladonna, Hepar sulphuris,** or **Mercurius vivus;** for chronic enlarged tonsils, *Baryta carbonica* or **Calcarea carbonica.**

Hydrotherapy

A hydrotherapist may recommend one or several of the following treatment techniques: tonsillar irrigation; a hot fomentation to the throat, neck, and mastoid; or a heating compress to the throat. Another remedy is known as warming socks: If your child's feet are cold, let her soak them in warm water for five to 10 minutes. Next, soak a pair of cotton socks in cold water and wring them out thoroughly. Place the cold, wet socks on her feet and cover them with dry wool socks. Let her go to bed, being careful to keep her from getting chilled. In the morning, the cotton socks should be dry.

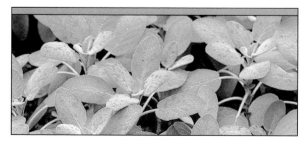

Sage • *The gray-green leaves of sage contain antiseptic and astringent components that may help fight the infection and relieve the discomfort of tonsillitis.*

Osteopathy

Osteopaths treat tonsillitis and tonsillar abscesses with the same surgical and drug therapies offered by conventional medical doctors but may also try gentle soft-tissue manipulation techniques to encourage lymphatic drainage.

Home Remedies

- A salt-water gargle can relieve soreness. Dissolve ½ tsp salt in a glass of warm water and let the child gargle as needed to ease pain. Tell your child not to swallow this solution.
- Ice cream or frozen yogurt after a tonsillectomy will relieve soreness.
- A cool-mist humidifier will increase moisture in the room and soothe a child's sore throat. Aim the mist away from your child so that it does not spray directly at her face, and change her clothes if they become damp. ■

The Tonsils

Tonsils are lymph nodes at the back of the mouth on either side of the uvula, or soft palate. These small, pinkish lumps of tissue redden and swell when infected, and may develop gray or yellow spots. During an attack of tonsillitis, the glands around the neck under the jaw may feel swollen and tender.

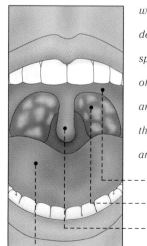

ROOF OF MOUTH

TONSILS

UVULA

TONGUE

Toothache

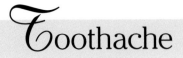

Symptoms

- Aching or sharp pain in tooth when biting or chewing.
- Soreness in teeth, gums, or jaw.

Call Your Dentist If

- your gums are painful, red, and swollen; you may have an impacted tooth or a gum disease. *(See Gum Problems.)*
- you experience continuous bouts of throbbing pain in a tooth, or the tooth is extremely sensitive to heat or cold; you may have tooth decay (a cavity) that requires a new or replacement filling. If the decay is advanced, you may need root canal work. You may also have a tooth abscess, a serious infection requiring emergency treatment.
- you have a sharp pain in your tooth, your tooth feels long or loose, and you have a fever. See your dentist immediately; you may have a tooth abscess.

A toothache can be caused by something as simple as a piece of food wedged between your gum and your tooth—in which case relief involves no more than rinsing or flossing away whatever is causing the pain. But if the pain is not so easily eliminated, you probably have a dental disorder that can cause serious problems if you don't visit your dentist.

The major cause of tooth decay is dental plaque—a substance composed of the bacteria, acids, and sugars in your mouth—which corrodes the protective enamel on your teeth. Initially, you may have no symptoms; but as decay develops, you may feel stabbing pain whenever you eat something hot, cold, sweet, or sour. If decay goes untreated, bacteria infect the underlying dentin and eventually the pulp, or fleshy core, of the tooth. To fight infection, pus floods the pulp, causing a painful tooth abscess. If left untreated, abscesses can damage the jawbone or sinuses and lead to blood poisoning.

Other causes of dental pain include impacted teeth and gum disease (see Gum Problems). Toothaches may also be caused by pressure from sinus congestion, by tooth grinding, or by a blow to the face.

Treatment Options

Alternative remedies may help alleviate the discomfort of symptoms, but conventional treatment is absolutely necessary to stop decay or infection from spreading. You must see a dentist for aches that you suspect may be related to tooth decay; in most cases, the dentist will remove the decayed portion and fill the cavity with a durable material. If the decay is serious, you may need a root canal, which involves removing the pulp, sealing the opening, and then capping the tooth with a crown. If the damage is so severe that a root canal is impossible, or if a tooth is impacted, extraction is the usual treatment. Alternative treatments may ease the pain in the meantime.

Acupressure

Apply deep pressure to the webbing between the index finger and the thumb (Large Intestine 4) to relieve dental pain *(see the Gallery of Acupressure Techniques, page 24)*. Do not press this point if you are pregnant. Massaging this area with an ice cube may also help.

OF SPECIAL INTEREST

Hypersensitive Teeth

If a tooth reacts just to heat or cold, you could have dentinal hypersensitivity. More than 40 million Americans feel pain caused by the wearing away of enamel and exposure of dentin. It's brought on by age, receding gums, dental surgery, or excessive brushing with whitening toothpastes or hard-bristled brushes. You can help relieve hypersensitivity by using a toothpaste made for sensitive teeth and a toothbrush with soft bristles.

Toothache

▪ Aromatherapy

The essential oils of clove and **niaouli** *(Melaleuca viridiflora),* applied to the area around the painful tooth, may help soothe a toothache. Be careful to avoid touching oil of clove to the skin, as it may irritate it or cause an allergic reaction.

▪ Ayurvedic Medicine

Applied directly to the affected tooth, the following remedies may bring pain relief: oil from the flowers of cloves; a mixture of ginger, cardamom, and licorice; or paste or oil of sesame seeds.

▪ Chinese Medicine

Acupuncture can often help soothe a toothache. Chinese herbal remedies frequently used for relief from acute dental pain include *Liu Shen Wan* (Six Spirit Pills), *Huang Lien Shang Ching Pien,* and Bezoar Antidotal Tablets.

▪ Flower Remedy

The Bach **Rescue Remedy** is often recommended for toothache. Consult a naturopath or other practitioner familiar with flower remedies.

▪ Herbal Therapies

Rubbing clove oil *(Syzygium aromaticum)* or **myrrh** *(Commiphora molmol)* on the gum around a painful tooth can help numb the area.

▪ Homeopathy

Homeopaths often recommend **Hypericum** (12x) and **Arnica** (12x) for relief of toothache. Consult your homeopathic practitioner for other remedies.

▪ Hydrotherapy

Depending on the circumstances of your case, a practitioner may recommend placing an ice pack or hot-water bottle on the jaw near the tooth.

▪ Massage

Gentle massage to the head and face can help relieve pain and tension associated with a toothache.

Home Remedies

Try the following remedies to relieve your pain:
- Rinse with salt water; if this doesn't work, floss gently to pry out any trapped particles.
- Numb your gums: Sucking on ice numbs the gum surrounding a painful tooth.
- Keep cool: Though a hot compress may ease pain, if your toothache is caused by an infection, heat will cause the disease to spread.

Prevention

- Brush and floss after eating; use a nonabrasive, fluoride-based toothpaste. Beware of so-called whitening agents; they often contain abrasives that can wear down enamel.
- Cut down on sweets and carbohydrates. ▪

Tooth Decay

Plaque buildup can erode a tooth's protective enamel, causing decay and infection of the underlying dentin. If left untreated, the infection can spread to the pulp, or fleshy core, of the tooth. As the body attempts to fight the infection, a painful, pus-filled abscess may form at the root of the tooth, possibly causing damage to the gum, jawbone, or even the sinuses.

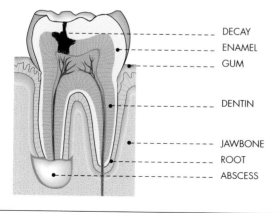

DECAY
ENAMEL
GUM
DENTIN
JAWBONE
ROOT
ABSCESS

V

$\mathcal{V}$aginal Problems

Symptoms

- Your vulva is inflamed and it itches; you may have vulvitis.

- The skin of the vulva is thick and has developed white patches; this may indicate a condition called lichen sclerosis or cancer of the vulva. See your doctor for diagnosis.

- Increased vaginal discharge with an offensive odor and burning, itching, and pain; you may have vaginitis.

- You have been sexually or psychologically abused and experience muscle constriction and pain at any attempt to penetrate the vagina; you may have vaginismus.

- An abnormal discharge, bleeding, and/or a firm lesion on any portion of the vagina; you may have vaginal cancer.

Call Your Doctor If

- your bleeding is not caused by menstruation. If you are taking oral contraceptives, it may only be breakthrough bleeding. Otherwise, you may have dysfunctional uterine bleeding. If you are pregnant, there may be a complication in the pregnancy. Postmenopausal bleeding sometimes indicates uterine cancer.

- you have lower abdominal pain along with fever, menstrual disturbances, abnormal discharge, and/or painful sex. You may have a pelvic infection.

- you use tampons, a diaphragm, or a contraceptive sponge and you develop a high fever or rash. You may have toxic shock syndrome.

*T*he vagina is the part of the female reproductive system that connects the cervix (the entrance to the uterus) with the vulva, the skin folds that enclose the urethral and vaginal openings. This elastic, muscular passage is lubricated by its own secretions and by mucus-producing glands in the cervix.

"Vaginitis" is an umbrella term meaning inflammation of the vagina. Yeast causes vaginal yeast infections, the most common form of the disorder. Other vaginal infections include bacterial vaginosis—in which a change in the balance of naturally occurring bacteria in the vagina allows disease-causing bacteria to dominate—and sexually transmitted diseases such as gonorrhea, trichomoniasis, and chlamydia.

The various types of vaginal cancer include squamous cell carcinoma and clear cell adenocarcinoma. Once cancer appears on the vagina, it may spread to surrounding tissues, including the bladder, rectum, vulva, and pubic bone.

Vaginismus is a sexually related psychological disorder. The spasming of the muscles may be painful, interfering with penile penetration or the insertion of other objects such as a speculum or tampon. Sufferers of this disorder usually fear sexual intercourse and associate it with pain.

Treatment Options

Treatment for most vaginal disorders is aimed at maintaining proper bacterial balance and soothing your discomfort. Alternative methods can often help relieve symptoms or ease recovery. But if you have vaginal problems, especially if they are severe or chronic, it is important that you see a doctor for diagnosis and care.

Herbal Therapies

Incorporate fresh **garlic** *(Allium sativum)* into your diet; it has antibacterial, antifungal, and antiviral properties and may be effective in treating vaginitis, including vaginal yeast infections. You can also try a douche made with **goldenseal** *(Hydrastis canadensis)* tea.

If itching or minor irritation is a symptom of your vaginitis, bathe with an infusion of fresh chickweed *(Stellaria media)* for relief. (Pour 1 cup of boiling water on 1 to 2 tsp of the herb, steep for

Vaginal Problems

five minutes, and let cool.) To reduce inflammation associated with vulvitis and infectious discharge of bacterial vaginosis, an herbal douche may bring relief. To make, pour 1 cup of boiling water over 1 to 2 tsp of **calendula** (Calendula officinalis) and steep for 10 to 15 minutes; let cool before using the tea as a douche.

Homeopathy

The following remedies taken three or four times a day for one or two days may be used for minor vaginal problems. A smelly, yellow discharge with severe burning, swelling, and soreness may be treated with Kreosotum (12c); for itching and a white or yellow discharge, **Sepia** (12c) is recommended; **Pulsatilla** (12c) may aid in treating a thick, creamy yellow-green discharge. See a professional homeopathic practitioner if your condition does not clear up.

Many over-the-counter homeopathic mixtures to treat vaginal yeast infections are available under brand names at your local drugstore.

Lifestyle

If you have recurrent vaginal infections, discontinue the use of tampons for six months. In addition, avoid sexual intercourse while your symptoms of vaginal yeast infection or bacterial vaginosis are still apparent.

OF SPECIAL INTEREST

Products That Can Irritate

Many women may not be aware that their itching and burning may be caused by irritation from products such as soaps, bath oils and crystals, spermicides, swimming pool chlorine, feminine-hygiene sprays, perfumed douches or lubricants, latex products, scented or colored toilet paper, or perfumed pads and tampons. If your physician cannot detect the cause of your irritation, then an allergy or sensitivity to these commercial products is the likely culprit. Stop using suspect items. Try cool soaks in a tub and add Epsom salt if desired.

Wearing cotton panties and avoiding pantyhose and tight clothing will aid in keeping the vagina cool and dry, which may help prevent vulvitis and certain forms of vaginitis.

Nutrition and Diet

If you are susceptible to yeast infections, eating yogurt containing active cultures may help to maintain the natural bacterial flora of the vagina.

Women with recurrent yeast infections should be checked for diabetes. Too much sugar in the diet—whether refined or natural—creates an environment in the vagina that is conducive to the growth of yeast. By removing sugar from your diet, you are in essence starving the yeast.

Home Remedies

Incorporating *Lactobacillus acidophilus* into your diet may be helpful for treating vaginal yeast infections. A paste can be made from refrigerated capsules, available at health food and nutrition stores. Pour the *Lactobacillus acidophilus* powder into your palm and add water to create a pasty substance that may be introduced into the vagina using a vaginal applicator or your finger.

Regular sexual intercourse in postmenopausal women may help prevent dryness and thinning of the vaginal walls, which could increase the likelihood of vaginitis. The activity stimulates blood flow in the area, which keeps vaginal tissue supple.

Prevention

Maintaining good hygiene and using condoms may help prevent vaginitis. If you suspect a vaginal infection, do not douche for 24 hours before seeing your physician, as this may wash away secretions that aid in the diagnosis of your disorder.

A true case of vaginismus is caused by fear rather than by physical abnormality. The best prevention for this disorder is a healthy home environment where sexuality is not made to seem dirty but rather, when appropriate, is discussed in an open, honest, and factual manner. If you have suffered sexual abuse or trauma, you should seek professional help.

$\mathcal{V}$aricose Veins

Symptoms

- Prominent dark blue blood vessels, especially in the legs and feet.

- Aching, tender, heavy, or sore legs, often accompanied by swelling in the ankles or feet after standing for any length of time.

- Bulging, ropelike, bluish veins indicate superficial varicose veins.

- Aching and heaviness in a limb, sometimes with swelling, but without any prominent or visible blue vein, may signal a deep varicose vein.

- Discolored, peeling skin; skin ulcers; and constant rather than intermittent pain are signs of severe varicose veins.

Call Your Doctor If

- swelling becomes incapacitating, or the skin over your varicose veins becomes flaky, ulcerous, discolored, or prone to bleeding. You may want to have the veins removed to avoid potentially worse problems.

- you have red varicose veins. This may be a sign of phlebitis, a serious circulatory condition.

- you have continuing pain with no outward signs. Contact a doctor at once about the possibility of deep varicose veins.

- you cut a varicose vein. Control the resulting burst of blood *(see Essential First Aid, page 394)* and have the vein treated to prevent complications.

V aricose veins usually announce themselves as bulging, bluish cords running just beneath the surface of your skin. They can appear anywhere in the body but most often affect legs and feet, particularly in women. Visible swollen and twisted veins—sometimes surrounded by patches of flooded capillaries known as spider-burst veins—are considered superficial varicose veins. Although they can be painful and disfiguring, they are usually harmless. On rare occasions, an interior leg vein becomes varicose. Deep varicose veins are usually not visible, but they can cause swelling or aching throughout the leg.

Treatment Options

Aromatherapy
Oils of cypress and **German chamomile** *(Matricaria recutita)* may soothe swelling and inflammation and help relieve pain.

Chiropractic
To treat varicose veins, chiropractic medicine combines diet and lifestyle therapy with physical manipulation of the skeletal system. Manipulation to relieve strain on the pelvis, for example, is intended to improve the flow of blood and other fluids through the body.

Exercise
Aerobic exercise totaling 30 minutes a day several times a week will help you keep your weight down while toning and strengthening veins. You might start your morning with a brisk walk, for example, or finish your day with a swim or bike ride.

Herbal Therapies
Ginkgo *(Ginkgo biloba)*, **hawthorn** *(Crataegus laevigata)*, and bilberry *(Vaccinium myrtillus)* are all reported to strengthen blood vessels and improve peripheral circulation. Tinctures or topical ointments of horse chestnut *(Aesculus hippocastanum)* and butcher's-broom *(Ruscus aculeatus)* are also recommended for toning veins while reducing inflammation; butcher's-broom can also be prepared as tea. For skin irritation associated with varicose veins, try a lotion made of distilled witch hazel *(Hamamelis virginiana)*.

Varicose Veins

Homeopathy

For immediate relief from specific symptoms, you can try over-the-counter homeopathic remedies: *Hamamelis,* or witch hazel, cream in a 6x to 15c solution applied to an area that is bluish and perhaps bruised may relieve soreness. *Hamamelis* 6x to 15c can also be taken internally as directed on the label for general relief. **Belladonna,** 12x or 12c potency four times a day, is recommended for red, hot, swollen, and tender varicose veins.

Hydrotherapy

Sponge or spray legs with cold water to relieve aches and pain from superficial varicose veins. Hot and cold baths may slow the progression of varicose veins on the feet and ankles: Dip your feet in warm water for one to two minutes, then cold water for half a minute, alternating this procedure for 15 minutes.

Massage

Regular massage can markedly alleviate discomfort associated with varicose veins. A massage therapist starts at the feet and massages your legs up to the hips and along the lymphatic system to mobilize congested body tissues. Use light pressure when massaging deep or severe varicose veins.

Nutrition and Diet

Extra body fat increases water retention and puts pressure on the legs and abdomen, aggravating varicosity. To decrease body fat, eat foods that are low in fat, sugar, and salt, and high in fiber. To promote a healthy flow of nutrients and waste through the body, make fruits, vegetables, and whole grains the mainstays of your diet, and drink plenty of fluids, especially spring water.

Home Remedies

To ease painful swelling and inflammation associated with varicose veins in your legs, rest frequently, wear support stockings, and take one or two aspirin or ibuprofen tablets daily until the condition clears. Cross your legs at the ankles rather than the knees for better circulation. Better yet, take a break and put your feet up; periods of rest with your feet

a few inches above your heart level help pooled blood drain from your legs. To further improve circulation, women should wear loose clothing and avoid high heels in favor of flat shoes.

Prevention

- If your daily routine requires you to be on your feet constantly, stretch and exercise your legs as often as possible to increase circulation and reduce pressure buildup.
- If you smoke, quit. Studies show that smoking may contribute to elevated blood pressure, which in turn can aggravate varicosity.
- If you're pregnant, be sure to sleep on your left or right side rather than on your back to minimize pressure from the uterus on the veins in your pelvic area. This position will also improve blood flow to the fetus. ■

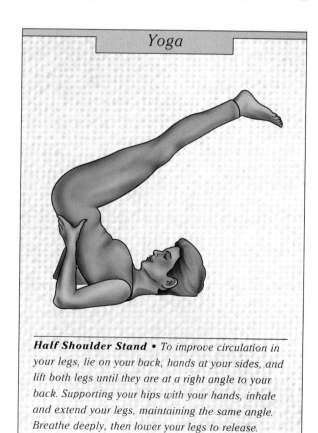

Yoga

Half Shoulder Stand • *To improve circulation in your legs, lie on your back, hands at your sides, and lift both legs until they are at a right angle to your back. Supporting your hips with your hands, inhale and extend your legs, maintaining the same angle. Breathe deeply, then lower your legs to release.*

Warts

Symptoms

- Common warts are small, hard, rough lumps that are round and elevated; they usually appear on hands and fingers and may be flesh colored, white, or pink, and either smooth or granulated.

- Digitate warts are horny and fingerlike, with pea-shaped bases; they appear on the scalp or near the hairline.

- Filiform warts are thin and threadlike; they commonly appear on the face and neck.

- Flat warts appear in groups of up to several hundred, usually on the face, neck, chest, knees, hands, wrists, or forearms; they are slightly raised and have smooth, flat or rounded tops.

- Genital warts are painless flesh-colored or grayish white growths on the vulva, anus, or penis that may develop a cauliflower-like appearance.

- Periungual warts are rough, irregular, and elevated; they appear at the edges of fingernails and toenails and may extend under the nails, causing pain.

- Plantar warts are small, bumpy growths on the soles of the feet, one-quarter inch to two inches in diameter, sometimes with tiny black dots on the surface.

Call Your Doctor If

- over-the-counter remedies or alternative therapies don't work.

- you are a woman and develop genital warts, which in rare cases may indicate cervical cancer.

- you are older than 45 and discover what looks like a wart; it may instead be a symptom of a more serious skin condition, such as skin cancer.

- you notice a change in a wart's color or size; this could indicate skin cancer.

Warts are among the most common dermatological complaints. A certain percentage of them may be caused by the human papilloma virus (HPV), which enters the skin through a cut or scratch and causes cells to multiply rapidly. Usually, warts spread through direct contact, but it is possible to pick up the virus in moist environments, such as showers and locker rooms. You can spread them to other parts of your body by touching them or shaving around infected areas. Children and young adults are more prone to getting warts because their defense mechanisms may not be fully developed, but it is possible to get a wart at any age.

Treatment Options

The best treatment for warts is often no treatment at all; most people develop an immune response that causes warts to go away by themselves. However, if your wart doesn't disappear, or if it's unsightly or uncomfortable, you can try the alternative treatments or home remedies listed here. Over-the-counter medications work by softening abnormal skin cells and dissolving them; your doctor can also remove warts surgically or by freezing or burning them off. Seek your doctor's care for genital warts.

Chinese Medicine
A doctor of Chinese medicine may place a slice of *ginger (Zingiber officinale)* root on top of the wart and cover it with smoldering **mugwort leaf** *(Artemisia argyi)*. The burning herb enables the ginger to release its antiviral constituents. This process is called indirect moxibustion.

Herbal Therapies
Several herbs contain chemicals thought to fight viruses and help treat skin conditions. Herbalists recommend applying the sticky juices of ***dandelion** (Taraxacum officinale),* milkweed *(Asclepias syriaca),* and celandine *(Chelidonium majus).* An ointment of thuja *(Thuja occidentalis)* applied four or five times a day may also help.

Whichever herbal remedy you try, first protect the surrounding skin with petroleum jelly and then cover the treated wart with a clean bandage. Repeat daily until the wart is gone.

Homeopathy

Homeopathic medicines for warts include *Causticum, Nitric acid,* and *Antimonium crudum.*

Mind/Body Medicine

Using guided imagery *(pages 133-134)* to relax may help speed the immune system's response to warts. Breathe deeply as you imagine the wart dissolving. Do this for five minutes, twice a day; some warts will disappear after one to two months.

Nutrition and Diet

Poor diet can be a factor in persistent or recurring warts. Foods high in *vitamin A*—eggs, cold-water fish, onions, garlic, and dark green and yellow vegetables—will help sustain your immune system, as will yogurt and other fermented-milk products. You can also consult a nutritional therapist about the potential benefits of supplemental *vitamins A, B complex, C,* and *E;* L-cysteine; and *zinc.*

Home Remedies

There are countless folk cures for warts. One that may have some validity is rubbing the wart with a slice of raw potato or the inner side of a banana skin; both contain chemicals that may dissolve the wart. You might also try any of the following applications:

- *Vitamins A* and *E,* which are generally good for skin conditions.
- A paste of crushed *vitamin C* tablets and water.
- Over-the-counter medicines or a paste of crushed aspirin; both contain wart-dissolving salicylic acid.
- *Aloe (Aloe barbadensis), dandelion,* or milkweed juices.
- Cotton soaked in fresh pineapple juice, which contains a dissolving enzyme.

Prevention

Practice good hygiene, and eat balanced meals high in *vitamins A, C,* and *E* to boost your immune system. Avoid stress, which can compromise your immunity, and learn to relax. ■

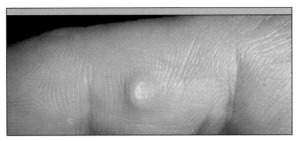

Common Wart • *Typically found on the hands and feet either singly or in clusters, common warts vary in size but average a quarter inch in diameter. The flesh-colored bumps tend to be circular and feel hard and rough to the touch. They pose no health risks and will eventually disappear, but they can also be removed with over-the-counter medications.*

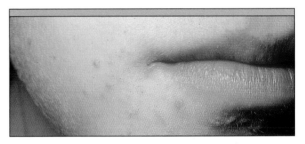

Flat Warts • *Children and young adults are those most likely to develop flat warts, which often occur in clusters of 10 to 30. The warts are slightly raised, smooth, and tan or flesh colored; they are often barely visible. Flat warts typically appear on the neck, face, wrists, backs of the hands, and knees. In children, they most often appear on the face.*

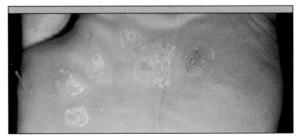

Plantar Warts • *Caused by the common wart virus, plantar warts appear on the sole of the foot, usually at pressure points such as the heel. They begin as small, painful warts that then become flattened and pressed into the skin. The soft core of the wart is surrounded by a hard, calluslike ring that may be peppered with tiny blood clots that appear as black dots.*

$\mathcal{Y}$east Infections

Symptoms

- In women, vaginal itching and irritation; redness and swelling of the vulva; unusually thick, white discharge; and pain during intercourse. These are signs of a vaginal yeast infection, also known as moniliasis.

- In men, red patches and blisters at the end of the penis and around the foreskin, possibly with severe itching and pain. These are symptoms of balanitis.

- Painless white patches in your mouth or throat that may come off when you eat or brush your teeth; this indicates oral thrush, which is most common in infants, the elderly, and AIDS patients.

- White patches in the mouth and throat, sometimes associated with painful swallowing; these are symptomatic of esophageal thrush, a potential complication of AIDS.

- Peeling skin on the hands, especially between the fingers; and swollen nail folds above the cuticle, possibly painful, red, and containing pus.

- Itchy or burning shiny pink rash with a scaly or blistered edge in the folds of the skin. This indicates intertrigo.

Call Your Doctor If

- you have any of the symptoms for the first time; you will need a professional evaluation before beginning treatment.

- the infection does not respond to treatment or recurs; you may have a more serious disorder such as diabetes or an HIV infection.

$\mathcal{Y}$east, or fungal, infection—sometimes called candidiasis—takes many forms. Yeast infections often develop where a moist environment encourages fungal growth, especially on the webs of fingers and toes, nails, genitals, and folds of skin. Oral thrush is a painless, often recurrent infection of the mouth and throat; it is common in babies, young children, and the elderly, but can affect all ages. Moniliasis is a painful vaginal yeast infection experienced by many women, most commonly during pregnancy or treatment with antibiotics. (See Vaginal Problems, pages 364-365.) Balanitis is a less common but equally irritating infection of the penis. Systemic yeast infections can occur in cases of diabetes, AIDS, and other ailments or drug treatments that suppress the immune system.

What Makes You Susceptible

Candida albicans is a fungal organism, or yeast, that thrives in your mouth, gastrointestinal tract, and skin; your body produces bacterial flora that keeps it in check. When fungal growth exceeds the body's ability to control it, yeast infection develops. This can happen when you are weakened by illness or upset by stress. Modern antibiotics that treat many ailments can actually kill the bacteria that otherwise control fungal outbreaks.

Yeast infections are common among dishwashers and people whose hands are often in water, in children who suck their thumbs or fingers, and in people whose clothing retains body moisture. Diabetics are especially prone to yeast infections because they have high levels of sugar in their blood and urine and a low resistance to infection—conditions that encourage yeast growth.

Treatment Options

Treatment depends on the specific kind of infection you have but should focus on counteracting the growth of the yeast organism. For vaginal yeast infections, an over-the-counter intravaginal cream containing miconazole or clotrimazole usually works well; an oral form is now also available. If over-the-counter medications are not effective, you may need to see a physician, who can prescribe a stronger medication.

Yeast Infections

Chronic Yeast Infection

Although the diagnosis is not universally accepted, some doctors recognize a condition called chronic candidiasis, or chronic yeast infection, that may affect the gastrointestinal, nervous, endocrine, and immune systems. Treatment focuses on eliminating predisposing factors, such as prescription or over-the-counter drugs, foods with high refined-sugar or yeast content, high-carbohydrate vegetables, and milk products. Your doctor may also test you for underlying conditions, such as diabetes or thyroid problems.

*An herbal remedy for chronic yeast infection is tea brewed from 2 to 3 tsp dried root of barberry (Berberis vulgaris) or **goldenseal** (Hydrastis canadensis) in a cup of boiling water, taken three times a day. With your doctor's approval, you may want to try taking daily supplements of 45 mg **iron**, 45 mg **zinc**, and 200 mcg **selenium** (avoid higher doses of selenium).*

Alternative remedies may also be effective. Some are targeted at strengthening the immune system so that your body will be better able to resist yeast infections; others provide symptom relief or aim to treat specific yeast infections and prevent them from recurring.

Ayurvedic Medicine

For vaginal yeast infections, tablets of the combination formula *Septilin* are sometimes given. Another Ayurvedic remedy is a vaginal douche made from an infusion of mugwort. Consult a qualified practitioner of Ayurvedic medicine to get specific information on these and other forms of Ayurvedic treatment.

Chinese Medicine

There are a variety of acupuncture and Chinese herbal treatments for yeast infections. Consult a practitioner of Chinese medicine for a specific diagnosis and treatment regimen.

Herbal Therapies

For healing yeast infections on your skin, apply full-strength **tea tree** (*Melaleuca* spp.) **oil** two to three times daily; a slight burning sensation is normal, but discontinue if the treatment is painful. An over-the-counter salve containing **calendula** (*Calendula officinalis*) is good for rashes in children over two years of age.

For infections caused by a fungus, try **pau d'arco** (*Tabebuia impetiginosa*). In tincture form, take 15 drops two times a day for a month or two; as a tea, drink 2 cups a day for two to three months. **Garlic** (*Allium sativum*) can also help fight yeast infections; try two capsules or pills two times a day for two or three months. These remedies may be helpful for chronic infection.

Homeopathy

Numerous homeopathic remedies are used to treat yeast infections; a licensed homeopathic physician will diagnose your condition and can then recommend the best remedies and course of treatment to match your symptoms.

Hydrotherapy

Alternating hot and cold sitz baths may provide symptom relief and help speed recovery from a vaginal yeast infection. To prepare a sitz bath, place a towel in the bottom of a washtub or bathtub, and fill the tub so that the water comes up to about ½ inch above your navel. For these baths, fill one tub with hot water and another with cold; sit in the hot water for about three minutes, then the cold water for about 30 seconds. Do this three times, making sure to end with the cold and dry yourself thoroughly after the treatment.

Prevention

- If work keeps your hands in water for long periods, wear rubber gloves. When you're done, wash your hands and apply a mild prescription or over-the-counter antifungal cream.
- Wear cotton or silk underclothes, which, unlike nylon and other synthetics, allow excess moisture to evaporate. Wash and dry your underclothes thoroughly; change them often. ■

Essential First Aid

F irst aid stabilizes an injured person's condition until trained emergency personnel can take over. In many instances, alternative therapies can augment first aid or can help the victim recover from injury. But in no circumstance should alternative therapies take the place of these critical first-aid steps.

ALTERNATIVE THERAPIES

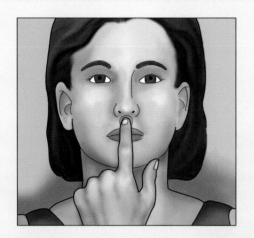

ACUPRESSURE

The acupressure point Governing Vessel 26, also called the first-aid revival point, may help stimulate the body's recovery from trauma or injury. Press this point, which is two-thirds of the way up from the upper lip to the nose, with your index finger for five to 15 seconds. Repeat as needed for up to one hour.

FLOWER REMEDIES

Bach flower remedy practitioners believe that the calming effects of **Rescue Remedy** can help speed a victim's recovery from trauma. Place 3 to 4 drops of Rescue Remedy under the conscious victim's tongue. If the victim is unconscious, rub a few drops onto the victim's lips, behind the ears, or on the wrists. Repeat every 10 to 15 minutes until the victim recovers.

WHAT TO DO IN AN EMERGENCY

1 **Call 911 or your emergency number, or tell someone nearby to do so.**

2 **Check the victim's ABCs** *(right).*

3 **Stop any severe bleeding** *(page 374).*

4 **Prevent shock** *(page 378).*

5 **Try to determine what happened.** Look around the scene for any clues, such as a Medic Alert tag on the victim or an open container of a poisonous chemical.

THE RECOVERY POSITION

Placing an unconscious victim who is breathing in the recovery position will keep the airway open. Support the victim's head and roll him onto his stomach. Bend the victim's arm and knee that are closest to you. Carefully tilt back the head so the airway remains open.

■ **Caution:** Do not place the victim in this position if you suspect a neck or back injury.

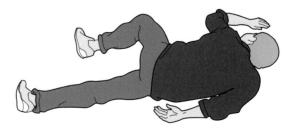

Emergency Basics

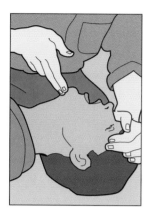

A irway

Open the victim's airway. Gently tilt back the victim's head and lift the chin.

■ **Caution:** If you suspect a head, neck, or back injury, just lift the chin.

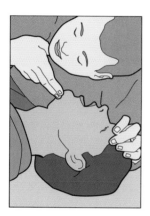

B reathing

Look, listen, and feel for breathing. Look for the victim's chest to rise. Put your ear to the victim's mouth and listen and feel for exhaled air; chest movement alone might not indicate breathing.

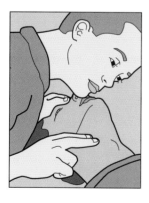

C irculation

Check for a pulse. Gently press two fingers, not your thumb, in the depression on the side of the victim's neck, next to the Adam's apple, and feel for a pulse.

If the victim is not breathing or does not have a pulse or heartbeat, call 911 or your emergency number now, or tell someone nearby to do so. Begin to give cardiopulmonary resuscitation *(right)* only if you have been trained in the procedure.

CARDIOPULMONARY RESUSCITATION

Treatment for cardiac or respiratory arrest is called cardiopulmonary resuscitation (CPR). The goals of CPR are to open the victim's airway, reestablish breathing, and reestablish circulation. Give CPR only if you have been trained in the procedure; call your local hospital or American Red Cross chapter to enroll in a CPR training course. Begin to give CPR after you are sure that the victim is unconscious, is not breathing, or does not have a pulse. To be sure, check the victim's ABCs *(left)*.

HEAD, NECK, AND BACK INJURIES

1   If you suspect a head, neck, or back injury, do not move the injured person unless it is absolutely necessary.

2   Check the victim's ABCs *(left)*. If you need to place the victim on his back, support his head, neck, and back together and carefully roll him onto his back. It is best to have someone else help you do this.

3   If the victim begins to choke or vomit or becomes unconscious, support his head, neck, and back together and carefully roll him onto his side. It is best to have someone else help you do this.

■ **Caution:** Make sure that the victim's head and neck move with his body.

CONTINUED

Bleeding

IMPORTANT

■ If the bleeding is severe, call 911 or your emergency number.

1 **Lay the victim flat on his back and check the victim's ABCs** *(page 373).* Raise the victim's feet several inches. If possible, elevate the wound above heart level.

2 **Remove any visible objects from the wound.**

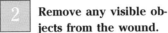

■ **Caution:** Do not remove any object stuck in the wound, probe it, or disturb it in any way.

Alternative aid. The Chinese formula *Yun Nan Bai Yao* may help stop the bleeding. Take two capsules, or sprinkle the powder on the wound.

3 **Apply direct pressure to the wound with a clean cloth or your hand.** Hold the edges of flesh together. If blood seeps through the cloth, put another cloth on top and keep pressing. You may need to apply firmer pressure if blood continues to seep through. For an embedded object, put pressure around the wound, not on the object.

4 **If the bleeding does not stop, apply pressure to the arterial pressure point that is closest to the wound, between it and the heart** *(left).* Keep direct pressure on the wound as you press the arterial point with your fingers held flat. Do not apply pressure to arteries leading to the head or neck unless bright red blood is spurting from an injured neck artery.

5 **When the bleeding stops, apply a bandage.** Do not remove any cloths placed on the wound to help stop the bleeding; wrap a clean cloth over the wound and tie it in place. If there is an object embedded in the wound, bandage around it to support it.

Alternative aid. To help prevent the victim from going into shock, homeopaths suggest giving the victim one **Arnica** (12x or 30c) tablet every 15 minutes until the victim's condition stabilizes.

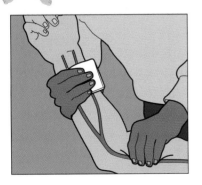

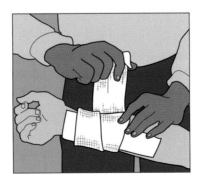

ALTERNATIVE AID FOR RECOVERY

HERBAL THERAPY
The herb **calendula** (*Calendula officinalis*) may help prevent the wound from becoming infected. Mix 1 tsp calendula tincture with ¼ cup water and apply the mixture to the cloth covering the wound.

HOMEOPATHY
Homeopathic practitioners recommend the following remedies: If the wound gets infected, try **Hepar sulphuris** (12x), *Pyrogenium* (12x), or **Silica** (12x); for pain, try *Staphysagria* (12x) or **Arnica** (12x); and for inflammation, try *Echinacea* (12x).

Choking

IMPORTANT

- If you suspect that an object is caught in a victim's throat and she cannot cough, breathe, speak, or cry, call 911 or your emergency number, or tell someone nearby to do so. Begin first-aid treatment for choking *(below)*. If you are the victim, see the box on page 376.

- If you suspect that an object is caught in a victim's throat but she is able to cough, breathe, speak, or cry, do not intervene. But be prepared to act if the situation worsens.

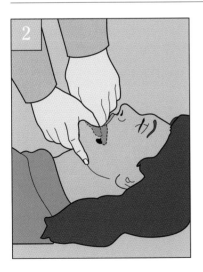

Give abdominal thrusts (the Heimlich maneuver). Place your arms around the victim's waist. Make a fist with one hand and place it in the middle of the victim's abdomen, just above the navel and below the ribs. Hold your fist with your other hand. Give quick, repeated thrusts, pushing inward and upward. Continue giving abdominal thrusts until the object is dis-lodged or until the victim loses consciousness.

- **Caution:** Do not try to retrieve an object lodged in the throat. This might force the object farther down the airway. If the victim is pregnant or obese, place your fist on the middle of the victim's breastbone; do not place your hands on the ribs or on the lower edge of the breastbone.

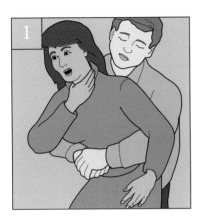

If the victim loses consciousness, lay her flat on her back. Sweep the victim's mouth. To sweep the mouth, hold the victim's tongue and lift the chin. Slide your index finger down the inside of the cheek and sweep out any loose objects. Then gently tilt back the victim's head and lift the chin to open the victim's airway.

- **Caution:** Do not try to retrieve an object lodged in the victim's throat.

3 **Look, listen, and feel for breathing**. Be sure to put your ear to the victim's mouth; chest movement alone might not mean breathing. If the object is dislodged and the victim is breathing, place her in the recovery position *(page 372)*.

ALTERNATIVE AID

Once the object is dislodged, and if the victim is breathing, homeopaths suggest crushing five or six ***Arnica*** (12x or 12c) tablets and placing them on the victim's tongue or gums; let them dissolve. This may help prevent the victim from going into shock as well as relieve any pain that may result from the abdominal thrusts. Pressing on the acupressure first-aid revival point *(page 372)* or administering ***Rescue Remedy*** *(page 372)* may also be helpful.

Choking

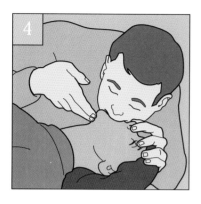

Breathe into the victim's mouth. Pinch the victim's nose shut and seal your lips tightly around the mouth. Give two slow breaths; remove your mouth between breaths. Watch for the victim's chest to rise with each breath; let the chest fall before you give the next breath. If the victim's chest does not rise with each breath, gently tilt the head farther back and try again to give two slow breaths.

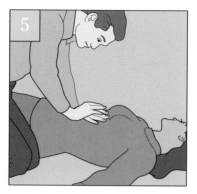

If the victim's chest still does not rise, give five abdominal thrusts. Position the heel of one of your hands against the middle of the victim's abdomen, just above the navel and below the ribs. Place your other hand on top of the first. Give quick thrusts, pressing your hands inward and upward.

■ **Caution:** Do not press to either side as you thrust.

6 **Sweep the victim's mouth, make sure the airway is open, and breathe twice again into the victim's mouth.**

7 **If the victim's chest still does not rise, give abdominal thrusts, sweep the mouth, and give breaths.** Give five abdominal thrusts. Sweep the victim's mouth and give two slow breaths. Repeat this sequence of abdominal thrusts, sweeps of the mouth, and slow breaths until the object is dislodged or until medical help arrives.

8 **If the object is dislodged but the victim is not breathing, call 911 or your** emergency number now. Begin to give CPR if you have been trained in the procedure.

SELF-HELP

Give yourself abdominal thrusts until the object is dislodged. Make a fist with one hand and place it in the middle of your abdomen, just above the navel and below the ribs. Hold your fist with your other hand, keeping your elbows out; bend over the back of a chair (below), countertop, or some other firm, hard object and press your fist with a quick, upward thrust into your abdomen.

■ **Caution:** If you feel or see an object lodged in your throat, do not try to retrieve it, as this might force the object farther down your airway.

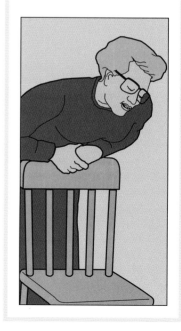

Poisoning

1 **Check the victim's ABCs *(page 373)*. Try to identify the poison**. Ask the victim what he swallowed or inhaled. Otherwise, look around for any open or nearby containers of chemicals or for any plants or household items that the victim may have swallowed; sniff the air for unusual odors.

2 **Call your local poison control center or 911.** Tell emergency personnel what chemical, plant, or household item the victim swallowed. Wait for further instructions.

3 **Follow the instructions given by the poison control center or by 911 personnel.** Depending on the poison, you may be instructed to give milk or water to drink, to give activated charcoal, or to induce vomiting by giving the victim syrup of ipecac. Save any vomit for medical personnel.

■ **Caution:** Do not try to induce vomiting unless told to do so; do not induce vomiting if it has been more than one hour since the victim ingested the poison. Do not give the victim anything to eat or drink unless told to do so. Do not rely on any instructions for counteracting the poison given on the container label.

4 **Place an unconscious victim in the recovery position** *(page 372)*.

Alternative aid. Pressing on the acupressure point Stomach 36 *(page 30)* may alleviate the nausea that accompanies poisoning.

ALTERNATIVE AID FOR RECOVERY

HERBAL THERAPY

Milk thistle *(Silybum marianum)* may help the body excrete poisons; take 30 drops of milk thistle tincture three to four times a day.

HOMEOPATHY

For persistent nausea, homeopaths suggest taking one ***Nux vomica*** (12x) tablet every 15 minutes, or two ***Ipecac*** (12x) tablets every four hours, until nausea subsides.

POISONOUS HOUSEHOLD ITEMS

In addition to the list of poisonous household items at right, many cleansers, detergents, deodorizers, disinfectants, and solvents are poisonous. Drugs, medications, herbal remedies, and vitamins, whether prescription or over the counter, may be poisonous if mixed together, mixed with alcohol, or taken in large quantities. Call your local poison control center about specific items.

POISONOUS PLANTS

There are hundreds of poisonous plants in the United States. Many plant parts, including seeds, berries, nuts, and bulbs, are potentially poisonous. If you have a question about a plant, call your local poison control center. Some of the most poisonous plants are listed at right.

■ Alcohol
■ Antifreeze
■ Fuels
■ Herbicides
■ Iron pills
■ Lye
■ Mothballs
■ Paints, polishes
■ Pesticides
■ Tobacco products
■ Turpentine
■ Windshield fluid
■ Castor bean
■ Dieffenbachia
■ Foxglove
■ Jimson weed
■ Oleander
■ Philodendron
■ Poison hemlock
■ Pokeweed
■ Pothos
■ Water hemlock

CONTINUED

Shock

1 **Check the victim's ABCs *(page 373)*. Position the victim so he is comfortable**. Unless the victim is more comfortable sitting up, lay him on his back with his head lower than the rest of his body. If you do not suspect any broken leg bones, elevate the legs eight to 12 inches. Recheck the victim's airway.

3 **Make the victim warm and comfortable.** Loosen any tight clothing and cover the victim with a blanket or additional clothing. Do not use an electric blanket or any other form of direct heat. If the victim is lying down, do not place a pillow under his head, as this might cause the airway to become blocked.

5 **If medical help is more than an hour away, give the conscious victim a clean cloth soaked in water to suck on.**

Alternative aid. Press the acupressure first-aid revival point *(page 372)* and give **Rescue Remedy** *(page 372).*

2 **Try to determine the cause of shock and perform first aid for the appropriate emergency.**

Alternative aid. To help treat shock, homeopaths recommend crushing five or six **Arnica** (12x or 12c) tablets into a powder and placing it onto the victim's tongue or gums to dissolve.

4 **Keep the airway open.** If the victim begins to choke or vomit, turn his head to one side so that the vomit will not block his airway.

ALTERNATIVE AID FOR RECOVERY

AROMATHERAPY
Inhaling the essential oil of **peppermint** *(Mentha piperita)* may help restore circulation and neural activity.

HERBAL THERAPIES
Herbal teas prepared with **sage** *(Salvia officinalis)* or **skullcap** *(Scutellaria lateriflora)* may help calm the nervous system, thus alleviating the symptoms of shock.

ANAPHYLACTIC SHOCK

IMPORTANT!

If you suspect a severe allergic reaction, the victim may be in anaphylactic shock.

SYMPTOMS:
■ Hives
■ Itching
■ Flushed face; warm skin
■ Dizziness
■ Swollen face or tongue
■ Nausea or vomiting
■ Abdominal cramps
■ Wheezing
■ Difficulty breathing
■ Unconsciousness

In addition to treating the victim as you would for shock, perform these steps:

1 Try to keep the victim calm.

2 Determine if the victim was stung by an insect. If so, carefully scrape the stinger off the victim's skin.
■ **Caution:** Do not use tweezers; this may push more venom into the skin.

3 Administer medicine. Some people are prone to anaphylactic shock and may have emergency supplies on hand. If this is the case, help the victim with his medicine; follow the instructions on the medication.

Alternative aid. The homeopathic remedy **Apis** (12x), one tablet given every few minutes until emergency medical treatment is available, may help open a swollen airway.

Conventional Medicine Chest

It is helpful to have some medications for common ailments on hand in your home so that when the occasional cold or flu strikes you'll be prepared. All of the items below are available over the counter (OTC) at most drugstores and supermarkets. When it comes to brand names among OTC classes, most preparations have the same active ingredients and differ only in packaging. Keep in mind that OTC products are still drugs and can have potentially dangerous side effects if misused.

All of these substances should be stored away from light, humidity, and the reach of children. Check expiration dates on all your medications periodically; many of these preparations have a limited shelf life. Members of your family may have other, specific needs, such as epinephrine for bee allergies. These medications should also be included in your home medicine chest.

MEDICATIONS

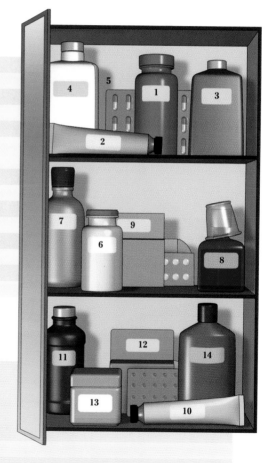

1 **Antacid:** indigestion.
2 **Antibiotic cream:** cuts, scratches.
3 **Antidiarrheal medication**
4 **Antifungal medication:** athlete's foot or jock itch.
5 **Antihistamine capsules:** allergies.
6 **Aspirin** or **acetaminophen:** pain such as headaches or muscle cramps.
7 **Calamine lotion:** itching of skin rashes and insect bites.
8 **Cough/cold/flu medicine**
9 **Dimenhydrinate tablets:** motion sickness.
10 **Hydrocortisone cream:** skin rashes and insect bites.
11 **Hydrogen peroxide:** antiseptic for cuts and scratches.
12 **Laxative:** constipation.
13 **Petroleum jelly:** chafing.
14 **Sunscreen**

FIRST AID

In addition to your home pharmacy, you should also keep a supply of bandages and first-aid materials on hand for emergencies. These items should be stored in clean, airtight containers.

- Adhesive bandages
- Adhesive tape
- Antiseptic wipes
- Butterfly bandages
- Cold packs (disposable)
- Cotton, both roll and balls
- Cotton-tipped swabs
- Elastic bandage

- First-aid manual
- Gauze bandages
- Hand wipes (disposable)
- Insect repellent
- Latex gloves
- Safety pins
- Scissors
- Sling (triangular bandage)

- Soap
- Sterile nonstick dressings
- Thermometer
- Tissues
- Tongue depressors
- Tweezers

CONTINUED

Alternative Medicine Chest

*N*atural preparations can be used for many common ailments. These herbs, oils, and homeopathic medications can usually be found at health food stores or specialized pharmacies. Oils and homeopathic pharmaceuticals are commonly prepackaged, but herbs may be purchased loose and combined at home to create specific preparations. Don't forget that herbs, like OTC drugs, are potent substances, to be used with care. See pages 107-116 and pages 74-103 for more information on most of the homeopathic remedies and herbs listed here.

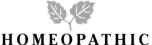

HOMEOPATHIC

1 **Aconite:** colds, croup, fever, shock.
2 **Apis:** bites and stings, hives.
3 **Arnica:** bruises, dislocated joints, shock.
4 **Arsenicum album:** colds, flu, food poisoning.
5 **Belladonna:** earache, fever, headache, infection, heatstroke.
6 **Bryonia:** back pain, fever, flu, headache.
7 **Hepar sulphuris:** abscesses, boils, croup, sore throat.
8 **Hypericum:** injury to nerves, insect bites.
9 **Nux vomica:** nausea, poisoning, diarrhea, migraine headache.
10 **Pulsatilla:** childhood infections, colds, fever, sinus problems.
11 **Rhus toxicodendron:** back pain, chickenpox, flu, sprains, strains.

HERBAL

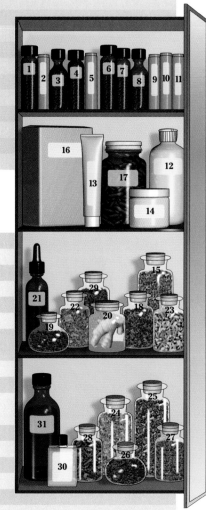

12 **Aloe** gel, applied externally, for bee stings, sunburn.
13 **Calendula** cream for relief of skin irritation and rashes.
14 **Calendula** ointment for cuts and bites but not puncture wounds.
15 **Catnip** hot tea to relieve indigestion.
16 **Chamomile** tea for indigestion.
17 **Dandelion** root decoction as a secretory laxative.
18 **Eyebright, peppermint,** and **yarrow** hot infusion of equal parts three times a day to relieve sinus pain.
19 **Flaxseed** *(Linum usitatissimum)* as a bulk laxative.
20 **Ginger** root hot infusion as needed to relieve nausea.
21 **Goldenseal** and **echinacea** tincture or glycerite formula for sore throat, cold, and flu relief.
22 **Horehound** *(Marrubium vulgare)* hot infusion as needed for coughs.
23 **Marsh mallow** cold infusion for bladder infections.
24 **Mullein** hot infusion three times daily for coughs; good for children.
25 **Nettle** infusion three times daily for hay fever.
26 **Peppermint** tea or infusion for indigestion, diarrhea, migraine.
27 **Psyllium** as a bulk laxative.
28 **Sage** gargle infusion for sore throat and congested sinuses.
29 **Skullcap** *(Scutellaria lateriflora),* **chamomile,** and **spearmint** infusion of equal parts for insomnia and nervousness.
30 **Tea tree oil** used externally for athlete's foot.
31 **Witch hazel** *(Hamamelis virginiana)* distilled, used externally for relief of itching and hemorrhoids.

Glossary

This glossary gives definitions of terms related to the alternative therapies listed in the A-Z Guide to Alternative Therapies. It also describes other therapies and remedies that are not included elsewhere in the book but that you may encounter if you pursue an interest in alternative medicine. Some of these therapies were not included in the main part of the book because they are controversial or have not proved to be beneficial; they are described here so that you can make yourself better aware of their pros and cons.

Adjustment: in chiropractic, a small controlled thrust that moves a joint slightly beyond its normal range of motion.

Allopathy: the treatment of disease by creating conditions that are opposite or hostile to the conditions resulting from the disease itself; from Greek roots meaning "other" and "disease." Drugs and surgery are allopathic treatments, for example. The term is sometimes used to refer to conventional Western medicine in general to contrast it with alternative therapies, particularly homeopathy, which is based on a philosophy of like curing like.

Amino acids: the chemical building blocks of proteins, which in turn are the primary constituents of the body's tissues and also control many of its processes. Amino acids that are not manufactured by the body are called essential amino acids and are obtained through diet or by taking supplements. Generally, supplementation is not necessary except for vegan vegetarians (those who eat no animal products), people on crash diets, or others who don't receive adequate protein in their diet. However, poorly nourished people also are more likely to experience adverse side effects from taking these supplements. Some supplements should not be taken by people with certain health problems: Check labels carefully.

Applied kinesiology: a diagnostic technique and therapy developed in the 1960s by a chiropractor named George Goodheart. Applied kinesiology posits that organ or gland dysfunctions show up as weaknesses in certain muscles. Using gentle pressure, applied kinesiologists test muscle strength to identify health problems and nutritional deficiencies. Applied kinesiology maintains that good health depends on three equally important elements: good nutrition, a positive mental outlook, and structural integrity, which refers to the relationship of the bones, mus-cles, and organs to one another. After diagnosis, treatment may involve exercises to strengthen a muscle, hands-on manipulation of the muscles and bones, and vitamin or mineral supplements. Practitioners are trained, licensed, and certified through the International College of Applied Kinesiology in Shawnee Mission, Kansas.

Biofield: an energy field that suffuses living bodies and extends several inches beyond the body. This concept is employed in therapies such as healing touch, medical qigong, therapeutic touch, and Reiki. In these therapies, the biofield from a practitioner's hands is joined to the recipient's biofield in order to treat an illness or to promote health. There is no consensus on what biofield is; some say it is spiritual energy, others say it is an electromagnetic field.

Blue-green algae: a type of algae that grows on some lakes and is cultivated commercially in Mexico, Japan, Thailand, and the United States as a nutritional supplement. Spirulina, one type of blue-green algae, is freeze-dried into powder or tablet form and sold and promoted as an energy booster, source of protein, appetite suppressant, and blood sugar stabilizer. According to the Food and Drug Administration, spirulina's appetite-reduction claims are unsubstantiated. Critics say that all the health claims are unfounded; they also note that many commercially prepared batches of spirulina have been seized because of contamination with toxins that can cause gastrointestinal distress and fatigue.

Chakras: in yoga, the seven vital energy centers of the body. The chakras extend from the base of the spine to the crown of the head. They are located in the rectal area, near the genitals, behind the navel, at the heart, at the neck, between the eyebrows, and on the crown of the head. According to yogic tradition, each chakra corresponds to certain colors, emotions, organs, nerve networks, and ruling deities.

Chelation therapy: a controversial treatment, used for atherosclerosis, angina, and Alzheimer's disease, that involves injecting the chemical EDTA into the bloodstream. EDTA—which stands for ethylenediaminetetraacetic acid, an amino acid—is FDA approved only for removing lead and other heavy metals from the bloodstream. But one theory holds that chelation removes the calcium in arterial plaque; another suggests that EDTA works as an antioxidant. Proponents say that chelation also reverses gangrene, relieves the pain associated with lupus and arthritis, and reverses memory loss. Many physicians have withheld judgment pending studies to determine the safety of chelation therapy. Potential side effects include kidney damage. Treatment typically requires from 10 to 40 sessions and may cost thousands of dollars. The American Board of Chelation Therapy in Chicago provides a list of practitioners certified in chelation therapy.

Chi: the Chinese concept of an invisible life force or energy that animates the universe and individuals alike. In humans, chi (sometimes spelled "qi") is said to flow through the body along an invisible network of branching channels called meridians. According to traditional Chinese medicine, illness occurs when chi is disrupted or blocked in some part of the body. Acupuncture and acupressure are two methods used to unblock chi.

Coenzyme Q10 (CoQ10): a cellular constituent involved in energy production. CoQ10 levels decrease as a person ages, leading to speculation that supplementation might slow down the aging process. In Japan, CoQ10 is used extensively to reduce the risk of heart attack, lower blood pressure, treat congestive heart failure, and boost the immune system. Some research shows it helps angina and congestive heart failure and prevents heart damage after surgery. CoQ10 is sold in the United States in capsule form as a dietary supplement.

Colon therapy: also known as colonic irrigation, a process that flushes up to 35 gallons of water through the entire five feet of the large intestine. According to proponents, this cleansing prevents toxins from accumulating in the colon and passing into the bloodstream and also helps restore regular bowel movements. Critics claim the procedure can do more harm than good. It may cause an electrolyte imbalance and can rupture the colon wall in people with certain intestinal diseases. Colon therapy should not be used by anyone with ulcerative colitis, diverticulitis, Crohn's disease, hemorrhoids, or tumors of the large intestine or rectum. Safer procedures include enemas (which use water to clean only the lower bowel) and fiber supplements, which also clean the colon.

Complementary medicine: another term for alternative medicine; may indicate therapies that are used in conjunction with conventional treatments—for example, using guided imagery and nutritional therapy to complement chemotherapy treatment for cancer.

Craniosacral therapy: a technique first developed by the American osteopath William Sutherland in the 1930s that involves manipulation of the bones of the skull and sometimes the spine. The manipulation is said to release tension that interferes with natural rhythmic oscillations in the craniosacral system, which includes the brain and the spinal cord, the cerebrospinal fluid and the surrounding membranes, and the bones of the skull and spine. The therapy is sought for relief of headache and TMJ syndrome, as well as chronic ear infection, vertigo, sinus pain, tinnitus, back and pelvis problems, and chronic pain.

Crystal therapy: the use of crystals or gems in healing. According to some Ayurvedic practitioners and others who practice crystal therapy, the energy vibrations of crystals can heal the body, balance the emotions, and increase spiritual sensitivity. Those who use this therapy believe that energy in the crystals and gems can activate energy centers in the body. The stones are worn as jewelry or placed on the chakras (major energy centers of the body) or throughout the house. Some proponents believe that the water that a gem has stood in for several hours contains the gem's energy and can be a tonic drink. Different properties are attributed to the various gems or crystals used, which include amethyst, quartz, malachite, pearl, agate, ruby, and diamond, among others. Crystal therapy is widely criticized as having no scientific basis.

Cupping: a Swedish massage percussion technique performed by striking the body with hands cupped so that only the fingertips and the heel of the palm touch the body. The term also applies to a traditional Chinese medicine technique of creating suction over specific points or regions of the body using small bamboo cups or glasses. To create a vacuum, a match is lit inside the cup and then removed as the cup is overturned on the body. As the hot air in the cup cools and contracts, the cup sticks tightly to the skin; it is left in place for about 10 minutes. Several cups are used at the same time in a specific area of the body. The technique is said to stimulate the circulation of the blood and is used to treat arthritis, bronchitis, and sprains.

Dance therapy: a form of therapy, also called dance/movement therapy or DMT, that uses spontaneous movement to promote healing. A dance therapist assesses a patient's movement and then uses movement therapeutically to address problems ranging from mental or emotional disturbances to a physical disability. Seen as a way to facilitate emotional expression, DMT has proved effective at improving self-esteem, reducing chronic pain, increasing communication, and decreasing isolation. Certification as a dance/movement therapist requires a master's degree and 700 hours of supervised clinical internship.

Designer food: according to the American Dietetic Association, processed foods that are supplemented with ingredients naturally rich in disease-preventing substances. This may involve genetic engineering of food. Orange juice fortified with calcium is an example of a designer food.

DHEA (dehydroepiandrosterone): a steroid hormone produced by the adrenal glands and synthetically manufactured for over-the-counter sale as a dietary supplement. DHEA levels tend to peak at age 30 and decline thereafter, leading some to speculate that reversing this decline in DHEA levels could produce an antiaging effect. Recent experiments in humans suggest that it can stimulate the immune system and prevent atherosclerosis and heart attacks in men by inhibiting platelet formation. However, since the body converts DHEA into testosterone and estrogen, DHEA supplements may increase the risk of prostate and breast cancers. In women, DHEA supplements may produce a masculinizing effect and increase the risk of heart disease.

Diathermy: deep-heat therapy that uses high-frequency electric currents to produce heat in body tissues. Physical therapists and sports physicians use diathermy to treat arthritis, bursitis, and fractures. It also may help treat gynecological diseases and sinusitis.

Dietary supplement: a product that is intended to supply nutrients and other healthful substances that may be lacking in a diet. The term used to apply only to vitamins, minerals, and proteins. In 1990, herbs were classified as dietary supplements, and the Dietary Supplement Health and Education Act of 1994 broadened the definition to include amino acids, glandulars (processed animal glands), enzymes, fish oils, and various extracts, such as flower essences. The 1994 act also relaxed the Food and Drug Administration regulation of dietary supplements: While their labels may not make any claims to cure, prevent, treat, or mitigate a disease, they can claim to help a structure or function of the body. Unlike food additives and prescription and over-the-counter drugs, dietary supplements do not require FDA approval to be sold on the market.

DMSO (dimethyl sulfoxide): a solvent capable of passing through body tissues and approved by the FDA to treat only one medical condition, an uncommon bladder inflammation called interstitial cystitis. However, proponents and manufacturers claim that DMSO heals a wider range of problems (including bruises, pimples, and herpes) and relieves pain from conditions such as muscle strains. They credit DMSO with the ability to kill bacteria and fungi, improve circulation, and stimulate the immune system. DMSO raises important safety concerns because it passes very quickly from the skin to the bloodstream and can bring other potentially harmful products along with it. DMSO produces a strong garlic breath in users, even when used topically or intravenously.

Environmental medicine: an approach to healing that concerns itself with the interaction of the body and the environment, looking especially at the role that allergies and normal exposure to chemicals in the environment play in illness. Doctors who practice environmental medicine say that in sensitive people environmental allergens can trigger such serious conditions as lupus, colitis, chronic fatigue syndrome, asthma, hyperactivity, psychosis, and high blood pressure, among others. Factors that trigger allergies include emotional or physical stress; infection; exposure to pesticides, and other chemicals in food or water; frequent use of antibiotics and steroids; electromagnetic disturbances in the environment; and poor nutrition. If someone's condition is exacerbated by allergies, treatment may involve lifestyle and diet changes to avoid exposure to allergens. The American Academy of Environmental Medicine in Denver, Colorado, trains physicians in environmental medicine.

Enzyme therapy: a form of therapy that employs supplements of plant and animal enzymes to improve digestive function and other conditions. During digestion, the body's own digestive enzymes are not the only ones at work; the enzymes present in raw fruits and vegetables also contribute to the breakdown of food in the stomach. Enzyme therapy advocates supplementation to reduce the work that the body has to do, and because plant enzymes are destroyed in cooking. Since enzymes can't be synthetically manufactured, supplements are derived from plants or from animal tissues. Some practitioners inject liquid enzymes to treat cancer and multiple sclerosis. Enzyme supplements are available over the counter, singly or in combination, and in capsule, tablet, powder, and liquid form.

Essential: a nutritional term applied to vitamins, minerals, and amino acids; refers to anything that the body does not manufacture and that must be obtained through the diet.

Feng shui: literally, "wind-water," an ancient Chinese practice involving the relationship of buildings, rooms, objects, and activities to the earth's vital energy (chi). Practitioners of feng shui (pronounced *fung shway*) study wind and water patterns, which are believed to indicate the flow of the earth's chi, and then design and place buildings so that they are harmoniously aligned with chi. This is believed to protect and enhance an inhabitant's health and good fortune.

Fixation: in chiropractic, an abnormality of motion said to interfere with the flow of nervous impulses and diminish the body's ability to stay healthy.

Functional food: according to the American Dietetic Association, any modified food or food ingredient that may provide a health benefit beyond the traditional nutrients it contains. The term is more common in Europe and Japan.

G

Glandulars: freeze-dried animal glands, processed into pill form and taken in the hope that they will give the body an extra dose of a hormone and improve the health of the user's own glands. Typically made from cow, sheep, or pig glands, glandulars on the market include adrenal, testicular, ovary, pancreas, pituitary, prostate, and thymus products. Critics point out that these supplements are unlikely to boost gland function because digestion breaks down and inactivates the DNA in a glandular. In addition, using glandulars may encourage your own glands to reduce hormone production. Other risks include bacterial contamination of the product, and the sometimes high levels of antibiotics and pesticides present in the glands of the livestock they were taken from.

Glucosamine sulfate: a natural amino sugar found in joint spaces. As a dietary supplement, it is said to stimulate the repair of arthritic joints by building up the protective cartilage that arthritis destroys.

H

Holistic: an adjective meaning targeted to the whole person—mind, body, and spirit. Holistic medicine considers not only the physical health but also the emotional, spiritual, social, and mental well-being of the person.

Hydrosol: in aromatherapy, the water that is obtained along with the essential oil after plant materials are distilled. In distillation, plant materials are heated in water to release the plant's oil, which vaporizes. The steam and vapor are channeled through a tube to a condensing coil, where they cool and return to liquid form. The essential oils float on top of the water. The hydrosol contains water-soluble plant constituents and trace amounts of essential oil. Hydrosols are sometimes used in aromatherapy together with the essential oils themselves and may be spritzed in the air and on the face and body.

L

Light box: a set of bright, broad-spectrum light bulbs inside a box with a reflective background and a diffusing screen. The box produces a light that's 10 to 20 times stronger than ordinary indoor light. Light boxes are used to treat winter depression, also known as seasonal affective disorder, or SAD. Treatment typically involves spending 15 minutes to three hours in front of a light box every day in the fall, winter, and early spring. Research suggests that bright lights help regulate the body's internal clock, which controls hormone secretion and sleep patterns. The amount of time a person needs to use a light box should be de-

termined by a practitioner. Light boxes are sold at special stores and by mail order. Depending on the manufacturer, the boxes may use either full-spectrum light bulbs with the ultraviolet light removed, or special high-intensity light bulbs. Experts advise against constructing a light box at home because of possible damage from ultraviolet light.

Light-emitting diodes (LEDs): tiny light sources frequently used in digital watches and electronic equipment. Recently, the devices have been used in the field of phototherapy. Their power output is low enough to be safe for human exposure but strong enough, say practitioners, to stimulate the biological responses involved in healing. Research indicates that LEDs may accelerate the healing of skin wounds and certain other conditions. A number of LED devices are available for self-treatment of minor skin conditions.

M

Manipulation: the application of manual force for healing. The term describes the techniques used in osteopathy, chiropractic, massage, and other bodywork therapies. Manipulation may involve various forms of massage, muscle pressure, and joint realignment or adjustment.

Megavitamin therapy: See Orthomolecular medicine.

Melatonin: a hormone produced by the pineal gland in the brain and released mainly at night in the absence of light on the retina. Melatonin regulates the onset and timing of sleep and such seasonal changes in the body as winter weight gain. Levels of melatonin decline with age, which may explain why many elderly people suffer from insomnia. Melatonin is being investigated as a sleep promoter and to prevent or reduce jet lag. Synthetic melatonin and melatonin derived from bovine pineal glands are available as over-the-counter dietary supplements. Melatonin occurs naturally in some foods but in fairly small amounts: 120 bananas provide only 3 mg melatonin. There are no studies on the health effects of long-term use, but reported side effects include reduced fertility, inhibition of male sexual drive, hypothermia, and damage to the retina. In the absence of clear research, some physicians and scientists advise against taking melatonin as a long-term supplement.

N

Neural therapy: a form of therapy based on the idea that illness is the result of disruptions in biological energy and that the disruptions are caused by changes in the electric activity of the autonomic nervous system, which controls involuntary functions like breathing. To recharge the body's flow of energy, anesthetics are injected into nerve sites of the autonomic nervous system and sometimes into acupuncture points, scar tissue, or painful areas. Neural therapy is said to help a wide range of conditions, from circulatory problems and hormonal imbalances to allergies and strained muscles. Neural therapy is not recommended for anyone with cancer, diabetes, renal failure, hemophilia, or allergies to anesthetics. For more information or referrals to practitioners, contact the American Academy of Neural Therapy in Santa Fe, New Mexico.

Neurotopic injection technique: a therapeutic procedure developed in 1982 by the German physician Volker Desnizza. Treatment involves dozens of injections of small amounts (0.5 cc or less) of sterile saline solution (0.9 percent salt) into the muscles at both sides of the spine near the places where the nerves enter into the back muscles. Over 20,000 patients have received the treatment in Germany. According to Desnizza's theory, salt injection helps the nerves function better, leading to improved circulation, control of pain, and healing of numerous disorders. Statistics on successful treatment of back and neck pain, sciatica, disk problems, headaches, arthritis, prostate and thyroid problems, asthma, and allergies have been presented at more than 15 international medical congresses since 1994. Not yet available in the United States, the technique is being evaluated in double-blind studies at the National College of Naturopathic Medicine in Portland, Oregon.

Nosode: a homeopathic remedy made from diseased tissue or bodily secretions rather than from a plant or animal. A nosode is like a homeopathic immunization, taken to build up an immune response against a specific disease. Like other homeopathic remedies, which are named for the plant or animal ingredient, nosodes are often named for the disease present in the material they were made from—for example, the flu nosode and the infectious mononucleosis nosode.

Nutriceutical: food products that provide medical or health benefits, including the prevention or treatment of disease. Foods rich in fiber could be called nutriceuticals because they are known to reduce the risk of colorectal cancer.

Orthomolecular medicine: a form of nutrient therapy that uses combinations of vitamins, minerals, and amino acids normally found in the body to maintain good health and to treat specific conditions, such as asthma, heart disease, depression, and schizophrenia. Coined by Linus Pauling, the term *orthomolecular* means an approach based on a correct (ortho) balance of substances present in the body.

Pet therapy: a therapeutic approach based on the idea that expressing affection for a pet helps people feel happier, maintain a positive outlook, and presumably, therefore improve their health. According to several studies, having a pet can reduce stress, lower blood pressure, and ward off loneliness and depression. Many nursing homes and some prisons have developed pet therapy programs, with excellent results.

Pharmafood: according to the American Dietetic Association, any food or nutrient that is purported to have medical or health benefits, including the prevention and treatment of disease.

Polarity therapy: a therapeutic technique based on a theory of energy flow in the body developed by Randolph Stone, a doctor of naturopathy, osteopathy, and chiropractic. According to this theory, energy flows along five predictable pathways, or currents, in the body. Specific points along the currents are said to hold either positive or negative energies. Polarity therapists use their own energy to treat a patient, placing their hands on points of the body with opposite charges and creating a current that is purported to balance the patient's energy flow. Back pain, headache, emotional problems, and stress are some of the conditions polarity therapists treat. For more information, contact the American Polarity Therapy Association in Boulder, Colorado.

Prana: the yogic concept of a cosmic energy or life force, similar to the Chinese idea of chi, that enters the body with the breath. Prana is thought to flow through the body, bringing health and vitality. It is considered the vital link between the spiritual self and the material self.

Pranayama: a term from yoga and Ayurveda meaning breath control.

Probiotics: substances such as acidophilus and bifidus that restore the beneficial bacteria normally present in the intestines. Stress, poor diet, antibiotics, and oral contraceptives can throw off the normal balance of bacteria and fungi. This imbalance may be manifested as a yeast infection, or in symptoms such as diarrhea or gastrointestinal disturbances.

Psychoneuroimmunology (PNI): the study of the ways the brain, the nervous system, and the emotions interact to affect the immune system. The term was coined by Dr. Robert Ader, a research psychologist who conducted experiments in 1974 showing that an animal's brain can influence its immune system. PNI became the cornerstone of subsequent efforts to demonstrate that mental attitude can affect the outcome of disease. Investigations have shown that negative approaches to life can interfere with immune system function, whereas positive expectations may actually help mobilize the immune system.

Qi: See Chi.

Shark cartilage: a controversial supplement touted as a cancer treatment. Sharks, whose frames are composed of cartilage rather than bone, get cancer infrequently, and proponents of this treatment claim it is because something in the cartilage inhibits the ability of tumors to create the blood supply they need to continue growing. Shark cartilage is also promoted as an immune system stimulant and a remedy for joint pain, swelling, and stiffness. Critics point to a lack of supporting scientific research and also warn that such controversial approaches should never substitute for conventional cancer treatment.

Shiatsu: a Japanese system of acupressure, developed in the early 20th century, that integrates ancient Chinese massage techniques with a modern understanding of anatomy and physiology. Shiatsu, which means "finger pressure," employs the principles of Chinese medicine to diagnose and treat such ailments as stress, circulatory problems, depression, asthma, headaches, diarrhea, and bronchitis. In a typical shiatsu session, the patient lies fully dressed on a floor mat while the practitioner applies thumb pressure to the body's meridian points to stimulate and balance the flow of chi in the body.

Sounding the body: a diagnostic and therapeutic technique used in sound healing. Sound healers read a patient's body by singing a series of tones and listening for imbalances in the natural frequencies of the body or its energy fields. Imbalances are said to be indicated by changes in the tone of the healer's voice. To correct a problem, the sound healer "applies sound" to the patient's body by singing certain tones near the affected organ, or by applying tuning forks or electronic vibratory instruments directly to the body.

Structural exam: an osteopathic diagnostic technique also known as structural diagnosis. The procedure involves a visual, hands-on assessment by an osteopathic physician of the skeleton, joints, muscles, ligaments, and tendons of the patient.

Subluxation: in chiropractic, a misalignment of bones within joints said to interfere with the flow of nervous impulses and diminish the body's ability to stay healthy.

Tonic: an herbal remedy made from mild herbs taken to maintain health or ward off illness, rather than to treat an illness. Also known as a normalizer.

Toning: in sound healing, the self-generated projection of a nonverbal sound inward to balance energy fields in the body.

Transcutaneous electrical nerve stimulation (TENS): the delivery of an electric current through the skin to the nerves. This procedure is used in physical therapy and to relieve painful conditions such as neuralgia, sciatica, and arthritis. The low-voltage electric current blocks the nerves' reception of pain signals and possibly stimulates the production of endorphins, the body's pain-killing chemicals. A typical TENS device consists of an electric generating unit attached by wires to electrodes, which are applied to the skin.

Vibrational medicine: sometimes known as energy healing; a holistic philosophy of medicine proposing that healing in the body begins on the energetic level. Vibrational therapies, which focus on unblocking or balancing the body's energy, include homeopathy, flower remedies, sound healing, color therapy, crystal and gem healing, Reiki, and therapeutic touch.

Yin and yang: according to ancient Chinese philosophy, the two polar, complementary forces that organize the universe: *Yang* is considered the sunny side of the mountain, *yin* the shady side. Yang aspects are said to be warmer, lighter, drier, and more activating; yin aspects are cooler, darker, moister, and more receptive. In good health, the individual's mind, body, and spirit reflect a blending of yin and yang. When the balance of these two forces is disturbed, either by immoderation—too much or too little of one factor—or by blockage of the flow of vital energy (chi), illness may result.

Zone therapy: another name for reflexology. The goal of this manual healing method is to eliminate energy blockages in the body by manipulating specific areas on the feet and hands that are thought to correspond to particular organs and body systems.

Bibliography

GENERAL

BOOKS

Alternative Medicine: Expanding Medical Horizons. Washington, D.C.: U.S. Government Printing Office, 1994.

Barrett, Stephen, MD, et al. *Health Schemes, Scams, and Frauds.* Mount Vernon, N.Y.: Consumer Reports Books, 1990.

Burton Goldberg Group. *Alternative Medicine.* Puyallup, Wash.: Future Medicine, 1993.

Butler, Kurt. *A Consumer's Guide to "Alternative Medicine."* Buffalo.: Prometheus Books, 1992.

Collinge, William. *The American Holistic Health Association Complete Guide to Alternative Medicine.* New York: Warner Books, 1996.

Fugh-Berman, Adriane, MD. *Alternative Medicine.* Tucson: Odonian Press, 1996.

Inlander, Charles B., et al. *The Consumer's Medical Desk Reference.* New York: Stonesong Press (Hyperion), 1995.

Kastner, Mark, and Hugh Burroughs. *Alternative Healing.* La Mesa, Calif.: Halcyon, 1993.

The Medical Advisor. Alexandria, Va.: Time-Life Books, 1996.

Micozzi, Marc S., MD (ed.). *Fundamentals of Complementary and Alternative Medicine.* New York: Churchill Livingstone, 1996.

Mills, Simon, and Steven J. Finando. *Alternatives in Healing.* New York: New American Library, 1988.

Nash, Barbara. *From Acupressure to Zen.* Alameda, Calif.: Hunter House, 1996.

Prevention Magazine Health Books: *Hands-On Healing.* Emmaus, Pa.: Rodale Press, 1989.
New Choices in Natural Healing. Emmaus, Pa.: Rodale Press, 1995.
The Prevention How-To Dictionary of Healing Remedies and Techniques. Emmaus, Pa.: Rodale Press, 1992.

Reader's Digest Association. *Family Guide to Natural Medicine.* Pleasantville, N.Y.: Reader's Digest Assn., 1993.

Stalker, Douglas, and Clark Glymour (eds.). *Examining Holistic Medicine.* Buffalo: Prometheus Books, 1985.

Walton, John, Jeremiah A. Barondess, and Stephen Lock (eds.). *The Oxford Medical Companion.* Oxford: Oxford University Press, 1994.

ACUPRESSURE

BOOKS

Bauer, Cathryn. *Acupressure for Everybody.* New York: Henry Holt, 1991.

Gach, Michael Reed. *Acupressure's Potent Points.* New York: Bantam, 1990.

Jarmey, Chris, and John Tindall. *Acupressure for Common Ailments.* New York: Simon & Schuster, 1991.

PERIODICALS

"Acupressure Band Prevents Nausea after Surgery." *Natural Health,* Mar./Apr. 1994.

Gach, Michael Reed. "Boost Your Energy with Acupressure." *Natural Health,* Nov./Dec. 1993.
"Press Away Your Arthritis Pain." *Bestways,* Sept. 1989.

Lipner, Maxine. "Different Strokes: Massage, Chiropractic, Acupuncture, and Acupressure Spell Relief for Many Athletes." *Women's Sports and Fitness,* May/June 1993.

Smith, Verena Johanna. "Acupressure Gives Relief during Pregnancy and Labor." *EastWest Natural Health,* Nov./Dec. 1992.

OTHER SOURCES

"Acupressure vs. Deep Tissue." Available on the World Wide Web at http://www.wildflower.com/deep.htm.

ACUPUNCTURE

BOOKS

Manaka, Yoshio, MD, and Ian A. Urquhart. *The Layman's Guide to Acupuncture.* New York: Weatherhill, 1986.

Mitchell, Ellinor R. *Plain Talk about Acupuncture.* New York: Whalehall, 1987.

Reid, Daniel. *The Complete Book of Chinese Health and Healing.* Boston: Shambhala, 1994.

PERIODICALS

Capp, Sheldon N. "So You're Going to an Acupuncturist." *Health News & Review,* Spring 1992.

"Pain Relief." *University of California at Berkeley Wellness Letter,* Aug. 1989.

OTHER SOURCES

American Academy of Medical Acupuncture and Medical Acupuncture Research Foundation home page. Available on the World Wide Web at http://www.olympus.net/dragons.

Ontario Breast Cancer Information Exchange Project. "Information on Unconventional Therapies." Available on the World Wide Web at http://aorta.library.mun.ca/bcuct/acu.htm.

APITHERAPY

PERIODICALS

Altomare, G. F., and G. L. Capella. " 'Bee Sting Therapy': The Revival of a Dangerous Practice" (letter to editor). *Acta Dermatovenereologica,* Sept. 1994.

Appleton, Elaine. "To Bee or Not to Bee?" *New Age Journal,* Jan./Feb. 1995.

Kim, Christopher M., MD. "Apitherapy (Bee Venom Therapy)." *Alternative Therapies in Clinical Practice.* July/Aug. 1996.

OTHER SOURCES

McCulloch, Michael. "Apitherapy: Frequently Asked Questions." Fact sheet. American Apitherapy Society.

"Questions & Answers: Frequently Asked Questions & Answers of the American Apitherapy

Society, Inc." Fact sheet. American Apitherapy Society.

Rothfeld, Glenn. "Bee Venom Therapy." *Spectrum Medical Arts.* Available on the World Wide Web at http://shore.net/~spectrum/apitherapy.html.

Wilkinson, Susan. "Is Bee Venom a Cure for Arthritis?" *Bee Culture Magazine,* American Apitherapy Society. Available on the World Wide Web at http://www.beesting.com/articles.html.

AROMATHERAPY

BOOKS

Davis, Patricia. *Aromatherapy: An A-Z.* Saffron Walden, Essex, England: C. W. Daniel, 1988.

Lawless, Julia. *The Encyclopedia of Essential Oils.* Rockport, Mass.: Element Books, 1992.

Price, Shirley. *Aromatherapy for Common Ailments.* London: Angus & Robertson, 1991.

Ryman, Danièle. *Aromatherapy.* New York: Bantam, 1993.

AYURVEDIC MEDICINE

BOOKS

Lad, Vasant. *Ayurveda.* Santa Fe, N.Mex.: Lotus Press, 1984.

Morrison, Judith H. *The Book of Ayurveda.* New York: Simon & Schuster, 1995.

PERIODICALS

"Ancient Ayurveda Still Effective against Many Ills." *Better Nutrition for Today's Living,* Mar. 1993.

Barnett, Robert, and Cathy Sears. "JAMA Gets into an Indian Herbal Jam." *Science,* Oct. 11, 1991.

Gormley, James J. "Ancient, Whole-Body Health Care Uses Powerful, Gentle Persuasion." *Better Nutrition,* Jan. 1996.

Greenwood, Michael T., et al. "Maharishi Ayur-Veda." *JAMA,* Oct. 2, 1991.

Hayhow, Sally. "The Ayurvedic Approach: The World's Oldest Medicine May Offer Hope for a Post-Antibiotic Era." *Vegetarian Times,* Aug. 1994.

Podolsky, Doug. "Big Claims, No Proof." *U.S. News & World Report,* Sept. 23, 1991.

OTHER SOURCES

Definitions and Descriptions of Complementary/Traditional Practitioners. Available as a link from the Complementary Medicine home page at http://fahc.vtmednet.org/im/gen/altlist1.htm ayur.

BODYWORK

BOOKS

Baginski, Bodo, and Shalila Sharamon. *Reiki: Universal Life Energy.* Mendocino, Calif.: LifeRhythm, 1988.

Brennan, Richard. *The Alexander Technique Workbook.* Rockport, Mass.: Element Books, 1992.

Krieger, Dolores. *The Therapeutic Touch.* New York: Prentice Hall Press, 1979.

Leibowitz, Judith, and Bill Connington. *The Alexander Technique.* New York: Harper & Row, 1990.

Morris, Joyce. *Reiki: Hands That Heal.* Encino, Calif.: Center Bookstore, 1993.

PERIODICALS

Collins, Tom. "Reiki: The Gift of Healing." *Whole Life Times,* May 1989.

Gallo, Nick. "Healing Hands: The Power of Touch Therapy." *Better Homes and Gardens,* May 1996.

Kotzsch, Ronald E.:
"The Alexander Technique: An Effective Therapy for Medical Problems?" *EastWest Natural Health,* Oct. 1990.
"The Feldenkrais Method." *EastWest Natural Health,* May/June 1992.
"Regain Grace: The Alexander Technique." *EastWest Natural Health,* Mar./Apr. 1992.
"Relieve Tension, Reduce Pain with Myotherapy." *EastWest Natural Health,* July/Aug. 1992.
"Restructure the Body with Rolfing." *EastWest Natural Health,* Nov./Dec. 1992.

Lally, Steven. "Massage: What It Can Do for You." *Prevention,* Dec. 1990.

Schecter, Melvin. "Healing Hands." *Psychology Today,* July-Aug. 1989.

Thomson, Bill. "Choosing a Qualified Bodyworker." *EastWest Natural Health,* July 1990.

OTHER SOURCES

Information packets from the following organizations: Aston Training Center, Incline Village, Nev.; Bonnie Prudden Pain Erasure, Tucson; Feldenkrais Guild, Albany, Oreg.; Hellerwork International, Mount Shasta, Calif.; North American Society of Teachers of the Alexander Technique, Champaign, Ill.; Rolf Institute, Boulder, Colo.; Trager Institute, Mill Valley, Calif.

CHINESE MEDICINE

BOOKS

Beinfield, Harriet, and Efrem Korngold. *Between Heaven and Earth.* New York: Ballantine, 1991.

Hsu, Hong-yen, and William G. Peacher. *Chinese Herb Medicine and Therapy* (rev. ed.). Los Angeles: Oriental Healing Arts Institute of U.S.A., 1982.

Hyatt, Richard. *Healing with Chinese Herbs.* Rochester, Vt.: Healing Arts Press, 1990.

Kaptchuk, Ted J. *The Web That Has No Weaver.* Chicago: Congdon & Weed, 1983.

Maciocia, Giovanni. *The Practice of Chinese Medicine.* New York: Churchill Livingstone, 1994.

Reid, Daniel P. *Chinese Herbal Medicine.* Boston: Shambhala, 1987.

CHIROPRACTIC

BOOKS

Beideman, Ronald P. "A Short History of the Chiropractic Profession." In *Fundamentals of Chiropractic Diagnosis and Management,* edited by Dana Lawrence. Baltimore: Williams & Wilkins, 1991.

PERIODICALS

Abrams, Maxine. "Chiropractic." *Good Housekeeping,* Mar. 1994.

"Chiropractors." *Consumer Reports.* June 1994.

Consumer Reports. Letters to the Editor, corrections. Mar. 1995.

Mead, Mark. "Chiropractic's New Wave." *EastWest Natural Health,* Nov. 1989.

ENERGY MEDICINE

BOOKS

Gerber, Richard. *Vibrational Medicine.* Santa Fe, N.Mex.: Bear & Co., 1988.

ESSENTIAL FIRST AID

BOOKS

Chancellor, Philip M. *Dr. Philip M. Chancellor's Handbook of the Bach Flower Remedies.* New Canaan, Conn.: Keats Publishing, 1971.

Kusick, James. *A Treasury of Natural First Aid Remedies from A to Z.* West Nyack, N.Y.: Parker Publishing, 1995.

Mayell, Mark, et al. *The Natural Health First-Aid Guide.* New York: Pocket Books, 1994.

Panos, Maesimund B., MD, and Jane Heimlich. *Homeopathic Medicine at Home.* New York: Jeremy P. Tarcher/Perigee, 1980.

FLOWER REMEDIES

BOOKS

Barnard, Julian. *A Guide to the Bach Flower Remedies.* Saffron Walden, Essex, England: C. W. Daniel, 1979.

Chancellor, Philip M. *Illustrated Handbook of the Bach Flower Remedies.* Saffron Walden, Essex, England: C. W. Daniel, 1971.

Kaminski, Patricia, and Richard Katz. *Flower Essence Repertory.* Nevada City, Calif.: Flower Essence Society, 1994.

Ramsell, John. *Questions and Answers Clarifying the Basic Principles and Standards of the Bach Flower Remedies.* Wallingford, Oxfordshire, England:

Bach Centre, 1986.

Wright, Machaelle Small. *Flower Essences.* Jeffersonton, Va.: Perelandra, 1988.

OTHER SOURCES

"Healing Herbs: English Flower Essences." Pamphlet. Nevada City, Calif.: Flower Essence Services, 1992.

Kaminski, Patricia, and Richard Katz. "Flower Essences: Nature's Healing Language." Pamphlet. Nevada City, Calif.: Flower Essence Society, 1986.

"1996-97 Perelandra Catalog." Warrenton, Va.: Perelandra Center for Nature Research, 1996.

"The Original Bach Flower Essences." Pamphlet. Philadelphia: Nelson Bach, 1995.

HERBAL THERAPIES

BOOKS

Tyler, Varro E. *The Honest Herbal* (3d ed.). New York: Pharmaceutical Products Press, 1993.

OTHER SOURCES

Hoffmann, David L. *Therapeutic Herbalism.* Unpublished course materials.

HOMEOPATHY

BOOKS

Castro, Miranda, *The Complete Homeopathy Handbook.* New York: St. Martin's Press, 1991.

Cummings, Stephen, and Dana Ullman. *Everybody's Guide to Homeopathic Medicines.* Los Angeles: Jeremy P. Tarcher, 1991.

HYDROTHERAPY

BOOKS

Moor, Fred B., et al. *Manual of Hydrotherapy and Massage.* Mountain View, Calif.: Pacific Press Publishing Assn., 1964.

LIGHT THERAPY

BOOKS

Amber, Reuben B. *Color Therapy.*

Santa Fe, N.Mex.: Aurora Press, 1983.

Perry, Susan, and Jim Dawson. *The Secrets Our Body Clocks Reveal.* New York: Ballantine, 1988.

PERIODICALS

Ericsson, Arthur D., and W. LaValley, "Pain Management and Wound Healing." *Explore! for the Professional,* 1993, Vol. 4, no. 6.

OTHER SOURCES

"Laser Therapy 101: The Basics—Part 2." *LLLT News Source.* Newsletter. Castle Rock, Colo.: Scott K. Deuel, n.d.

"Questions and Answers about the Use of Light Therapy in Winter." Information sheet. New York: Winter Depression Program, Columbia-Presbyterian Medical Center. Research Foundation for Mental Hygiene, 1995.

MASSAGE

BOOKS

Massage. Alexandria, Va.: Time-Life Books, 1987.

Tappan, Frances M. *Healing Massage Techniques: A Study of Eastern and Western Methods.* Reston, Va.: Reston Publishing, 1978.

Thomas, Sara. *Massage for Common Ailments.* New York: Simon & Schuster, 1989.

MIND/BODY MEDICINE

BOOKS

Benson, Herbert, MD:
The Relaxation Response. Avenal, N.J.: Random House Value, 1992.
Timeless Healing. New York: Scribner, 1996.

Dossey, Larry, MD. *Healing Words.* San Francisco: HarperSanFrancisco, 1993.

Goleman, Daniel, and Joel Gurin (eds.). *Mind/Body Medicine.* Yonkers, N.Y.: Consumer Reports Books, 1993.

Gordon, James S., MD. *Manifesto for a New Medicine.* Reading, Mass.: Addison-Wesley, 1996.

PERIODICALS

Hochman, John, MD. "Recovered Memory Therapy and False Memory Syndrome." Altadena, Calif.: *Skeptic,* 1994.

Wallis, Claudia. "Healing." *Time,* June 24, 1996.

NATUROPATHIC MEDICINE

BOOKS

Murray, Michael T., and Joseph Pizzorno. *An Encyclopedia of Natural Medicine.* Rocklin, Calif.: Prima Publishing, 1991.

OTHER SOURCES

Pizzorno, Joseph E., et al. *Naturopathic Medicine.* Report to Task Force on National Health Reform. Seattle: American Assn. of Naturopathic Physicians, Apr. 1993.

NUTRITION AND DIET

BOOKS

Carper, Jean. *The Food Pharmacy.* New York: Bantam, 1989.

Haas, Elson M., MD. *Staying Healthy with Nutrition.* Berkeley, Calif.: Celestial Arts, 1992.

Keeping Well. Amsterdam: Time-Life Books, 1996.

PERIODICALS

Krey, Susanna H. "Alternate Dietary Lifestyles." *Primary Care,* Sept. 1982.

OTHER SOURCES

"Facts about Olestra." Nutrition fact sheet. American Dietetic Assn., 1996.

"Olestra and Other Fat Substitutes." FDA Backgrounder BG95-18. Washington, D.C.: U.S. FDA, Nov. 28, 1995.

"What is Macrobiotics?" Available on the World Wide Web at http://www.macrobiotics.org.

OSTEOPATHY

BOOKS

Peterson, Barbara A. "Major Events in Osteopathic History." In *Foundations for Osteopathic Medicine,* edited by Robert C. Ward. Baltimore: Williams & Wilkins, in press.

PERIODICALS

Fitzgerald, Nancy. "DOs Bring Unique Philosophy, Treatment to Practice of Medicine." *The DO,* June 1994.

Page, Leigh. "Osteopathic Physicians Moving into Mainstream." *American Medical News,* June 26, 1995.

OTHER SOURCES

"OMT: Hands-On Care." Educational brochure. Chicago: American Osteopathic Assn., 1996.

QIGONG

BOOKS

McGee, Charles T., MD, with Qigong Master Effie Poy Yew Chow. *Miracle Healing from China . . . Qigong.* Coeur d'Alene, Idaho: MediPress, 1994.

PERIODICALS

Sancier, Kenneth M. "Medical Applications of Qigong." *Alternative Therapies,* Jan. 1996.

REFLEXOLOGY

BOOKS

Byers, Dwight C. *Better Health with Foot Reflexology.* St. Petersburg, Fla.: Ingham Publishing, 1983.

Carter, Mildred, and Tammy Weber. *Body Reflexology.* West Nyack, N.Y.: Parker Publishing, 1994.

Ingham, Eunice D. *The Original Works of Eunice D. Ingham.* St. Petersburg, Fla.: Ingham Publishing, 1984.

SOUND THERAPY

PERIODICALS

Clark, Michael E., and Peter Kranz. "A Survey of Backgrounds, Attitudes, and Experiences of New Music Therapy Students." *Journal of Music Therapy,* Summer 1996.

Crowe, Barbara J., and Mary Scovel. "An Overview of Sound Healing Practices." *Music Therapy Perspectives,* 1996, Vol. 14, no. 1.

Mandel, Susan E. "Music for Wellness: Music Therapy for Stress Management in a Rehabilitation Program." *Music Therapy Perspectives,* 1996, Vol. 14, no. 1.

OTHER SOURCES

Information packet from the National Association for Music Therapy, Silver Spring, Md.

T'AI CHI

BOOKS

Liang, T. T. *T'ai Chi Ch'uan for Health and Self-Defense.* New York: Vintage Books, 1977.

Managing Stress. Alexandria, Va.: Time-Life Books, 1987.

Reid, Howard. *The Book of Soft Martial Arts.* London: Gaia Books, 1994.

PERIODICALS

Hudgens, Dallas. "Tai Chi: Slow but Sure." *Washington Post,* Aug. 23, 1996.

"Meditation in Motion." *University of California at Berkeley Wellness Letter,* Feb. 1994.

YOGA

BOOKS

Iyengar, B. K. S. *Light on Yoga* (rev. ed.). New York: Schocken Books, 1979.

Lidell, Lucy. *The Sivananda Companion to Yoga.* New York: Simon & Schuster, 1983.

Monro, Robin, R. Nagarathna, and H. R. Nagendra. *Yoga for Common Ailments,* New York: Simon & Schuster, 1990.

PERIODICALS

"That's Abusing Your Head!" *Medical Update,* Oct. 1992.

OTHER SOURCES

"Finding a Yoga Teacher." Information sheet. Sarasota, Fla.: American Yoga Assn., 1994.

Index

Page numbers in italics refer to illustrations or illustrated text.

A

Abana (Ayurvedic remedy), 200, 231
Abdominal thrusts, *375, 376*
Abscesses: tonsillar, 360; tooth, 362, *363*
Achillea millefolium (yarrow), *69*, 103; in combinations, 77, 81
Aconite, 107
Acupressure, 16-17, *18-31, 34-35;* Bladder 10, *18;* Bladder 13, *18;* Bladder 23, *18;* Bladder 25, *18;* Bladder 32, *19;* Bladder 40, *19;* Conception Vessel 4, *19, 305;* Conception Vessel 6, *19, 261;* Conception Vessel 12, *20;* Conception Vessel 17, *20;* Conception Vessel 22, *20;* first-aid revival point, *372;* Gall Bladder 2, *20;* Gall Bladder 20, *21, 256;* Gall Bladder 21, *21;* Gall Bladder 34, *21;* Gall Bladder 39, *21;* Governing Vessel 4, *22;* Governing Vessel 14, *22;* Governing Vessel 20, *22;* Governing Vessel 24.5, *22, 268;* Governing Vessel 25, *23;* Governing Vessel 26, *372;* Heart 3, *23;* Heart 7, *23;* Hiccup 1, *31;* Kidney 1, *23;* Kidney 3, *24;* Large Intestine 4, *24, 273, 343;* Large Intestine 10, *24;* Large Intestine 11, *24, 255;* Large Intestine 20, *25, 256, 343;* Liver 2, *25;* Liver 3, *25;* Liver 8, *25;* Lung 1, *26;* Lung 5, *26, 243;* Lung 7, *26, 309;* Lung 10, *26, 345;* Pericardium 3, *27;* Pericardium 6, *27, 200, 259, 311, 317;* Small Intestine 3, *27;* Small Intestine 17, *27, 311;* Spleen 3, *28, 264;* Spleen 4, *28;* Spleen 6, *28, 277, 285;* Spleen 8, *28;* Spleen 9, *29;* Spleen 10, *29;* Spleen 12, *29;* Stomach 2, *29;* Stomach 3, *30, 273;* Stomach 7, *30, 358;* Stomach 25, *30;* Stomach 36, *30, 277;* Stomach 44, *30;* Triple Warmer 3, *31;* Triple Warmer 5, *31, 197;* Triple Warmer 6, *31;* Triple Warmer 17, *31*
Acupuncture, 32-33, *34-35,* 58, 59, 60
Aesculus, 283
Aesculus hippocastanum (horse chestnut), 366
Agastache *(Agastache rugosa),* 276
Agrimony (flower remedy), 68
Alanine, 331
Alcohol use, 145-146, 209, 235
Aletris farinosa (true unicorn root), 330

Alexander, Frederick Matthias, 47, 50
Alexander technique, 47-48
Alfalfa, 209, 231, 320
Allergies, 196-197; bee sting, 37; conjunctivitis, 238, 239; food, 146, 196, 197; hay fever, 268-269; and otitis media, 251; poison ivy, oak, and sumac, 326-*327;* vaginal, 365
Allium cepa (homeopathic remedy), 107
Allium cepa (onion), 247, 284
Allium sativum (garlic), 83, *88;* in combination, 80
Aloe *(Aloe barbadensis),* 74
Aloe (Ayurvedic remedy), 352
Aloe vera, 249, 341
Althaea officinalis (marsh mallow), 91
Alveoli, *325*
Amala, 250
Amenorrhea, 304-305, 306, 307
Anaphylactic shock (anaphylaxis), 196, 197, 378
Anemia, 198-199; iron deficiency, 159; megaloblastic, 152; pernicious, 155
Anemone pulsatilla (pasqueflower), 331
Angelica sinensis (dong quai), 81; in combinations, 74, 95, 101
Angina, 200-201
Aniseed, 221, 243, 260; oil, 206, 220
Antacids, 276, 346, 347
Anthemis nobilis (Roman chamomile), 266, 292, 314, 348
Antibiotics, 250, 287
Antimonium crudum, 369
Antimonium tartaricum, 243, 325
Antioxidants, 156, 161, 209, 227, 287
Antiprostaglandins, 253
Apis, 107
Apitherapy, 36-37
Apium graveolens (celery), 223, 264
Arctium lappa (burdock), 77; in combination, 93
Arctostaphylos uva-ursi (uva ursi), 102; in combination, 81
Argentum nitricum, 239
Arnica, 108
Aromatherapy, 38-41
Arrhythmias, heart, 278
Arsenicum album, 108
Artemisia argyi (mugwort), 92
Artemisia dracunculus (tarragon), 41
Artemisia vulgaris (mugwort), 92, 371
Arteries: atherosclerosis, 208-*209;* coronary, disease of, 279; high blood pressure, 284-285; pressure points, *374*
Arthritis, 202-205, *203;* gout, 264-*265*
Asclepias syriaca (milkweed), 368, 369
Ascorbic acid (vitamin C), 155
Asian diet, 148
Asparagus racemosus (shatavari), 255, 291, 303, 315
Aspen (flower remedy), 68

Aspiration (herbs), 245
Asthma, 206-*207*
Aston, Judith, 49
Aston-Patterning, 49
Astragalus *(Astragalus membranaceus),* 74; in combinations, 81, 101
Astragalus Ten Formula, 233
Atherosclerosis, 208-*209*
Athletic injuries, 210-213
Atopic dermatitis (eczema), 332, 333
Autogenic training, 139
Autoimmune disorders, 286. *See also* Arthritis, Diabetes, Multiple sclerosis (MS)
Avena sativa (oat), 245, 319, 327, 335
Ayurvedic medicine, 42-46
Azadirachta indica (neem), 310, 317

B

Bach, Edward, 66
Bach flower remedies, 66-69
Back problems, 210-211, 214-215, 373
Balanitis, 370
Baptisia tinctoria (wild indigo), 309
Barberry, 238, 291, 371
Baryta carbonica, 361
Basal cell carcinoma (BCC), 333, *334*
Basil, 244; Indian, 255, 351
Bayberry, 266, 267, 295, 299
Bay laurel, 40
Ba Zhen Wan (Chinese remedy), 199
B-complex vitamins, 152-155
Bdellium, Indian (gugulipid), 209, 231, 354, 360
Beech (flower remedy), 68
Bee pollen, 36, 37, 197
Bee products, 36-37, 107, 197
Bee venom therapy, 36, 37
Beijing Absolute Red, 353
Belladonna, 108
Benign prostatic hyperplasia (BPH; enlarged prostate), 330, *331*
Benson, Herbert, 138, 139
Benzoicum acidum, 265
Berberis (barberry), 238; *B. vulgaris,* 291, 371
Berberis vulgaris (homeopathic remedy), 331
Bergamot, 308
Beriberi, 153-154
Beta carotene, 153
Betony, wood, 272
Bezoar Antidotal Tablets, 363
Bilberry, 262, 306, 366
Biofeedback, 132, 245
Biofield therapeutics, 64-65
Bioflavonoids, 197, 209, 231, 251, 267, 269, 343

Biotin, 152
Bi Yan Pian (Chinese remedy), 196
Black haw, 253, 306
Bladder: incontinence, 288-289; infections, 216-217
Bladder wrack, 357
Bleeding, first aid for, *374*
Blood pressure, high, 284-285
Bloodroot, *74, 75*
Blood vessels and heart. *See* Cardiovascular problems
Bodywork, 47-56; chiropractic, 61-63; massage, 48, 121-123, *124-129*
Boerhaavia diffusa (punarnava), 231
Bones. *See* Musculoskeletal problems
Boneset, *76;* in combinations, 77, 88
Bonnie Prudden Myotherapy, 52
Bonnisan (Ayurvedic remedy), 248, 291, 310, 316
Botulism, 258
Bowel movement abnormalities: constipation, 240-241; diarrhea, 248-249; irritable bowel syndrome, 294-295
BPH (benign prostatic hyperplasia; enlarged prostate), 330, *331*
Brain wave biofeedback, 245
Breast health, *218-219*
Breathing, reestablishing, *376*
Breathing exercises, 139, 293
Breathing problems. *See* Respiratory problems
Broken bones, 210
Bromelain (pineapple enzyme), 209, 235, 306, 342, 355, 369
Bronchial tubes (bronchioles), 220, *221;* and asthma, *207*
Bronchitis, 220-*221*
Bryonia, 109
Buckthorn, 241
Bugleweed, 357
Bupleurum *(Bupleurum chinense),* 76
Burdock, 77; in combination, 93
Bursitis, 222-223
Bushmaster snake, 112
Butcher's-broom, 235, 366
Butter, 145
Bu Zhong Yi Qi Wan (Chinese remedy), 233
B vitamins, 152-155

Cactus grandiflorus, 201
Cajuput, 216
Calcarea carbonica, 109
Calcarea fluorica, 321
Calcarea phosphorica, 321
Calcium, 157; carbonate, 109; pantothenate, 154; sulphide, 111

Calculus Bovis Clear the Upper Pills, 238
Calendula *(Calendula officinalis),* 77
Calendula (homeopathic remedy), 335
Calming Essence (Rescue Remedy), 69
Cananga odorata (ylang-ylang), 41
Cancer, 224-227; diet and, 148, 149; prostate, 330; skin, 332-333, *334,* 335; vaginal, 364
Candidiasis (yeast infection), 364, 365, 370-371
Cannabis sativa (marijuana), 262-263
Cantharis, 109
Capsaicin, 78, 341
Capsella bursa-pastoris (shepherd's purse), 306
Capsicum annuum var. *annuum* (cayenne), *78;* in combinations, 75, 77, 90
Carbohydrates, 144
Carbo vegetabilis, 261, 277
Carcinogens, 225
Cardamom, 363
Cardiac glycosides, 280
Cardiomyopathy, 279-280
Cardiopulmonary resuscitation (CPR), 373
Cardiovascular problems: angina, 200-201; atherosclerosis, 208-*209;* cholesterol, 230-231; circulation, 234-235; heart, 278-281; high blood pressure, 284-285; varicose veins, 282-283, 366-367
Carob, 295
Carotenoids, 153
Carpal tunnel syndrome (CTS), 228-229
Cartilage, breakdown of, *203*
Caryophyllus aromaticus (clove), 298, 363
Cassia senna (senna), 241
Castor-oil packs, 219, 223
Catnip, 77
Caulophyllum thalictroides (blue cohosh), 306
Causticum, 289, 369
Cavities, dental, 362, *363*
Cayenne, *78;* in combinations, 75, 77, 90
Cedarwood oil, 216, 335
Celandine, 368
Celery seed, 223, 264
Centaury (flower remedy), 68
Centella asiatica (gotu kola), 87; as Ayurvedic remedy, 348
Cerato (flower remedy), 68
Ceratonia siliqua (carob), 295
Chaenomeles speciosa (Japanese quince), 315
Chalazions, 350, 351
Chamaemelum nobile (chamomile), 291
Chamomile, 78, *80;* Ayurvedic remedy,

291; in combinations, 84, 86, 102, 103; homeopathic remedy from, 110; oil, 40, 328, 337; Roman, 266, 292, 314, 348
Chamomilla, 110
Charcoal, 249, 259, 277
Charley horse, 210, 213
Chaste tree, 79, *82*
Chelation therapy, 200, 234, 280
Chelidonium majus (celandine), 368
Cherry: wild black, 324; winter, 348
Cherry Plum (flower remedy), 68
Chestnut (flower remedy): bud, 68; red, 69; sweet, 69; white, 69
Chi (energy), 16, 32, 57, 59, 165, 166, 172, 173
Chicken soup for colds, 237
Chickweed, 364-365
Chicory (flower remedy), 68
Children: athletic injuries, 212; depression, 244; growing pains, 211; otitis media, 250, 251; rheumatoid arthritis, juvenile, 202; tonsillitis, 360-361
Chills and fever, 254-255
Chimaphila umbellata (pipsissewa), 330, 339
Chinese angelica root (dong quai), 81; in combinations, 74, 95, 101
Chinese foxglove root, 79; in combinations, 80, 81, 90
Chinese medicine, 57-60; acupuncture, 32-33, *34-35,* 58, 59, 60; herbs, 58-59, 70-71, 72; qigong, 165-166. *See also* Acupressure
Chinese yam, 79
Ching Wan Hung (Chinese remedy), 353
Chiropractic, 61-63
Chloride, 157
Choking, first aid for, *375-376*
Cholecalciferol, 156
Cholesterol problems, 230-231
Chromium, 157
Chronic Epstein-Barr virus (CEBV), 232-233
Chronic fatigue syndrome (CFS), 232-233
Chrysanthemum flower *(Chrysanthemum indicum),* 284
Chrysanthemum parthenium (feverfew), 83, *86*
Cimicifuga *(Cimicifuga foetida),* 215
Cimicifuga racemosa (black cohosh), 71, 75; in combination, 103
Cinnamon bark *(Cinnamomum cassia),* 80; in combination, 101
Cinnamon twig *(Cinnamomum cassia),* 82, 101, 207
Circulatory problems, 234-235. *See also* Cardiovascular problems
Citrus reticulata (tangerine), 100; in combination, 95
Clay, 261, 326, 327

Cleavers, 77, 309, 361
Clematis (flower remedy), 68
Clove, 298, 342, 363
Clover, red, *71, 96*; in combinations, 77, 92
Club moss, 113
Cluster headaches, 270, *271*, 272, 273
Cobalamin (vitamin B₁₂), 155
Cobalt, 158
Cocculus, 301
Coenzyme Q10 (CoQ10), 227, 233, 281, 313
Coffea, 293
Cohosh, black, *71, 75*; in combination, 103
Cohosh, blue, 306
Colchicum, 264
Cold, common, 236-237
Cold laser therapy, 119, 120
Colocynthis, 249, 295
Color therapy, Ayurvedic, 45
Coltsfoot, 80; in combinations, 88, 92
Comfrey, 355
Commiphora molmol (myrrh), 93; in combinations, 77, 78
Commiphora mukul (gugulipid; Indian bdellium), 209, 231, 354, 360
Congenital heart defects, 278-279
Conium, 301
Conjunctivitis, 238-239
Constipation, 240-241
Contact dermatitis, 332, *333*; poison plants, 326-*327*
Convallaria majalis (lily of the valley), 280
Copper, 158
Coptis, 98; *Coptis chinensis*, 339
Coriander *(Coriandrum sativum)*, 317
Coronary heart disease, 279
Cough, 220, 242-243
Cough syrups, 243
CPR (cardiopulmonary resuscitation), 373
Crab Apple (flower remedy), 68
Cramp bark, 103, 205, 215, 223, 253, 272, 306
Cramps: menstrual, 305, 306, 307; muscle, 314-315
Cranberry, 217
Cranesbill, wild, 306
Crataegus laevigata; Crataegus oxyacantha (hawthorn), 87
Crocus, autumn, 264
Cross-fiber stroking, *127*
Cuprum metallicum, 315
Curcuma longa (turmeric), *71, 101*, 315, 340
Cuttlefish ink, 116
Cyanocobalamin, 155
Cymbopogon martinii (palmarosa), 41
Cyperus rotundus (nut grass), 303

Cypress, 298, 306, 344, 366
Cystitis, 216-217

Dandelion, *71, 81*
Deadly nightshade, 108
Decongestant, 269
Deep-heat therapy, 222
Deep-tissue massage, 319
Degenerative joint disease (osteoarthritis), 202-*203*
Dental problems: gum problems, 266-*267*; TMJ syndrome, 358-359; toothache, 362-*363*
Dentinal hypersensitivity, 362
Depression, 244-245; seasonal affective disorder, 336-337
Dermatitis, 332, *333*, 334-335; poison plants, 326-*327*
Diabetes, 246-247
Diarex (Ayurvedic remedy), 248
Diarrhea, 248-249
Diathermy, 222
Diet and nutrition, 144-151, *147*, 152-162
Digestive problems. *See* Gastrointestinal problems
Digitalis purpurea (foxglove), 280
Dioscorea opposita (Chinese yam), 79; in combination, 79
Dioscorea villosa (wild yam), 103
Dislocations, 210
Dong quai, 81; in combinations, 74, 95, 101
Doshas, concept of, 42-43
Dragon bone, 356
Drosera, 243
Du Huo Ji Sheng Wan (Chinese remedy), 205
Duodenal ulcers, 346, *347*
Dysmenorrhea, 304, 305, 306, 307
Dysthymia, 244

Ear, *251*
Earache, 250-251
Ear problems, 250-251; hearing loss, 274-275; Ménière's disease, 300-301
Echinacea *(Echinacea* spp.), 81, *84;* in combination, 80
Echinacea (homeopathic remedy), 374
Eczema, 332, *333*
EDTA (chemical), 200, 234
EEG biofeedback, 245
Effleurage, *124-125*
Eicosapentaenoic acid (EPA), 335

Eight Flavor Pills, 303
Eight Treasure Pills, 199
Elbow injuries, 210
Elder, 77, 82, 88, 92, 197, 237, 255, 257, 308, 343
Elecampane, 207, 221; in combination, 75
Eleutherococcus senticosus (eleuthero; Siberian ginseng), 86
Elm (flower remedy), 68
Elm, slippery, 99
Emergencies. *See* First aid
Emotions, flower remedies for treating, 66, 67, 68-69
Endocrine problems: diabetes, 246-247; thyroid, 356-*357*
Endometriosis, 252-*253*
Energy medicine (energy therapy), 64-65
Enokidake, 286
EPA (eicosapentaenoic acid), 335
Ephedra *(Ephedra sinica)*, 82
Epicondylitis, 210
Equisetum arvense (horsetail), 87
Ergocalciferol, 156
Esophagus in heartburn, 276
Essential oils, 38-41
Estrogen: decrease in, 302; plant estrogens, 303, 321
Eucalyptus *(Eucalyptus)*, 39, *71*; eucalyptus globulus *(E. globulus)*, 40; lemon-scented *(E. citriodora)*, 40
Eucommia *(Eucommia ulmoides)* bark, 284; in combination, 90
Eupatorium perfoliatum (boneset), *76;* in combinations, 77, 88
Eupatorium purpureum (gravelroot), 264
Euphrasia, 269
Euphrasia officinalis (eyebright), 82
Evening primrose oil, 219, 306, 329, 331, 334
Everlasting, 40
Exercises: hamstring stretch, *213;* Kegel, *289;* weight-bearing, *320. See also individual* ailments
Expectorants, 242, 243, 324-325
Eye, *239, 263, 351*
Eyebright, 82
Eyelid infections, 350-*351*
Eye problems: conjunctivitis, 238-239; glaucoma, 262-*263;* sties, 350-*351*

Fasts, juice and water, 287
Fatigue, chronic, 232-233
Fats, dietary, 144, 145, 150, 231, 295
Feet: athletic injuries, 211-212; gout, *265;* plantar warts, 368, *369;* reflexology areas, 167-168, *169, 301*

Feldenkrais, Moshe, 50
Feldenkrais method, 50
Female health. *See* Women
Fennel, 260, 291
Fenugreek, 231, 247
Ferrum phosphoricum, 110
Fever and chills, 254-255
Feverfew, 83, *86*
Feverwort (boneset), *76;* in combinations, 77, 88
Fiber, dietary, 145, 241, 295
Filipendula ulmaria (meadowsweet), 86, 259, 291, 317
First aid, 372-378; ABCs, checking, *373;* acupressure, *372;* back injuries, 373; bleeding, *374;* choking, *375-376;* CPR, 373; head and neck injuries, 373; poisoning, 377; recovery position, *372;* shock, 378; supplies, 379
Fitzgerald, William, 167
Five Flower Formula (Rescue Remedy), 69
Flammulina velutipes (enokidake), 286
Flavonoids, 197, 209, 231, 251, 267, 269, 343
Flaxseed, 241, 380
Fleeceflower (polygonum), 95
Flint, 116
Flower remedies (flower essences), 66-69
Flu, 256-257
Fluoride, 158
Foeniculum vulgare (fennel), 260, 291
Folic acid (folacin; folate; vitamin B$_9$), 152
Food Guide Pyramid, *147*
Food intolerances, 146, 196, 197
Food poisoning, 258-259
Fo-ti (polygonum), 95
Foxglove, 280
Fractures, 210, 211, 212
Free and Easy Wanderer Pills, 306, 329
Friction (massage), *127*
Fritillaria and Loquat Cough Mixture, 243
Fritillary bulb *(Fritillaria cirrhosa),* 343
Fucus spp. (kelp), 89
Fucus vesiculosus (bladder wrack), 357
Fungal (yeast) infections, 364, 365, 370-371

Galium spp. (cleavers), 77, 309, 361
Ganoderma *(Ganoderma lucidum),* 83
Gardenia *(Gardenia jasminoides),* 354
Gargles, homemade, 345
Garlic, 83, *88;* in combination, 80
Gas and gas pains, 260-261

Gasex (Ayurvedic remedy), 291, 310, 316
Gastric ulcers, 346, *347*
Gastritis, 316
Gastroenteritis, 248, 316
Gastrointestinal problems: constipation, 240-241; diarrhea, 248-249; food poisoning, 258-259; gas and gas pains, 260-261; heartburn, 276-277; hemorrhoids, 282-283; indigestion, 290-291; irritable bowel syndrome, 294-295; nausea, 316-317; stomach ulcers, 346-*347*
Gather Vitality (herbs), 245
Gattefossé, René-Maurice, 38
Gaultheria procumbens (wintergreen), 236, 271, 323
GBE (ginkgo biloba extract), 85
Gelsemium, 110
Genetic factors in cancer, 225
Gentian (flower remedy), 68
Gentian *(Gentiana lutea),* 198, 291
Gentiana *(Gentiana scabra),* 84
Gentiana Drain the Liver Pills, 340
Geranium, 323; oil, 300, 302, 306, 328
Geranium maculatum (wild cranesbill), 306
Geriforte (Ayurvedic remedy), 231, 302, 348
German chamomile, 40, 78, *80,* 110; in combinations, 84, 86, 102, 103
Ginger, 84; Ayurvedic remedy, 248, 298, 303, 315, 363; in combinations, 90, 92, 103; oil, 322
Ginkgo *(Ginkgo biloba),* 85, *90*
Ginseng, American, 85
Ginseng, Asian, 85; in combinations, 74, 80, 95, 100
Ginseng, Siberian, 86
Glaucoma, 262-*263*
Glutamic acid, 331
Glutamine, 347
Glycine, 331
Glycosides, cardiac, 280
Glycyrrhiza glabra (licorice), 89; Ayurvedic use, 298, 363
Glycyrrhiza uralensis (licorice), 82, 84, 207, 233, 339, 356
Goiter, 356, *357*
Goldenrod, 82, 197, 269, 343
Goldenseal, 86; in combinations, 77, 82
Gonorrhea treatment, 339
Gorse (flower remedy), 68
Gotu kola, 87, 348
Gout, 264-*265*
Grape skins, 209, 231
Graphites, 335
Gravelroot, 264
Growing pains, 211
Guduchi (Ayurvedic remedy), 255
Gugulipid (Indian bdellium), 209, 231, 354, 360

Guided imagery, 133-134
Gum problems, 266-*267*
Gum tree, 40

Hahnemann, Samuel, 104
Half bath, hot, 249
Hamamelis (homeopathic remedy), 283, 367
Hamamelis virginiana (witch hazel), 86, 93, 283, 327, 366, 380
Hamstring stretch, *213*
Hare's ear (bupleurum), 76
Hawthorn, 87
Hay fever, 268-269
Hayfever (herb mixture), 196
HDL (high-density lipoprotein), 230, 231
Headache, 270-273, *271*
Head injuries, 373
Hearing problems, 274-275
Heart, *279*
Heartburn, 276-277
Heart problems, 278-281; angina, 200-201
Heart valve disease, 279
Heat cramps, 314, 315
Heather (flower remedy), 68
Heating compress, 299
Heat therapies, 118
Heimlich maneuver, *375, 376*
Helichrysum italicum (everlasting), 40
Helicobacter pylori (bacterium), 290, 291, 346, 347
Heller, Joseph, 51
Hellerwork, 51
Hemoglobin, 198
Hemorrhoids, 282-283
Hepar sulphuris, 111
Herbal oils, 38-41
Herbal therapies, 58-59, 70-103; medicine chest, *380*
Herpes zoster virus, 340
High blood pressure, 284-285
High-carbohydrate, high-plant-fiber (HCF) diet, 247
Histamine, 196, 269
Holly (flower remedy), 68
Homeopathy, 104-116; medicine chest, *380*
Honey, 36, 37, 269
Honeybee products, use of, 36-37, 107, 197, 269
Honeysuckle, 81, 343; flower remedy, 68
Honeysuckle and Forsythia Powder, 360
Hops, 293; wild, 109
Horehound, 75, 80, 88, 92, 324, 380
Hormonal problems: diabetes, 246-247; thyroid, 356-*357*
Hormone replacement therapy, 302, 320

Hornbeam (flower remedy), 68-69
Horse chestnut, 366
Horsetail, 87
Hot compresses, 315, 351, 355, 357
Hou Yan Wan (Chinese remedy), 298
Howard, John, 62
Huang Lien Shang Ching Pien (Chinese remedy), 363
Humidifying devices, 221; cool-mist humidifier, 361
Humulus lupulus (hops), 293
Hydrastis canadensis (goldenseal), 86; in combinations, 77, 82
Hydrotherapy, 117-118
Hypericum (homeopathic remedy), 111
Hypericum perforatum (St.-John's-wort), 100, 111
Hypersensitive teeth, 362
Hypertension, 284-285
Hyperthyroidism, 356, 357
Hypnotherapy, 135
Hypoglycemia, 246
Hypothyroidism, 356, 357
Hyssop *(Hyssopus officinalis)*, 88, *92;* oil, 39, 220

Ice packs, 213
Ignatia, 111
Imagery, guided, 133-134
Immune problems, 196, 286-287. *See also individual names*
Impatiens (flower remedy), 69
Impatiens (jewelweed), 326
Incontinence, 288-289
Indian basil, 255, 351
Indian bdellium (gugulipid), 209, 231, 354, 360
Indian country mallow, 352
Indian tobacco (lobelia), 90; in combination, 92
Indigestion, 290-291
Indigo, wild, 309
Infections: bladder, 216-217; and bronchitis, acute, 220; conjunctivitis, 238-239; ear, 250-251, 274-275; eyelid, 350-*351;* food poisoning, 258-259; gum, 266-*267;* pneumonia, 324-325; prostatitis, 330-331; sexually transmitted diseases, 338-339; sinusitis, 342-343; tonsillitis, 360-361; tooth, 362, *363;* and ulcers, 346, 347; vaginal, 364-365, 370, 371; yeast, 364, 365, 370-371. *See also* Viral infections
Infectious arthritis, 202
Influenza, 256-257
Injuries: athletic, 210-213; repetitive stress, 228-229; tendon, *355. See*

also First aid
Insomnia, 292-293
Intermittent claudication, 234
Intestinal flu (gastroenteritis), 248, 316
Intestinal problems. *See* Gastrointestinal problems
Inula helenium (elecampane), 75, 207, 221
Iodide and thyroid, 357
Iodine, 159
Ipecac, 112
Irish moss, 356
Iron, 159
Iron phosphate, 110
Irritable bowel syndrome (IBS), 294-295

Jasmine *(Jasminum grandifolia),* 238
Jasmine oil, 244, 333, 349
Jaw, *359;* TMJ, 358-359
Jewelweed, 326
Joint mobilization, *129*
Joints. *See* Musculoskeletal problems
Jostling (massage), *129*
Juglans nigra (black walnut), 75
Juniper: *Juniperus communis,* 88; oil, 216, 306, 328, 335
Juvenile rheumatoid arthritis, 202

Kali bichromicum, 112
Kegel exercises, *289*
Kelp, 89
Ketoacidosis, 246
Kidney disease, 296-297
King To's Natural Herb Loquat Flavored Syrup, 243
Knee problems, 211
Kneipp, Sebastian, 117
Kreosotum, 365
Krieger, Dolores, 55, 65

Lachesis, 112
Lactobacillus acidophilus, 259, 365
Larch (flower remedy), 69
Larch moss (usnea), 101
Larch needles, 235
Laryngitis, 298-299
Laryngitis Pills, 298
Larynx, *299*
Latrodectus mactans, 201

Laurus nobilis (bay laurel), 40
Lavender *(Lavandula angustifolia),* 40
Lavender *(Lavandula officinalis), 68,* 89
L-carnitine, 231, 281
L-cysteine, 369
LDL (low-density lipoprotein), 230, 231
Lecithin, 233, 313
Ledum, 113
Lemon balm, 291, 317, 341, 348
Lemon oil, 256, 335
Lemon-scented eucalyptus, 40
Lentinus edodes (shiitake), 231, 232, 233, 286
Leonurus cardiaca (motherwort), 280, 303, 357
Licorice *(Glycyrrhiza glabra),* 89; Ayurvedic use, 298, 363
Licorice *(Glycyrrhiza uralensis),* 82, 84, 207, 233, 339, 356
Life root, 253, 306
Light therapy, 119-120
Ligusticum porterii (osha), 327
Lily of the valley, 280
Lime blossom, 293
Linden, 272
Ling, Pehr Henrik, 121-122
Ling zhi (ganoderma), 83
Linoleic acid, 313
Linum usitatissimum (flaxseed), 241, 380
Lipoproteins, 230, 231
Liu Shen Wan (Chinese remedy), 360, 363
Liu Wei Di Huang Wan (Chinese remedy), 303, 321
L-lysine, 341
Lobelia *(Lobelia inflata),* 90; in combination, 92
Long Dan Xie Gan Wan (Chinese remedy), 340
Lonicera japonica (honeysuckle), 81, 343
L-tryptophan, 245
Lumps, breast, 219
Lung problems. *See* Respiratory problems
Lust, Benedict, 141
Lycium fruit *(Lycium barbarum; L. chinense),* 90; in combination, 95
Lycopenes, 331
Lycopodium, 113
Lycopus spp. (bugleweed), 357

Macrobiotic diet, 149
Mad dog weed (skullcap), 99
Magnesium, 159-160
Magnolia flower *(Magnolia liliflora; M. denudata),* 91
Maharishi Ayur-Veda, 44, 46

Mahesh Yogi, Maharishi, 44, 136
Mahonia aquifolium (Oregon grape), 291
Ma huang (ephedra), 82
Malignancies. *See* Cancer
Mandarin orange (tangerine) peel, 100; in combination, 95
Manganese, 160
Margarine, 145
Marijuana, 262-263
Marjoram oil, 291, 292, 348
Marrubium vulgare (horehound), 75, 80, 88, 92, 324, 380
Marsh mallow, 91
Marsh tea, 113
Massage, 48, 121-123, *124-129*
Matricaria recutita (German chamomile), 40, 78, *80;* in combinations, 84, 86, 102, 103
Meadowsweet, 86, 259, 291, 317
Medicago sativa (alfalfa), 209, 231, 320
Medicine chest, *379, 380*
Meditation, 136-137
Mediterranean diet, 150
Megaloblastic anemia, 152
Melaleuca spp. (tea tree oil), 101; *M. alternifolia,* 41; *M. viridiflora* (niaouli), 41
Melanoma, 332-333, *334*
Melatonin, 293
Melissa officinalis (lemon balm), 291, 317, 341, 348
Melittin, 36
Menadione, 156
Ménière's disease, 300-301
Menopause, 302-303
Menorrhagia, 304, 305-306, 307
Menstrual problems, 304-307
Menstruation, 304-307; end of, 302-303; premenstrual syndrome, 328-329
Mental disorders: depression, 244-245; seasonal affective disorder, 336-337; stress, 348-349
Mentat (Ayurvedic remedy), 348
Mentha (mint), Ayurvedic use, 255, 291, 298, 360
Mentha piperita (peppermint), *68,* 95, *98;* in aromatherapy, 41; in combinations, 88, 102
Mentha spicata (spearmint), 99, *102*
Menthol, 95, 103, 248, 342
Mercurius corrosivus, 217
Mercurius vivus, 113
Meridians, 16, 32, *34-35,* 57
Mesmer, Franz, 64-65
Middle ear infection, 250-251
Migraines, 270, 272, 273
Milk as remedy, misconceptions about, 277, 293, 347
Milk thistle, 91
Milk-vetch root (astragalus), 74

Milkweed, 368, 369
Mimulus (flower remedy), 69
Mind/body medicine, 130-140
Mindfulness meditation, 136, 137
Minerals, 144, 146, 157-162
Minor Bupleurum Pills, 233, 287, 308
Mint: Ayurvedic use, 255, 291, 298, 360; and heartburn, 277
Moles, *334*
Molybdenum, 160
Moniliasis (vaginal yeast infection), 364, 365, 370, 371
Monkshood, 107
Mononucleosis (mono), 308-309
Moss: club, 113; Irish, 356; larch (usnea), 101
Motherwort, 280, 303, 357
Motion sickness, 310-311
Mountain daisy, 108
Moxibustion, 33, 92, 294, 368
MS (multiple sclerosis), 37, 312-*313*
Mugwort leaf, 33, 39, 92, 371
Mulberry Chrysanthemum Pills, 237
Mullein, 92; in combinations, 80, 86
Multiple sclerosis (MS), 37, 312-*313*
Muriaticum acidum, 293
Muscle cramps, 314-315
Muscle tear, *355*
Musculoskeletal problems: arthritis, 202-205, *203;* athletic injuries, 210-213; back problems, 210-211, 214-215; bursitis, 222-223; carpal tunnel syndrome, 228-229; gout, 264-*265;* muscle cramps, 314-315; osteoporosis, 320-321; tendinitis, 210, 211, 354-*355;* TMJ syndrome, 358-359
Music therapy, 170, 171
Mustard (flower remedy), 69
Mustard poultice, 325
Myalgic encephalomyelitis (ME; chronic fatigue syndrome), 232-233
Myelin loss, 312, *313*
Myofascial pain dysfunction (TMJ syndrome), 358-359
Myotherapy, 52
Myrica spp. (bayberry), 266, 267, 295, 299
Myrobalan: beleric, 248, 298, 360; emblic, 348
Myrrh, 93; in combinations, 77, 78
Myrtle hydrosol, 238
Myxedema coma, 356

Naja tripudians, 201
Narcolepsy, 292
Natrum muriaticum, 114
Natrum sulphuricum, 207

Naturopathy, 141-143
Nausea, 316-317
Neck injuries, 373
Neem, 310, 317
Negative ionizers, 336
Nepeta cataria (catnip), 77
Neroli, 292
Nervous system: carpal tunnel syndrome, 228-229; headache, 270-273, *271;* multiple sclerosis, 312-*313;* neuralgia, 318-319, 340
Nettle, *71,* 93
Neuralgia, 318-319; postherpetic, 318, 340
Neural therapy, 235
Neutrophils, 236
Niacin (vitamin B₃), 152-153
Niacinamide, 273
Niaouli, 41
Nightshades: and arthritis, 205; deadly, 108
Nitric acid, 369
Niu Huang Shang Qing Wan (Chinese remedy), 238
Nonmelanomas, 333, *334*
Notoginseng root, 93
Nut grass, 303
Nutrition and diet, 144-151, *147,* 152-162
Nux vomica, 114

Oak (flower remedy), 69
Oak, white, 299
Oat, preparations, 245, 319, 327, 335; wild (flower remedy), 69
Ocimum (Indian basil), 255, 351
Oenothera biennis (evening primrose oil), 219, 306, 329, 331, 334
Ohsawa, George, 149
Oils, essential, 38-41
Olestra, 145
Olive (flower remedy), 69
OMT (osteopathic manipulative therapy), 164
Onion, 231, 247, 284; red, 107
Ophthalmia neonatorum, 238
Oregano, 360
Oregon grape, 291
Origanum majorana (marjoram), 291, 292, 348
Osgood-Schlatter disease, 211
Osha, 327
Osteoarthritis, 202-*203*
Osteopathy, 163-164
Osteoporosis, 320-321
Otitis media, 250-251
Oxygen therapy, 273

PABA (para-aminobenzoic acid), 335, 353
Paeonia lactiflora (peony) root, 284
Pain, chronic, 322-323
Palmarosa, 41
Palmer, Daniel David, 61, 62
Palmetto, saw, 98
Panax ginseng (Asian ginseng), 85; in combinations, 74, 80, 95, 100
Panax notoginseng (notoginseng root), 93
Panax pseudoginseng (pseudoginseng root), 93
Panax quinquefolius (American ginseng), 85
Panchakarma therapy, 45, 356
Pantethine, 231
Pantothenic acid, 154
Parsley, *94;* oil, 216
Pasqueflower, 331
Passionflower *(Passiflora incarnata),* 94
Pau d'arco, 95, *96*
Pedicularis canadensis (wood betony), 272
Pelargonium odoratissimum (geranium), 323
Pellagra, 153
Peony, 76, 81, 207, 284, 356
Peppermint, 41, *68,* 95, *98;* in combinations, 88, 102
Peptic ulcers, 346-*347*
Percussion (massage), *128-129*
Pericardial disease, 279
Periodontal disease, 266-*267*
Pernicious anemia, 155
Petrissage, *125-126*
Petroselinum crispum (parsley), *94*
Phosphorus, 160-161
Phosphorus (homeopathic remedy), 114
Phototherapy (light therapy), 119-120
Phytoestrogens (plant estrogens), 303, 321
Phytonadione, 156
Phytosterols, 231
Piles (hemorrhoids), 282-283
Pilewort, 282-283
Pill Curing, 259, 291
Pimpinella anisum (aniseed), 206, 220, 221, 243, 260
Pine: flower remedy, 69; oil, 206, 216, 220, 324, 342
Pinkeye, 238, 239
Pinus sylvestris (pine) oil, 206, 216, 220, 324, 342
Pipsissewa, 330, 339
Plantago major (plantain), 326
Plantago psyllium (psyllium), 96

Plantain, common, 326
Plant estrogens, 303, 321
Plaque, dental, 267
Plaques, arterial, 208, *209*
PMS (premenstrual syndrome), 328-329
Pneumonia, 324-*325*
Po Chai (Chinese remedy), 259, 291
Podophyllum, 259
Poisoning: first aid for, 377; food, 258-259
Poison ivy, 115, 326-*327*
Poison nut, 114
Poison oak and sumac, 326, *327*
Polarity therapy, 64
Polygonum *(Polygonum multiflorum),* 95
Polyporus *(Polyporus umbellatus),* 287
Pomegranate, 238
Poria *(Poria cocos),* 79, 276
Postherpetic neuralgia, 318, 340
Posture, 215
Po Sum On Medicated Oil, 354
Potassium, 161; broth, 249
Potassium bichromate, 112
Potato poultice, 239
Practitioner, choosing, 15
Prayer, 140
Premenstrual syndrome (PMS), 328-329
Prickly ash, 223, 266, 267
Priessnitz, Vincenz, 117
Primary myocardial disease, 279-280
Progressive muscle relaxation, 139
Prostaglandins, 253, 305
Prostate problems, 330-*331*
Prostatitis, 330-331
Protease inhibitors, 148
Proteins, 144
Prudden, Bonnie, Myotherapy, 52
Prunella *(Prunella vulgaris),* 284
Prunus serotina (wild black cherry), 324
Pseudoginseng root, 93
Psoriasis, 332, *333,* 334-335
Psychoneuroimmunology, 287
Psyllium, 96
Pulsatilla, 115
Pulse, checking for, *373*
Punarnava root, 231
Punica granatum (pomegranate), 238
Pygeum *(Pygeum africanus),* 330
Pyridoxine; pyridoxamine; pyridoxal (vitamin B₆), 154-155
Pyrogenium, 374

Qigong, 165-166
Quercetin, 269
Quercus alba (white oak), 299
Quince, Japanese, 315

Ranunculus ficaria (pilewort), 282-283
Rashes, 332, *333-*335; from poison plants, 326-327
Raspberry, red, 97
Recovery position, *372*
Red blood cells, 198
Reflexology, 167-168, *169, 301*
Rehmannia glutinosa (Chinese foxglove root), 79; in combinations, 80, 81, 90
Reiki, 53
Reishi (ganoderma), 83
Relaxation techniques, 138-139
Repetitive stress injuries (RSI), 228-229
Repressed memories, 133
Rescue Remedy, 69
Respiratory problems: allergies, 196, 197; asthma, 206-*207;* bronchitis, 220-*221;* cough, 242-243; flu, 256-257; pneumonia, 324-*325;* sinusitis, 342-343
Retinol (retinene; retinoic acid; retinyl palmitate; vitamin A), 153
Rhamnus purshiana (buckthorn), 241
Rheumatoid arthritis (rheumatism), 202, *203*
Rhus toxicodendron, 115
Riboflavin (vitamin B₂), 154
RICE treatment (rest, ice, compression, elevation), 355
Rock Rose (flower remedy), 69
Rock Water (flower remedy), 69
Rolf, Ida, 49, 51, 54
Rolfing, 49, 51, 54
Roman chamomile, 266; oil, 292, 314, 348
Rose, oil of, 244, 292; wild (flower remedy), 69
Rosemary *(Rosmarinus officinalis),* 97; in combination, 89; oil, 41
Royal jelly, 36, 37, 197
Rubus idaeus (red raspberry), 97
Rue (rue bitterwort), 115
Rumex crispus (homeopathic remedy), 243
Rumex crispus (sourdock), 320, 339
Ruscus aculeatus (butcher's-broom), 235, 366
Ruta, 115
Rutin, 263

Sabadilla, 197
SAD (seasonal affective disorder), 336-337
Sage, *69,* 97, *100;* clary, 40; in combination, 88; oil, 39, 40, 298, 302; red, 75, 298

Salix spp. (willow), 205, 223; *S. alba* (white willow), 103
Salt, 114, 145
Salvia officinalis (sage), *69, 97, 100;* in combination, 88; oil, 39, 298, 302; var. *rubia* (red), 75, 298
Salvia sclarea (clary sage), 40
Sambucus nigra (elder), 77, 82, 88, 92, 197, 237, 255, 257, 308, 343
Sandalwood, 216, 300, 352
Sang Ju Yin Pian (Chinese remedy), 237
Sanguinaria canadensis (bloodroot), *74, 75*
San She Dan Chuan Bei Ye (Chinese remedy), 243
Santalum album (sandalwood), 352
Sarsaparilla, 339
Saw palmetto, 98
Scalp massage, 273
Scleranthus (flower remedy), 69
Scutellaria baicalensis (skullcap), 98
Scutellaria lateriflora (skullcap), 99; in combination, 89
Seasonal affective disorder (SAD), 336-337
Selenium, 161
Self-hypnosis, 323
Senecio aureus (life root), 253, 306
Senna, 241
Sepia, 116
Septilin (Ayurvedic remedy), 360, 371
Serenoa repens (saw palmetto), 98
Sesame seeds *(Sesamum indicum),* 363
Sexually transmitted diseases (STDs), 338-339
Shatavari (Ayurvedic remedy), 255, 291, 303, 315
Shen Nung, Emperor (China), 58
Shepherd's purse, 306
Shiatsu, 17, 123, 126, 284
Shiitake, 231, 232, 233, 286
Shingles, 340-341
Shi Quan Da Bu Wan (Chinese remedy), 199
Shock, 378; anaphylactic, 196, 197, 378
Shoulder injuries, 210
Sida cordifolia (Indian country mallow), 352
Silica, 87, 116
Silica (homeopathic remedy), 116
Silybum marianum (milk thistle), 91
Sinus headaches, 270-*271,* 273
Sinusitis, 342-343
Sitz baths, 283, 371
Six Flavor Pills, 303, 321
Six Spirit Pills, 360, 363
Skin cancer, 332-333, *334,* 335
Skin problems, 332-335, *333, 334. See also individual names*
Skullcap *(Scutellaria baicalensis),* 98
Skullcap *(Scutellaria lateriflora),* 99;

in combination, 89
Sleep disturbances, 292-293
Slippery elm, 99
Smilax spp. (sarsaparilla), 339
Smoking: and colds, 237; and pneumonia, 325
Snake venom (lachesis), 112
Sodium, 161-162
Sodium chloride, 114
Solidago virgaurea (goldenrod), 82, 197, 269, 343
Sore throat, 344-345
Sound therapy, 170-171
Sourdock, 320, 339
Spanish fly, 109
Spastic colon (spastic colitis; irritable bowel syndrome), 294-295
Spearmint, 99, *102*
Spiritual healing, 140
Spongia tosta, 299
Sports injuries, 210-213
Squamous cell carcinoma (SCC), 333, *334*
Stable (Type II) diabetes, 246, 247
Stannum metallicum, 325
Staphysagria, 217, 331, 374
Star-of-Bethlehem (flower remedy), 69
STDs (sexually transmitted diseases), 338-339
Steam, use of, 220, 221, 236, 257, 343, 345
Stellaria media (chickweed), 364-365
Sties, 350-*351*
St. Ignatius bean, 111
Still, Andrew Taylor, 163
Still's disease, 202
St.-John's-wort, 100, 111
Stomach flu (gastroenteritis), 248, 316
Stomach ulcers, 346-*347*
Stress, 348-349; and relaxation, 130, 138
Stress incontinence, 288, 289
Structural integration, Rolfing called, 54
Sty, 350-*351*
Sulfites, 207
Sulfur, 116, 162
Sulphur, 116
Sunburn, 352-353
Sun protection, 335, 353
Sunscreens, 353
Superior Sore Throat Powder, 360
Swank Diet, 313
Sweat plant (boneset), *76;* in combinations, 77, 88
Swedish massage, 122, *124-129*
Swimmer's ear, 250, 251
Symphytum officinale (comfrey), 355
Syndrome X, 281
Synovitis (rheumatoid arthritis), 202, *203*
Syphilinum, 339
Syphilis, 338, 339
Syzygium aromaticum (clove), 342, 363

Tabacum, 311
Tabebuia impetiginosa (pau d'arco), 95, *96*
T'ai chi, 172-173, *174-181*
Tanacetum parthenium (feverfew), 83, *86*
Tangerine peel, 100; in combination, 95
Tannins, 75, 92, 97, 102, 199
Tapotement, *128-129*
Taraxacum officinale (dandelion), *71,* 81
Tarragon, 41
Teak tree, 291
Tea tree oil, 41, 101
Tectona grandis (teak), 291
Teeth, problems of, 362-*363*
Temporomandibular joint, *359;* TMJ syndrome, 358-359
Ten Complete Great Tonifying Pills, 199
Tendinitis, 210, 211, 354-*355*
Tension headaches, 270, *271,* 272, 273
Terc, Phillip, 36
Terminalia bellirica (beleric myrobalan), 248, 298, 360
Therapeutic touch, 55
Theridion, 301
Thermal biofeedback, 273
Thiamine (vitamin B$_1$), 153-154
Thistle, milk, 91
Thorowax root (bupleurum), 76
Throat: laryngitis, 298-299; sore, 344-345; tonsillitis, 360-361
Throat Irritation Pills, 298
Thrush, 370
Thuja *(Thuja occidentalis),* 39, 331, 339, 368
Thyme *(Thymus vulgaris),* 41, 235, 339
Thyroid, 357
Thyroid problems, 356-*357*
Tieh Ta Yao Gin (Chinese remedy), 212, 354
Tilia spp. (linden), 272; *T. cordata* (lime), 293
TMJ syndrome, 358-359
Tocopherols, 156
Tongue, Chinese view of, 60
Tonify the Middle and Augment the Chi Pills, 233
Tonsillitis, 360-361
Tonsils, 360, *361*
Toothache, 362-363
Tooth decay, 362, *363*
Trager, Milton, 56
Trager approach, 56
Transcendental meditation (TM), 136
Traumatic Injury Medicine, 212, 354
Traveler's diarrhea, 248
Trench mouth, 266
Trifolium pratense (red clover), *71,* 96; in

combinations, 77, 92
Trigeminal neuralgia, 318, 319
Trigger points, 52
Trigonella foenum-graecum (fenugreek), 231, 247
Trikatu pills, 356
True unicorn root, 330
Trumpet (pau d'arco) tree, 95, *96*
Tryptophan, 100, 152, 245, 293
Tui na (massage), 354
Tumors, kinds of, 224
Turmeric, *71*, 101, 315, 340
Tussilago farfara (coltsfoot), 80; in combinations, 88, 92
Tyrosine, 100, 357

Ulcers, stomach, 346-*347*
Ulmus fulva (slippery elm), 99
Ultraviolet (UV) radiation, 335, 352, 353
Unicorn root, true, 330
Urethra and prostate, *331*
Uric acid and gout, 264, *265*
Urinary tract problems: bladder infections, 216-217; incontinence, 288-289; kidney disease, 296-297; prostate problems, 330-*331*
Urtica dioica (nettle), *71, 93*
Urtica urens, 265
Usnea (*Usnea* spp.), 101
Usui, Mikao, 53
Uva ursi, 102; in combination, 81
UV (ultraviolet) radiation, 335, 352, 353

Vaccinium myrtillus (bilberry), 262, 306, 366
Vaginal problems, 364-365, 370, 371
Vaginitis, 364-365; yeast infection, 364, 365, 370, 371
Vaidya (Ayurvedic doctor), 46
Valerian *(Valeriana officinalis)*, *71*, 102
Valves, heart, disease of, 279
Vanadium, 162
Vaporizers, use of, 221
Varicose veins, 366-367; hemorrhoids, 282-283
Vegetarian diet, 151
Veins, varicose, 366-367; hemorrhoids, 282-283
Venereal (sexually transmitted) diseases, 338-339
Veratrum album, 259
Verbascum thapsus (mullein), 92; in combinations, 80, 86

Vervain (flower remedy), 69
Vervain *(Verbena officinalis),* 215, 293, 309
Vibration (massage), *129*
Viburnum opulus (cramp bark), 103, 205, 215, 223, 253, 272, 306
Viburnum prunifolium (black haw), 253, 306
Vincent's angina, 266
Vine (flower remedy), 69
Vinegar pack, 315, 355
Viral infections: common cold, 236-237; flu, 256-257; mononucleosis, 308-309; shingles, 340-341; warts, 368-*369*
Visualization, 133-134
Vitamins, 144, 146, 152-156; A, 153; B_1 (thiamine), 153-154; B_2 (riboflavin), 154; B_3 (niacin), 152-153; B_5 (pantothenic acid), 154; B_6 (pyridoxine), 154-155; B_7 (biotin), 152; B_9 (folic acid), 152; B_{12} (cobalamin), 155; B complex, 153; C (ascorbic acid), 155; D, 156; E, 156; H (biotin), 152; K, 156
Vitex agnus-castus (chaste tree), 79, 82
Vocal cords, 298, *299*
Vulva, problems of, 364, 365

Walnut (flower remedy), 69
Walnut, black, 75
Warming socks, 361
Warts, 368-*369*
Water therapy, 117-118
Water Violet (flower remedy), 69
Wear-and-tear arthritis (osteoarthritis), 202-*203*
White blood cells, 236
Willow, 205, 223; white, 103
Willow (flower remedy), 69
Windflower, 115
Wintergreen, 236, 271, 323; interaction with, 103
Witch hazel, 86, 93, 283, 327, 366, 367, 380
Withania somnifera (winter cherry), 348
Wolfberry (lycium fruit), 90; in combination, 95
Women: bladder infections, 216, 217; breast health, *218-219;* endometriosis, 252-*253;* heart disease, 281; incontinence, stress, 289; menopause, 302-303; menstrual problems, 304-307; osteoporosis, 320, 321; PMS, 328-329; vaginal problems, 364-365, 370, 371
Wrist, *229*
Wristbands, acupressure, 310

Xanthium fruit *(Xanthium sibiricum),* 91, 343
Xiao Chai Hu Wan (Chinese remedy), 233, 287, 308
Xiao Yao Wan (Chinese remedy), 306, 329

Yams: Chinese, 79; wild, 103
Yarrow, *69,* 103; in combinations, 77, 81
Yeast infections, 370-371; vaginal, 364, 365, 370, 371
Yellow jasmine, 110
Yin and yang states, 57-58
Yin Qiao Pian (Chinese remedy), 237
Ylang-ylang, 41
Yoga, 182-183, *184-193;* Abdominal Massage, *184,* 294; Boat, *184,* 252; Bow, *184, 329;* Bridge, *184;* C, *185, 204;* Camel, *185, 307;* Cat, *185, 204;* Child, *185, 225, 287;* Cobra, *186, 240, 331;* Corpse, *186, 348;* Dog, *186;* Dog, Downward, *187, 307;* Dog, Upward, *193;* Half-Moon, *187, 233;* Hand and Thumb Squeeze, *187, 204;* Head to Knee, *187;* Hero, *188;* Knee Down Twist, *188;* Locust, *188, 252;* Lotus, *189;* Mountain, *189, 233;* Pigeon, *189, 206;* Plow, *189;* Posterior Stretch, *190;* Rag Doll, *190, 233;* Seated Angle, *190;* Shoulder Crunch, *190;* Shoulder Stand, *191, 282, 357;* Shoulder Stand, Half, *191, 275, 367;* Sphinx, *191, 280;* Spider, *191, 204;* Spinal Twist, *191;* Standing Angle, *192;* Tree, *192;* Triangle, *192;* Warrior, *193;* Yoga Mudra, *193, 225;* Yoga Mudra, Standing, *192*
Yun Nan Bai Yao (Chinese remedy), 306-307, 374

Zanthoxylum americanum (prickly ash), 223, 266, 267
Zheng Gu Shui (Chinese remedy), 212, 354
Zhi Bai Ba Wei Wan (Chinese remedy), 303
Zinc, 162
Zingiber officinale (ginger), 84; Ayurvedic use, 248, 298, 303, 315, 363; in combinations, 90, 92, 103; oil, 322

Acknowledgments

The editors wish to thank the following individuals and institutions for their valuable assistance in the preparation of this volume:

American Chiropractic Association, Arlington, Va.; Lucille Arcouet, National Education Coordinator, Nelson Bach USA, Wilmington, Mass.; Denise Bowles-Johnson, LMT, Creative Body Therapies, New Haven, Conn.; Al Bumanis, National Association for Music Therapy, Silver Spring, Md.; Patricia Kaminski, Flower Essence Society, Nevada City, Calif.; William J. Lauretti, DC, Bethesda, Md.; Barbara Mitchell, National Acupuncture and Oriental Medicine Alliance, Olalla, Wash.; Joyce Morris, Reiki Center of Los Angeles, Encino, Calif.; Perelandra, Jeffersonton, Va.; Holly H. Shimizu, Lewis Ginter Botanical Garden, Richmond, Va.; James P. Swyers, MA, Takoma Park, Md.

Picture Credits

Abbreviations

c	in homeopathic dosages, indicating a dilution ratio of 1 part to 99 parts	**IU**	international units, measurement used for fat-soluble vitamins	**pt** pint
cal	calorie	**lb**	pound	**qt** quart
F	Fahrenheit	**mcg**	microgram	**spp.** various species, often used with botanical names of herbs to indicate that more than one species of a plant may be used medicinally
gal	gallon	**mg**	milligram	**tbsp** tablespoon
in	inch	**ml**	milliliter	**tsp** teaspoon
		oz	ounce	**x** in homeopathic dosages, indicating a dilution ratio of 1 part to 9 parts